UNDERSTANDING AND INTERPRETING EDUCATIONAL RESEARCH

Understanding and Interpreting Educational Research

Ronald C. Martella
J. Ron Nelson
Robert L. Morgan
Nancy E. Marchand-Martella

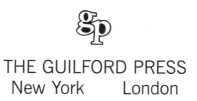

THE GUILFORD PRESS
New York   London

© 2013 The Guilford Press
A Division of Guilford Publications, Inc.
72 Spring Street, New York, NY 10012
www.guilford.com

Printed in the United States of America

This book is printed on acid-free paper.

Last digit is print number: 9   8   7   6   5   4   3   2   1

Library of Congress Cataloging-in-Publication Data is available
from the publisher.

ISBN: 978-1-4625-0962-1 (paperback)
ISBN: 978-1-4625-0974-4 (hardcover)

Portions of this book are drawn from *Research Methods: Learning to Become a
Critical Research Consumer*, published by Pearson Education, Inc.

Preface

OBJECTIVES OF THIS BOOK

Our primary purpose in writing this book is to provide a comprehensive coverage of research design issues that students find throughout the educational and psychological research literature. For example, group designs are found in psychological and educational research, but other designs, such as qualitative methods and single-case research designs, are also common. It is critical for readers to understand our approach to these different methods. We do not discount the importance of one or more methods, or claim that one type of methodology is superior to another. Our approach is that there are several different types of research methodologies. The choice of methodology should be based not on some preconceived notion of the superiority of one over another but on an assessment of which methodology is best suited to answer the research question or to test the hypothesis at hand. Therefore, the selection of a particular methodology should be based not on personal bias but on a thorough knowledge of the different methodologies.

Few other research methods books provide the depth of coverage of the wide array of designs covered here. For instance, whereas most research methods books provide superficial coverage of single-case designs as part of a chapter, we provide three chapters on these important designs, which are prevalent in behavioral and special education research. Researchers may find the coverage of these designs particularly useful when conducting field studies in which experimental control is required. However, we do not provide expanded coverage of one methodology at the expense of other approaches. We attempt to provide equal depth of coverage of the common methods found in the research literature, including the latest research techniques on mixed-methods research, grounded theory development, phenomenology, and conducting literature reviews including online searches. We have also fully covered survey research, as a stand-alone chapter in the quantitative research methods section of the text.

ORGANIZATION OF THE BOOK

The organization of this book reflects our primary goal in writing it: to aid students in becoming consumers of research. In our opinion, before a student is ready to conduct independent research, he/she needs an understanding of the research process, including the decisions researchers make and why they make them. Therefore, we placed material on variability and threats to internal and external validity near the beginning of the book (Chapter 2). This material is typically located much later in other textbooks. However, given that variability, and the control of variables that contribute to variability, is so critical in the research endeavor, placing the material early on is more suitable.

We have also attempted to reduce the redundancy found in many books by presenting information in a sequenced format, the material in each chapter building on material covered in previous chapters. Therefore, it is best to present the material in the book in the sequence provided. Students will find that the sequence is logical and will aid in their mastery of the concepts.

Among the more important aspects of the book are the sample articles at the end of each of the research design chapters. Since the main purpose of our book is to teach students how to consume and understand research, these are provided to give students opportunities to practice interpreting an article that covers techniques discussed in the chapter. Each article is followed by questions to prompt class discussion of the article and guide students through a critique of how the research was conducted, why it was conducted that way, and whether the researchers' conclusions were warranted. It is important for students to read these articles and to complete the activities associated with them to enhance their learning.

TOPIC COVERAGE

The book includes seven major parts comprising 16 chapters, reflecting the fact that many universities cover research methods as a 16-week course. Following is a description of the contents associated with each of the parts.

Part I discusses skills in learning how to become a critical research consumer (Chapter 1). Information needed to think critically about research includes descriptions of science, what science is, the process of science, and the purpose of science.

Part II covers critical issues in research, including the concept and sources of variability. Internal and external validity are keys to understanding much of the educational and psychological research produced. Therefore, a great deal of time is spent on these concepts. Statistical and social validity are also described. A discussion of the differences in these important forms of validity is presented (Chapter 2). The concepts of reliability and validity from quantitative and qualitative perspectives are also discussed in Part II. Interobserver agreement, a special form of reliability and validity that is used in single-case research, is presented. Finally, factors to consider when assessing measurement devices in the context of an investigation are discussed (Chapter 3). Several examples and nonexamples are presented throughout the chapter to help students learn key concepts.

Part III concerns quantitative research methods. Part III begins with a presentation of some basic statistical concepts. Knowledge of these concepts is critical for an understanding of many quantitative designs. Sampling methods are also discussed at length. The method of sampling is important in determining the type of design used, as well as claims that can be made about the generalizability of the results (Chapter 4). The different methodologies are covered, including true experimental, factorial, quasi-experimental, and preexperimental designs (Chapter 5). Additionally, causal–comparative research methods (Chapter 6), correlational research methods (Chapter 7), and survey research (Chapter 8) are presented. At the end of each chapter, we describe when to use each form of research method. Finally, Chapters 5–8 present sample articles for students to critique, including rating forms to analyze various aspects of the studies.

Part IV focuses on qualitative research methods (Chapter 9) and data collection and designs (Chapter 10). Methods of sampling are discussed. Chapter 10 closes with a discussion about when different qualitative research methods should be used. A sample article for students to analyze and an analysis form are included in the chapter.

Part V presents a detailed discussion of single-case methods. We show how single-case methods may be thought of as a combination of quantitative and qualitative designs. Methods of graphing and withdrawal and associated designs are discussed in Chapter 11. Multiple-baseline designs (Chapter 12) and additional single-case designs (Chapter 13) are presented. Each chapter discusses when to use the various types of single-case designs. A sample article for critique, along with a rating form, is presented at the end of each of the chapters.

Part VI focuses on evaluation research, including program evaluations (Chapter 14) and a detailed discussion of research syntheses (Chapter 15). We discuss when each form of research is conducted. We also present a sample article for critique at the end of each chapter.

Part VII covers issues to consider when planning and conducting a research project (Chapter 16). Recall that the book is designed to teach students to think critically about research; however, we also want to produce scientist-practitioners. Practitioners can, and in some instances should, produce data to make informed decisions. Practitioners who produce such data are engaging in action research. A discussion of how to conduct action research is presented. When a decision is made to conduct an investigation, ethical issues must then be considered. These ethical issues are described. "Action researchers" should also know the process one goes through to write and submit an article for publication. We describe that process. Finally, a sample article is presented at the end of the chapter to critique.

PEDAGOGICAL FEATURES

This book has several pedagogical features to aid instructors with material presentation and to help students understand the multitude of concepts they encounter. Following is a brief description of the major features of our book:

- **Objectives.** Each chapter begins with a numbered list of objectives. These serve as an anticipatory set allowing students to obtain a quick snapshot of the contents of the chapter.
- **Chapter-opening graphic organizers.** Each chapter contains a graphic organizer. These enable students to see the contents of each chapter in an organizational framework.

- **Overviews.** An overview provided at the beginning of each chapter allows students to understand the importance of the material that follows.
- **Main headings in the form of questions.** All main headings are framed as questions in order to facilitate student note taking. Students should be taught how to list each question heading, then to read the materials under each heading to answer the question. This approach is important in helping students better understand chapter content.
- **Figures and tables.** Several illustrations and tables in each chapter present a visual representation of concepts or provide a summary of critical material.
- **Running glossary.** In each chapter, a running glossary box defines key terms introduced on a two-page spread.
- **Research examples.** Throughout each chapter, research examples highlight key concepts. Additionally, each research methods chapter contains boxes with research questions. Descriptions of investigations that answer these questions are provided throughout the chapters. These boxes are designed to prompt students to think about how they would answer the questions and then provide a description of how researchers would answer them. These activities give students a way to evaluate their understanding of the material.
- **Bulleted summary.** Each chapter ends with a bulleted summary. These summaries serve as a review of material and a study aid for tests and quizzes.
- **Discussion questions.** Questions provided at the end of each chapter allow for rich discussion of chapter material. These questions also help students evaluate their understanding of concepts presented throughout the chapter.
- **Additional exercises.** Additional (i.e., interpretation, practice) exercises are provide in Chapters 2 and 3 to highlight important concepts needed as a foundation for later material.
- **Journal articles as illustrative examples.** Each research methods chapter (Chapters 5–8 and 10–16) provides an illustrative example from published peer-reviewed articles. These examples give students opportunities to read authentic research articles and to critique them with guidance from the instructor. This feature is perhaps the one that best exemplifies the purpose of the book— to teach students how to read and consume research. Each illustrative example has questions to prompt discussion of the article and activities to guide students through the critiquing process. For example, several chapters include threats to internal validity and external validity forms.
- **Additional research examples.** Lists of additional research examples are provided in Chapters 5–8 and 10–16 for instructors or students who want to access further readings on the concepts within each chapter.
- **End-of-book glossary.** The book includes a detailed glossary of key terms. This glossary provides an additional resource for students to access when defining terms.
- **Complete list of references.** A complete list of references is found at the end of the book, as opposed to the end of each chapter. The placement of the references makes it easier for instructors and students to find cited material.
- **Author index.** An author index at the end of the book aids in the search of particular authors of interest to students.
- **Subject index.** A subject index at the end of the book helps students locate specific information in the book.
- **Supplementary electronic instructor's resource manual.** This comprehensive

aid for course preparation includes a detailed outline of each chapter for lecture notes (also available in downloadable PowerPoint format); answers to within-text discussion questions, interpretation/practice exercises, and illustrative example questions; and an extensive test bank of multiple-choice questions and short-answer/essay questions readable to most test management software. A link to this electronic manual is sent automatically via e-mail to any professor who orders an exam copy directly from The Guilford Press. Please contact customer service (*info@guilford.com*) for further information.

AUDIENCE FOR THE BOOK

The book is designed to be used across several different levels of instruction. The primary audience for the book is upper-level undergraduate or master's students. However, the book may also be used (and has been used in the past) at the doctoral level with supplementary materials. With this in mind, we attempted to use language that is appropriate not only for advanced undergraduate students but also for students at more advanced levels of study.

Given the sequencing of the material in the book, it may also be used for self-study. We have had success in the past with students studying the material in the book on their own. If the book is used for self-study, we recommend reviewing the Objectives to each chapter, answering the Discussion Questions at the end of each chapter, and also completing any additional exercises that are available. It is especially important for the self-study student to read the sample articles at the end of each research design chapter carefully and to complete the indicated activities.

ACKNOWLEDGMENTS

We would be remiss not to acknowledge the individuals who have affected our educational careers. First and foremost, we wish to thank our families for their support. We would especially like to thank our children for allowing us to take the time to complete the project.

In order to complete this text, several individuals were involved. We wish to thank everyone at The Guilford Press for their continued support of the entire project, especially C. Deborah Laughton, without whom this project would not have come to fruition. We would also like to thank Ryan Sain for taking the lead on developing the instructor's manual. Finally, we are grateful to the reviewers whose criticisms were highly constructive: Melody Whiddon, College of Education, Florida International University; Anthony Salvatore, Department of Speech–Language Pathology, University of Texas, El Paso; Tracy Walker, School of Liberal Arts and Education, Virginia State University; Hisako Matsuo, Department of Sociology and Anthropology, Saint Louis University; and Hansel Burley, College of Education, Texas Tech University.

Brief Contents

Extended Contents

PART III ■ QUANTITATIVE RESEARCH METHODS

PART V ▪ SINGLE-CASE RESEARCH METHODS

11 ▪ Withdrawal and Associated Designs   369

12 ▪ Multiple-Baseline Designs   408

PART VI ▪ EVALUATION RESEARCH

PART VII ▪ ACTION RESEARCH

The electronic instructor's resource manual with test bank is available via a link automatically e-mailed to any professor who orders an exam copy directly from The Guilford Press. Contact customer service (*info@guilford.com*) if you have not received this e-mail.

PART I

- - - -

Understanding Research

CHAPTER 1

∎ ∎ ∎ ∎

Thinking Critically
about Research

OBJECTIVES

After studying this chapter, you should be able to . . .

1. Outline the elements that must be considered to develop critical thinking skills.
2. Describe what is meant by science and the scientific method.
3. Illustrate the purposes of science.
4. Explain what is meant by a scientific theory.
5. Outline the types of scientific logic.
6. Describe the ways we gain information.
7. Illustrate the constraint levels in educational and psychological research.
8. Explain the differences between basic and applied research.
9. Clarify what is meant by replication research.

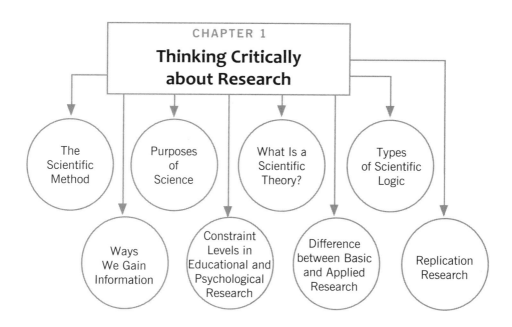

OVERVIEW

In our view, one of the most important skills areas to be developed is becoming a critical research consumer. *Critical thinking* is the ability to take an issue, consider all sides, and make an informed decision. For example, when reading educational and psychological research, we must read what the researcher has written, consider how the research was conducted, determine whether there were any plausible alternative explanations, and make a decision on the believability of the claims made by the researcher. Unfortunately, many professionals seem to skip the middle steps. They read what the researcher has written and accept the conclusions made by the researcher as fact. Or they dismiss the conclusions outright because the findings compete with their philosophy or current conceptualization.

How the research was conducted may have impacted the findings. A modification in the procedures may have produced different results. The researcher may have been invested in his/her procedures and overlooked alternative explanations. Focusing on these and other issues is a step toward becoming a critical research consumer.

Due to the possible difficulties in making an impact on education through educational and psychological research, we should teach educational and psychological professionals how to become critical research consumers. Educational and psychological professionals should be able to read and understand what research is and interpret research findings. Professionals who learn to consume research learn how to conduct research. Thus, the primary purpose of teaching about research is to *develop critical thinking skills*.

Our purpose in this chapter is to learn to think critically about research to make informed decisions about a researcher's methods, findings, and conclusions. We describe science and its purpose, method, theory, and logic; how we gain information; what constraint levels have to do with information we gain; what differences distinguish basic and applied research; and why replication is important. We want readers to learn how to process and analyze research, so this chapter begins the journey. In doing so,

readers will see research as something exciting to drive their professional practice, not as something that must be feared and avoided.

HOW IMPORTANT IS CRITICAL THINKING?

Francesco Sizzi, an Italian astronomer in the 17th century, was credited as the first scientist to detect the annual rotation of sunspots. Unfortunately, he is also remembered by many scientists for failing to recognize Galileo's discovery of the four moons of Jupiter (Drake, 1958). Apparently, the documentation provided by Galileo from his astronomical experiments ran counter to Sizzi's conventional thinking, compelling Sizzi to write:

> Just as in the microcosm there are seven "windows" in the head (two nostrils, two eyes, two ears, and a mouth), so in the macrocosm God has placed two beneficent stars (Jupiter, Venus), two maleficent stars (Mars, Saturn), two luminaries (sun and moon), and one indifferent star (Mercury). The seven days of the week follow from these. Finally, since ancient times the alchemists had made each of the seven metals correspond to one of the planets: gold to the sun, silver to the moon, copper to Venus, quicksilver to Mercury, iron to Mars, tin to Jupiter, lead to Saturn. From these and many other similar phenomena of nature . . . we gather that the number of planets is necessarily seven. . . . Now if we increase the number of planets, this whole system falls to the ground. . . . Moreover, the satellites are invisible to the naked eye and therefore can have no influence on the earth, and therefore would be useless, and therefore do not exist. (Drake, 1958, p. 155)

Soon, the European astronomical community had confirmed Galileo's discovery and chastised Sizzi for failing to recognize the new evidence. Galileo was quick to forgive Sizzi and even defended him as a leading scientist in telescopic astronomy (Drake, 1958). But Sizzi had exposed his lack of critical thinking in analyzing Galileo's discovery. The implications for his mistake were to follow him throughout his career.

Being a critical research consumer could have assisted Sizzi in making a better, more informed decision and allowed him to avoid the scrutiny of history. But all of us who read research confront these decisions. And all of us struggle at times to make critical decisions about research.

WHAT ARE THE ELEMENTS TO BECOMING A CRITICAL RESEARCH CONSUMER?

In order to develop critical research consumer skills, several elements must be learned (see Figure 1.1). As a foundation, research consumers must be familiar with different research methodologies. However, it is not enough to know the different designs. Critical research consumers know why different designs are used and what types of research questions are answered.

First, critical research consumers must learn what science is, how it works, and why it works. Science means different things to different people. Therefore, it is critical to come to some understanding of what we mean by the term. We present a definition of science, describe how science works, and discuss the purposes of science.

Second, critical research consumers should know what constitutes a scientific theory. There are many theories put forth. In order to discriminate between a theory that is scientific and one that is not, we must understand the distinctions between the two types. We discuss what constitutes scientific theories.

Third, it is important to understand the different types of logic used in science. The method of logic one uses will determine how one approaches the study of a particular phenomenon. We describe the two types of scientific logic and discuss how the logic forms can be combined.

Fourth, some methods of establishing knowledge fit within a scientific framework and others do not. Unfortunately, many people do not understand or appreciate the differences between scientific sources of information and sources that are not scientific. In fact, Sandbek (2010), commenting on the Public Opinion Laboratory Poll from the mid-1990s, claims that many Americans are "scientific illiterates." He asserts that scientific illiteracy has accelerated in the last few years, indicating that while everyone takes advantage of scientific progress, very few people understand how science moves forward by gathering information, raising questions, testing alternatives, drawing conclusions, and generating new questions. Some individuals cannot make a distinction between valid sources of information and sources that are suspect. We present various sources of information and explain which are considered scientific and which are not.

Fifth, critical research consumers must know how to discriminate between research methods

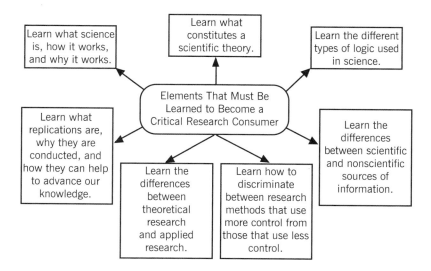

FIGURE 1.1. Elements that must be learned to become a critical research consumer.

that use more control (i.e., high constraint levels) and those that use less control (i.e., low constraint levels). Different constraint levels can
affect our ability to draw conclusions about the
effects of variables, and whether those effects
occur in real-world settings. Variables that can
affect the interpretation of research must be
clear to consumers. Issues of reliability and
validity are critical aspects of research and are
presented in this chapter.

Sixth, the differences between research that
focuses on more theoretical issues (i.e., basic)
and research that addresses educational–psychological problems (i.e., applied) should be
understood as well. Some research findings
may not have an immediate impact on society.
However, the value of research does not depend
on its immediate impact on society. The differences between basic and applied research are
discussed in this chapter.

Seventh, science does not advance with single, isolated bits of research findings. In order
to make advances in a field of inquiry, we must
see the same results several times (called *replications*) through different research investigations.
Thus, critical research consumers must know
what replications are, why they are conducted,
and how they can help to advance our knowledge. Replication research is discussed later in
this chapter.

WHAT ARE SCIENCE
AND THE SCIENTIFIC METHOD?

As we scan the literature, we do not find one
completely agreed upon definition of science.
According to Cooper, Heron, and Heward
(2007), *science* is a systematic approach to seeking and organizing knowledge about the natural world. Gall, Gall, and Borg (2007) define *scientific research* as a continual process of rigorous
reasoning supported by a dynamic interplay
among methods, theories, and findings. Generally, science is the search for understanding of
the world around us. Science is the attempt to
find order and lawful relations in the world. It
is a method of viewing the world. Finally, science is testing of our ideas in a public forum in a
series of five steps (Humphreys, 2004; see Figure
1.2).

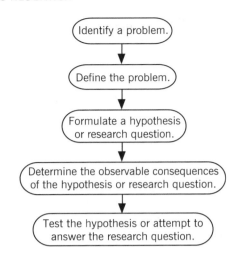

FIGURE 1.2. Steps in the scientific method.

The first step of the **scientific method**, to
identify a problem, involves an awareness on
the part of the researcher that something is
missing in a knowledge base. The desire, then,
is to find information to fill the gap or move the
information forward. For example, there may be
a gap of knowledge in how a teacher's reaction
to disruptive behavior encourages future disruptive behavior.

Second, the researcher must define the problem. The attempt here is to become clear about
what exactly the problem is. For example, a
problem such as "disruptive behavior in the
classroom" is not well defined. Students may be
engaging in serious problem behavior such as
fighting or minor problems such as whispering
or exchanging notes. The term *disruption* must
be defined in a way that develops a clear picture
of what is meant by it. Therefore, the problem
must be identified and defined.

Third, the researcher must formulate either
hypotheses or research questions. *Hypotheses* are
statements about the tentative relation between
two or more concepts (Gall et al., 2007). For example, we can hypothesize that if a teacher attends
to disruptive behavior, then the disruptive behavior will get worse. *Research questions* are queries
about events, not attempts at predicting what
will occur. For example, instead of the hypothesis
stated earlier, we could ask, "What happens if a
teacher attends to disruptive behavior?"

The fourth step in the scientific method is to determine the observable consequences of the hypothesis or research question. For instance, for the previous example, we could conclude that "teachers who do not attend to disruptive behaviors, but instead, attend to students behaving appropriately, will have better classroom management than teachers who attend to disruptive behavior."

The final step, to test the hypothesis or attempt to answer the research question, requires the actual collection of data. Once they are gathered, the data are analyzed to determine whether the hypothesis is correct or whether the data answer the research question in the expected way. For example, the data indicate that teachers who attend to disruptive behaviors in the classroom experience higher levels of disruptions than do teachers who do not attend to such disruptive behaviors.

Although the scientific method is powerful in filling gaps in knowledge, critical research consumers must understand that even though the data are gathered and the hypothesis is tested or the research question is answered, errors may occur in the investigation, some of which place the researcher's conclusions in question. Additionally, any isolated observable event obtained from a single investigation can support several theories, sometimes, even conflicting theories. Therefore, as we see later in the chapter, we can never prove a theory; we can only provide support for it due to errors made by researchers or the possibility that isolated, observable events are due to the presence of only chance findings.

WHAT ARE THE PURPOSES OF SCIENCE?

Generally, we can assume that science has several purposes: to describe phenomena, to predict events or outcomes, to improve practice, and to explain phenomena (Gall et al., 2007; see Figure 1.3). Each purpose is described below.

Description

Throughout the scientific process, we attempt to describe an event or phenomenon. For example, Piaget described certain abilities in children at different points in their lives. From his

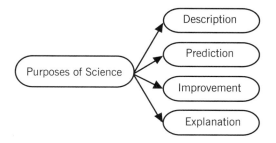

FIGURE 1.3. The four purposes of science.

observations, he developed a theory of child development that has different developmental stages, each with its own set of abilities.

Describing events is something we all do on a daily basis. In education, we describe how classrooms are situated, what methods of instruction are effective, and how students attend to the teacher. The descriptions we make allow us to draw some conclusions. We can think of description as the first step in science. Scientific inquiry begins with descriptions of the phenomenon that can lead to future research questions. For example, in describing how third-grade students achieve in a school using a math program, we might ask, "How much more would students achieve if we dedicated an additional 15 minutes a day to independent practice with Math Program A lessons?" Descriptions can also lead to important discoveries. For example, if every time the teacher turns away a student begins to disrupt the class, it may seem as if the student is displaying the disruptive behavior to get the teacher's attention.

Through description, educators have gathered and organized substantial amounts of information about our schools and how they are doing. For example, information such as students' achieved levels of reading is descriptive

> The **scientific method** involves (1) identifying the problem, (2) defining the problem, (3) formulating a hypothesis (a researcher's expectations about what data will show) or research question, (4) determining the observable consequences of the hypothesis or research question, and (5) testing the hypothesis or attempting to answer the research question.

information. Percentages of students who drop out of school, take drugs, and commit crimes comprise descriptive information. Policymakers can use this descriptive information to make decisions. The federal government, state, and/or local school districts may use this information to set priorities for grant funds or instructional programs. Whether the funded interventions (e.g., instructional programs) work is a question for another purpose (i.e., improvement).

Essentially, all research provides some form of a description. However, certain research methods are geared to provide only descriptive information. These methods, presented in Chapters 9 and 10, generally come under the heading of qualitative research and ideally provide a description of the observed phenomenon.

Prediction

A second purpose of science is to make predictions about what will happen in the future. If you are studying this text, you likely have taken standardized tests such as the *American College Testing* (ACT) program or the *Scholastic Aptitude Test* (SAT). If you want to go to graduate school, you may take the *Graduate Record Exam* (GRE); if you go to law school, you will most likely take the *Law School Aptitude Test* (LSAT); and if you want to go to get an advanced degree in business, you may need to take the *Graduate Miller Analogies Test* (GMAT). The purpose of all of these tests is to predict how you will do in school. The results of these tests, along with other information such as grades in high school or college, are used to select students who predictably will achieve in a program.

Professionals also use predictions to identify students who are more likely to do poorly in school. Children with low socioeconomic status (SES) backgrounds may be admitted into Head Start Programs. These programs are aimed at increasing the chances for success of students whose backgrounds might otherwise decrease their chances of succeeding in school. Variables that may place children at higher risk of failure include coming from a single-parent household, having parents who lack educational background, being a member of a minority group, coming from a family with few economic resources, and coming from the inner

> ### *Predictions Gone Awry*
>
> - Computers in the future may . . . perhaps only weigh 1.5 tons (from *Popular Mechanics*, 1949).
> - There is no reason for any individual to have a computer in their home (from Kenneth Olson, President and Founder of Digital Equipment Corp., 1977).
> - This "telephone" has too many shortcomings to be seriously considered as a means of communication. The device is inherently of no value to us (from Western Union internal memo, 1876).
> - The wireless music box has no imaginable commercial value. Who would pay for a message sent to nobody in particular? (David Sarnoff's associates, in response to his urgings for investment in the radio in the 1920s).
> - While theoretically and technically television may be feasible, commercially and financially it is an impossibility (from Lee DeForest, inventor).
>
> Retrieved from *http://personalitycafe.com/science-technology/46575-bad-science-technology-predictions.html.*

city. When these risk factors are combined, the risk of school failure is increased. A caution here is in order. With prediction studies, the probability of something such as school failure is increased when variables are combined; however, the probability will not reach 100%. However, an inner-city African American child from a single-parent household, with a parent who has a fifth-grade education and earns less than the poverty threshold, may not fail in school. The prediction simply means that, proportionally, more children from this background fail in school compared to, for example, a European American child who lives in the suburbs with two college-graduate, middle-class parents. Thus, the importance of making predictions of this sort is to identify a probable outcome and provide some sort of intervention to produce an alternative outcome.

As with descriptive research, most research methods allow the prediction of something in the future. The more we know about a phenomenon, the better able we are to make future predictions. However, specific research methods are developed to provide predictions; these methods, presented in Chapters 6 and 7, include causal–comparative and correlational research methods. These methods provide an indication of the strength of relationship between or among variables.

Improvement

The third purpose of science is to make improvements in the subject matter. When discussing these improvements, interventions are at issue. Essentially, one purpose of science is to determine the best or most effective interventions to bring about desirable changes. Examples of interventions range from drug therapies to engineering procedures for behavioral treatments. For example, in determining how best to instruct students, we are attempting to determine which interventions are most appropriate. This purpose is the basis for the effective teaching literature developed over a number of years.

Inherent in their quest for improvement researchers also attempt to determine the variables (e.g., type of instruction, method of behavior management) that control how children respond (e.g., amount of material learned, on-task behavior). These are called *independent variables* (we also use the terms *interventions* and *treatments* throughout the text to refer to independent variables), and responses to these independent variables are called *dependent variables*.

What Works Clearinghouse (WWC)

The WWC was created in 2002 by the U.S. Department of Education's Institute of Education Sciences (IES) to show scientific evidence for what works in education. WWC teams review research critically to assess the available evidence. They apply rigorous criteria to what constitutes well-designed research demonstrating positive effects of educational interventions. The outcome is a list of interventions that have been repeatedly documented to improve educational practice. Topics include academic achievement, career readiness and college access, dropout prevention, early childhood education, educational technology, and many others.

Retrieved from *http://ies.ed.gov/ncee/wwc*.

The question becomes "What causes this to occur, or how can we control this response to bring about desired changes?"

Unlike the previous two purposes of science, the goal of making improvements is somewhat more difficult to achieve, because of *extraneous variables* that can interfere with accurate conclusions. These variables are presented in Chapter 2. Three research categories allow for the investigation of improvement methods. First, experimental research requires a manipulation of the independent variable to determine the effects on participants' behavior (also called the *dependent variable*), such as changing the type of instruction or comparing groups receiving different types of medication. Experimental research allows for the demonstration of cause-and-effect relationships. Experimental methods are presented in Chapter 5.

Second, causal–comparative methods provide a comparison of participants on some existing condition such as the academic achievement of high-SES compared to low-SES students. The independent variable (i.e., SES) is predetermined, in that it is not possible randomly to assign some students to low-SES status and others to high-SES status (see Chapter 6).

Third, correlational research can provide information on how to make improvements as the relationship between two or more variables is measured. Similar to causal–comparative research methods, correlational methods can help to determine how students with different SES levels perform in school. Correlational research takes advantage of how natural variations in one variable (e.g., not all children come from identical SES backgrounds) are related to natural variations in a second variable (e.g., not all children have the same achievement levels). Correlational research is presented in Chapter 7.

Explanation

The final purpose of research is to explain why a phenomenon occurs. To achieve this purpose, researchers develop theories. However, not everyone agrees that we can explain fully why phenomena occur, because there is an infinite number of possible reasons why something occurs. We can never really isolate all of the variables that are potential causes of an event.

Therefore, some researchers argue that we can demonstrate relationships among variables but never truly know what causes something to occur. Whether we can truly explain a phenomenon is up for debate.

Explanation of a phenomenon requires knowledge from the other three purposes of science. To explain a phenomenon, we must first describe it, predict when it will and will not

---

Causation or Correlation?

Correlation is a term that indicates the extent to which two or more variables are related. It identifies the strength of the relationship between/among variables. Causation indicates that when one variable is introduced, it causes another to occur or change. The terms are often confused in popular media, and sometimes in research as well. Correlation does not imply causation. Instead, any of a number of explanations may account for the relationship. Variable A may be the cause of B. Variable B may be the cause of A. Some unknown third factor (C) may cause either A or B. Or the effects may simply be coincidental. Consider the following statement: "As ice-cream sales increase, the rate of drowning deaths increase. Therefore, eating ice cream causes drowning." Clearly, this is not a causal relationship. Additional variables, such as hot weather and summer vacation, are associated with both increased ice-cream sales and drowning, and probably account for the relationship. Other spurious relationships are more deceptive and harder to detect. Consider the following research conclusion: Numerous medical studies showed that women taking hormone replacement therapy (HRT) had lower-than-average coronary heart disease, which prompted researchers to conclude that HRT reduced heart disease (Rozenberg, Vasquez, Vandromme, & Kroll, 1998). Yet later studies showed the reverse effect; that is, HRT increased risk of heart disease. A reexamination of the data revealed that the initial conclusion was unwarranted, because women who participated in the research were from higher socioeconomic strata, with better diet and exercise routines (Lawlor, Smith, & E... accounted more... HRT. Educators... examine statem... other ways that v...

Theory
Purpose ↗

---

occur, and finally be able to change the direction of the phenomenon. Once we are able to do all three of these things, we can begin to explain why something occurs. Again, our explanation is not necessarily correct, since we could make a mistake along the way. We can gain a sufficient amount of confidence in our explanation, but we can never prove that it is correct. Not being able to prove that our explanation is correct can be better understood by knowing what a scientific theory is.

WHAT IS A SCIENTIFIC THEORY?

A theory is an explanation of a certain set of observed phenomena about constructs and how they relate to one another (Gall et al., 2007). A theoretical construct is a concept inferred from observing events. Generally accepted constructs based on repeated research include verbal fluency, depression, anxiety, and intelligence (Jackson, 2011), among many others. In a more specific example, we might present a theory that teaching alternative, or replacement, behaviors to children is an effective way to decrease problem behavior when that behavior serves as an attempt to communicate something. Such a theory is consistent with functional communication training (Tiger, Hanley, & Bruzek, 2008). Replacement and problem behaviors that serve as an attempt to communicate qualify as theoretical constructs, which are developed through observation of events that yield some predictable outcomes. For example, if a researcher observes that after teaching a child to use the replacement behavior, the child asks for help instead of displaying a tantrum, then he or she has evidence for the construct of a replacement behavior. A variable is a quantitative expression for a construct (Graziano & Raulin, 2010). Observing that the child asked for help three times and did not display tantrums, all after being taught to engage in a replacement behavior, would be a variable providing evidence for the construct.

Theories have three purposes (Gall et al., 2007). First, they identify commonalities in otherwise isolated phenomena. Darwin's copious and repeated observations of various species led to his theory of the descent of man (Ruse, 2009).

Darwin's work linked commonalities regarding development across species. Second, theories enable us to make predictions and to control phenomena. Scientists can make relatively accurate predictions by observing weather patterns, geological events, space travel, chemical reactions, and even human behavior. "Control" to scientists refers to a functional relation, or when an experiment reveals that a change in one event reliably produces a change in another event (Cooper et al., 2007). Third, a theory may refer to an explanatory system that describes the data gathered before the theory was developed. A theory attempts to determine regularities in the phenomenon. For example, after data are gathered, the researcher takes all of the data into consideration and looks for uniformities. Once these uniformities are found, the constructed theory is based on these uniformities. These theories do not rely on guessing or speculation in the absence of observation. The theories are derived *from* experimentation; they do not come *before* experimentation. Theories are grounded in the data that were generated.

Examining theories as we have presented them is quite different from the popular notion of a theory as something like a thought or an idea without observation or data. Scientific theories grounded on a solid foundation of systematically collected data contrasts sharply from what Popper (2002) calls *psychologism*, or merely generating ideas.

Now that we see there are three purposes of theories, we must determine whether a theory is a scientific one. According to Popper (1957/1996), a *scientific theory* is one that is falsifiable or refutable. In other words, a scientific theory must be able to be disproven. This sounds counterintuitive until we realize that technically, a scientific theory can only be disproven, not proven. The reason we are not able to prove a theory is that we never know all of the variables that can affect the results of an experiment supporting the theory, or from which the theory was developed. Simply stated, errors are always made in scientific research conclusions. We do not know where or when those errors will occur, only that they can occur at some point. If we make an error in a research conclusion and say that we have proven a theory, we are placing trust

in a potentially false theory. Thus, we say that we have confidence in a theory. For instance, we might use 100 studies to develop or support an existing theory, but if data gathered from one additional study do not fit with the theory, the theory can be disproven.

So we set out to disprove theories, not to prove them; in order to disprove a theory, we must be able to test it. Many psychological theories are untestable. For example, Popper (1957/1996) indicated that the psychoanalytic theories of Freud and Jung were not testable. It is not possible, for example, to disprove the existence of the id, ego, and superego. Thus, Popper indicates that we must look to refute a theory through testing. As stated by Popper:

1. It is easy to obtain confirmations, or verifications, for nearly every theory—if we look for confirmations.
2. Confirmations should count only if they are the result of risky predictions; that is to say, if, unenlightened by the theory in question, we should have expected an event which was incompatible with the theory—an event which, had it happened, would have refuted the theory.
3. Every "good" scientific theory is one that forbids certain things to happen; the more a theory forbids, the better.
4. A theory that is not refutable by any conceivable event is nonscientific. Irrefutability is not a virtue of a theory (as people often think) but a vice.
5. Every genuine test of a theory is an attempt to falsify it, or to refute it. Testability is falsifiability, but there are degrees of testability: some theories are more testable, more exposed to refutation, than others; they take, as it were, greater risks.
6. Confirming evidence does not count except when it is the result of a genuine test of the theory; and this means that it can be presented as an unsuccessful but serious attempt to falsify the theory.
7. Some genuinely testable theories, when found to be false, are still upheld by their admirers—for example, by introducing ad hoc some auxiliary assumption, or by reinterpreting the theory ad hoc in such a way that it escapes refutation. Such a procedure is always possible, but it rescues the theory from refutation only at the price of destroying or at least lowering its scientific status. (1957/1996, pp. 159–160)

Consider each of Popper's (1957/1996) statements. The first statement refers to what many people do today. We can find research to support virtually every theory. However, this is not critical thinking. Thinking critically about science is attempting to find alternative explanations for research findings (i.e., theories).

The second statement is a caution about accepting research that supports a theory as a confirmation of the theory. Confirmations may occur when we are not looking for them. If we are looking for confirmation, we can usually find them in any set of data.

The third statement refers to placing restrictions on what is expected based on the theory. For example, if we have a prediction that instructing students based on a discovery format will result in improved skills but we do not specify these skills, the theory is weaker than one that predicts that the instruction will improve specific skills. The more specific one is, the easier it is to refute the theory.

The fourth through seventh statements allude to the fact that scientific theories must be disprovable. Essentially, we must not look for confirmations, since we will usually find them. We must look for falsifications instead. However, some scientists may attempt to protect or rescue their theories from being disproven. These attempts do not constitute science. Critical research consumers should attempt to determine whether the theory can be tested and disproven. If a theory cannot be tested or disproven, it does not fall under the category of scientific theory.

"Good" versus "Bad" Scientific Theories

Thomas (1996) discusses how to distinguish a good theory from a bad one. He describes 14 different standards with which to compare theories in child development. Table 1.1 summarizes each of these standards from Thomas (pp. 17–26). The importance of these standards is that a critical research consumer can use them to determine the utility of the theory. Essentially, all theories that impact education, such as those proposed by Skinner, Piaget, Vygotsky, Goodman, Goodlad, and Gardner, can be assessed in terms of their utility by considering these standards.

TABLE 1.1. Standards to Determine Whether a Theory Is Good or Bad

- Standard 1. Theory accurately reflects the facts of the real world.
- Standard 2. Theory is stated in a way that makes it clearly understandable to anyone who is reasonably competent (i.e., *anyone who has an adequate command of language, mathematics, and logical analysis*).
- Standard 3. Theory not only explains why past events occurred but also accurately predicts future events.
- Standard 4. Theory offers practical guidance in solving daily problems.
- Standard 5. Theory is internally consistent (i.e., *all of the parts fit together logically*).
- Standard 6. Theory is founded on as few unproven assumptions as possible and requires the simplest possible mechanisms to explain all the phenomena it encompasses.
- Standard 7. Theory can be *disproven*.
- Standard 8. The evidence supporting it is convincing.
- Standard 9. Theory is able to accommodate new data.
- Standard 10. Theory provides a novel or original view of the phenomenon.
- Standard 11. Theory offers reasonable answers to questions about all educational phenomena.
- Standard 12. Theory stimulates the creation of new research techniques and the discovery of new knowledge.
- Standard 13. Theory continues to attract attention and enlist adherents over an extended period of time.
- Standard 14. Theory explains the phenomenon in a manner that fits with one's way of viewing the world (e.g., *behaviorally, cognitively, humanistically*).

Note. The *italicized* words are modifications of Thomas (1996).

Science or Pseudoscience?

A website called "Quackwatch" (*www.quackwatch.com/01quackeryrelatedtopics/pseudo.html*) attempts to distinguish between science and pseudoscience. The first recommendation is to know as much as possible about science, including how evidence is produced, what design is used in experiments, how hypotheses are tested, and so forth. Specific knowledge of the scientific method makes the distinction clearer. Advice is offered on how to spot pseudoscience. A brief summary follows:

1. Pseudoscientific research is described in general and ambiguous terms. Rather than provide details on their scientific methods, pseudoscientists usually report information from unreliable sources. They rarely conduct their own investigation.

2. Pseudoscientists begin with a hypothesis and look only for items that appear to support it. Evidence that might conflict with the hypothesis is ignored.

3. Pseudoscience relies on subjective "validation." Pseudoscientists seek out testimonials from individuals rather than findings from controlled research involving groups.

4. Pseudoscientists avoid solid criteria or valid evidence. Rather than describe repeatable scientific experiments, pseudoscientists rely on unverifiable testimony, hearsay, and anecdote.

5. Pseudoscience attempts to persuade rather than provide results of tested hypotheses. The objective of pseudoscientists is to convince consumers of a point of view and bring them on board as supporters.

6. Pseudoscientific literature is aimed at the general public. There is no review by scientific peers or demand for accuracy, precision, and specific definition of terms.

7. Results cannot be verified or reproduced. If studies are conducted, they are described vaguely.

Testability of a Theory

The ability of a scientific theory to be tested is the most important criterion to be met (Roberts & Pashler, 2000). The requirement for a testable theory, like other areas of philosophy, can be interpreted in a number of ways. Consider the question: Can a person's intelligence be tested directly? Some researchers would say that intelligence is a theoretical construct used to explain how people behave in different contexts. Others see intelligence as something real that cannot be directly measured. However, intelligence can be indirectly measured through intelligence tests. The responses to questions on intelligence tests are measures that allow the testing of intelligence. What about long-term memory? A theory about long-term memory may not be testable according to some researchers, since the term *long-term memory* means being able to remember something for a given period of time. Others see long-term memory as a construct that exists and can store information for later recall. However, can we test long-term memory directly? At the present time, we may lack the physiological instruments to measure long-term memory directly. However, we may be able to test what long-term memory is able to do indirectly. At issue, then, is the thing that is being tested. With a theory of long-term memory, we must be testing long-term memory. Others may argue that long-term memory is not being tested, only responses to certain environmental events at a later time. Thus, there is a lack of agreement as to what constitutes the testing of a theory. Ultimately, it is left up to critical research consumers to determine whether the theory was tested.

WHAT ARE THE TYPES OF SCIENTIFIC LOGIC?

Simply, scientific theories are constructed one of two ways depending on the scientific logic one uses. First, theories are constructed after a large number of investigations are conducted and researchers develop a theory based on past research results. Second, theories are constructed, then used to predict what will occur in future investigations. In other words, theories may be constructed after data have been collected (*induction*) or before data are collected (*deduction*). Thus, scientific logic takes two basic forms—induction and deduction (see Figure 1.4). There are also combinations of the logic forms, and these constitute how most theories are constructed.

Inductive Logic

Inductive logic involves moving from the specific to the general. For example, we offer an inductive hypothesis: Every student who has taken this class has learned how to think critically about research; therefore, all students in future classes will also learn how to think

Inductive Logic:
Moving from specific (individual
study findings) to general (theory)

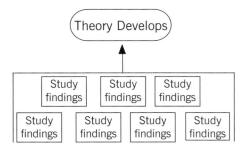

Deductive Logic:
Moving from general (theory) to
specific (individual study findings)

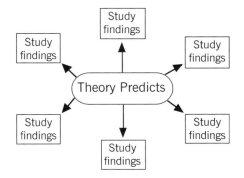

FIGURE 1.4. Inductive and deductive forms of scientific logic.

critically about research. Inductive logic is the process used in the formulation of theories. Theories involving inductive logic are developed after supporting research data are collected in a systematic fashion. For example, some researchers see the scientific method as comprising three steps (Kitchener, 1994). The first step involves the collection of data. Data that are to be collected are based on observable events. The second step involves the formation of scientific regularities, which lead to the development of generalizations and laws. For example, Thorndike's Law of Effect involves the collection of observable data across a large range of organisms and finding consistencies. The Law of Effect states that the effects of our actions will determine whether the actions will be repeated. In the third step, formulated theories are collections of earlier laws and include previously collected data. Several investigations are required that lead to the demonstration of scientific regularities, which then lead to the development of a theory. Thus, the development of a theory takes a great deal of time. The critical aspect of inductive logic is that theories are grounded in the data, and investigations are not guided by the theory.

Inductive logic has the advantage of grounding the theory in data. Once a theory is constructed, it will have a great deal of empirical support. Proponents of inductive logic also argue that it allows for research that is

not theory-laden. In other words, there are no hypotheses that the researcher is attempting to disprove. There are only research questions that allow the researcher to move in a number of directions due to a lack of constraint by hypotheses. Johnston and Pennypacker (1993) explain:

> Actually, researchers do not need to state hypotheses if they are asking a question about nature. When the experimental question simply asks about the relationship between independent and dependent variables, there is no scientific reason to make a prediction about what will be learned from the data. Whatever is learned will describe something about that relation that was presumably not known

before, and whether it matches anyone's expectations has nothing to do with its truth or importance (Sidman, 1960). (p. 48)

Being able to demonstrate lawful relations is a critical aspect of a science of human learning. Although inductive logic sounds "logical," not everyone agrees with this premise. Popper (2002) offers this view of induction:

> It is usual to call an inference "inductive" if it passes from singular statements . . . such as accounts of the results of observations or experiments, to universal statements, such as hypotheses or theories. Now it is far from obvious, from a logical point of view, that we are justified in inferring universal statements from singular ones, no matter how numerous; for any condition drawn in this way may always turn out to be false: no matter how many instances of white swans we may have observed, this does not justify the conclusion that *all* swans are white. (p. 27)

Among the arguments against induction are the following: (1) The future will not likely be exactly like the past; (2) a limited number of tests or observations will not provide enough evidence that a universal theory is true; and (3) there is no justification for inductive inferences (i.e., making generalized statements based on limited data). The first concern, for many researchers, is the assumption that human learning is consistent and orderly, which is not likely true. There is a great deal of variation between and among individuals. The second concern involves the amount of evidence needed to develop a theory. In essence, there will never be enough evidence to show that a theory is true. Thus, the question becomes "When do we move from collecting data to constructing a theory?" The final concern is that there is no real justification for induction, since it cannot be shown to be correct on logical grounds or on the basis of the success it has shown (Popper, 2002).

Deductive Logic

<u>Deductive logic</u> moves from the general to the specific. For example, we offer a deductive hypothesis: All students who take this class become proficient critical research consumers;

Student A took the class; therefore Student A is a proficient critical research consumer. Deduction in research essentially involves constructing a theory containing a set of postulates (i.e., assumptions), making predictions or hypotheses based on the theory, then the testing of parts of the theory to determine whether the results uphold the theory. If the results of an investigation do not support the theory, the theory may need to be either discarded or modified when taking into consideration the results. As stated by Johnston and Pennypacker (1993):

> To the extent that experimental outcomes verify the predictions, the experimenter may have increased confidence in the validity of the postulates. However, if the experiment fails to support a logically valid prediction from the postulate, then one or more of the postulates have been falsified. The appropriate action is then to revise the postulate set until the obtained results can be predictable and to confirm the new prediction by repeating the experiment. (p. 51)

Therefore, the difference between inductive and deductive logic is that the theory is developed last in inductive logic and first in deductive logic. The assumption is that with inductive logic, the theory is correct or valid due to the empirical evidence that builds up before theory construction. With deductive logic, the assumption is that the theory is valid, or that confidence in the validity of the theory is increased, due to the data supporting the theory or predicted by the theory.

According to its proponents, the primary advantage of deductive logic is that it has explanatory power. A major purpose of science is to explain phenomena. Theories are developed to

---

Inductive logic *involves moving from the specific to the general. It is the type of logic used in the formulation of theories after supporting research data are collected in a systematic fashion.*

Deductive logic *moves from the general to the specific. It is the type of logic that involves the construction of a theory followed by testing parts of the theory to determine whether the results of the testing uphold the theory.*

The Principle of Deductive Logic

All X are Y. All Y are Z. Hence, all X are Z. Examples of deductive logic:

1. All oranges are fruits. All fruits grow on trees. Hence, all oranges grow on trees.
2. All bachelors are single. Johnny is single. Hence, Johnny is a bachelor.

Retrieved from *www.buzzle.com/articles/deductive-reasoning-examples.html*.

explain phenomena. Explanatory theories in turn are supported by research. Deductive logic also enables researchers to provide evidence that can increase the confidence in a theory. If, upon successive testing, the theory is not refuted, confidence in that theory is heightened. Deductive logic also allows the researcher, based on the existing theory, to make predictions of what should be observed in the future, guiding the researcher in making and testing constructs or ideas. Finally, deductive logic allows the production of hypotheses, a critical part of scientific inquiry. In educational and psychological research, the majority of research relies on the development of hypotheses.

Although deductive logic has several advantages, several limitations are also noteworthy. First, deductive logic essentially "locks" a researcher into testing certain constructs or ideas. For example, in general, a researcher may be interested in testing the statement "When less teacher-directed structure is implemented in a classroom setting, more in-depth learning will result." Unfortunately, if more in-depth learning does not result, little note is taken as to what occurred instead (Johnston & Pennypacker, 1993). Inductive logic, on the other hand, requires asking questions rather than making deductive statements. Rather than predicting what will occur when discovery learning is implemented, an inductionist would ask, "What is the relation between teacher directedness and learning?"

Second, a deductive approach to science cannot rely on itself. Deductive conclusions are essentially elaborations on previous knowledge.

Deductive logic takes what is already known and points to new relationships among known variables, but it cannot be a source for new truth.

Finally, a deductive approach has the tendency to make researchers more interested in "proving" their hypotheses or predictions than in exploring new information that was previously unknown.

Combination of Logic Forms

Induction and deduction actually do not occur in isolation, but in some combination. Johnston and Pennypacker (1993) call this combination a fusion of induction and deduction, and Graziano and Raulin (2010) call the combination a functional theory. Science essentially involves a combination of the two and does not advance using a single strategy of logic (Johnston & Pennypacker, 1993). Think of it this way: When we engage in deductive logic, the source of the original formulation of the theory comes from induction. In other words, the researcher must build on something when formulating the theory. This "something" involves the experiences and prior knowledge about the phenomenon under consideration. Once the theory is constructed, the researcher can make hypothetical statements or predictions about expected results in future investigations of the phenomenon. This hypothesis testing is deductive. Let's return to the hypothesis that teacher-directed instruction is critical for in-depth learning. When we are attempting to affirm the original hypothesis, we verify that in-depth learning did occur. Once we determine that in-depth learning has occurred, we engage again in induction by concluding that teacher-directed instruction is critical for in-depth learning to occur. However, as noted by Cooper et al. (2007):

> When the independent variable is present (*A*), the data show that the behavior has changed (*B* is true). Therefore, the independent variable is the controlling variable for the behavior (*A* is true). The logic, of course, is flawed; other factors could be responsible for the truthfulness of *A*. (p. 171)

To logicians, this relationship (i.e., if *A* is true, *B* is true; *B* is true; therefore *A* is true) is a fallacy called *affirmation of the consequent* (Schroyens &

Schaeken, 2003). Other factors could have been responsible for *A*. For example, if we entertain the hypothesis that the "Power-Packed Reading Program" (*A*) will increase reading scores (*B*) and scores increase, then the "Power-Packed Reading Program" accounted for the increased reading scores (induction). But *B* may have occurred for a variety of reasons. However, from the perspective of inductive reasoning, no fallacy exists; that is, the truth of the antecedent, *A*, can be established only by observation of the consequent, *B*. Cooper et al. (2007) recommend that researchers establish several if, *A*, then *B* possibilities to reduce the likelihood that factors other than the independent variable accounted for the change.

A discussion of the problems and paradoxes of confirming theories is beyond the scope of this book; however, suffice it to say that not all researchers agree with the use of induction, since it requires regularities observed today to be projected into the future. A consensus on either side of the debate will most likely never occur. Therefore, the main concern for critical research consumers is probably less what type of logic a researcher uses and more what the research was attempting to do. If a researcher sets out to "prove" a theory and finds supporting evidence for it, critical research consumers should be cautious. It is not difficult to find support for one's theory; it is much more difficult to show how incremental findings add to confidence in the theory, or to show how, after many serious attempts, falsification of the theory has not been achieved. In other words, before critical research consumers accept the validity of claims about a theory, large amounts, not isolated bits, of data must be taken into consideration.

Critique of Both Deduction and Induction

As we critically examine scientific logic, we should note that some researchers (e.g., Fischer, 1998; Galison, 1997) argue that neither deduction nor induction provide logical methods leading to defensible conclusions. Fischer (1998) begins by describing the neopositivist approach as the epistemological doctrine that physical and social reality are independent of those who observe it. Fischer describes empiricism (the *neopositivist perspective*) as failing to establish itself

as a predictive science or a source of solutions to social problems. He notes that in researchers' attempts to explain the physical world, the position of the observer influences what is observed and what conclusions are drawn. He describes the *postpositivist approach*, in which science is viewed as more of a sociocultural activity than a technical one.

IN WHAT WAYS DO WE GAIN INFORMATION?

Try to answer the following question: You are teaching fourth-grade students and an administrator approaches you and asks, "Are your students learning?" You answer the question with "yes." From where will you get your information? We are asked questions all the time about many topics, such as "Will the economy get better or worse in the next 5 years?"; "What are the best methods to teach reading or math?"; "What is the possibility of life on distant planets?"; "Do we have a good relationship with our family?"; and "What is the effectiveness of the death penalty in deterring violent crimes?" We usually answer these questions readily and in some instances automatically. But where does the information come from that allows us to answer these questions? And are the sources of this information valid? Finally, depending on the sources of information we use, how sure are we that our answers are correct?

We all use various sources of information, usually without actually being aware of them. Whether we accept the information we receive depends on our experiences throughout our lives, including our educational, familial, religious, and social backgrounds. To be a critical research consumer entails questioning sources of information we once accepted and accepting information from sources we once refused to consider. In a sense, we will be providing experiences throughout this volume that will change how readers gain information and what they do with it once it is in their possession. To this end, there are five ways of obtaining information to consider—three that are nonscientific (i.e., tenacity, intuition, authority) and two that are scientific (i.e., empiricism, and rationalism; see Figure 1.5).

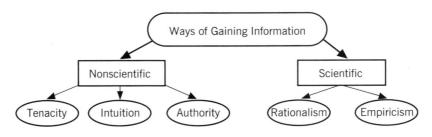

FIGURE 1.5. Nonscientific and scientific methods of gaining information.

Tenacity

The first way we acquire knowledge is through *tenacity,* the persistence of a certain belief or way of thought for a long period of time. We essentially accept the information as being correct since, if it were not correct, it would not have lasted such a long time. For example, Francisco Sizzi tenaciously held to the belief that there could be only seven planets, because there were seven windows of the head, seven days of the week, and seven metals. Here is a more common and timely example. We may ask people about what they consider to be the best method of child discipline. Some people indicate that it is preferable to spank children when they behave poorly. Others believe in this method of child discipline because it has been around for as long as we can remember. Arguments such as "I was spanked, my parents were spanked, and my grandparents were spanked, and we all turned out okay" are used to defend the practice. Spanking may be the most effective disciplinary method devised, but do we really know this from tenacity? The answer is "no." Just because beliefs have been around for a long time does not make them correct. Recall that for centuries the world's population, including many scholars, believed that the world was flat. Just because the belief was held by many for so long does not make the information correct. At some point, research will either support or refute long-held beliefs. However, long-held beliefs tend to be resistant to contrary evidence. Tenacity is not considered a source of scientific information. Tenacity can aid us in asking research questions, such as "What is the best way of disciplining children?" It is not an adequate source of confirming or refuting information.

Intuition

The second way we acquire knowledge is through so-called *intuition,* which is a "feeling" one gets about a topic. For example, suppose we are exposed to two options in teaching a child how to spell. One method is through teaching about *morphographs* (i.e., the smallest unit of language that carries meaning) and the other is a sight word–only method. We look at both methods and have a feeling that the sight word method would be more successful because it seems easier to teach. We make our decision based on our intuition. Intuition most likely comes from our past and current experiences rather than some form of extrasensory perception. We may have been taught ourselves via the sight word method or had more familiarity with it. Thus, our decisions based on intuition are supported by previous information on the same or similar topics.

Some curriculum developers have indicated to us that intuition is the most important source of information. One writer in particular indicated that curricula she writes do not need to be field-tested to assess their effectiveness, since she just *knows* they will work. However, if intuition is based on past experiences, our intuition may not be altogether accurate, since accuracy depends on the occurrence of past information. Possibly more problematic with intuition is that its accuracy is usually not assessed in any meaningful manner.

There is a lack of feedback regarding the accuracy of our intuition. If we do not get feedback, there is no way to adjust our intuition. In other words, if our intuition is based on faulty information from the past, our intuition will always be based on this faulty information unless we have feedback to let us know the information is incorrect. If this feedback does not occur, our intuition will continue to be incorrect. Intuition is not a way to obtain scientific information. As with tenacity, intuition can help us raise research questions, but it is not a way of confirming or refuting information.

Authority

One of the skills college students should develop is *critical thinking*, which means taking into consideration all available information and making an informed decision about a topic. Unfortunately, college educators may be faced with a dilemma. On the one hand, it would be wonderful if students developed critical thinking skills. On the other hand, the development of critical thinking skills may mean that students challenge educational authority. If we want students to accept everything we tell them, students must rely on our authority for information.

For example, students are frequently confused about the best way to teach reading to elementary-age schoolchildren. Unfortunately, the debate has created an "us versus them" mentality. Some college faculty members may tell students to use a whole-language or literature-based approach to reading. Others tell students to use a systematic approach that emphasizes learning phonics first. Students come away unclear and wonder who is correct. Many students align themselves with the faculty members who seem most authoritative. Thus, accepted information is based on the person or persons providing the information. But what are the pitfalls of acquiring information from authorities? First, many authorities may simply be wrong in the information they are providing. Second, authorities provide information based on their particular biases; therefore, the information is rarely objective. Third, even if the information provided by an authority is correct, one would have to rely on that authority or other authorities to tell one so. Critical research consumers may rely on authorities but also must search out confirming evidence. Again, as with tenacity and intuition, authority requires an active attempt on the part of critical research

Why Question Authority? Why Not?

- Unthinking respect for authority is the greatest enemy of truth. (from Albert Einstein)
- No provision in our Constitution ought to be dearer to man than that which protects the rights of conscience against the enterprises of the civil authority. (from Thomas Jefferson)
- The ultimate authority must always rest with the individual's own reason and critical analysis. (from the Dalai Lama)
- Anyone who conducts an argument by appealing to authority is not using his intelligence, he is just using his memory. (from Leonardo da Vinci)
- Men in authority will always think that criticism of their policies is dangerous. They will always equate their policies with patriotism, and find criticism subversive. (from Henry Steele Commager)
- The teacher, like the artist and the philosopher, can perform his work adequately only if he feels himself to be an individual directed by an inner creative impulse, not dominated and fettered by an outside authority. (from Bertrand Russell)
- I have as much authority as the Pope. I just don't have as many people who believe it. (from George Carlin)

Retrieved from *http://thinkexist.com/quotes/with/keyword/authority/2.html.*

consumers to gather supporting or refuting evidence of the obtained information. Authority is a source for developing research questions, but it cannot provide us with information to help confirm or refute a scientific theory.

Empiricism

The three aforementioned ways of acquiring information all have the same weakness: They do not require the level of rigor that is needed in scientific inquiry. This level of rigor is what separates science from other endeavors; science requires a level of evidence that is not required in everyday life. The fourth source of information is one that we all use in our lives but most likely not to the extent and systematic manner in which a scientist uses it. This source is

empiricism. Empiricism involves gaining information from our senses. If we say that a student in a classroom is sad, we most likely infer an emotional state based on what we observe, such as a frown, a lowered head, or a quiet demeanor. If we wished to test the effectiveness of a reading program, we might observe how well students read before and after the program. Empiricism, then, is the foundation on which science functions. Instead of relying on what has been around for a long time, what we feel to be correct, and what others tell us, we actually go out and see for ourselves. It is like saying, "Show me that it works."

Empiricism must meet a higher level of rigor than the previous three ways of obtaining information, simply because it is public. Others must observe the same phenomenon before we can come to any acceptable conclusions in regard to our research results. However, empiricism is not infallible. Mistakes can be, and often are, made. Observations require some repeatability over a period of time. In other words, if we observe something only once, we cannot be sure that a real phenomenon is taking place unless we see it again. If we observe something only once and make conclusions based on some isolated incident, we run the risk of making incorrect conclusions, since an isolated incident does not provide enough evidence to allow us to make correct or adequate conclusions.

Rationalism

Rationalism is the interpretation and understanding of the world through our reasoning processes. An example of this is the process of deductive logic described earlier. We first begin with a general statement, such as "All students who read this book will learn how to think critically about research." Then, we have a second statement, such as "This student just finished reading the book." Finally, we make a logical conclusion based on our previous statements, such as "This student has learned how to think critically about research." Unfortunately, we cannot know from rationalism alone whether the statement is true. For instance, in the example about reading the textbook on research, we do not actually know whether every student who reads the book will be able to think critically

about research. We must make some type of assessment to determine whether, indeed, every student who read the book learned how to think critically about research. Thus, what is needed is the addition of empiricism to rationalism. When we add the two together, we have a method of gathering information in a scientific context.

Rationalism and empiricism can be combined in three ways. First, we can use deductive reasoning in which we first make a general statement, then make observations, and finally conclude whether the general statement is supported. Thus, we use rationalism in making the general statement, empiricism in making the observations, and rationalism again in making the conclusion.

Second, we can use the combination of rationalism and empiricism when we engage in inductive reasoning, in which we make observations, then develop general statements about the phenomenon. In this case, we first use empiricism when making the observations, then rationalism when taking the research findings into consideration, to make general statements about the phenomenon.

Third, we can combine the two when we fuse induction with deduction. We first make observations, develop general statements based on these observations, then continue to make observations to test the accuracy of the general statements. We use empiricism to make the initial observations, rationalism to make general conclusions about the phenomenon, empiricism to make further observations of the phenomenon, and, finally, rationalism to determine whether the observations support the general statements.

WHAT ARE CONSTRAINT LEVELS IN EDUCATIONAL AND PSYCHOLOGICAL RESEARCH?

All empirical research methods are not created equal, and as we demonstrate throughout the text, all research methods do not address the same questions or serve the same purposes. A major difference between or among research methods is the **level of constraint** placed on the participant and/or setting. The level of constraint has to do with the level of limits or control one has over the research process (Graziano & Raulin, 2010). Level of constraint in research does not make a particular research method good or bad. Instead, the questions asked by the researcher or the purpose of the research should determine the level of constraints placed on the participants. For example, if we wanted to determine whether X (the independent variable) caused Y (the dependent variable), we would need to use high constraint in the research, because we are attempting to determine the effects of one variable on another, while excluding the effects of other variables on the dependent variable. (*Note. Cause* can mean one thing resulted due to something else; *cause* can also mean that there is a functional relationship between variables, such as when X occurs, it is reliably followed by Y.) For example, suppose we want to determine whether the physical arrangement of a classroom (independent variable) affects the on-task time (dependent variable) of students. We would need some way to remove or at least control for the effects of other variables, such as the type of task in which the students engage, the way the teacher presents the task, and the level of distractions in the hallway. In other words, this research would have a high level of constraint.

If we use a research method that does not control for these other variables, we would have a difficult time determining the effects of the physical arrangement on student behavior independent of everything else. On the other hand, if we wish to measure how students feel when engaged in a classroom activity, we could use a lower constraint type of research.

The advantage of high-constraint research is that it allows us to make cause-and-effect determinations. The main disadvantage is that high constraints may make the context artificial. Thus, to say variable X causes Y in a research context with high constraint is not to say that variable X will cause Y in a different situation. The ability to generalize the results of high-constraint research to other contexts is limited. Low-constraint research can tell us what will happen in an applied context, such as a classroom. We can say that in this situation, something happened. However, we cannot say that variable X will cause Y in that or any other context. Thus, there are trade-offs in research. If

we want to know what occurs in a participant's life, we could use low-constraint research. If we want to know what causes the participant to do what he/she does, we could use high-constraint research.

A description of the constraint levels in educational and psychological research follows. Generally, there are five levels of constraint—experimental, causal–comparative, correlational, case study, and naturalistic or descriptive research (see Figure 1.6 for a continuum of constraint levels). We consider each of these constraint levels in turn, moving from highest to lowest constraint level research. Additionally, we describe each of the five constraint levels in more detail throughout the text.

Experimental Research

Experimental methods are considered the highest level of constraint research due to the attempt to isolate the causal variable. In order to do this, the impact of all other variables outside of the investigation must be kept to a minimum so the researcher can determine whether the independent variable caused the changes in a participant's behavior and not some other, uncontrolled variable. Thus, an investigation with the highest level of constraint would be one that is conducted in a laboratory setting. In this type of setting, the sights, sounds, smells, and so forth, can be controlled, ensuring that as many outside variables as possible are eliminated. As investigations move from high-constraint settings, such as laboratories, to more natural settings, such as classrooms, the constraint level decreases due to an inability to control for many of the variables outside of the investigation that could impact the participant. Therefore, there is

Empiricism *involves gathering information by gaining knowledge through the observation of our world.*

Rationalism *involves interpreting or understanding the world around us through our reasoning processes.*

Level of constraint *is the degree to which a researcher imposes limits or controls on the research process.*

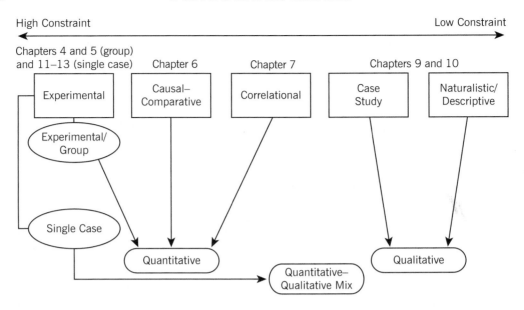

FIGURE 1.6. Continuum of constraint levels for different research methods. *Note.* The categories of quantitative and qualitative methods are for general guidance only, since case study and naturalistic and descriptive research methods can also fall under the category of quantitative research, depending on how the data are collected and analyzed. Survey research (Chapter 8), program evaluations (Chapter 14), and action research (Chapter 16) can also have aspects of both quantitative and qualitative research methods.

a continuum of constraint levels within experimental research methods.

Although **experimental research methods** differ in terms of their respective levels of constraint, all have three things in common. First, experimental research methods involve attempting to gather information in an objective manner. Second, experimental researchers most likely come from a scientific–rational perspective. Finally, the method of gathering data is strictly prescribed. The researcher attempts to remain as separate from the participants as possible, interacting with the participants only when it is absolutely necessary. The data gathered are operationally defined. In other words, the dependent variable (what is being measured) is defined in an observable manner. Numbers are attached to these observations, such as the percentage of math questions answered correctly or the score achieved on a standardized test.

Researchers using experimental methods usually believe that the results of an investigation can be generalized to a larger number of individuals.

Thus, they see that there is variability between and within each individual but assume that, as a whole, the group, culture, or population is relatively consistent. Experimental researchers typically deal with variability among individuals by calculating an average score for the group. The average score is then used to make conclusions. For example, the researchers may conclude that a higher average score for Writing Group A compared to Writing Group B means that the writing program used by Group A is superior. The goal of many experimental researchers is to find general laws that hold true for large numbers of people. Thus, the attempt is to gather a sample of participants for an investigation that is representative of the entire population or some target population. (*Note.* Sampling methods are discussed in Chapter 4.)

Experimental Methods

A major feature of much experimental or group research is the attempt to find cause-and-effect relationships. In order to do this, researchers manipulate the independent variable. Recall that an independent variable may have an effect on the dependent variable. For example, a computer tutorial used in your class can be considered an independent variable, and the knowledge the students gain is the dependent variable. An experimental researcher may provide the computer tutorial to your class and not to another, and make comparisons on a test at the end of some specified period of time. Thus, the assumption is that the researcher can determine whether the independent variable (i.e., computer tutorial) caused changes in the dependent variable (i.e., knowledge gained). Chapter 5 describes several different experimental designs.

Single-Case Methods

Single-case research involves one or a limited number of participants and is designed to identify causal relationships between variables employing within-participant comparisons across conditions (Horner et al., 2005). Although some professionals may see experimental research as requiring random assignment of participants (e.g., each participant selected for a sample has an equal chance of being assigned to experimental and control groups), experimental designs do not have to include this procedure. Experimental designs are experimental because they are designed to control for variables outside of the experiment; that is, experimental designs attempt to find cause-and-effect relationships. Single-case designs do this as well. Although experimental designs are typically quantitative, single-case designs may be thought of as a combination of quantitative and qualitative designs (see Chapters 11–13). Single-case designs rely on the intensive investigation of a single individual or a group of individuals. The studies develop, and experimental decisions are made as they progress. For example, researchers may record the number of problem behaviors of each of three children with autism spectrum disorder over several days, then implement positive reinforcement for the absence of problem behaviors. Researchers continue to record problem behaviors during the reinforcement phase to see whether problem behaviors are eliminated.

Single-case methods rely on objective rather than subjective data collection methods, and the experimenter does not attempt to interact with the participants in a manner that would affect their performance. Finally, the data collected are quantified and are based on direct observation of the subject matter.

Researchers conduct single-case studies for reasons that fall into two general categories—because of the limitations of group research and the research question under investigation. First, many single-case researchers consider group designs to have ethical problems (because one group of participants does not receive an intervention), practical problems (it is difficult, if not impossible, to randomly assign students in a classroom to two groups or to obtain a large enough sample of students), averaging of results (loss of information on the outcomes for individual participants), generality of findings (it is difficult to generalize results to individual participants with particular characteristics), and intersubject variability (some participants improve, whereas others deteriorate) (Cooper et al., 2007).

Second, single-case researchers view the variability in individuals as being important from a scientific viewpoint; that is, single-case investigators assume that much of the variability seen within participants is due to environmental or contextual circumstances. Therefore, single-case researchers collect repeated data on the performance of individual participants over time to analyze variability as opposed to averaging scores across participants. Single-case designs are presented in Chapters 11 through 13.

Causal–Comparative Research

Causal–comparative research looks very similar to experimental research (i.e., group research), with two main differences. First, participants are not randomly assigned to one of at least two

> **Experimental research methods** *are quantitative in nature. The designs typically require a number of participants placed into one or several groups. Thus, these designs are also called* group designs.

groups. Second, the independent variable is not manipulated. Causal–comparative research is conducted for one of two reasons: (1) when the independent variable of interest cannot be manipulated, such as in comparing an instructional technique for students with and without Down syndrome (independent variable), since it is not possible to assign Down syndrome to some participants; or (2) when it would be unethical to manipulate the independent variable, such as the effects on students who receive proper and improper nutrition (independent variable). With causal–comparative research, the main independent variable is called a *classification, subject,* or *organismic* variable, since it is something that resides within the individual or is due to some characteristic the individual possesses (e.g., ethnicity, disability, gender). Thus, participants are already assigned to a group due to some innate characteristic. Independent variables may be presented, such as instruction, but the comparisons are based on the nonmanipulated independent variable (e.g., how individuals with and without Down syndrome respond to the same instruction). The main function of causal–comparative research is to determine relationships between or among variables. Causal–comparative research is discussed further in Chapter 6.

Causal–comparative research is considered to have a lower constraint level than experimental research, because no attempt is made to isolate the effects of a manipulable independent variable on the dependent variable. Thus, the level of control or the ability to determine the effects of an independent variable is more limited than that for experimental research.

Correlational Research

Correlational research has the same goal as causal–comparative research, in that relationships between or among variables are sought. There is no manipulation of an independent variable. Unlike causal–comparative research, there is usually just one group, or at least groups are not compared. For this reason, correlational research has a lower constraint level than causal–comparative research. There is not an active attempt to determine the effects of the independent variable in any direct way.

Examples of Correlation Research Questions in Education

1. Is there a relationship between the number of students in a class and student educational achievement in a subject area?

2. Is there a relationship between the number of teachers in a hallway during junior high passing periods and incidents of student problem behavior?

3. Is there a relationship between how many times students have opportunities to respond in class and their educational achievement?

4. Is there a relationship between early childhood educational involvement and kindergarten readiness?

5. Is there a relationship between self-determination for one's special education program in high school and post–high school adjustment?

6. Is there a relationship between a college student's scores on the GRE and performance in graduate school?

With correlational research, measurements are taken in a single group of two or more variables. One of the variables is called the independent variable and the other, the dependent variable, although the distinction many times is not critical. Researchers seek to determine relationships between variables, such as whether a relation exists between grades and SAT scores. Correlational research is discussed further in Chapter 7.

Case Study Research

Case study research may be considered to be qualitative in nature, since the effort is to study a single participant or group of participants in depth. Qualitative researchers do not believe that everything to be studied can be operationally defined to permit observation. Therefore, it is critical to get to know the context in which the individuals interact and to become acquainted with the individuals themselves to study them adequately. Qualitative researchers do not attempt to reduce the phenomenon under study to operational definitions that may limit what can be studied. They believe that if we count the number of correct math problems, for example, we overlook a great deal of other information regarding the process of learning. Thus, in order to get a comprehensive understanding of the participants, we must not be limited to specific and precise definitions of what is being observed.

Case studies are not the same as single-case research. Single-case research attempts to manipulate the independent variable. Qualitative research does not actively attempt to manipulate variables. Case studies have a lower constraint level than correlational research, since there is no attempt to determine how variables are related systematically to one another. Case studies may be conducted in less constrained settings, such as a therapist's office or in the community. The most important characteristic of a case study, however, is the attempt to learn about individuals by studying them in an in-depth manner.

Naturalistic or Descriptive Research

Naturalistic research is concerned with the ecological validity of research (i.e., the extent to which the findings reflect the behaviors that actually occur in natural settings; Carey, 1980). Naturalistic research is considered to have the lowest level of constraint, since an independent variable is not defined and manipulated in any manner, and identifying a cause-and-effect relationship is not the purpose of the research. The research is conducted in the participant's natural setting; case study research may be conducted in an artificial setting that raises the amount of control over the participants' environment, thereby raising the level of constraint.

Naturalistic or descriptive research can also be considered qualitative; however, some may argue that descriptive research can also be quantitative, depending on how the data are collected (i.e., in a qualitative manner, such as through field notes [see Chapter 10], or quantitatively, such as counting the occurrences of a particular behavior). For our purposes, we consider descriptive research to be primarily qualitative in nature. Since descriptive research is typically conducted in the natural setting, we use the term *naturalistic research* for the remainder of the chapter.

Naturalistic research makes no attempt to determine cause-and-effect relationships. However, qualitative researchers are not always in total agreement as to what one can and cannot study with this approach. Some believe that cause-and-effect relationships can be drawn from naturalistic research; others believe that naturalistic research only provides descriptions of what one observes. There may not be an attempt to generalize the findings of naturalistic research, since the participant under study is observed in his/her context, which will not exactly match the context of other individuals. However, some qualitative researchers believe that it is possible to generalize the findings of research studies to a larger population (see Chapter 9).

Whereas quantitative research has defined designs, qualitative research may not have specified design types, since the research design develops throughout the investigation. Thus, the definition of qualitative research is more difficult to agree upon than that of quantitative research. Philosophical discussions of qualitative research methods are presented in Chapter 9.

Ethnographic Research

Another type of qualitative research, ethnographic research, involves the intense and in-depth study of a culture. Thus, ethnographic research is a type of naturalistic research that is more intense than other forms of qualitative research. A culture can be as wide as a nation or as narrow as a classroom. A key feature of ethnographic research is that multiple data collection methods are used to obtain as complete a picture as possible of the phenomenon under study. For example, interviews and observations may be used in combination, or information may come from a variety of sources, such as the teacher, researcher, student, and administrator. Several types of interview methods are available, as are participant and nonparticipant observation methods. The major difficulty with ethnographic research is summarizing and interpreting the vast amount of data generated. Ethnographic research has a low constraint level due to the natural setting in which it is conducted and the lack of attempt to isolate the effects of an independent variable on a dependent variable. Ethnographic research, types of observation research, and types of interview methods are presented in Chapter 10.

WHAT ARE THE DIFFERENCES BETWEEN BASIC AND APPLIED RESEARCH?

It is important to understand the difference between basic and applied research. Recall that basic research focuses on more theoretical issues than does applied research, which focuses on educational–psychological problems. It is especially important for educators to understand the importance of each, because the distinction bears on educational practice.

Basic Research

Basic research helps to develop a new theory or refine an existing one. Unfortunately, there seems to be a movement away from valuing basic research. Today, people in the community want to know how a research study impacts their school or family. However, basic research does not work this way. Basic research may not seem to have any relevance for us at all, since its primary purpose is the development of theory. Consider early research on behavioral principles, when much of the data were collected on rats in a small experimental chamber called a Skinner box. What is the relevance of a rat pressing a bar to receive a piece of food for children learning to read in the classroom? Other types of basic research may have more obvious links with the applied setting. Consider the research on multiple intelligences by Gardner (2006), who proposed that there are eight intelligences, and that instruction should build on the type of intelligence a particular child may have. Similarly, Piaget's research led to a theory of human development. Initially, Piaget set out to describe the development of children. He did not set out to seek the best way to facilitate student learning. However, later research by developmentalists aimed at developing educational practices based on Piaget's theory of human development (Lourenco & Machado, 1996). This later research was of the applied nature. The immediate relevance of basic research results may not be obvious or even known for a number of years. However, basic research is critical for applied research to survive. Basic research provides the foundation for applied researchers in future endeavors.

Applied Research

Applied research attempts to solve real-life problems or to study phenomena that directly impact practitioners or laypeople, using a theory developed through basic research, for example, a phenomenon in education, such as how to teach mathematics in a manner that is efficient and facilitates problem solving. The results of the research can have a direct impact on how we educate children in mathematics. A few years ago, two of the authors of this volume (Nancy Marchand-Martella and Ronald Martella) and their colleagues began to study the best method to teach problem solving that would result in participants' ability to use the skill in other contexts. The participants, adults with traumatic brain injuries, were placed in independent or semi-independent living arrangements. The difficulty these individuals encountered was an inability to solve everyday problems that most people may take for granted, such as what to do when the electricity goes out. The first step was to find out what had been done in the past with regard to teaching problem solving. Next, the typical method of teaching problem solving had to be modified, since participants had limited memory abilities. A problem-solving program was developed and tested. The results of the investigation led to further investigations that would ultimately improve and refine the teaching method. The problem-solving investigations that were applied sought to improve the lives of individuals having difficulties.

One of the other authors of this volume (Ron Nelson) was involved in applied research on a different topic: disruptive behavior in schools. A major problem today in schools is the level of student disruption in and out of the classroom. Thus, current research has focused on how to improve the school climate by setting up a schoolwide management system to decrease the level of disruptive behaviors. Therefore, applied research attempts not only to gather information on human behavior but also to provide information that is immediately useful to practitioners in applied settings.

Action Research

Action research, probably the purest form of applied research, involves the application of the scientific method to everyday problems in the classroom. The difference between action research and other research is that the research is conducted in real-life settings, with less control than one may have in a more artificial setting, school personnel are involved directly with the implementation of the research, and there is less impact on the field as a whole than is possible with other methods. Think of action research as research on a micro level. Suppose that a teacher has difficulty gaining the attention of some members of her class. An action research study involves implementing a different instructional technique, for example, and measuring the effects. The results of the research are limited to the classroom, since there is lack of information about how the class is similar to other classes, and how the students are similar to other students. This limitation does not imply that action research is less important than other research; in fact, for that teacher, action research may be more important, since the findings can lead to improvement in her classroom. Action research promotes the use of the scientific method to improve the classroom environment, so that teachers find out for themselves what works and does not work for them.

The exciting aspect of action research is that teachers and practitioners who conduct research not only learn more about their settings and those with whom they serve but they also help to inform other educational and psychological professionals. There are opportunities for teachers and practitioners to publish written accounts of their action research investigations. Action research, ethical research practices, and information on how to write a research report are presented in Chapter 16.

WHAT IS REPLICATION RESEARCH?

Replication "is the primary method with which scientists determine the reliability and

usefulness of their findings and discover their mistakes" (Cooper et al., 2007, p. 6). Throughout this book, we discuss different research methods, how research is conducted, and for what purposes. However, you will not likely become a critical research consumer unless you understand the importance and purpose of replications. Unfortunately, many research textbooks allocate a few pages to replication and do not typically discuss its importance to science.

Reasons for Replication

Essentially, replicating a research study involves doing it over again. Replications have been called a critical aspect in the advancement of science (Cooper et al., 2007; Sidman, 1960; Yin, 2009). Thus, replications are necessary when investigating a phenomenon. There are two primary reasons for the importance of replications—reliability and generalizability (see Figure 1.7).

Reliability

Replications allow us to determine the reliability or consistency of previous findings (Johnston & Pennypacker, 1993; Thompson, 2002). Suppose that you read a study on the effectiveness of using *manipulatives* (i.e., physical objects that help to represent a concept) in teaching mathematics and there are no other studies regarding the use of manipulatives at that time. The investigators indicate that the improvement of the students is significant and that teachers should use manipulatives when teaching mathematics. What is your reaction? If you had finished this volume before reading the study but had not read this section on replications, you most likely

> **Basic research** *focuses on more theoretical issues; it is used to develop a new theory or refine an existing one.*
>
> **Applied research** *attempts to solve real-life problems or to study phenomena that directly impact what practitioners or laypeople do.*
>
> **Replication**, *or repeating procedures used in a previous study, aids in determining the reliability and usefulness of findings.*

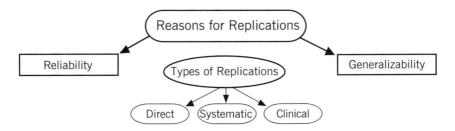

FIGURE 1.7. Reasons for replication and the types of replications.

would consider the type of design used and how the researchers measured the dependent variable (i.e., math skills, such as counting) and applied the independent variable (i.e., manipulatives). You also might have considered whether there are possible reasons for the improvement in the math skills of the students other than the independent variable. Once you completed all of these considerations, you might have concluded that the study was well conceived and designed, and that the study showed that manipulatives have the desired effect on the math skills. Furthermore, you might have even concluded that the findings are valid, or at least supported by the results of the study. Would your conclusion have been correct?

In most, if not all, applied research, researchers make mistakes or are forced to do things that weaken the investigation. These weaknesses are seen by critical research consumers and create questions about the validity of the researchers' claims. The concern here is whether an aspect of the investigation made the researchers' claim incorrect. Will you know this based on one investigation? Most likely not. Unfortunately, not everyone thinks critically about research. A great deal of money and professional respect has been lost because people do not consider the importance of replicating previous research. See the following example.

Cold Fusion

As you consider the importance of replication, read the following passage from Hernan and Wilcox (2009):

> On 23 March 1989, Fleischmann and Pons claimed they had achieved nuclear fusion in a jar of water at

room temperature (Fleischmann, Pons, & Hawkins, 1989). Their claim was met with disbelief mixed with excitement. If cold fusion was possible, it could solve the energy crisis. It would revolutionize energy exploration. It would change everyone's habits in using energy. In the following weeks, physicists from the best research centers in the world sought to replicate the Pons–Fleischmann experiment. They failed.

On 3 May 1989, while Pons was in Washington waiting to meet with President Bush's advisors, the American Physical Society concluded that every possible variant of the Pons–Fleischmann experiment had been tried without success. The claim of cold fusion was declared invalid. [The American Physical Society] provided dramatic accounts of the failure of cold fusion. . . . The cold fusion story shows the importance of replication to the scientific process. Scientists could not replicate the cold fusion claim, and so—regardless of the reputations of the investigators or the journal involved—the claim was rejected. (p. 167)

The news of cold fusion was exciting. Think of having as much energy as we want. We could essentially generate energy from a glass of water. If the results were correct, our lives would be forever changed. The state of Utah moved to help fund further research, as did the federal government. But the replication process was unsuccessful. If we endorse the scientific assumption that we can find order in natural phenomena, we would expect the original results to be reliable. But they weren't. Over the period of a few years, the general conclusion was that the researchers who discovered an excess of energy misinterpreted their readings. The excitement over cold fusion died. It looked as if money was wasted because people did not wait until successful replications were conducted.

One should not place too much confidence in the results of a single investigation. The articles that generally are published are about successful research. Unsuccessful investigations rarely make it into print. Also, consider the percentage of articles selected for publication. It may surprise some students that not all articles written by researchers are published. Some journals publish fewer than 10% of all articles submitted for publication. Therefore, the articles that are published represent a biased sample of all studies actually conducted. So the concern is that if articles that are printed represent a biased sample, and if unsuccessful investigations are rarely published, then how is one to know whether the published article represents data that are reliable? The answer is, you can't. The only way to determine the reliability of the findings of an investigation is to conduct replications.

We hope that researchers are honest. It is probably safe to assume that the overwhelming majority of researchers are. But it is also safe to assume that some researchers interpret their results to be consistent with their hypotheses, fail to attend adequately to alternative explanations for their results, or in extreme cases, report fraudulent data. The National Research Council (2002) encourages researchers to disclose research publicly and to invite professional scrutiny and critique, stating:

> Scientific studies do not contribute to a larger body of knowledge until they are widely disseminated and subjected to professional scrutiny by peers. This ongoing, collaborative, public critique is an indication of the health of a scientific enterprise. Indeed, the objectivity of science derives from publicly enforced norms of the professional community of scientists, rather than from the character traits of any individual person or design features of any study. (p. 5)

Generalizability

The second reason that replications are important is that information on the generalizability or transferability of the results of one investigation is enhanced. In Chapter 2 we discuss in more detail the concern of generalizability of research results. Suffice it to say that a single investigation, no matter how complex or how many individuals are involved, cannot equal the weight of several investigations of the same phenomenon.

Hendrick (1990) indicates that seven aspects must be considered in understanding the generalizability of a study's results. The following is a discussion of each of the seven aspects.

1. *Participant characteristics.* Researchers and critical research consumers must be aware of the participant characteristics. Suppose that you are a teacher working with children in the fourth grade. You read an investigation on the effectiveness of a curriculum aimed at improving the self-esteem of students. You are interested in using the curriculum in your class. What should you consider? The first question you must ask yourself is "Are these participants similar to my students?" If there are differences, you should consider whether the differences are significant enough to make the curriculum ineffective for your students. Students differ in terms of age, gender, culture, language, family and socioeconomic background, and personality characteristics. You must be aware of the differences among your students and determine whether participants in the investigation represent your students. Replications aid in this determination, particularly if multiple investigations have been conducted with students of different ages, from different socioeconomic backgrounds, and with different behavioral or personality characteristics.

2. *Research histories of participants.* A second concern for teachers and practitioners as critical research consumers involves histories of the participants. For example, if participants were volunteers, they may be very different from your students. Participants may also have received incentives to participate, such as payment, which may have made them more willing to continue in the program than unpaid students. Participants may also have been involved in other investigations. This involvement is not unusual in some situations, such as laboratory schools associated with universities. Students involved in research investigations as participants may be fairly sophisticated and may respond to an independent variable differently than naive students. Replications can help to decrease this concern by involving students with varying histories. If you were to see an intervention that was effective with a wide range of students with different histories, you might be more confident that the investigation's results would hold true with your students.

3. *Historical context.* Historical context refers to the particular sociocultural settings that research participants represent. The question is that if research is conducted with participants from the inner city, for example, will the results hold true for participants who live in the suburbs? Historical context is not limited to the geographic setting. In fact, the geographic setting is less important than social experiences or the cultural backgrounds of the participants (Klingner, 2006). For example, suppose that you worked on a Native American reservation teaching secondary age school-youth. You determine that the students must learn social skills to increase the chances they will be successful once they get out of school and/or leave the reservation. To develop social skills you select a curriculum that was shown to be effective in one research investigation containing mostly European American students from a large city. One skill taught is to establish eye contact when interacting with others. The problem here is that in some cultures, such as in many Native American tribes, making eye contact with elders or persons of authority is a sign of disrespect. The social skills curriculum would have a difficult time achieving the same types of outcome as those in the research study. Replications can aid by determining the effectiveness of interventions or independent variables within and across historical contexts, such as cultures or social situations.

4. *Physical setting of the research.* Variables such as the amount of light in the room, the level of noise, participants' familiarity with the surroundings, and the color of the setting may affect the interventions. In classrooms, variables such as the room arrangement and whether there are windows may differentially affect what works in the classroom. For example, if the participants in the original investigation were in a classroom without windows, the level of distraction would be minimal. However, a teacher's concern might pertain to how windows in her classroom affect her students' classroom performance. Would her students respond to the same type of instruction the participants in the study received even with the added distraction of windows? Replications could help to answer this question to a certain extent if the physical surroundings of different investigations were varied.

5. *Control agent.* We know that the characteristics of different teachers can interact with student characteristics. One student may be difficult to teach for one teacher but fairly easy for another, even when both use the same instructional techniques. Consider what would happen if you had someone (i.e., control agent) come into the setting in which you work to observe what you are doing. If you liked, trusted, and knew the person well, you might be relaxed. If, on the other hand, you were being observed by someone you disliked (i.e., control agent) or someone you did not know, you might act differently. Another potential difficulty is the skills level of the person involved in the research. Many investigations are not going to use poor teachers when attempting to determine the effectiveness of an instructional technique. Teachers or control agents may be, and often are, very well trained and masters at what they do. Critical research consumers should be concerned with the skills level and characteristics (e.g., gender) of the person actually interacting with the participants in an investigation. The question we should ask is "Do my skills (or characteristics) match those of the persons involved in the study?" Replications involving different control agents can provide valuable information on the effectiveness of the intervention when persons with varying skills levels and characteristics are involved.

6. *Specific task variables.* Specific task variables involve the details of the methods used in research. As with several of these other aspects, the effect of different task variables is not always known. Variables such as the format in which information is presented (e.g., single-sided or double-sided pages), the formatting of materials (e.g., font sizes and styles), and the "look" of the materials (e.g., gray cover without designs or colorful covers with appealing artwork, type of paper) may be important. Interestingly, business marketers have known for years the importance of specific details. The manner in which items are packaged can determine the success or failure of a new product, for example. Unfortunately, most educational and psychological researchers are not as sophisticated in these small details.

For example, suppose that you had to select a textbook and you had two choices—one that had few or no pictures and a bland cover, and another with pictures throughout and a sparkly cover. Chances are, you would be more likely to select the one that is more appealing to you (i.e., the flashy one). Participants can be affected the same way. They may respond differently to the way materials are designed and/or presented. Successful replications using materials that are formatted differently and presented in a number of different ways can increase our confidence that these small details are not critical. However, if replications reveal that participants respond differently to how the material is presented, we have information that is critical to our success.

7. *Primary information focus.* A final concern with generalizability is the methods by which information is transmitted to participants. This information is the independent variable. Essentially, primary information focus involves the methods by which the independent variable is implemented. For example, suppose that you are teaching a sex education class and wished to teach secondary students about disease prevention techniques during sexual activity. You read an article explaining how to teach about "safe sex." The results of the investigation show that the instruction was successful in changing the students' opinions about abstinence and disease prevention techniques (i.e., they were more likely to refrain from sexual activity or, if they were going to become or stay sexually active, they stated that they would be more likely to use "safe sex" techniques). The authors described the intervention, which included verbal information on the problem of teenage pregnancies and AIDS, a film showing the negative effects of sexually transmitted diseases, and class discussions. Based on the information, you decide to implement the intervention with your class. You acquire the written documents used in the study, as well as the film. You implement the independent variable exactly as it was described in the investigation. The question is "Will your students acquire the same information as the participants in the investigation?" Students may interpret the information differently based on their past and present experiences, their

characteristics, the person leading the discussion, or the manner in which they are seated.

Another potential problem occurs when the researchers do not fully describe the independent variable, or a historical event that could have affected the independent variable is left out of the description. Details can be left out if they are considered to be unimportant or if the researchers are unaware of information, such as a student in the class who has a family member with AIDS and the other participants are aware of this. In this case, the effects of the independent variable or the information received by your students may not be the same as that shown in the investigation. Replications can increase our confidence in the primary information focus if the results across investigations are consistent even though there are possible additions to or deletions from the independent variable.

Types of Replications

Now that we know why replications should be conducted, we should learn about the different types of replications. Sidman (1960) described two types of replications—direct and systematic—and Barlow, Nock, and Hersen (2008) described a third type—clinical (see Figure 1.7).

Direct Replications

Probably the most straightforward type of replication is the direct replication. Simply stated, *direct replications* are investigations in which an experiment is conducted in the same manner as a previous experiment. The replication is also conducted by the same researcher. Obviously, one difference in the replication study and the original study is the change in participants; however, the participants in the two investigations are homogeneous (i.e., essentially alike on critical attributes). All other variables remain essentially unchanged. For example, suppose that a researcher wanted to determine the effectiveness of a safety program at the elementary level. The researcher would define the participants, set up the assessment methods, present the independent variable, and so on. The same researcher would then perform the same procedures during a second investigation with students who were similar in all important respects (age, grade level, previous safety training, etc.).

The information gained from a direct replication reflects generality across groups of individuals with identical characteristics. Essentially, all that direct replications do is add to the total number of participants exposed to the intervention. Thus, if the results of the replication are consistent with the original study, we gain more confidence that the same procedures will work with other individuals with the same or similar characteristics as the participants in the investigation. Therefore, the utility of direct replications is somewhat limited. In order for replications to provide the largest amount of information possible, the replications should be independent of one another.

Systematic Replications

Direct replications are important in that they allow us to determine whether the same results will be found under the same conditions. Unfortunately, direct replications are not independent replications, in that they rely on the same researcher to conduct the investigation. **Systematic replications** allow for the generalization of a procedure to other individuals, as do direct replications, but also generalization across other situations. Thus, systematic replications are investigations by different researchers and/or different people implementing the independent variable, involve participants with different characteristics than those in the original investigation (e.g., secondary students without disabilities vs. students with disabilities), and/or are conducted in different settings (e.g., the classroom vs. the community). For example, suppose that a researcher wanted to determine the efficacy of a problem-solving program designed for individuals with traumatic brain injuries when individuals with mild intellectual and developmental disabilities serve as the participants. The researcher is different, but the independent and dependent variables are the same. Additionally, the participants differ on important characteristics. First of all, the participants from the two investigations do not have the same impairments. The participants may also be different ages. We can change the example by stating that

different teachers were involved in the investigations. We can also say that different measures of the dependent variable were used. We can use a different variation of the independent variable, such as peer tutors presenting the problem-solving program instead of having a teacher present it. We can also replicate the original investigation's procedures exactly, with the exception of making some change in part of the procedures, such as spending 5 days rather than 2 days per week to teach children a skill, as in the original investigation, to speed up the program.

Systematic replications aid in increasing the independence of investigations. Their obvious advantage over direct replications is that the generalization of the original study's results can be demonstrated across more variables than the number of participants. However, if too many variables are modified in a systematic replication, a researcher may be unable to account for a failure to replicate the original findings. For example, if participants with intellectual or developmental disabilities were a different age and trained by peer tutors, and the problem-solving program yielded different results from the original research, failure to replicate could have been due to several factors. Manipulation of a limited number of specific variables and careful adherence to procedures used to implement and measure effects of a treatment are important in systematic replication.

Clinical Replications

Clinical replications essentially come about as a result of direct and systematic replications. As explained by Barlow et al. (2008), direct and systematic replications essentially involve one independent variable, whereas clinical replications involve the combination of two or more independent variables to form an intervention package. Barlow et al. have also used the term *field testing* to describe the same process. For example, suppose we wanted to study the most effective method of classroom management. Some direct replications over the years have shown the effectiveness of using a behavioral procedure called *time-out* with elementary-school-age children. Systematic research has also shown that time-out is effective in settings other than the classroom and with different teachers. Children from different age groups have shown reductions in problem behavior due to the procedure. Other investigations have shown that classroom structure and procedures, such as rules and routines, also can have a positive impact on student behavior. Investigations have been replicated with both direct and systematic approaches. If we combined these independent variables (i.e., time-out and classroom structure), we would have an intervention package that teachers could use. Clinical replications, then, involve applying the intervention package to elementary-school-age children.

The obvious advantage of clinical replications is that they allow a researcher to build on previous replications in a manner that is more representative of what actually occurs outside of the typical research setting. In a research setting, one independent variable may be provided to the participants. However, in real life, many things are going on that can affect the student.

Thus, combining variables and assessing their combined effect more closely represents the dynamics that occur in an applied setting.

Replication as the "Big Picture"

The purpose of presenting this information on replication research early in the text is to stress the importance of looking at the "big picture." Throughout the text, issues and concerns of research investigations and types of research methods are presented. The presentation of these issues, concerns, and methods is similar to looking at each tree in a forest. We can tell how healthy each tree is in isolation. However, if we look at only one tree, we cannot determine the overall health of the forest. The remainder of this book will aid you in determining the health of individual trees, but you must remember that the goal of science is to determine the overall health of the forest.

SUMMARY

❖ The seven elements that must be considered to develop critical thinking skills include (1) learning what science is, how it works, and why it works; (2) knowing what constitutes a scientific theory; (3) understanding the different types of logic used in science; (4) learning that some methods of establishing knowledge fit within a scientific framework and others do not; (5) knowing how to discriminate between research methods that use more control (i.e., high constraint levels) and those that use less control (i.e., low constraint levels); (6) understanding the differences between research that focuses on more theoretical issues (i.e., basic) and research that addresses educational–psychological problems (i.e., applied); and (7) learning that science does not advance with single, isolated bits of research findings.

❖ Science is a systematic approach to seeking and organizing knowledge about the natural world. Science is the attempt to find order and lawful relations in the world. It is a method of viewing the world. Finally, science is the testing of our ideas in a public forum that takes a series of five steps—(1) identifying a problem,

(2) defining the problem, (3) formulating a hypothesis (a researcher's expectations about what data will show) or research question, (4) determining the observable consequences of the hypothesis or research question, and (5) testing the hypothesis or attempting to answer the research question.

❖ Science has four primary purposes: (1) to describe phenomena, (2) to predict events or outcomes, (3) to improve practice, and (4) to explain phenomena.

❖ A theory, which is an explanation of a certain set of observed phenomena about constructs and how they relate to one another, has

> **Systematic replication** *is an investigation conducted by different researchers and/or different people implementing the independent variable, involving participants with different characteristics than those in the original investigation (e.g., secondary students without disabilities vs. students with disabilities) and/or different settings (e.g., in the classroom versus in the community).*

three purposes: (1) identifies commonalities in otherwise isolated phenomena, (2) enables us to make predictions and to control phenomena, and (3) refers to an explanatory system that describes the data gathered before the theory was developed. A scientific theory is one that is falsifiable or refutable (i.e., a scientific theory must be able to be disproven).

❖ Scientific theories may be constructed in one of two ways—(1) after researchers conduct a large number of investigations and develop a theory based on past research results (inductive logic, or moving from the specific to the general) or (2) when theories are constructed, then used to predict what will occur in future investigations (deductive, or moving from the general to the specific). Each form of logic has several advantages and disadvantages. There are also combinations of the logic forms which is how most theories are constructed.

❖ There are five ways of obtaining information we must consider—three that are nonscientific (i.e., tenacity [persistence of a certain belief or way of thought], intuition [the feeling one has about a topic], authority [belief because of the influence of a person in power]), and two that are scientific (i.e., empiricism [gaining information through observation], and rationalism [use our reasoning processes to make decisions]).

❖ Level of constraint is the degree to which a researcher establishes limits or controls on the research process. High-constraint research allows us to make cause-and-effect determinations but may make the context artificial. Low-constraint research can tell us what will happen in an applied context, such as a classroom, but cannot inform us about cause-and-effect relationships. Generally, there are five levels of constraint on a continuum from high to low—experimental (high), and causal–comparative, correlational, case study, and naturalistic or descriptive research (low).

❖ Basic research focuses on more theoretical issues; it is conducted to develop a new theory or refine an existing one, while applied research attempts to solve real-life problems or study phenomena that directly impact what practitioners or laypeople do by using a theory developed through basic research.

❖ Replicating a research study involves doing it over again. Replications have been called a critical aspect in the advancement of science and have two main purposes: (1) to determine the reliability or consistency of previous findings, and (2) to provide information on the generalizability or transferability of the results of one investigation. There are three basic types of replications: (1) direct (conducting an experiment in the same manner as a previous experiment), (2) systematic (investigations by different researchers and/or different people implementing the independent variable, involving participants with different characteristics than those in the original investigation and/or in different settings), and (3) clinical (the combination of two or more independent variables to form an intervention package).

DISCUSSION QUESTIONS

1. Do you agree with the following statement? "One reason why educators are not much affected by scientific research is that they have not developed critical thinking skills about research." Why or why not? In your answer, indicate how we can develop critical thinking skills about research.

2. What are the steps taken in the scientific method? Describe each.

3. Is it possible to "prove" any scientific theory by finding evidence in support of the theory? Explain.

4. What is meant by the term *science*? In your response, describe the different purposes of science.

5. What do the terms *inductive* and *deductive logic* mean? How are they different, and how can they be combined?

6. What are the different ways of gaining information? Of these, explain which ones are scientific and why.

7. How are quantitative and qualitative research different? Which type of research allows researchers to make cause-and-effect claims?

8. What is the importance of basic and applied research? How is applied research dependent on basic research?

9. What is action research? Why is it important for teachers and other professionals to know how to conduct action research?

10. What is replication research? In your answer, describe why science is dependent on replication research, and define the three different forms of replication research.

PART II

....

Critical Issues
in Research

CHAPTER 2

Fundamental Issues for Interpreting Research

OBJECTIVES

After studying this chapter, you should be able to . . .

1. List the two primary roles of individuals involved in research, and outline what these roles involve.
2. Illustrate the concept of variability.
3. Describe what is meant by the term *internal validity*, and outline the different threats to internal validity.
4. Explain what is meant by the term *external validity*, and outline the different threats to external validity.
5. Clarify the terms *statistical validity* and *social validities*.

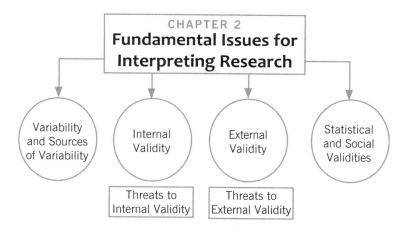

OVERVIEW

Researchers face several methodological issues when conducting research. These issues vary depending on the type of research conducted; however, we discuss general methodological issues in this chapter and revisit them as we move through the text.

We focus on two primary roles of individuals involved with research. The first role is that of the researcher. Researchers' roles include (1) developing the research question(s) they will attempt to answer and/or the research hypothesis (i.e., a test of the assumptions made by researchers), (2) using an appropriate methodology to answer the research question and/or test the hypothesis, (3) interpreting the results, and (4) making conclusions based on the results of the study. Researchers attempt to use the most appropriate methodology to form their conclusions. However, some researchers make a mistake in the selection or implementation of the methodology. Applied research is difficult to conduct in many instances, because there are some things we simply may not be able to do in applied situations (e.g., randomly assigning a classroom of students to two different instructional procedures) that we can do in a laboratory setting. Therefore, many limitations to the methodology of a study are the result of the constraints placed on researchers.

The second role of an individual involved in research is that of the critical research consumer. The critical research consumer's role involves review of the methodology used to determine whether it was appropriate, whether it had any weaknesses, and whether the researcher's conclusions are valid. This consumer must also understand that some methodological flaws are the result of the applied environment rather than a mistake or omission made by the researcher. (We discuss this throughout the text.)

Our purpose in this chapter is to provide a general framework of information necessary for the chapters that follow. In doing so, this chapter gives critical research consumers the necessary skills to think critically about various types of research methodologies and to make decisions with regard to the validity of the researchers' conclusions. Of course, the types of skills used to critique a study depend on the methodology used; in some cases, the tools are not appropriate for the task, and in other cases, the tools are absolutely critical. Methodological issues faced by researchers fall into at least five general categories: variability, internal validity, external validity, statistical validity, and social validity. These five general categories are discussed throughout this chapter.

WHAT IS VARIABILITY?

Variability, the amount of dispersion in a distribution of scores (Gall et al., 2007), generally refers to the extent to which things differ from one another. Variability is in every part of daily life. We do not always feel the same every day. Some days we are happy, and other days we are sad. Those around us also vary in the way they feel. However, variability is not restricted to the way we feel. When we play basketball, we do not shoot the ball the same way every time. When we write a paper, we do not use the same words each time or even hold the pencil the same way. There is variability in everything we do. This variability can have many different effects on research results. In some cases, we want variability to occur; in other cases, variability can have a negative effect on our research results. Thus, variability can be either friend or foe. When it is our friend, we want to encourage and support it. When it is our foe, we want to reduce or eliminate it. The methods by which researchers attempt to encourage some sources of variability and reduce other sources of variability associated with each specific design are discussed in detail in later chapters.

Sources of Variability

There are several sources of variability in research. If researchers can learn where these sources are, then they can attempt to control them. Sources of variability can be placed in two general categories—unsystematic variance and systematic variance (see Figure 2.1).

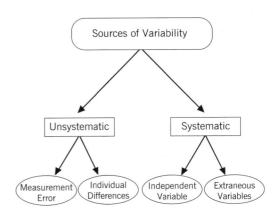

FIGURE 2.1. Sources of variability. *Note:* Extraneous variables can also be termed *confounding variables* and *threats to internal validity.*

Unsystematic Variance

Unsystematic variance is variability within individuals and/or groups of individuals. This variability is essentially random: Some individuals change in one direction; others, in another direction; and still others do not change at all. For example, some individuals may feel better than they did yesterday, others may feel worse, and still others may feel the same as they did yesterday. Another example occurs when taking tests. Some individuals perform better on a test one day than the next, others' performance declines, and still others have essentially the same test performance. When taken together, the overall result of this variance is little overall change. Most researchers would consider unsystematic variance a fact of life that cannot be totally eliminated or accounted for at this time. However, it may be possible to account for some unsystematic variance at a later time, when our understanding of human behavior and our measurement systems evolve enough to allow for such accountability (Sidman, 1960). There are two major sources of unsystematic variance—*measurement error* and *individual differences* (see Figure 2.1).

Measurement Error. Measurement error exists because a measurement device (e.g., a test, a person doing an observation) does not measure an attribute the same way every time (Kubiszyn & Borich, 2007). Measurement error occurs frequently and comes from many sources. In fact, we can assume that all measurements have some measurement error. For example, if a person weighs 150 pounds but the scale weighs him at 148 pounds, then there is measurement error of 2 pounds on that scale. In other words, the scale has an error of measurement built into it. In order for this measurement error to be considered unsystematic, the scale would have to weigh him at 148 pounds one time, 153 pounds another, and 150 pounds a third time. The sum of all his weight differences from the average weight (the sum of all weighings divided by the number of weighings) would be zero if we did an infinite number of weighings. In the end, the measurement error would be a wash, and that average would be the best estimate of this person's true weight.

We can never weigh ourselves an infinite number of times. Therefore, measurement error must be estimated. Measurement error is directly related to the reliability of the measurement instrument (i.e., how consistent the device measures an attribute)—the less reliable the measurement device, the larger the measurement error. Researchers are concerned with the reliability of their measurement devices, since they desire to reduce their measurement error. This issue is discussed in more detail in Chapter 3.

Individual Differences. Another source of unsystematic variance is individual differences (Cohen, Manion, & Morrison, 2007). Most researchers assume that intrinsic factors, or unaccounted for factors, cause people to be different from one another. For example, one reason why you do well in math and a peer does not may be due to an inborn ability to achieve at math or to factors of which the researcher is unaware, such as past learning histories. Therefore, whereas some people respond favorably to math instruction, others may not.

Systematic Variance

Systematic variance is variability that we can account for between or among groups of people (Cohen et al., 2007); that is, something is occurring that makes a group of individuals move in the same direction. Some individuals may improve, others may worsen, and still others may remain approximately the same; however, on the whole, the group's performance will change. On the other hand, all individuals may move in the same direction, with the amount of change differing among the individuals. Think of systematic variance as moving your hand through water. You cup your hand and push the water in a certain direction. Some water will escape and not move in the direction you wish. Some of it may move in the opposite direction. But on the whole, much of the water will move in the direction you desire. Using the same

> **Variability** *is the amount of dispersion or fluctuation in a set of scores. It refers to the extent to which things differ from one another.*

example, if you move your hand through a narrow trough, you may be able to move virtually all of the water. If you attempt to move water in a lake, the amount of water you move may be small. The amount of water you move on the whole depends to a large extent on the amount of control you can exert on the body of water. This occurrence is similar to what researchers attempt to do. They want to see what moves individuals in a certain direction. They understand that some individuals will not be affected as intended, but on the whole, the group will be affected. In order to have a larger effect on individuals, researchers may attempt to exert as much control over the environment of those individuals as possible.

Take the previous example of weighing the man on a scale. If he were to get on the scale an infinite number of times and the scale weighed him at 148 pounds every time he stood on it, we would have an example of systematic measurement error. In order to find his actual weight we would simply add 2 pounds to the scale reading. Thus, if we were to measure a group on some attribute and we measured individuals consistently lower on that attribute, we would have systematic variance. Now take two groups of individuals. If we consistently measured one group lower on an attribute and the other group higher on the attribute, we would see differences between the two groups. Unlike unsystematic variance, whose influence researchers attempt to decrease, researchers attempt to increase one source of systematic variance. The difference between the two groups would be due to this type of systematic variance.

Researchers are primarily concerned with two sources of systematic variance—the *independent variable* and *extraneous variables* (Graziano & Raulin, 2010; see Figure 2.1). The systematic variance associated with the independent variable is desirable to quantitative researchers; the systematic variance associated with extraneous variables is not desirable to quantitative researchers, and an attempt is usually made to decrease the impact of extraneous variables on the dependent variable (i.e., what we are trying to impact or change).

Independent Variable. The method that quantitative researchers use to achieve systematic variance is to manipulate (e.g., present then withdraw) the **independent variable** or to have at least two levels (e.g., high degree of a treatment, low degree of a treatment) or forms of the independent variable (i.e., presence and absence of treatment). Qualitative researchers do not attempt to manipulate the independent variable as do quantitative researchers but they nevertheless have a concern for detecting the source(s) of systematic variance. The approach used by qualitative researchers differs from that used by quantitative researchers (Marshall & Rossman, 2011; Silverman, 2005) and is discussed in Chapters 9 and 10.

Extraneous Variables. A second source of systematic variance is from factors that are not designed (i.e., unplanned) to be in a study. Researchers frequently refer to these extraneous variables as *confounding variables* or as threats to internal validity (Gersten et al., 2005).

WHAT IS INTERNAL VALIDITY AND ITS THREATS?

The relationship between dependent and independent variables is sometimes referred to as a *functional relationship*. **Internal validity** simply addresses the question, "Did the individual change as a result of what I did/observed, or was the change due to something else?" Extraneous variables, like independent variables, may affect individuals in a similar manner.

The effects of extraneous variables on the dependent variable are a major concern of researchers and constitute threats to the internal validity of a study. One purpose of the research design is to control for these extraneous variables. Thus, it is important for critical research consumers to determine whether threats to the internal validity of the study are present, and if they are, what their affect on the results of the study may be. Think of the critical research consumer's role as that of a detective. His/her job is to find out what else may have accounted for the results. It is important to realize that few research studies are free from threats to internal validity; thus, critical research consumers must assess the results of a study and the conclusions made by the researcher based on those results, since those conclusions may be faulty. They must weigh these factors before drawing any conclusions about the significance or importance of the study.

There are several possible threats to the internal validity of a study (see Cook & Campbell, 1979; Gall et al., 2007; Gersten et al., 2005). These threats, shown in Table 2.1, can be separated into two categories: (1) threats that result in differences within or between individuals (i.e., maturation, selection, selection by maturation interaction, statistical regression, mortality, instrumentation, testing, history, and resentful demoralization of the control group), and (2) threats that result in similarities within and between individuals (i.e., diffusion of treatment, compensatory rivalry by the control group, and compensatory equalization of treatments). Each threat is described in detail, along with examples and nonexamples and their effects on a study.

Internal validity threats are different depending on the type of research design; that is, internal validity threats vary depending on the type of study. Table 2.2 refers the reader to tables throughout the book showing internal validity threats related to various quantitative designs. Use this table to guide you to the information you need on potential internal validity threats for different types of designs.

TABLE 2.1. Threats to Internal Validity

Results in differences within or between individuals

Maturation—Changes in the dependent variable may be due to biological or psychological processes.

Selection—Differences between groups may be due to differential selection or assignment to groups.

Selection by maturation interaction—Similar to selection, but the main focus is the maturation of the participants.

Statistical regression—Changes in the dependent variable may be due to the movement of an attribute to the mean of that attribute.

Mortality—Differences between groups may be due to a differential loss of participants.

Instrumentation—Changes in the dependent variable may be due to changes in how the dependent variable is measured.

Testing—Changes in the dependent variable may be due to the effect of the first testing on the second.

History—Changes in the dependent variable may be due to events other than the independent variable that occur between the first and second measurement or during the application of the independent variable.

Resentful demoralization of the control group—Differences between groups may be inflated due to a lack of effort on the part of the control group.

Results in similarities within or between individuals

Diffusion of treatment—Differences between or within groups may be decreased due to unintended exposure to the independent variable.

Compensatory rivalry by the control group—Differences between groups may be decreased due to increased effort on the part of the control group to keep pace with the experimental group.

Compensatory equalization of treatments—Differences between groups may be decreased due to unintended compensation of the control group for not receiving the independent variable.

Threats That Result in Differences within and between Individuals

There are nine threats to the internal validity of an investigation that result in differences within and between individuals. These threats include maturation, selection, selection by maturation interaction, statistical regression, mortality, instrumentation, testing, history, and resentful demoralization of the control group (see Figure 2.2).

Maturation Threat

Maturation may threaten the internal validity of a study when, over time, biological or

When trying to determine whether X caused Y, the X is what the researcher manipulates or is interested in observing, and is thus the **independent variable**.

Internal validity indicates a functional relationship between the independent variable and the dependent variable; associated or correlated with the implementation of the independent variable and not something else.

A **maturation threat** involves a passage of time in which biological or psychological changes in participants take place.

TABLE 2.2. Tables of Internal Validity Threats for Various Quantitative Designs

Design	Chapter	Table
Experimental designs		
True experimental	5	5.2
Pretest–posttest control-group		
Posttest-only control-group		
Solomon four-group		
Quasi-experimental designs	5	5.6
Static-group comparison		
Nonequivalent control-group		
Counter-balanced		
Time-series		
Preexperimental designs	5	5.8
One-shot case study		
One-group pretest–posttest		
Causal–comparative design	6	6.1
Correlational research	7	7.4
Single-case research methods		
Withdrawal and associated designs	11	11.3
A-B design		
A-B-A design		
A-B-A-B design		
B-A-B design		
A-B-C-B design		
Multiple-baseline designs	12	12.1
Across behaviors		
Across participants		
Across settings		
Multiple-probe design		
Additional single-case designs	13	13.1
Changing-criterion		
Multitreatment		
Alternating treatments		
Combination		

psychological changes in participants take place. For example, suppose we wanted to improve the motor skills of a group of 4-year-old children with physical limitations through a technique called *patterning*, which involves using exercises that supposedly help individuals relearn each stage of motor learning. Let's say we gave a pretest to measure the childrens' motor skills and compared these results to a posttest measurement taken 2 years after the application of the pretest. The findings indicate that the motor skills of the children improved markedly. It would be difficult to claim that the improvement was due *only* to the patterning; it may have been affected by the natural maturation of the children due to the time lapse between the pretest and posttest assessment.

Maturation may also be a threat depending on the time at which measures were taken. For example, if we were to take measurements early

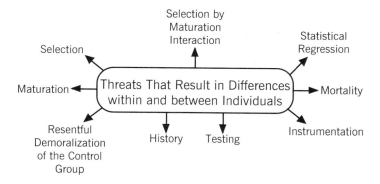

FIGURE 2.2. Threats to internal validity that result in differences within and between individuals.

in the morning and again in the afternoon, we might see changes in individuals' responses simply due to the passage of time. Likewise, if we took measurements prior to lunch and then after lunch, we might see that changes had taken place. Maturation is always a concern when we see that measurements were taken at different times for two different groups. Say we wanted to test the effectiveness of a new curriculum. The difference between two groups of students in fourth grade was measured. One group received the new curriculum, and the other received the standard curriculum. We noticed that the group that received the new curriculum outperformed the group that received the standard curriculum. However, the time the measurement was applied must be taken into account. The measurement was given to the students who received the standard curriculum just before they left for home, and it was given to the students who received the new curriculum the next morning. Therefore, we concluded that at least some of those observed differences may have been because students are usually more tired at the end of the day than when they arrive at school in the morning.

A nonexample of this threat can be illustrated by the following. Suppose we wanted to determine whether the types of instruction (i.e., phrased as questions vs. directives) provided to children with a high level of noncompliance affect the probability of following directions. Students were provided with instructions in the form of questions (e.g., "Can you put the book on the shelf?") the same time each morning.

Then, after some period of time had elapsed, the form of instructions changed to directives (e.g., "Please put the book on the shelf"). These instructions were presented at the same time each morning as before. The time of measurement of compliance was important, since the passage of time (i.e., morning vs. afternoon) could have differentially affected the probability of following instructions. Thus, maturation is not a threat in this example, since the time at which instruction was provided was the same before and after the implementation of the independent variable.

Selection Threat

Selection may threaten the internal validity of a study if groups of individuals are selected in a differential manner. The key word here is *differential*. What makes groups of individuals different from one another is how they were selected in the first place. This threat is common when we select preexisting groups to be involved in an experiment and do not attempt to demonstrate how they are similar on critical variables. Even if we can demonstrate that the groups are equivalent on critical variables, we may still have a selection threat, since it would be hard to imagine an instance where we would be aware of all of the critical variables that could account for group differences.

> A **selection threat** *occurs when groups of individuals are selected in a differential manner.*

Say we wanted to compare two types of mathematics curricula. To do this, one group of individuals that received the standard curriculum was compared to a group that received the new curriculum. Now suppose that the first group was from a remedial classroom for students who have difficulty in mathematics and the second group was students in a classroom for gifted and talented children in mathematics. After the instruction, we found that the second group that received the new curriculum outscored the first group. Obviously, the second group would be expected to outscore the first group, because the students were initially better at mathematics. In this case, we would be unable to assess which curriculum was more effective, because the groups were different from the outset.

An instance in which selection would not be a threat might involve a situation where we wanted to study the effects of play therapy on the aggressive behavior of students with behavior disorders. Students were randomly assigned to two groups (see Chapter 4). The experimental group received play therapy, and the control group received the normal classroom routine. The experimental group's level of aggressive behavior was compared to that of the control group. After the play therapy intervention was finished, we found that the experimental group's level of aggressive behavior was considerably lower than the level for the control group. Selection would not be a strong threat, since we assumed that the two groups were equivalent on important variables before the implementation of the independent variable. In other words, the only difference between the two groups should have been the independent variable.

Selection by Maturation Interaction

This threat to the internal validity of a study is similar to the maturation and selection threats described earlier; however, the main concern here is the maturation of the individuals selected for involvement in the study.

For example, say we worked with several individuals with articulation problems. Participants were assigned to two groups (i.e., experimental and control) on a nonrandom basis. The average age of the experimental group was 5 years, and the average age for the control group was 8 years. The experimental group was provided with an independent variable designed to improve articulation by teaching the participants how to emit specific speech sounds. The control group received group support. The articulation skills of participants in both groups were measured 1 year later; we found that the experimental group made greater gains than the control group in articulation abilities. Our conclusion that the independent variable improved the experimental participants' articulation may have been erroneous, since we failed to see whether the groups were initially equivalent on critical variables. They were similar to each other except on the basis of age. We would expect that younger children would make greater gains than the older children simply by growing older and having more experience with language. Thus, many of the gains made may have been due to the maturation of the participants in the experimental group, and not due to the independent variable.

Selection by maturation interaction would not be a threat in the following investigation. Suppose we wanted to measure the attitudes of students toward their teachers after a grading period. Two groups of students were selected and compared. The first group of students was enrolled in a discovery–learning classroom, and the second was enrolled in a skills-based classroom. The students were the same age (12 years) and in the same grade (seventh). They came from similar socioeconomic backgrounds and had parents with similar educational levels. We compared the attitudes of the two groups after the grading period and detected a major difference between their attitudes. The skills-based group had more positive overall attitudes about its educational experiences than the discovery–learning group. Based on this information, we concluded that students favored the skills-based classroom. The students were measured within the same period of time after the study. The equalization of time of measurement was important, since attitudes can change over time. Thus, we can rule out a selection by maturation interaction as a threat, since both groups were similar on all critical variables and were exposed to the same passage of time.

Statistical Regression

Statistical regression may be a threat to the internal validity of a study if we select participants who are extreme on some attribute. It is a phenomenon that occurs when individuals deviate from the norm. When these individuals are selected, a change in that attribute toward the mean can be expected. The greater or more pronounced the difference between the participants and the norm, the greater the expected change in some attribute toward the mean. Let's assume for a moment that there is no genetic relationship between physical height and one's offspring, or intelligence and one's offspring. Consider the following: If your parents are taller than the mean height (e.g., the father is 6 feet, 9 inches and the mother is 6 feet, 2 inches), we would expect you to be shorter, on average, than your parents. The opposite is true for shorter individuals. If your parents are shorter than the mean height (e.g., the father is 5 feet, 3 inches and the mother is 4 feet, 7 inches), we would expect you to be taller than your parents. This phenomenon also occurs with other human attributes, such as intelligence. For example, if your mother were gifted, say, with an IQ of 150, we would expect your IQ to be less than 150. Your IQ would "regress" toward the mean IQ of the population, which is 100.

Statistical regression is a threat to the internal validity of an experiment if our choice of participants is based on extreme scores (e.g., intellectual disability) and we see a change from one test to the next. For example, suppose that we gave a pretest, such as an intelligence test, to a group of children and found that the average IQ for the group was 65. After a metacognitive strategy was implemented to improve mental processing, the group's average IQ increased to 75. We could not conclude that the metacognitive strategy was effective in improving IQs, since an increase in the group's posttest average intelligence would be expected to move toward 100 simply because of statistical regression to the mean. (*Note.* Regression toward the mean would be expected here, since most intellectual disabilities are considered to be due to socioeconomic disadvantage, not inherited traits; Emerson, 2003; Olsson & Hwang, 2008.) We would likely have seen an improvement in the group's scores without any independent variable being implemented. If we were not aware of statistical regression, we might have mistakenly concluded that the independent variable was effective when, in reality, it might not have been effective at all.

A nonexample of this threat is a comparison of two groups of participants with low IQ scores (i.e., 50). The first group is exposed to the independent variable, and the second group is not. The only difference between the two groups should be the independent variable. So, if any differences are noticed between the groups, we can safely conclude that statistical regression did not contribute to the cause of the change, since any statistical regression to the mean would have occurred with both groups. Any noticeable difference can be attributed to the independent variable.

Mortality

Mortality can be a threat to the internal validity of a study when there is a differential loss of participants. This differential loss could be from death (thankfully an unusual occurrence), selectively eliminating scores of some group members, or the withdrawal of participants. The key to the definition of mortality is the term *differential*.

Consider the following example. Suppose we were attempting to see whether a new metacognitive skill could enhance the learning rates of students. We set out to determine the learning rates of students through timed trials of oral responses to mathematics facts. Twenty students were randomly assigned to one of two groups. The metacognitive skill was taught to one group of students (experimental) but not to the second group (control). On the pretest, we saw that both groups of students had an average time of getting through all of their required math facts in 90 seconds. Upon posttest, we saw that the experimental group made it through the math facts in 75 seconds on average; the control group answered the math facts in 88

A **statistical regression** *threat occurs when individuals who are selected for the study deviate from the norm.*

seconds on average. At this point, we concluded that the metacognitive skills enhanced learning. However, only seven students were left in the experimental group after the posttest, whereas the control group had all 10 students. Therefore, the experimental group's change from pre- to posttest was attributed to mortality, not to the metacognitive skills. We concluded that mortality was a threat, because the students who dropped out of the experimental group were the slower students in the first place. So, if we remove the slower students from the group, the learning times should decrease. Now, suppose that on seeing that the number of students in both groups differed, the data of three students in the control group were thrown out randomly. There is still a problem with mortality, since three students is still a differential loss of participants. Thus, it really does not matter if the number of participants lost from both groups is the same; whether the participants lost from each group are similar to each other is the critical question.

Mortality is not a threat in the following scenario. Suppose two groups of individuals were involved in a study of short-term memory. On the pretest, the two groups scored similarly on the number of nonsense symbols they could remember after a passage of 5 seconds from the time they saw the symbols to when they were requested to recall the symbols. The experimental group was provided with a newly discovered memory strategy aimed at enhancing short-term memory. At posttest, it was discovered that the experimental group retained 50% more words than did the control group. However, 10% of the participants were lost from each group. Information on the characteristics of those lost from each group was gathered, and it was determined that the individuals lost in each group had similar characteristics on variables considered important for the study (e.g., intelligence, age, experience). Thus, there probably was not a differential loss of participants, and mortality was an unlikely threat.

Instrumentation Threat

Instrumentation can be a threat to the internal validity of a study when there are changes in the calibration of the instrument(s) used

in measurement. If the measurement device changes throughout or at any time during the study, we cannot be sure whether the change was due to the independent variable or to changes in the way the dependent variable was measured.

For example, suppose we wanted to see how a certain behavior management procedure works to decrease the self-injurious behavior of a young child. Self-injury involving direct harm to body tissue is sometimes associated with autism spectrum disorders. A frequency count (i.e., tally of every instance of a behavior) was used for 4 hours before the independent variable was implemented; then we changed the way we measured the dependent variable to count only if the behavior occurred at least once in eight half-hour intervals. We presented data to suggest that the behavior decreased from an average frequency of 100 behaviors in a 4-hour period before the independent variable was implemented to eight behaviors in 4 hours while the independent variable was in effect. Although this result was impressive, changes in the measurement device rather than the independent variable accounted for the results. Consider that the maximum number of behaviors (i.e., at least once per half-hour interval) was eight.

A nonexample of instrumentation as a threat would involve using observers who did not know whether the independent variable (i.e., assertiveness skills) was in effect for each participant. Assertiveness involves standing up for one's rights without being aggressive. During a period in which the normal occurrence of the behavior was observed, we saw a somewhat stable response pattern of low assertiveness skills. The participants were then taught how and when to be assertive; the observers continued to measure the level of assertiveness demonstrated by participants. Throughout this time, the observers did not know whether we were teaching the skills to the participants. We saw that during the assertiveness training, participants' skills improved significantly. In this case, instrumentation is less likely to be a concern, since any change in the manner of measurement would not likely be the result of knowledge the observer possessed about how the participant(s) should respond. Likewise, if we made sure that the dependent variable was measured in a consistent fashion (i.e., no major changes took place in how the device was used in measuring the dependent variable or in how behaviors were counted), instrumentation would be less of a threat to the internal validity of the study.

Testing Threat

Testing threatens the internal validity of a study when participants show improvement on a posttest simply due to the effects of taking the pretest. If the two tests are alike, participants may have learned some things from the first test (i.e., they had become test wise), thus improving their scores on the second test. In other words, the independent variable may not have accounted for a change in participant behavior; the change may have been due to pretest exposure.

For example, say we wanted to compare two groups. The experimental group was provided with a pretest and a posttest; the control group was provided with only a posttest. We saw that the experimental group outperformed the control group. Testing may be a major problem here. The two groups were different not only with regard to the independent variable but also with regard to exposure to the test. The experimental group had an advantage over the control group, since the experimental group had the opportunity to learn about how the test was conducted and was able to perform at a higher level because of previous experience with the test.

Testing would not be a threat in the following situation. Suppose a pretest measuring concern for multicultural issues were provided to an experimental group and also to a control group. In this instance, the two groups would be equated on all variables, including the past exposure to the pretest. A training seminar was provided to the experimental group on multicultural awareness, whereas the control group was provided a seminar of equal length on social skills. If previous exposure to the test on multicultural issues resulted in improved performance on the posttest, we would have seen an improvement in the control group's performance. The difference between the control group and the experimental group on the posttest would most likely have been due to the independent variable, since the threat of testing was removed as an alternative explanation. (A

simpler solution would be to assign participants randomly to two groups and give both groups only the posttest. By removing the pretest altogether, we would remove testing as a threat to the internal validity of the study.)

History Threat

History may well be one of the threats to the internal validity of a study that gives researchers the most concern. *History* is defined as anything other than the independent variable that is occurring between the pretest and the posttest, or during the implementation of the independent variable, that may affect the participants' performance.

For example, suppose we wished to teach students how to perform cardiopulmonary resuscitation (CPR). A CPR training program was developed to teach the students this important skill. We conducted a pretest to determine whether the students knew how to do CPR. The CPR training program was implemented, then the posttest was conducted. We found that the students' posttest performance improved and concluded that the program was successful. However, we did not realize that the students were involved in the Boy Scouts at the same time as our training program. We also learned that as part of their experiences in the Boy Scouts, the students received first-aid training that included CPR around the same time that we were teaching them how to perform CPR. There is a problem of history in this scenario. We cannot conclude that our program was successful—that is, that changes were due to the independent variable (the training we provided).

A nonexample of history as a threat follows. Suppose we wanted to decrease the

---

An **instrumentation threat** *occurs when there is a change in the calibration of the measurement device.*

A **testing threat** *occurs when scores on a posttest are affected by the experience of taking the pretest.*

A **history threat** *occurs when anything other than the independent variable affects the participant's performance.*

hyperactivity of several students. Half of the students were randomly assigned to an experimental group and half to a control group. For the experimental group, we used a self-management program to teach the students how to control their own behavior. The control group received time on a computer equal to the amount of time the control group was involved in the program. Upon completion of the study, we determined that the experimental group had a significantly lower level of hyperactivity than did the control group. History was less of a threat to the internal validity of this study, since the control group was exposed to the same history as the experimental group. Thus, any change in the experimental group as a result of history would have also been seen in the control group.

Resentful Demoralization of the Control Group

Resentful demoralization can be a threat to the internal validity of a study when a group of individuals believes that another group is receiving something desirable that is not given to everyone involved. Thus, individuals not receiving that "something" may feel demoralized and resentful toward the other individuals, since they believe that something desirable is being withheld from them. They may put forth less effort than they would have ordinarily in tasks such as a posttest.

For example, suppose that a number of low-performing students were assigned to an experimental group to receive help in math that incorporated a new remedial instructional technique. Other low-performing students did not receive the special remediation (control). When the students in the control group realized that the other students had access to special help, they felt cheated. Their effort in completing homework diminished, as did their efforts in class. At the end of the grading period, these individuals had fallen behind the experimental group participants. The results seemed to indicate that the independent variable was more powerful than it actually was. If the control group participants had continued trying as they had before the study, they might not have fallen as far behind.

The following investigation illustrates a non-example of this threat. Say we had two groups of individuals involved in a program designed to decrease their episodes of depression. The experimental group received a new drug, and the control group received a placebo. Since the control group was blind to the type of "drug" it was receiving, it was unlikely that the group would become demoralized by not receiving the new drug. We saw large differences between the two groups' responses to the independent variable; thus, it was unlikely that the difference was due to the control group becoming upset with what it could have considered an inequity that might have led to further depression.

Threats That Result in Similarities within and between Individuals

There are three threats to the internal validity of an investigation that result in similarities within and between individuals: diffusion of treatment, compensatory rivalry by the control group, and compensatory equalization of treatments (see Figure 2.3).

Diffusion of Treatment

Diffusion of treatment is a threat to the internal validity of a study when the independent variable is applied when it is not intended. If this occurs, the effectiveness of the independent variable may be diminished.

For example, suppose we had an experimental group that received the independent variable and a control group that did not. The experimental and control group participants were in close proximity to one another (i.e., in the same class). During the delivery of the independent

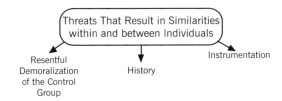

FIGURE 2.3. Threats to internal validity that result in similarities within and between individuals.

variable, the experimental group participants noticed that they were learning new and exciting things. They called their friends, who included some of the control group participants, and told them what they were learning. The control participants wanted to change just as much as the experimental group participants, so they tried doing what their counterparts were doing. The control participants also began to learn these new and exciting things based on discussions with friends exposed to the independent variable. Given the posttest, we noted that the differences between the two groups were minimal. We concluded that the independent variable was not very effective, when it may in fact have been very effective.

Diffusion of treatment would not be a threat in the following situation. We counseled a participant in his marital relationship. Participant was taught a set of interpersonal skills that we thought would help his marriage. His social interactions with peers were also assessed, and we planned to teach other skills to help him get along with others. We noticed that his relationship with his wife improved, but his relationships with friends did not. The independent variable seemed to have been effective, since the other relationships did not change. Later, he was taught how to improve other relationships, and we noticed that these improved as well. In this case, we ruled out diffusion as an alternative explanation for the results of the study, since his relationships with others did not improve until the independent variable was implemented.

Compensatory Rivalry by the Control Group

This internal validity threat is also called the *John Henry effect*. If you remember the story of John Henry, recall that he fought against the use of a steam-powered railroad spike driver. John Henry increased his efforts to keep up with the power tool. A similar thing may happen in research. If individuals who are not exposed to the independent variable believe they are in competition with the experimental group, they may increase their effort to keep up with or surpass their peers. The results of this increased effort may mask the effects of the independent variable.

For example, suppose we took two classrooms and decided to implement a new form of reading instruction in one of them (experimental). The other classroom (control) received a standard reading curriculum. The teacher in the control classroom, wanting to look as competent as the other teacher, increased the intensity of her instruction. At the end of the term, the students in both classes took a standardized reading test. We found that the differences between the classrooms were minimal. This lack of difference may have been due not to an ineffective independent variable but to the increased effort exercised by the teacher in the control classroom.

A nonexample of compensatory rivalry by the control group involved a situation in which we wished to study the effects of a new math curriculum in one of two classes. The first class (experimental) received the new curriculum, and the other class (control) received the standard curriculum. Before the independent variable was in effect, several observations were conducted in both classes to determine the normal routine in each class. Then, we implemented the independent variable and continued to observe the routines in both classrooms. The observations confirmed that the teacher in the control classroom did not alter her routine. There were only minimal differences between the two groups at posttest; thus, we were fairly confident that there was no compensatory rivalry by the teacher in the control classroom.

Compensatory Equalization of Treatments

This threat to internal validity may occur if individuals not receiving the independent variable receive as compensation from people within or outside of the study something additional to what is normally received.

For example, say we provided special counseling services to a group of individuals with depression (experimental) and no counseling services to others with depression (control). When we compared the groups' scores on a depression inventory, we found that the two groups did not differ much. It seemed that the special counseling was ineffective. However, we received additional information that the caseworker for those in the control group received money for a special outing once a week, since these individuals were not afforded the opportunity to receive counseling. Essentially, we were comparing counseling and special outings as compared to counseling and no counseling. Both groups received different independent variables. Both variables may have been effective or ineffective. The problem arose from making conclusions based on the understanding that the control group did not receive a special intervention.

Compensatory equalization of treatments would not be a threat in the following study. Say we studied the effects of pretraining of job skills on on-the-job training. The group that received the pretraining met two times a week for approximately 1 hour. An attempt was made to ensure that the other group received the prescribed independent variable and did not receive additional training. This additional training could have occurred if the second group received two workshops per week lasting 1 hour each to supplement the on-the-job training. The implementation of the prescribed independent variable was monitored. Little difference between the two training methods was noticed; thus, we concluded that there was little difference between pretraining and on-the-job training of vocational skills. We were confident that there was little chance for a compensatory equalization of treatments threat.

WHAT IS EXTERNAL VALIDITY AND WHAT ARE ITS THREATS?

We may never know exactly whether a particular threat to internal validity affects the results of a study. However, there must always be an attempt to determine all of the possible causes or functional relationships that exist between the independent and dependent variables. Once the possible extraneous variables that may affect the outcomes of a study are determined, our attention must then turn to the generalizability of the results. Critical research consumers must ask, "What does this mean for me and the individuals with whom I work, in my setting, at this particular point in time?" This question refers to *external* validity.

External validity asks, "What is the generalizability of the results of a study?" This question is a crucial one for those of us who are concerned with translating research into practice. If a study has sound internal validity but little external validity, we might consider the results to be of little value to us at this point in time. Having limited external validity does not mean that the results are not important. Basic research may seem to have little relevance for practitioners; however, basic research is critical to us at later times. Applied researchers take findings from basic research studies and attempt to apply the information gained to everyday situations.

Practitioners are especially concerned with external validity, because their situation dictates that they apply the best practices from research. If research results cannot be generalized from the laboratory to the field, they have little relevance to practitioners. Thus, applied researchers must be especially concerned with the external validity of their results if those results are to be generalized to other individuals and situations. There are two general categories of threats to the external validity of an investigation: *population* and *ecological validity* (Onwuegbuzie & Johnson, 2006; Shadish, Cook, & Campbell, 2001; see Table 2.3).

Note that external validity threats differ depending on the type of research design. Table 2.4 refers the reader to tables throughout the book showing external validity threats related to various quantitative designs. Use this table to guide you to the information you need on potential external validity threats for different types of designs.

Population Validity

Population validity concerns the ability to generalize results of a study from a sample to a larger group of individuals. It answers the question, "Will the independent variable change the performance of the individuals with whom I work?" Population validity is usually what we think of as external validity. Population validity can be separated into two types—generalization across participants and interaction of personological (i.e., related to characteristics of people in the sample) variables and treatment effects (see Figure 2.4).

TABLE 2.3. Threats to External Validity

Population

Generalization across subjects—The extent to which we can generalize from the experimental sample to the accessible population.

Interaction of personological variables and treatment effects—The extent to which the intervention differentially affects experimental participants based on their characteristics.

Ecological

Verification of the independent variable—The extent to which one can reproduce the exact implementation of the independent variable.

Multiple treatment interference—The extent to which one can generalize the effects of a single independent variable when participants are exposed to several independent variables.

Hawthorne effect—The extent to which the extra attention provided to the participants during the study limits generalization to situations in which the extra attention is not present.

Novelty and disruption effects—The extent to which the novelty or disruptive aspects of an independent variable limit generalization to situations in which these novelty or disruptive aspects are not present or fade away.

Experimenter effects—The extent to which the study's results are limited to the individual(s) implementing the independent variable.

Pretest sensitization—The extent to which the study's results are limited to situations in which only a pretest is utilized.

Posttest sensitization—The extent to which the study's results are limited to situations in which only a posttest is utilized.

Interaction of time of measurement and treatment effects—The extent to which the effects of the independent variable on the dependent variable will maintain through time.

Measurement of the dependent variable—The extent to which the generalizability of the study's results are limited to the particular dependent measure used.

Interaction of history and treatment effects—The extent to which the study's results can be generalized to a future time period.

Generalization across Participants

When we speak of generalization across participants, we must define the participants targeted for generalization. Gall et al. (2007) address this point when they discuss two levels of generalization. First, researchers want to generalize results from the study participants (e.g., 50 students with attention deficits in a school district) to the accessible population (e.g., all students with attention deficits in a school district). The *accessible population* is selected participants who are available to the researcher. Gall et al. refer to the accessible population as a "local" one. Second, there is the generalization from the accessible population to the target population. The target population is a much larger group, such as all individuals with attention deficits in the United States. This type of validity is difficult to achieve, since the accessible population must be similar in all respects to, or representative of, the larger population.

Generalizing across participants usually involves the generalization of results from the study participants to the accessible population. The best and possibly only valid way to achieve generalization from the accessible population to the target population is through several replications of a study (see Chapter 1).

For example, say we wanted to compare a drug intervention for middle school students with attention deficit disorders and no-drug intervention. From an advertisement placed in the local newspaper for volunteers to become involved in the study, 50 such individuals responded. These volunteers were randomly assigned to one of two groups. At the end of the study, the group that received the drug was compared to the no-drug control. It was concluded that the drug had some positive effects. A concern arose as to whether these results could be generalized to other individuals in the same area where the advertisement was placed (accessible population). Because we knew that

> **External validity** *is concerned with the generalizability of the results of a study.*
>
> **Population validity** *is concerned with generalizing the results of a study from a sample to a larger group of individuals.*

TABLE 2.4. Tables of External Validity Threats for Various Quantitative Designs

Design	Chapter	Table
Experimental designs		
True experimental Pretest–posttest control-group Posttest-only control-group Solomon four-group	5	5.3
Quasi-experimental designs Static-group comparison Nonequivalent control-group Counterbalanced Time-series	5	5.7
Preexperimental designs One-shot case study One-group pretest–posttest	5	5.9
Causal–comparative design	6	6.2
Correlational research	7	7.5
Single-case research methods		
Withdrawal and associated designs A-B design A-B-A design A-B-A-B design B-A-B design A-B-C-B design	11	11.4
Multiple-baseline designs Across behaviors Across participants Across settings Multiple-probe design	12	12.2
Additional single-case designs Changing-criterion Multitreatment Alternating treatments Combination	13	13.2

volunteer participants differ in some important respects from nonvolunteer individuals (Rosenthal & Rosnow, 2009), we concluded that generalization across participants was a threat to the external validity of the study.

A nonexample of this threat would be randomly sampling individuals from an accessible population. Random sampling would allow us to generalize the results from the sample to the accessible population, because everyone in the accessible population would have an equal chance of being selected to participate in the study. Say we wished to find out the working memory capacity of individuals with attention problems. The target population was defined as all individuals diagnosed as having an attention

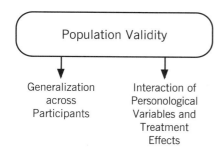

FIGURE 2.4. Threats to external validity related to population validity.

deficit disorder, as defined by the *Diagnostic and Statistical Manual of Mental Disorders*, fourth edition, text revision (DSM-IV-TR). Next, those individuals who were accessible for the study were selected. Once this was done, the number of individuals to include in the study was determined. Finally, this number was randomly selected from the accessible population. When the results were interpreted, we were better able to generalize these results to others in the accessible population, since we assumed that the study's participants were representative of the accessible population.

Interaction of Personological Variables and Treatment Effects

An **interaction of personological variables and treatment effects** exists when the independent variable has differential effects on the members of the experimental group based on the characteristics (sometimes referred to as *personological variables*) of each group member.

For example, suppose we paid participants in an experimental group $1 for every book read (independent variable). The number of books read was measured; we found that the experimental group read three more books on average than a group of individuals who did not receive payment (the control group). We decided to take a closer look at the members of the experimental group and found that some members were from high socioeconomic status families and others were from low socioeconomic status families. Thus, we asked the additional question of

whether the money paid for reading books was more or less effective depending on the socioeconomic status of the group members. If there were an interaction, we would have had to be careful with our claims of the generalizability of the results to the accessible population, since the socioeconomic status of participants may differentially affect how they responded to the independent variable.

A nonexample of interaction of personological variables and treatment effects as a threat involves one type of interaction—aptitude-by-treatment interaction. A popular theory in education is that of learning styles. This theory indicates that if we match styles of teaching (e.g., lecture, use of media, hands-on activities) to each student's unique style of learning (e.g., auditory, visual, tactile/kinesthetic), we can teach students more effectively. This theory rests on the interaction of a student's aptitude (i.e., style of learning) and the intervention used. We set up a study with an experimental and a control group. Two independent variables were defined—(1) the style of teaching, and (2) the style of learning. This illustration is an example of a factorial design (see Chapter 5). The results indicated that the style of teaching had strong effects on the achievement of students; hands-on activities seemed to produce higher levels of academic achievement compared to the other methods of instruction. The style of learning was also shown to interact with the type of instruction (e.g., auditory learners outperformed other learners when the lecture format was used; visual learners outperformed other learners when instructional media was used; tactile/kinesthetic learners outperformed other learners when hands-on activities were used). We made conclusions with regard to the type of instruction that was most effective with each type of learner. (*Note.* Such an interaction has not been consistently demonstrated; Slavin, 1994; Willingham, 2005.)

> An **interaction of personological variables and treatment effects** *threat occurs when the independent variable has a differential effect on members of the experimental group dependent on their characteristics.*

Ecological Validity

Ecological validity is concerned with the generalization of results to other environmental conditions (Gall et al., 2007; Shadish et al., 2001). When reading a research report, we must be concerned with the ability to generalize the results of the investigation to other situations, outside of the investigation. Ecological validity is concerned with 10 threats to the external validity of a study—**verification of the independent variable**, multiple treatment interference, the Hawthorne effect, novelty and disruption effects, experimenter effects, pretest sensitization, posttest sensitization, interaction of history and treatment effects, measurement of the dependent variable, and interaction of time of measurement and treatment effects (see Figure 2.5).

Verification of the Independent Variable

A frequently ignored but important concern of ecological validity is whether the independent variable was implemented as described (Lane, Bocian, MacMillian, & Gresham, 2004). Measuring the extent to which the independent variable was implemented as described has been referred to as *treatment integrity* (Lane et al., 2004). A slightly broader term referring to implementation of all experimental procedures is *procedural integrity/fidelity* (Belfiore, Fritts, & Herman, 2008). Researchers spend a great deal of time making sure that the dependent variable is measured consistently, but they may fail to ensure that the independent variable is

implemented consistently. If the independent variable is not implemented in a consistent and verifiable fashion, we cannot determine what was done to produce a change in the dependent variable. In at least some cases, inconsistencies are found in implementation of the independent variable (Wolery & Garfinkle, 2002).

Hagermoser-Sanetti, Gritter, and Dobey (2011) reviewed the research literature in four school psychology journals from 1995 to 2008 to determine the extent to which procedural integrity/fidelity data were reported; that is, they sought to determine whether operational definitions of the independent variable were included in treatment outcome research studies, and whether researchers monitored implementation of the treatment(s). Overall, 223 studies were examined, and 31.8% included an operational definition of the independent variable, 38.6% provided reference to another source for information, and 29.1% did not define the independent variable. Over one-third reported neither quantitative data nor on monitoring intervention implementation. From 1995 to 2008, a slight trend was evident in percentage of studies with definitions and procedural integrity/fidelity monitoring (39.7 [1995–1999] to 59.1% [2004–2008]).

A critical aspect of science is replicating the findings of previous research. We cannot replicate a study and obtain the same results when the independent variable has not been implemented as intended.

For example, suppose we attempted to find the effects of specific praise on the motivation of

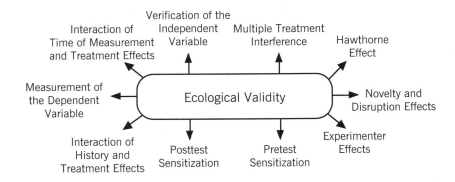

FIGURE 2.5. Threats to external validity related to ecological validity.

a student. *Specific praise*, defined as a verbal indication of desirable behaviors that the student exhibited (e.g., "Good job, Billy. You put the book on the shelf" vs. "Good job"), was provided for every fifth desirable behavior on average. However, the implementation of the independent variable was not documented. Our results indicated that the student's motivation improved; this improvement seemed to be due to the independent variable. However, if we were to implement the same techniques used in this study in another setting, we might obtain different results. The person implementing the independent variable may have praised every desirable behavior, not every fifth behavior on average. If this occurred, we would need to know about it to replicate the study and understand its results.

The following scenario provides a nonexample of this threat. Suppose we wanted to determine the effects of problem-solving training on a group of individuals with cognitive delays. A teacher implemented the independent variable, and the effects on the dependent variable were measured. At the same time, data were collected on whether or not the teacher provided appropriate praise and appropriate error correction procedures. Thus, we were more confident that the independent variable was implemented as described, and we increased the chances that if others implemented problem-solving training in the same manner, they would obtain similar results.

Multiple Treatment Interference

If **multiple treatments** are used together, we are prevented from claiming that any one independent variable produced the effects. We would have to take into consideration that all independent variables were used together. To make any claims for ecological validity, we would have to describe the combined effects of the independent variables.

For example, say we exposed a group of students to a phonics-based reading program and measured decoding and reading comprehension performance. The same participants were then assessed on how they performed when taught with a whole-language approach. The results indicated that the whole-language approach was superior to the phonics approach. However,

the two independent variables were not separated. The results might have been different if the approaches had been implemented in isolation, or if the whole-language approach had been implemented before the phonics approach.

If only one level of the independent variable were implemented with each group, multiple treatment interference would not be a threat. Suppose we wanted to initiate counseling for individuals with eating disorders and to determine the impact of three counseling techniques (e.g., behavioral, cognitive, and familial counseling). Participants were assigned to one of three groups, with one of the techniques implemented in each group. The behavioral technique was found to be more effective in reducing the occurrence of the behaviors associated with eating disorders. Notice that we did not expose each group to more than one technique, since we wanted to generalize the results to situations in which only one technique would be used.

Hawthorne Effect

The **Hawthorne effect** gets its name from several studies carried out at the Hawthorne Plant of the Western Electric Company (Grimshaw, 1993; Jones, 1992). Essentially, when the experimenters increased lighting in the plant, the productivity of the workers increased over time. However, in later studies, when the lights were turned down, productivity increased. In fact, no matter what the researchers did, the productivity of the workers increased. It seemed that the critical variable was not what the researchers

---

Ecological validity *involves generalizing the results of a study to other environmental conditions.*

Verification of the independent variable *refers to measuring the extent to which the independent variable was implemented as described.*

A **multiple treatment interference** *threat occurs when multiple independent variables are used together.*

The **Hawthorne effect** *occurs when participants are aware that they are in an experiment and/or are being assessed.*

did but the extra attention employees were receiving. However, some scholars debunk the effects of attention on employee behavior (e.g., Jones, 1992). The Hawthorne effect is a potential problem whenever the participants are aware that they are in an experiment and/or are being assessed.

For example, say we wanted to assess the effects of lowering the sugar intake of individuals considered to be hyperactive. Two groups of individuals diagnosed with attention deficit disorder (ADD) were formed. The individuals were randomly assigned to one of two groups. One group (experimental) had its diet planned and was strictly monitored, whereas the other group (control) was allowed to eat in a normal fashion. The control group's diet was not planned, nor was the group's diet monitored as closely as that of the experimental group. A large reduction in the experimental group's level of hyperactivity was observed; however, there was not a change in the control group's behavior. We concluded that the sugar restriction aided in decreasing hyperactive behavior. However, this decrease may not be replicated in situations where we were not present or when the individuals did not receive the same level of monitoring as the experimental group.

If a control group is provided with the same amount of attention as the experimental group, then the Hawthorne effect would not be a threat to the external validity of the study. Suppose we wanted to see the results of family counseling on the levels of physical and emotional abuse suffered by family members. Rural families who had little contact with others were included in the investigation. Instructors went into some homes and provided training on effective behavior management techniques. A goal was to find out whether the training sessions were effective; therefore, the level of abuse of families exposed to the training was compared to that of families who did not receive the training. One possible difficulty was that the families who were visited and received training improved simply due to greater outside contact. Thus, to decrease this threat, we made visits to the other families for approximately the same length of time but provided no training. If the Hawthorne effect were present, we would have likely seen it in the second group of families.

Novelty and Disruption Effects

Novelty and disruption effects may occur when the experimental variables introduced into an investigation change the situation in such a manner that the participants react to the changes in the situation in general rather than the presentation of the independent variable in particular. In other words, being part of an investigation itself may change the impact of the independent variable. When novelty effects are present, the effect of the independent variable may be enhanced. Thus, it is difficult to generalize the initial results if the investigation brings something into the environment (in addition to the independent variable; e.g., more people, recording instruments) that is different from the ordinary routine. The initial effects may not hold true if the novelty wears off or the independent variable is assimilated into the normal routine. The opposite is true for a disruption threat. When the experimental variables of an investigation are implemented, the investigation may disrupt the normal routine of the participants. When this occurs, the effectiveness of the independent variable may be suppressed if the participants fail to respond to the independent variable, or if they respond to it negatively due to having their routine broken or disrupted.

For example, suppose we wanted to study the effects of teaching styles on students in a high school class. The teaching styles used in the classroom were evaluated, and the teacher was questioned on what she was doing and why. The teacher was given feedback, and she made some changes in instructing her students. The students responded positively (i.e., their academic progress accelerated) to the change in teaching style. We left the classroom, confident that what we taught the teacher was effective and could generalize to other classrooms. If our presence and/or the novelty of the independent variable affected the students, we would have had a problem with the external validity of the study. When other teachers attempt to use the new teaching style, they may not get the same results, because novelty effects may not be in effect. The opposite would hold for disruption effects. Our presence in the classroom may have caused a disruption in the class routine, thereby making the independent variable less effective.

In this example, the disruption caused by the study may have interfered with students' concentration and, thus, decreased the academic progress they were making before we became involved with the class.

A nonexample of these threats involves investigating the effects of an instructional procedure that produces high rates of responding on the disruptive behaviors of students in a middle school classroom. We entered the classroom for 2 weeks before the implementation of the independent variable. During this time, the level of disruptions decreased and then returned to the level before we were present. After the students became accustomed to our presence, the independent variable was implemented. The data revealed that the independent variable was effective in decreasing the students' disruptions. Since we stayed in the class for an extended period of time to allow students to get used to our presence, novelty and disruption threats were reduced.

Experimenter Effects

Experimenter effects are also referred to as *generalization across behavior change agents*. Just because we have certain findings with one person implementing the independent variable does not mean that others implementing the independent variable will have the same success. Studies are usually well planned, and the individuals conducting the studies are usually well trained and typically have some expertise in the area they are investigating. Thus, it may be difficult to claim that the results of a study will generalize to other individuals who implement the independent variable without the same level of training, the same motivation, or the same personological variables that were present in the original experiment. These are referred to as experimenter effects.

Consider the following example. Teaching is a profession that is affected by a variety of factors. What makes one teacher effective and another ineffective depends not only on the curriculum they are using but also on other factors, such as the excitement they exhibit toward the subject matter. Suppose we developed a better way of teaching social interaction skills to students with behavior disorders. The new technique

used scenarios in which the participants had to respond (e.g., "You see a person you dislike at a store and that person approaches you. How would you react?"). Our findings on the new program indicated that we were effective in teaching social skills to students with behavior disorders. A teacher purchased the program to use with her students who also had difficulties interacting with others. She began the program but believed that the scenarios were too juvenile for her students. She took them through the program but did so in a very subdued and unexcited fashion. After the program, she found that the students did not improve and concluded that the program did not work. Critical research consumers must be concerned with the possibility that the manner in which the independent variable is presented, and by whom, may make a difference in the replicability of the results.

A nonexample of experimenter effects involves implementing a program to improve the productivity levels of employees at an assembly plant. The plant was one division of a large corporation. The plant managers brought in a motivational speaker, who discussed the importance of a productive workforce, improvement in self-esteem for workers, and the increased pride of being associated with a productive workforce. The managers measured the productivity levels of the workforce before and after the speaker. They found that the productivity level increased significantly. The managers recommended that other divisions of the corporation bring in motivational speakers. In the other divisions, speakers focused on the same topics as the first speaker, and the reaction of the workforce was measured. They, too, found that productivity levels increased after each speaker. Experimenter effects were not a strong threat, since other speakers exhibiting

---

Novelty and disruption effects *are threats when participants react to changes in the experimental situation as opposed to the independent variable.*

Experimenter effects *are threats in which there is a lack of information that someone other than the person implementing the independent variable will have the same success.*

different presentation styles but speaking on the same topics had similar results.

Pretest Sensitization

Many times researchers provide a pretest when attempting to determine the effects of the independent variable on the dependent variable. After this pretest, they provide the independent variable, followed by the posttest. The difference between the pretest and the posttest may then be determined to be the result of the independent variable. However, the pretest may make the independent variable more effective than it would have been without the pretest. This is referred to as **pretest sensitization**.

For example, suppose we wanted to see the effects of a class on developing students' self-esteem. A questionnaire was provided before class to determine how each individual felt about him-/herself in terms of popularity, ability, and physical appearance. The independent variable that was then implemented involved teaching students how each was unique and could have an impact on other people. The class lasted approximately 2 weeks. At the end of the 2-week period, a posttest was conducted. The data indicated that participants' self-esteem improved from pretest to posttest assessment. A teacher read about the study and decided to replicate the procedure in her classroom. She taught the self-esteem class and conducted a posttest to determine the effects. She found that the students still had relatively low levels of self-esteem. One possible reason for her failure to replicate the results of the previous study might be that she did not implement a pretest. When a pretest is implemented, it may become part of the independent variable. The pretest might have altered participants' perceptions of the upcoming class and made the class more effective. Although researchers frequently use a pretest to assess the effectiveness of an independent variable, practitioners may not do so.

Pretest sensitization would not be a threat if a pretest were not provided. Suppose we tested the effectiveness of a drug prevention/drug awareness program. Sixty participants from an accessible population of middle school children were randomly selected. The children were then matched based on age, socioeconomic status of their parents, parental educational level, and whether they had previously been exposed to drugs. Matching on these variables helped to ensure that the groups were equal or similar on what we considered to be important variables. A pretest was not provided, since there was less need to see whether there were initial differences between the groups. The experimental group was exposed to the drug prevention/drug awareness program; the control group was not exposed to the program. A posttest measured attitudes about the acceptability of experimenting with illegal drugs. The results indicated that the experimental group participants were less inclined than the control group participants to experiment with drugs. Since a pretest was not used, this threat was removed.

Posttest Sensitization

Posttest sensitization is similar to the pretest sensitization threat. The application of a posttest may make the independent variable more effective, since the posttest essentially synthesizes the previously learned material. This threat is referred to as **posttest sensitization**.

For example, suppose we wanted to find out how much information students in a statistics class remember. A pretest was given, and the results indicated that the students' knowledge levels were low, with students scoring an average of 20% on the test. The students were instructed throughout the semester, then given a posttest at the end of the term. Students taking the test indicated that they began to realize how to put together all of the information they learned during the semester; that is, they realized how to use statistics to answer research questions and to see the "big picture." The students did well on the posttest by answering an average of 85% of the questions correctly. We concluded that the independent variable was effective. However, the extent to which the posttest improved the effectiveness of the independent variable was not known.

Posttest sensitization would not be a threat in the following study. Say we were interested in researching the effectiveness of teaching cognitive skills to adults with learning disabilities. The independent variable involved helping the adults become aware of how they go about solving a problem and teaching personal speech, or self-talk. A group of adults diagnosed as having a specific learning disability in reading comprehension was selected. Half of the adults were randomly assigned to an experimental group and the other half to a control group. The independent variable (cognitive skills instruction) was implemented, and a posttest was conducted after 10 weeks of instruction. The posttest, which measured the ability to comprehend a series of written passages, revealed that the experimental group outperformed the control group. In this example, the posttest may have brought everything learned in training to the surface or helped the information fall into place. Since this was a potential problem, we indicated that the posttest was part of the independent variable, and if others were to implement the same procedure, the posttest should be added to the intervention package.

Interaction of History and Treatment Effects

All research is conducted in some time frame. This time frame can affect the generalization of the findings if the environment has changed. We live in a different world compared to that in which a study is conducted, no matter how slight the difference is between the worlds of today and yesterday. If these differences are major, we might have an especially difficult time in making external validity claims. This difficulty is why researchers attempt to use the most up-to-date references available to set up the purpose or importance of their study. If we see a researcher who cites a study from 1900, for example, we may be very concerned about the generalizability of those results. However, if there is a particular need to set the context for the current investigation (e.g., to set a historical context) and an investigation conducted long ago is so important that it is needed to set such a context, an older reference may be appropriate. The key here is to determine the purpose of such a reference and how it is used. If the reference has historical significance, it is probably appropriate; if the reference is not used for such a purpose, it may be not appropriate.

For example, suppose we assessed the effect of condom use for adolescents in a particular high school. The use of condoms was promoted, and free samples were provided to all who requested them. Results of a survey conducted before and after the program indicated that safe sex practices increased during the program. We concluded that our intervention had the desired effect and promoted the program on a wider scale. However, any number of events that occurred at the same time as the program may have enhanced its effectiveness. Say we found that just after the program began, reports of an increase in the number of individuals diagnosed with HIV were made public. There was also a nationwide media campaign on the importance of safe sex. The program's effectiveness probably increased as a result of this event. That event may or may not be repeated again in other high schools. Therefore, the generalizability of the results would be limited to certain historical events.

A nonexample of interaction of history and treatment effects might involve the following. Suppose we wanted to demonstrate the efficacy of a group counseling procedure with adults with depression. Six individuals who met the criteria for clinical depression were recruited. Self-reports of their level of depression were measured on a rating scale before and after group counseling. Before the group counseling began, the average self-rating for feelings of depression was 7 out of 10 (with 10 being *very severe* and 1 being *no depression*). After 2 months, we administered a posttest to measure the effects of group counseling. The average self-rating decreased to 4. However, the events in each person's life (e.g., illnesses of a family member, employment) as well as the general environment (e.g., economy, weather), were also tracked. We noticed that at the same time as our counseling, a general feeling of optimism hit the country. The economy improved, the job outlook was very positive, and Congress was discussing increased funding for rehabilitative

---

Pretest sensitization *occurs when the pretest makes the independent variable more effective than it would have been without the pretest.*

Posttest sensitization *occurs when the posttest makes the independent variable more effective than it would have been without the posttest.*

services that might impact participants directly. These events are documented, and conclusions are made with these factors in mind. We did not claim that counseling *alone* was effective, but we stated that counseling seemed to be effective during this particular time in history (i.e., describing what occurred at the time). Since our claims were restricted to a limited time span, the threat of history and treatment was minimized.

Measurement of the Dependent Variable

When reviewing a study, the method of measuring the dependent variable must be viewed closely. There should be some assurances that the results are not limited to particular measures. A concern arises as to whether the results may differ if other measures are used.

For example, suppose we were teaching individuals how to engage in problem solving. They are taught how to go through a series of problem-solving steps. At the end of the sequence of steps, the individuals generate a possible solution to a given problem. We assess the individuals' problem-solving skills by asking them to describe problem situations and say how they would solve the problem. We found that the problem-solving skills of these individuals improved as a result of the independent variable. We claimed that these results could be generalized to the actual environment, and that these individuals were prepared to solve the real problems they faced in everyday life. However, our problem was that we could not be sure what happened when these individuals were faced with real-life problems. There was no way of knowing whether they could respond to situations that were similar to or different from the problems used in training. Generalizability of results would be restricted to only those measures used in the study.

Measurement of the dependent variable would not be a threat in the next scenario. Say we wanted to determine the effects of self-instructional training on adults with developmental disabilities involved in supported employment situations. It was commonly believed that self-instructions would aid these employees in completing work tasks. The employees were taught how to talk themselves through a work task. During the assessments, employees were asked to describe verbally how they would complete a work task. We measured employees' self-instructions by having them state the self-instructions aloud. After the program ended, the level of self-instructions improved. However, a more critical measurement is whether each person's actual correct completion of work tasks improved during training. Thus, the ability to complete work tasks appropriately before and after the self-instructional training was assessed. We found that the correct completion of work tasks improved during self-instructional training. Measurement of the dependent variable was less of a threat, since we assessed not only employees' self-instructional abilities but also their actual completion of work tasks.

Interaction of Time of Measurement and Treatment Effects

The interaction of time of measurement and treatment effects is a problem when we consider that the time the measurements are taken may determine the outcomes of a study. Most skills taught to individuals may be expected to diminish over time if these individuals are not given sufficient opportunities to perform or practice the behavior. However, the effect of the independent variable might decrease, stay the same, or even increase over time. Most researchers (e.g., Biemiller & Boote, 2006; Wolfe & Chiu, 1999) take posttest measures immediately after the completion of the study. Critical research consumers must also be concerned with the maintenance of the independent variable's effects or the generalization across time. If maintenance is assessed, it is usually for the short term (e.g., less than 6 months). Long-term maintenance (often more than 6 months) occurs much less frequently.

For example, suppose we wanted to assess the effects of a weight-loss program. Several individuals were weighed before and after the program was completed. The results indicated that those individuals who completed the program lost more weight than those who were not involved in the program. It seemed as if the program was successful in reducing the weight of individuals who were overweight. However, program effects must stand the test of time. Thus, we should have continued to assess whether participants maintained their weight loss for an extended period of time.

A nonexample of this threat might involve investigating the efficacy of teaching abduction prevention skills to children. The independent variable that was implemented involved teaching the children to say "no" when approached by a stranger attempting to lure them away from a park, to walk or run away from the stranger, and to tell an adult about the encounter. A posttest that was then conducted involved having a "stranger" approach the children and attempt to lure them away from a park. All of the children performed the skills at the criterion level (i.e., they said "no," walked or ran away, and told an adult about the encounter). The interaction of time of measurement and treatment effects is an important consideration when teaching such skills. Thus, maintenance data were taken at 1 month, 3 months, 6 months, and 1 year after the program ended. The children's skills were found to maintain at acceptable levels through the 3-month assessment, but they deteriorated during the 6-month and 1-year assessments. We concluded that ongoing booster training is required to maintain abduction prevention skills for more than 3 months. Our claims of external validity were enhanced, since we were able to determine the interaction between the time of measurement and treatment effects.

WHAT ARE STATISTICAL AND SOCIAL VALIDITIES?

Researchers are concerned about the validity (i.e., the degree to which *accurate* inferences may be based on the results of a study) of their work. A study that is valid will be deemed important by others in the field. We may even say that the ultimate purpose of any study is to achieve a high level of validity. Different types of validity must be considered. Two critical types are *statistical* and *social* validity. In education and psychology, most research is determined to have statistical validity if the results reach a certain level of confidence (e.g., $p < .05$; i.e., the probability of obtaining the results of the investigation by chance—not due to a systematic variable). With social validity, researchers must determine whether the results of a study are important to society.

Statistical Validity

Statistics are mathematical models that provide evidence for some types of research questions. Suppose we use the analogy of digging a hole. A shovel is an appropriate tool for such an activity. With a shovel, we can dig a deep hole and do so efficiently. However, if we wish to rake the yard, a shovel is not the most appropriate tool to use. If we attempt to use a shovel to rake the yard, we face a rather difficult task. A shovel is not an efficient tool, any more than a rake is appropriate to dig a hole. The same thing happens in research. Statistics should be used in a manner that is consistent with their purpose. For example, if we wish to find the average score for a group of students, a descriptive statistic called the *arithmetic mean* is used. If we wish to find out how individual scores on a dependent measure are distributed around the mean, a descriptive statistic called a *standard deviation* is used. If we want to make inferences back to the accessible population, we use *inferential statistics*. Likewise, we use inferential statistics if we want to determine the probability that our results occur due to chance. Statistics are not mysterious devices; they are simply tools that help us to determine the effect of systematic variables on the dependent variable and interpret our data.

Inferential statistics can be used to argue against one special threat to internal validity—*chance*. Suppose we took a sample of two groups from a target population to use in an investigation. Both groups were found to be the same at the beginning of the study but different at the end of the study. It was assumed that this difference was due to chance. If our results reached a level of statistical significance (e.g., $p = .05$), we would be able to determine how likely that chance finding is. The difference between the groups was an unlikely chance finding (e.g., less than five times in 100), so we concluded that the results were statistically significant. In other words, the probability of committing a Type I error (i.e., incorrectly concluding that there was systematic variance that affected the dependent variable when there was no systematic variance—the results were a chance finding) was 5%.

Suppose we implemented a process to increase the intellectual functioning of individuals with intellectual disability. On the pretest, the experimental and control groups had average IQs of 60. The independent variable was implemented with the experimental group. A statistically significant difference (at the .05 level) was found in the IQs of the experimental group (mean = 65) compared to the control group (mean = 60) on the posttest. That is, the probability of differences this large or larger, assuming that all results were due to chance, was about 5 in 100. Research is considered to have **statistical validity** if the results reach a certain *level of confidence* (pertaining to the probability of obtaining the results of the investigation by chance and not some systematic variable).

Social Validity

If our research results are to be used outside of the research setting, we must achieve some level of **social validity**. Research is considered to have social validity when society deems it to be important (Finn & Sladeczek, 2001; Wolf, 1978). According to Wolf, social validity was once seen as a difficult area of inquiry for those who wished to use only objective measurement in research. Social validity is subjective, since it cannot be operationally defined in a manner that allows it to be observable. However, social validity is ultimately a critical aspect of any research study, especially in applied research.

There are three concerns of social validity (Wolf, 1978). First, critical research consumers must determine the social validity of the goals of a study. If the goals are not socially relevant, the purpose of our research is suspect. For example, suppose we had the goal of determining whether students in a mathematics classroom acquired and maintained information better if the teacher used only a drill-and-practice format compared to a discovery–learning format. On the one hand, this research question seemed desirable, since the acquisition of mathematics knowledge is critical for future success. On the other hand, suppose we had a goal of determining whether children can be taught to read before the age of 4 years. Many educators may not see this as a desirable goal. Thus, even if we were able to demonstrate reading ability in children under age 4, the techniques used to teach these children (and the age at which instruction

begins) may not be adopted by educators, since the outcomes are not seen as socially desirable and, to some, are counterproductive.

Second, critical research consumers must determine whether the procedures used in the study were worth the findings that resulted. That is, do the ends justify the means? Suppose we wanted to improve the independent living skills of adults with traumatic brain injuries. The cost of rehabilitation may add up to hundreds of thousands of dollars. Since the long-term outlook of these individuals is likely dim without such services, the long-term costs may outweigh the short-term costs. Society may value the rights of individuals to receive the most appropriate services available no matter the cost; therefore, the high cost of rehabilitation may be justified. On the other hand, suppose that our goal was to get students to not disturb others during instruction. We set out to determine whether having the students wear mouthpieces decreases the disruptions they make during instruction. We may have a desirable goal, but the procedures we use to achieve that goal are likely to be less than socially acceptable.

Third, critical research consumers should determine the social validity of the study's effects. For example, we again had the goal of keeping students from disrupting others during instruction. To achieve this, students were taught how to monitor their own disruptive behavior. Upon completion of the study, the students' level of disruptive behavior decreased from 80% of the instructional session to 5% of the instructional session (which was the average level of comparison students). We probably would consider this to be a large improvement. On the other hand, suppose we wanted to improve the intelligence (as measured by an IQ test) of 7-year-old children with intellectual disability. We enhanced the children's academic stimulation in the home by asking parents to read to their children selected children's books every evening. The children's IQs were measured 6 months after the program began. The results indicated the children's IQs improved an average of 5 points (from an average of 62 to 67). This finding may not be seen as important since such a small improvement probably will not result in improved academic performance.

SUMMARY

❖ There are two primary roles of individuals involved with research. The first role, that of the researcher, includes (1) developing the research question(s) the researcher will attempt to answer and/or the research hypothesis (i.e., a test of the assumptions made by the researcher), (2) using an appropriate methodology to answer the research question and/or test the hypothesis, (3) interpreting the results, and (4) making conclusions based on the results of the study. Researchers attempt to use the most appropriate methodology to form their conclusions. The second role of individuals involved in research is that of the critical research consumer, which includes reviewing the methodology and determining whether it was appropriate, whether the methodology had any weaknesses, and whether the researcher's conclusions were valid.

❖ Variability is the amount of dispersion in a distribution of scores (Gall et al., 2007). Generally, it refers to the extent to which things differ from one another. There are several sources of variability in research. If researchers can learn where these sources are, they can attempt to control them. Sources of variability can be placed in two general categories—*unsystematic variance* (variability within individuals and/or groups of individuals that is essentially random and includes measurement error and individual differences) and *systematic variance* (variability that we can account for between or among groups of people, because something that occurs makes a group of individuals move in the same direction, and includes the independent variable and extraneous variables).

❖ Internal validity indicates that we are confident that a change in the dependent variable is associated or correlated with the implementation of the independent variable. There are several possible threats to the internal validity of a study. These threats can be separated into two categories: (1) threats that result in differences within or between individuals (i.e., maturation, selection, selection by maturation interaction, statistical regression, mortality, instrumentation, testing, history, and resentful demoralization of the control group), and (2) threats that result in similarities within and between individuals (i.e., diffusion of treatment, compensatory rivalry by the control group, and compensatory equalization of treatments).

❖ External validity concerns the generalizability of the results of a study. There are two general categories of threat to the external validity of an investigation: *population validity* (generalization across participants and interaction of personological variables and treatment effects) and *ecological validity* (verification of the independent variable, multiple treatment interference, the Hawthorne effect, novelty and disruption effects, experimenter effects, pretest sensitization, posttest sensitization, interaction of history and treatment effects, measurement of the dependent variable, and interaction of time of measurement and treatment effects).

❖ Two critical types of validity are *statistical* (the probability of getting differences this large or larger, assuming that all results were due to chance) and *social* (society deems the results of an investigation to be important).

DISCUSSION QUESTIONS

1. Explain variance and provide an example of how you demonstrate variability in your daily life.

2. Explain how unsystematic variance and systematic variance are related.

3. Systematic variance moves a group in the same direction. Do all individuals in a group move in the same direction with systematic variance? Explain your response.

4. Suppose you are a practitioner working with individuals with a particular need. What

Statistical validity *occurs when the results of a study are unlikely to be the result of chance factors (an unsystematic variable).*

Social validity *occurs when the results of a study are deemed important by society.*

would be more important to you, internal validity or external validity? Why?

5. Is it possible to have external validity without internal validity? Explain your response.

6. What threats to internal validity are likely to make groups exposed to the independent variable different than those not exposed to the independent variable? Which threats are likely to make the groups more alike?

7. Is it true that the larger the number of participants in a group, the greater the ability to generalize to the target population? Why or why not?

8. If statistical validity only controls for chance events, why do people still place so much emphasis on it?

9. Is it appropriate to interpret statistical validity as a difference between groups due to the independent variable? In your answer, describe what makes up systematic variance.

10. Should applied researchers be required to report some form of social validity in their research? Why or why not?

INTERPRETATION EXERCISES

Internal Validity

For the following scenarios, indicate the major threat to internal validity that is present and provide a justification for your answer. (*Hint:* Use a process of elimination to determine the major threat.) There may be more than one correct response; what is important here is the justification.

1. Fifty infants, born to mothers on welfare who were receiving child care services, were randomly assigned to either an enrichment (experimental) group or to a normal regimen of child care (control). The experimental group was tested monthly to follow the progress of the children. The groups were tested by examiners who did not know the group affiliations of the children. Both groups were assessed at the end of the study at age 2. The mean IQ scores of the experimental and control groups were 130 and 90, respectively. It was concluded that the enrichment program was effective in raising IQ scores.

2. Students involved in extracurricular activities were compared to children not involved in such activities at the end of 12th grade. The SAT was used for comparison purposes. It was found that students involved in extracurricular activities scored on average 100 points above those not involved in the activities. The school principal decided that she would implement a schoolwide program to get more students involved in extracurricular activities, since involvement can increase SAT scores by an average of 100 points.

3. A psychologist investigating the incidence of child abuse trends realizes that the incidence of physical abuse is increasing at an alarming rate. The psychologist believes that the cause of this increase must be due to the increased stress parents are under as a result of economic pressures. He decides to implement a counseling program to reduce the stress on parents.

4. Children who were born to mothers with IQs less than 70 were placed in an early intervention center that offered special sensory stimulation. At 3 years of age, the children were found to have an average IQ of 85 (on average 15 points higher than their mothers). The examiners were not aware of the purpose of the study. The researchers pointed out that children born to mothers with low IQs will likely have low IQs themselves. Thus, the researchers concluded that the special sensory stimulation was effective, and that all early intervention centers should implement this program.

5. Ten children with articulation problems were placed in a special speech development program at age 4. They were assessed with a reliable instrument before the program began. After a period of 4 years, the children were again assessed with a parallel form of the first assessment. The researchers found that the posttest level of articulation problems decreased substantially from the pretest level. They concluded that the program should be implemented on a wide scale due to the positive results of this study.

6. Twenty individuals with head injuries and memory difficulties were matched on age, length of time since injury, educational level, and socioeconomic status. Each pair was randomly assigned to one of two groups and provided a pretest. One group (experimental) was given a memory-enhancing drug, and the other group (control) received a placebo drug. Both groups received 10 hours of rehabilitation services (e.g., vocational and independent living skills) per week during the study; the experimental group received an additional 2 hours of memory training per week. At the end of 3 months, the groups were tested again. The researchers found that the experimental group outperformed the control group by 25%; this result was statistically significant. The researchers argued for the use of the drug with all individuals with both head injuries and memory difficulties.

7. A sociologist studying the effects of a government program designed to get homeless people off the street and into shelters followed a random sample of 100 homeless individuals. At the beginning of the study, 20% of the individuals regularly used shelters, 50% used the shelters in cold weather only, and 30% never used the shelters. After 2 years in the program, the sociologist could only contact 80 of the individuals. The sociologist found that 25% of the individuals regularly used the shelters, 60% used the shelters only during cold weather, and only 15% never used the shelters. The sociologist indicated that the program increased the regular use of the shelters by 5%, and 85% of the individuals used the shelters during cold weather, compared to 70% before the implementation of the program. The sociologist concluded that the program was successful.

External Validity

For the following scenarios, indicate the major threat to external validity and provide a justification for your answer. (*Hint:* Use a process of elimination to determine the major threat.) There may be more than one correct response; what is important here is the justification.

1. A psychologist decided to study the effects on cognitive ability of college students facing a task, with and without someone watching. He hypothesized that the response rate of individuals would be slower when they were being watched. The results of the study confirmed the hypothesis, and the psychologist claimed that these results were important to supervisors of employees and student teachers. He indicated that if we expect individuals to perform at their best, we must not interfere by using obtrusive observation methods. He believed that since there is no reason to suggest that college students in an introductory psychology class who volunteer to become participants in the study are any different than others, we can generalize these findings to others in the target population.

2. A researcher demonstrated that the best way to teach individuals how to use covert verbalizations to control their respective phobias was through direct instruction of the skills. The results of the study indicated that individuals who go through this direct instruction learn how to engage in covert verbalizations and are better able to reduce their phobias. The teacher, a PhD-level therapist who had 20 years of experience working with individuals with phobias, was the codeveloper of the Direct Instruction method and very excited about its potential. The researcher claimed that almost any person working with individuals with phobias could experience success with this method of intervention.

3. A health psychologist interested in increasing the use of seat belts among high school student drivers provided a driver training workshop and discussed the possible benefits and dangers of driving without a seat belt. She provided to participants a pretest that included watching films of cars involved in serious accidents. After watching the film, she asked participants to rate the likelihood that they would use a seat belt. She also provided a posttest in the same manner as the pretest. She found that after the workshop participants were much more likely than before to indicate they would wear seat belts. She concluded that the study indicated that a similar workshop should be provided in high schools around the country (she mentioned nothing about the pretest and posttest).

4. An educator researched the best way to teach young children sight words. She compared two training programs, one based on learning words in context and the other based on phonics. After the students learned all of the words, she provided a posttest in which all of the words were presented

in context; however, she did not test the words out of context. She found that the students who learned the words in context outperformed the students who learned the words through a phonics-based approach. She concluded that teaching words in context was superior to teaching words through phonics.

5. An educational psychologist attempted to show the best way to set up a classroom to promote appropriate behavior. He met with the teacher before going into the classroom and taught her several effective teaching techniques. The teacher indicated that she hoped the new techniques would work, since she was having increased difficulty with the class. After the first week of implementing the new technique, the teacher recorded a 90% decrease in disruptive behavior. The psychologist suggested that all of the teachers in the school should try the new technique, since it was so effective.

6. An educator, frustrated with the limited retention of information his students demonstrated, noticed that the students remembered little after the summer break, and that he spent too much time reviewing what students had learned the previous year. Thus, during the new school year, he decided to use less lecture in classes and more hands-on experiences. He used this teaching style

up to Christmas break and tested how much of the material students retained over the break. To his delight, the students retained nearly 80% of the information they had learned (he estimated that students only retained 50% of the information over the summer break). He concluded that the hands-on approach was far superior to the lecture method in helping students retain learned information, and that his colleagues should use the same technique.

7. A school counselor working with depressed students decided to determine the effects of a comprehensive counseling package on feelings about committing suicide. As part of the counseling, she began a support group for not only students but also their families. She also gave the students homework that involved finding reinforcing activities or hobbies. Additionally, she used group counseling techniques and one-on-one counseling in an attempt to change their negative thinking processes. After 1 year, she found that students' suicidal thinking had decreased. She believed that the critical part of the package was the group and individual counseling. She indicated that other school counselors should use these procedures to decrease the suicidal thoughts of students suffering from depression.

CHAPTER 3

■ ■ ■ ■

Reliability, Validity, and Interobserver Agreement

OBJECTIVES

After studying this chapter, you should be able to . . .

1. Describe the primary goal of measurement and explain how quantitative, single-case, and qualitative researchers attempt to achieve this goal.
2. Outline the reliability and validity issues in quantitative research.
3. Describe how researchers assess the reliability of measurement devices.
4. Explain how researchers determine the validity of measurement devices.
5. Clarify reliability and validity issues in qualitative research.
6. Illustrate interobserver agreement methods.
7. Describe the methods of establishing interobserver agreement.
8. Outline the factors that influence interobserver agreement.
9. Clarify the factors to consider when assessing measurement devices in the context of a study.

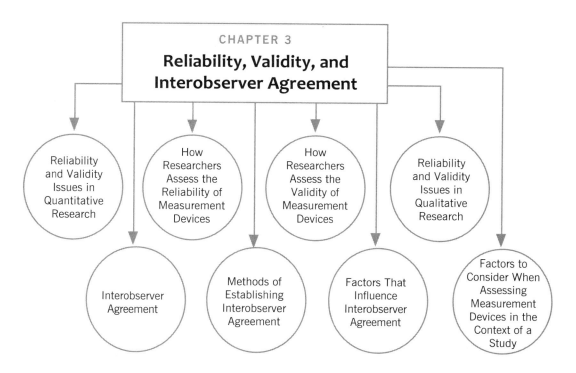

OVERVIEW

Of all the decisions made by researchers, determining how to measure the variable of interest may be the most important. The goal of measurement in research is to turn the complexity of the environment in which the study is being conducted into a set of data that represents only those features in which the researcher is interested. All features of the participants, as well as all aspects of the environment not key to the purpose of the research, are intentionally ignored as far as measurement is concerned. In this way, measurement is a process in which targeted features of the participants and study environment are selected from among all possible features and recorded. This process involves generating a set of numerical data for quantitative researchers and a narrative description for qualitative researchers.

The primary goal of measurement is to obtain a complete and accurate record of the targeted features of the participants and study environment. The ideal goal of measurement is that the resulting data represent all instances of these targeted features. Implicit in the idea of completeness is that the recorded data should reflect what has actually happened. If the measurement procedures used by researchers do not detect all instances of the targeted features of the participants and study environment, the resulting data cannot be said to be accurate. On the other hand, even if the measurement procedures provide a complete record of these targeted features, the data may still be inaccurate through the recording of nontargeted features. Thus, because it is impossible to obtain a totally accurate record of the targeted features of the participants and study environment, measurement procedures or devices provide estimates of these targeted features.

It should be clear that a primary concern of quantitative researchers is the completeness and accuracy of their findings. The concepts of reliability, validity, and interobserver agreement (in the case of the direct observation of behavior) not only constitute the framework to guide the design and implementation of measurement procedures but also the framework to judge the trustworthiness of the findings.

The concepts of reliability and validity are interrelated. *Reliability* centers on the question of whether the measurement device produces consistent results across observations, providing the researcher a way of assessing the trustworthiness of the findings. *Interobserver agreement* can be considered a special case of reliability in which the degree of agreement between independent observers provides a measure of the trustworthiness of the data. *Validity* generally focuses on the question of whether the measurement device indicates what it purports to measure. More accurately, it is not the measurement device that is valid, but the inference made by the researcher based on this measurement device (Messick, 1994). It may be helpful to remember that the word *validity* has the same root as *valor* and *value*, referring to strength or worth.

Reliability and validity have traditionally been defined in educational and psychological research concerned with the indirect measurement (e.g., rating scales, checklists, interviews that rely on informants) of the targeted features of the participants and study environment. For example, one indirect assessment of children's conduct problems in the classroom, the Behavior Assessment Scale for Children (2nd ed.), requires teachers, parents, and the individual to rate various behaviors of an individual child (Reynolds, 2010). In comparison, interobserver agreement has been defined in educational and psychological research concerned with the direct measurement (e.g., observations of actual participant performance) of the targeted features of the participants and study environment. For example, a direct assessment of children's conduct problems in the classroom would measure the frequency (number) of conduct problems exhibited in the classroom rather than a teacher's rating of conduct problems on a checklist or rating scale.

Questions about the validity of a measurement device and the resulting data are not typically a concern when researchers directly assess the behavior about which they intend to draw conclusions. For example, although validity would be an issue if a researcher used a questionnaire to measure the study habits of students at risk for school failure, it would not be a concern if the researcher directly observed how these students study. In other words, validity is considered to be inherent in direct observations.

In the case of qualitative research, reliability is viewed differently than it is in quantitative research (Seale, 1999). This difference arises primarily because qualitative researchers produce a narrative rather than a numerical record of the targeted features of the participants and study environment. Qualitative researchers view reliability as the fit between what actually occurs in the setting under study and what is recorded as data, whereas quantitative researchers view reliability as the consistency across different observations (Marshall & Rossman, 2011). Both qualitative and quantitative researchers consider their findings valid if the inferences they draw about the matter under study are accurate.

This chapter begins with a discussion of the concepts of reliability and validity within the context of quantitative research. This discussion includes a description of three methods used for determining reliability and their relationship to standard error of measurement, as well as three types of validity. Next, the concepts of reliability and validity are discussed within the context of qualitative research, including the procedures used to determine them. This chapter concludes with a presentation of interobserver agreement and a discussion of guidelines on how to assess measurement device(s) in the context of a research study.

WHAT ARE RELIABILITY AND VALIDITY ISSUES IN QUANTITATIVE RESEARCH?

Different types of reliability vary based on the evidence gathered. Similarly, there are different types of validity, depending on the intended function of the measurement device used by the researcher. Most researchers view reliability as the consistency of the results over time (e.g., Henson, 2001). In other words, most researchers believe that reliability indicates whether the participants would essentially respond the same way at different times. This type of reliability, referred to as *stability*, constitutes only one of three methods researchers use to secure estimates of the stability of measurement devices. However, critical research consumers should consider the relationship between reliability and validity before looking more closely at the three procedures for estimating the reliability of measurement devices.

If a measurement device is reliable, is it valid? If a measurement device is valid, is it also reliable? Answers to these questions depend on the relationship between reliability and validity. Reliability has traditionally been considered a necessary but insufficient condition in measurement use (e.g., Feuer, Towne, & Shavelson, 2002; Johnson & Onwuegbuzie, 2001). In order for a measurement device to be valid, it must be reliable. Unreliable measurement devices cannot be valid. Yet a measurement device's reliability does not guarantee that it is valid. For example, a highly reliable standardized academic achievement test might be valid for assessing children's academic competence but not for predicting their success in college.

Again, it is not the measurement device that is valid, but the inferences made by the researcher based on this measurement device. Put another way, a measurement device may yield both valid and invalid scores depending on the inferences drawn by the researcher. On one hand, the measurement device may be considered valid if the researcher draws inferences for which the device is designed. On the other hand, the measurement device may be considered invalid if the researcher draws inferences for which the device is not designed. The measurement device would also be considered invalid if the researcher draws inaccurate conclusions.

The validity of inferences drawn from tests is sometimes referred to as *consequential validity* (Gall et al., 2007). Problems arising from these inferences are not surprising given that many of the constructs of interest within education and psychology (e.g., intelligence, personality) are value-laden. See the example in the following box.

Inappropriate Inferences Made in the Area of Intelligence

Gould (1996) chronicles the range of inappropriate inferences made in the area of intelligence. For example, in the late 1800s, some researchers believed that intelligence was a function of brain size, and thereby drew inappropriate conclusions. For example, in 1879, Gustave LeBon concluded:

> In the most intelligent races, as among the Parisians, there are a large number of women whose brains are closer in size to those of gorillas than the most developed male brains. This inferiority is so obvious that

no one can contest it for a moment; only its degree is worth discussion. All psychologists who have studied the intelligence of women, as well as poets and novelists, recognize today that they represent the most inferior forms of human evolution and that they are closer to children and savages than to an adult, civilized man. They excel in fickleness, inconstancy, absence of thought and logic, and incapacity to reason. Without doubt there exist some distinguished women, very superior to the average man, but they are as exceptional as the birth of any monstrosity, as, for example, of a gorilla with two heads: consequently, we may neglect them entirely. (Gould, 1996, pp. 136–137)

Can you imagine LeBon describing his views to today's audiences? Gould (1996) noted that the claim was, of course, unfounded, because gender differences in brain size can be easily explained by other factors, such as height and weight.

Do valid tests have to be reliable? As discussed in Chapter 2, researchers must be concerned with measurement error, because it is directly related to the reliability of the measurement device. Measurement devices provide estimates (true value plus measurement error) of the attribute under study. Measurement devices that yield unreliable or inconsistent scores have large unsystematic measurement error. (Systematic error does not affect the reliability of measurement devices.) When the score fluctuates even though the attribute under study does not, the problem rests with the measurement device. The measurement device yields results that are influenced by unsystematic measurement error. Such a device cannot yield a consistent measurement of a variable. Thus, it is not possible to demonstrate the validity or accuracy of something that cannot be measured consistently.

For example, suppose we wish to make an inference about a person's intelligence using an intelligence test. We administer the test the first time and obtain a score of 115. A second test produces a score of 95; a third, a score of 105. What is the person's intelligence score? It is not possible to make an inference due to the inconsistency or unreliability of the scores. Thus, we cannot have validity without reliability. On the other hand, we can measure foot size fairly consistently. We can say that the measure of foot size is reliable. However, can we then say that

foot size represents that person's intelligence? We would have a problem with the inference we made or the validity of the statement. Therefore, we can have reliability without validity.

HOW DO RESEARCHERS ASSESS THE RELIABILITY OF MEASUREMENT DEVICES?

Reliability is an extremely important characteristic of measurement devices and should be examined closely. In short, we are concerned with estimating the precision with which one may generalize from one sample of behavior to other samples when considering the reliability of measurement devices.

There are different ways of securing evidence of the reliability of the measurement device used by quantitative researchers. We now consider the three most commonly used approaches to assess the reliability of measurement devices. These approaches include the *coefficient of stability*, the *coefficient of equivalence*, and the *coefficient of internal consistency* (Ponterotto & Ruckdeschel, 2007). With the exception of the coefficient of internal consistency (where comparisons are made among the items on the measurement device), each of these approaches involves comparison of one administration of the measurement device with another, using the same people. This comparison is followed by the calculation of a correlation coefficient that measures the degree of relationship between two sets of scores.

Types of Reliability Coefficients

There are three types of reliability coefficients—**coefficient of stability**, coefficient of equivalence, and coefficient of internal consistency.

Coefficient of Stability

A reliable measurement device is one in which each participant's score is reasonably the same on the second assessment as on the first, relative to the rest of the group. In other words, it is not necessary for a measurement device to produce essentially the same score for each participant on the second occasion as on the first. In the case of a measurement device with a high degree of test–retest reliability, if scores change (move up or down) from one administration to the next, they do so in a relatively systematic manner (i.e., on average, all participants' scores tend to go up or down the same degree).

The coefficient of stability is expressed numerically by determining the correlation or relationship between the scores obtained from two or more administrations of the measurement device; this coefficient provides an estimate of the stability or consistency of the measurement device over time. The sequence for obtaining the coefficient of stability is depicted in Figure 3.1. As shown, the measurement device is provided, there is a time delay, then the same measurement device is applied a second time to the same participants.

This sequence is depicted in the following example. Let's say we want to establish the coefficient of stability for a survey of teachers' attitudes toward students with disabilities. The same survey is administered to the same teachers on two different occasions. A reasonable time delay between the first and second administration is approximately 4 weeks. This period of time ensures that teachers will be unable to recall their responses on the first survey and not be influenced by other factors such as training or experience. Participant scores on the first and second occasion are then correlated to establish the coefficient of stability for the survey.

If the coefficient of stability has been used by the researcher to assess the reliability of the measurement device, it is important to consider the period of time delay. On the one hand, if the retest is administered too quickly after the initial test, participants' recall of their responses to many of the items tends to produce a spuriously high reliability coefficient. On the other hand, if the retest is delayed too long after the initial

test, participants' abilities may have changed, producing an indeterminable effect on the reliability coefficient. Between-test intervals of 3 to 6 weeks are common with measurement devices that can be influenced by maturation (e.g., growing older) or instruction (e.g., achievement tests). Longer between-test intervals are often programmed with intelligence or aptitude measurement devices that are not easily influenced by development or instruction.

Coefficient of Equivalence

A reliable measurement device using the **coefficient of equivalence** is one in which each participant's score is reasonably the same on the second form of the measurement device as on the first, relative to the rest of the group. It is computed by administering two analogous forms of the measurement device to the same group of individuals. Again, it is not necessary for a measurement device to produce a corresponding score for each participant on the second form of the measurement device as on the first. In the case of a measurement device with a high degree of alternate forms reliability, if scores change (move up or down) from one form of the measurement device to another, they do so in a relatively systematic fashion.

The correlation coefficient is expressed numerically and derived by correlating the two sets of scores obtained on the alternate forms of the measurement device. This correlation provides an estimate of stability or consistency of the measurement device between samples of the targeted feature under study. Alternate forms reliability is important in cases in which there is a need to eliminate the potential influence of practice effects on participants' scores.

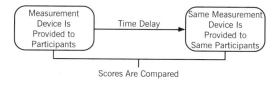

FIGURE 3.1. The sequence for obtaining the coefficient of stability.

> The **coefficient of stability**, sometimes called test–retest reliability, is computed by administering the measurement device to a sample of individuals, and then readministering the device to the same sample after some time delay.
>
> The **coefficient of equivalence**, sometimes called alternate forms or parallel forms reliability, is a measure of the magnitude of the relationship between participants' scores on two analogous forms of the measurement device.

For example, let's say we are interested in studying the effects of an intensive instructional
approach in science over a 1-week period. In
this case, it would be necessary to use parallel
forms of the measurement device, because there
is a high probability that there will be practice
effects. The sequence for obtaining the coefficient of equivalence is depicted in Figure 3.2.
Form A of a measurement device is administered to individual participants, and Form B of
the same measurement device is provided to the
same participants without a delay.

Researchers sometimes include a time delay
when calculating the coefficient of equivalence,
essentially combining stability and equivalence.
In this case, the sequence for obtaining the
coefficient of equivalence is depicted in Figure
3.3. Form A of measurement device is administered, followed by a time delay, then Form B
of the same measurement device is provided to
the same individuals. The following example
depicts this sequence. Suppose we want to establish the alternate forms reliability of a measurement device for the science program we wish to
conduct. The first form would be administered
to a group of students on Monday. Given that
the study period is 1 week, the second form of
the measurement device would be administered
on Friday of the same week. Participants' scores
on the two forms of the measurement device
would be correlated to establish the coefficient
of equivalence.

If the coefficient of equivalence has been used
by the researcher to assess the reliability of the
measurement device, it is important to consider
the equivalence of the sample items used for each
form of the measurement device. Because measurement devices typically include only a small
sample of all potential items, they are likely to
discriminate in favor of some participants and

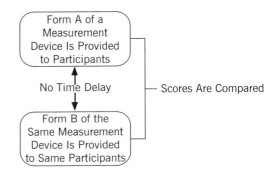

FIGURE 3.2. The sequence for obtaining the coefficient of equivalence.

against others. If the researcher has included
items on the two forms of the measurement
device that are very similar in nature, each
form will discriminate in favor of the same participants, which tends to produce a spuriously
high reliability coefficient. If the researcher has
included on the two forms of the measurement
device items that are not similar in nature, each
form discriminates in favor of different participants, which tends to produce a conservative
reliability coefficient.

Coefficient of Internal Consistency

In contrast to the two methods discussed earlier, the coefficient of **internal consistency** is
determined from a single administration of
the measurement device. Internal consistency
establishes how unified the items are in a measurement device. In other words, it provides a
measure of the degree to which items on the
measurement device are functioning in a homogeneous (similar) fashion. For example, let's say
we want to establish the internal consistency

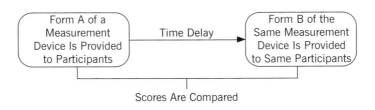

FIGURE 3.3. The sequence for obtaining the coefficient of equivalence with a delay.

of a personality measure containing 40 items. Because each of these items is believed to be measuring the same construct (i.e., personality), we want each item to reflect an individual's personality. This point is also true for measurement devices that contain subscales reflecting different aspects of a construct or entirely different constructs. The sequence for obtaining the coefficient of internal consistency is depicted in Figure 3.4. Subtest A and Subtest B of the measurement device are provided at the same time.

There are three commonly used methods for computing internal consistency: split-half correlation, the Küder–Richardson method of rational equivalence, and Cronbach's coefficient alpha (Basham, Jordan, & Hoefer, 2009). The split-half correlation is computed by administering the measurement device to a group of individuals. The measurement device is then split into two subtests to obtain two sets of comparable items. This division is typically accomplished by placing odd-numbered items in one subtest and even-numbered items in another subtest. The scores of the two subtests are then computed for each individual and correlated with one another. Of course, calculating split-half reliability demands that the items comprising the two subtests be as similar as possible. Otherwise, the estimate of reliability will be complicated by a change in the content of the two subtests. This demand is more likely to be met by a measurement device with homogeneous items than by a device that is designed to measure multiple attributes. Additionally, whereas the correlation obtained is an estimate of the reliability for only *half* the measurement device, the Spearman–Brown prophecy formula estimates the reliability of the *entire* measurement device (Gall et al., 2007).

The method of rational equivalence is the only technique used by researchers that does not require the computation of a correlation coefficient (Basham et al., 2009). This method assesses the internal consistency of the measurement device through analysis of the individual items. As such, it requires only a single administration of the test. A number of formulas have been developed to provide an estimate of the internal consistency of measurement devices that are scored dichotomously (i.e., right or wrong) and for those not scored dichotomously. The Küder–Richardson formulas (K-R20 and K-R21) are used in measurement devices that are scored dichotomously, and Cronbach's coefficient alpha is used in devices not scored dichotomously (Gall et al., 2007). Each of these formulas can be thought of as representing the average correlation from all possible split-half reliability estimates.

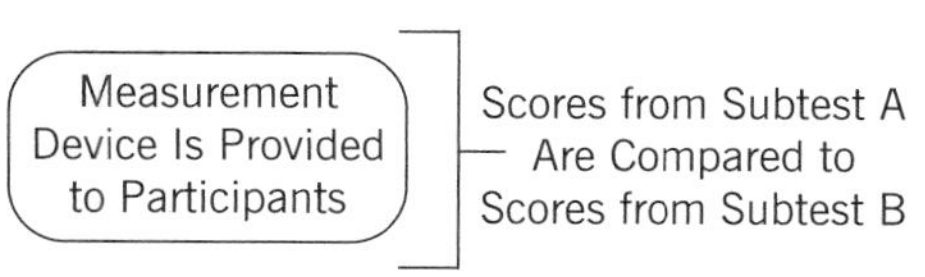

The basic rationale underlying the measures of internal consistency is that if the items on a measurement device are relatively homogeneous, then there will be a great deal of variance across individuals on the measurement device. This variance occurs on any given measurement device, because some participants will score high and others will score low, if the items are measuring the same thing. The internal consistency formulas incorporate this rationale by stressing the impact of score variance, with minor adjustments made for test length.

Interpretation of Reliability Coefficients

In general, reliability coefficients provide an estimate of the effect of unsystematic measurement error on the findings. In other words, the reliability coefficient provides an estimate of the extent to which the measurement device is free of unsystematic measurement error. Reliability coefficients vary between values of 0.00 and 1.00, with 1.00 indicating perfect reliability and 0.00 indicating no reliability (see Figure 3.5). The higher the reliability, the smaller the influence of measurement error. Although it is difficult to assess what constitutes high and low reliability in research, some guidance is necessary

FIGURE 3.4. The sequence for obtaining the coefficient of internal consistency.

> **Internal consistency** *refers to the tendency of different items to evoke the same response from any given participant on a single administration of the measurement device.*

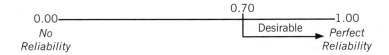

FIGURE 3.5. Continuum of reliability coefficients.

to assess the quality of the measurement device used by researchers. Reliability coefficients of .70 or above are usually considered respectable regardless of the type of reliability calculated or the method of calculation used. Reliability coefficients of .90 and above are not unusual for standardized achievement tests. Although reliability coefficients of .70 and higher are certainly desirable among many measures, lower coefficients can be tolerated; of course, this will reduce the level of confidence in the findings.

Researchers need to look closely at the reliability of commonly used measurement devices. The use of projective personality tests is a case in point. Projective personality tests such as the Rorschach Inkblot Test, the Thematic Apperception Test (TAT), the Children's Apperception Test (CAT), and the Draw-a-Person Test (D-A-P) have been derived from the psychoanalytic model of personality in which *projection* is defined as a primary defense mechanism against anxiety (Bornstein, 1999). For example, the Rorschach Inkblot Test comprises 10 inkblot designs, of which five are black and white, and five are in full or partial color. The cards are presented in a specific order, and the client is asked to report whatever he/she sees in the inkblot. The results are scored according to one of several standardized systems. Reliability studies of the Rorschach Inkblot Test have yielded low reliabilities (e.g., ranging from .20 to .64) that are similar to those of other projective personality tests (Wood, Nezworski, & Stejskal, 1997). These low reliability figures led Anastasi (1982) to conclude:

> Projective techniques are clearly found wanting when evaluated in accordance with test standards. This [conclusion] is evident from the data summarized . . . with regard to standardization of administration and scoring procedures, adequacy of norms, reliability, and validity. The accumulation of published studies that have "failed" to demonstrate any reliability and validity for such

projective techniques as the Rorschach and the D-A-P is truly impressive. (p. 589)

Relationship among Reliability Coefficients and Sources of Unsystematic Measurement Error

Participants' responses on a measurement device are influenced by many things other than the matter under study by the researcher. These other things are called measurement error. As mentioned in Chapter 2, some measurement error is systematic and some is unsystematic. The reliability methods described before provide an estimate of the degree to which unsystematic error affects the findings, and different methods take into account different sources of error. The five primary sources of unsystematic measurement error that affect reliability include the following:

1. *Variations in individuals,* such as fluctuations in mood, alertness, and fatigue, and recent good or bad experiences. For example, changes in the performance of participants from pretest to posttest might be influenced if the pretest is given early in the day, when participants are alert, and the posttest is given at the end of the day, when participants are fatigued.

2. *Variations in the conditions of administration from one administration to the next,* such as unusual noise or inconsistencies in the administration of the measurement device. For example, differences in pretest and posttest performance of participants might be influenced if the individual administering the tests uses different administration procedures (e.g., participants read the instructions independently on the pretest, while the individual administering the posttest reads the instructions and solicits questions).

3. *Biases associated with the measurement device,* such as items that discriminate in favor

of some individuals and against others. There are numerous biases that may be encountered in measurement devices, including those based on gender, religion, geographic location, linguistic ability, and race. An example of racial bias in intelligence testing was punctuated by Robert L. Williams (1974), an African American psychologist, who noted:

> Is it more indicative of intelligence to know Malcolm X's last name or the author of *Hamlet*? I ask you now, "When is Washington's birthday?" Perhaps 99% of you thought February 22. That answer presupposes a white norm. I actually meant Booker T. Washington's birthday, not George Washington's. (p. 222)

Another type of bias occurs when the researcher uses a measurement device that discriminates in favor of the experimental group and against the control group. For example, a researcher is interested in assessing the effects of a mnemonic strategy (i.e., a memorization aid) designed to help students recall science-related facts. To do so, the researcher compares the performance of the experimental group that receives the mnemonic strategy with that of the control group that receives instruction on global science concepts rather than factual information, using a measurement device that includes only factual questions. In this case, it would not be surprising that the experimental group would outperform the control group, because the measurement device is likely to discriminate in favor of the experimental group.

4. *Biases associated with participants*, such as cheating, help given to participants by the administrator of the measurement device, guessing, marking responses without trying to understand them, practice effects, and anticipation of participants regarding the results expected by the researcher. For example, differences in pretest and posttest performance of participants might be influenced if they are monitored closely during the pretest but not the posttest. This lack of monitoring would provide participants the opportunity to assist one another.

5. *Biases associated with the administrator of the measurement device*, such as differences in

scoring or interpreting results, errors in computing scores, and errors in recording scores. These types of biases tend to occur across both experimental and control groups, introducing error variance in their scores.

These five sources of unsystematic measurement error affect reliability of the findings by introducing unaccounted error; therefore, researchers are unable to determine the effect of sources of error on the findings of their investigation. The effect of the first three sources of unsystematic measurement error can be estimated by applying the different methods of estimating reliability described previously. The last two sources of unsystematic measurement error cannot be accounted for by the different methods of estimating reliability. Rather, the researcher must take steps to ensure that biases associated with the participants and the administrator of the measurement device do not affect the findings.

Table 3.1 summarizes the sources of unsystematic measurement error relative to each of the methods of estimating reliability. The different methods of estimating the reliability of measurement devices take into account different sources of error. Reliability coefficients based on a single administration of the measurement device (i.e., *internal consistency*) do not account for two important sources of error—variations in individuals and conditions. Individuals vary from day to day on many subtle attributes such as mood, fatigue, and attitude toward the measurement device. Similarly, it is difficult for researchers to maintain standard conditions when the measurement device is administered on different occasions.

Reliability coefficients based on the administration of the same measurement device on two different occasions (i.e., *coefficient of stability*) do not account for biases associated with the measurement device. The specific items on a measurement device are likely to discriminate in favor of some participants and against others, because the items typically constitute a limited sample of all of the items that could be included on the device.

Each of these sources of unsystematic error is only estimated when reliability coefficients are based on the administration of two different

TABLE 3.1. Sources of Unsystematic Measurement Error Estimated by Each Reliability Method

Method of estimating reliability	Sources of unsystematic measurement error estimated
1. Coefficient of stability	• Variations in individuals • Variations in conditions

2. Coefficient of equivalence
  • Single administration of both forms
  • Time delay between administrations
    of both forms
	• Biases associated with the measurement device
	• Variations in individuals
	• Variations in conditions
	• Biases associated with the measurement device

3. Coefficient of internal consistency	• Biases associated with the measurement device

forms of the measurement device with a time delay between administrations (i.e., *coefficient of equivalence*). Additionally, this method of estimating reliability tends to reflect more closely the conditions in place in applied settings. Critical research consumers should consider which of the aforementioned sources of unsystematic measurement error is present in the setting to which they wish to generalize the findings, and take these sources of error into account when assessing the reliability of the measurement device.

Standard Error of Measurement

The methods for estimating the reliability of measurement devices have centered on providing an overall estimate of the consistency in a group of participants' scores on the measurement device. However, these methods do not tell us much about the consistency of an individual's score. The **standard error of measurement** is used to provide an estimate of the consistency (or accuracy) of an individual's score. This estimate of the variability of an individual's score, based on data from the group, enables the researcher to estimate the range within which an individual's true score probably falls. The formula for the standard error of measurement is as follows:

$$SEM = SD\sqrt{1 - r_{xx}}$$

where *SEM* is the standard error of measurement, *SD* is the standard deviation of the scores or responses, and r_{xx} is the reliability of the test.

An example illustrating use of the *SEM* follows. Suppose we are working with a measurement device that has an *SD* of 8.0 and a reliability

coefficient of .92. We make substitutions in the formula and solve as follows:

$$SEM = 8.0\sqrt{1 - .92}$$
$$= 8.0$$
$$= 8.0(.28)$$
$$= 2.24$$

How does one interpret what 2.24 means? Based on the properties of the normal probability curve, the value of ±2.24 can be used to make some confidence-band assertions about the accuracy of an individual's scores. The relationship between errors and the normal probability curve is depicted in Figure 3.6. About 68% of all test scores are within ± 1 *SEM* of their true score, and about 95% will be within ± 2 *SEM* of their true score. In the preceding example, if a participant obtains a score of 50 on a measurement device, then there are 68 chances in 100 that his/her true score will be between 47.76 and 52.24 (i.e., 50 ± 2.24), and 95 chances in 100 that his/her true score will lie between 45.52 and 54.48 (i.e., 50 ± 4.48).

The size of the *SEM* is inversely related to the reliability coefficient. That is, as the reliability of the measurement device increases, the *SEM* decreases. Thus, measurement devices of low reliability are subject to large errors, whereas devices of high reliability are subject to small errors. For example, if the measurement device in the preceding example had had a reliability of .98, the *SEM* would have been 1.12; whereas, if the reliability had been .52, the *SEM* would have been 5.52.

Although researchers do not often report the *SEM*, it can be easily calculated from the information provided (i.e., reliability of the

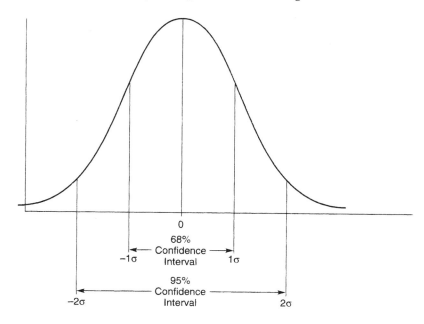

FIGURE 3.6. Normal probability curve depicting 68 and 95% confidence intervals (σ is the population *SD*).

measurement device and *SD*). The *SEM* is typically more useful to the researcher, because it is very stable across populations. The *SEM* is more useful in interpreting test scores than are reliability coefficients (Gall et al., 2007). Additionally, the *SEM* helps the researcher understand that the scores obtained on measurement devices are only estimates and can differ considerably from the individual's "true score."

HOW DO RESEARCHERS DETERMINE THE VALIDITY OF MEASUREMENT DEVICES?

Validity and reliability refer to different aspects of a measurement device's "believability." It should be clear that reliability coefficients answer the question "Does the measurement device yield consistent results?" Judgments of validity answer the question "Is the measurement device an appropriate one for what needs to be measured?" These are questions critical research consumers must ask about any measurement device researchers select to use.

Consider the report by Weinstein (1990) regarding the impact of teacher preparation programs on prospective teachers' beliefs about teaching. Weinstein concluded that teacher preparation programs do not change prospective teachers' beliefs about teaching. She indicated that despite coursework and field experiences, prospective teachers' beliefs about teaching and themselves remain unchanged. However, Weinstein found that there was a significant decrease in optimism ($p < .05$), a 13% decrease in the number of candidates who stressed caring, an 8% increase in the number of candidates enthused about teaching, a 13% increase in the number of candidates who believed they had the ability to maintain discipline, a 16% decrease in the number of candidates who believed they had the ability to motivate students, and a 14% increase in the number of candidates who believed they could meet the diverse needs of individual students. This case illustrates how researchers can misrepresent and invalidate their data. This case also punctuates the notion that there is an

> The **standard error of measurement** *can be viewed as an estimate of the variability of an individual's score when the measurement device is administered over and over again.*

uncritical acceptance of researchers' conclusions by others; this lack of skepticism is extremely problematic.

It is important to note that validity deals with not only the measurement device's representation of the construct under study but also the circumstances of its administration. The validity of the measurement device is affected by the manner in which it is administered. If the measurement device is administered improperly, the interpretation of the results, and hence the validity of the measurement device, will be adversely affected.

Like reliability, there are a number of procedures used to validate a measurement device (see Figure 3.7). We deal with three types of validity—construct, content, and criterion. Each type of validity provides a different view of whether the measurement device is fulfilling its purported purpose. It is important to note that we do not discuss *face validity* (simply looking at items on a measurement device and judging the device to measure what it is supposed to measure) directly, because it is not an approved form of validity according to the *Standards for Educational and Psychological Testing* (American Educational Research Association [AERA], 1999). Despite the fact that face validity is not an accepted form, the validity of many measurement devices is based on it. Indeed, the standards were originally developed to stifle the proliferation of claims regarding face validity.

Types of Validity

There are three types of validity—construct validity, content validity, and criterion-related validity.

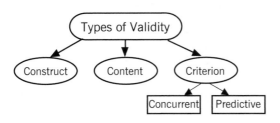

FIGURE 3.7. Three types of validity (including two forms of criterion validity).

Construct Validity

The word *construct* refers to the skills, attitudes, or characteristics of individuals that are not directly observable but are inferred on the basis of their observable effects on behavior. The extent to which it can be shown that a measurement device has **construct validity** depends largely on the specificity of the construct itself. Sometimes the construct measured is one for which representative items can be written with reasonable ease, such as the ability to compute mathematical problems correctly. In this situation, there is a high degree of agreement about what demonstration of the construct would look like. However, in many psychological constructs, such as intelligence, attitude, and personality, there may be little agreement about what demonstration of the construct would look like. Demonstrating construct validity when there is no clear, widely accepted definition is problematic.

There is no single way to demonstrate the construct validity of a measurement device. The authors of the *Standards for Educational and Psychological Testing* (AERA, 1999) make clear that the construct validity of a measurement device cannot be established with a single study. Rather, construct validity is based on an accumulation of research studies. More often than not, the construct validity of a measurement device is inappropriately based on face validity claims. One common face validity procedure involves using the opinions of judges or experts in an area to establish the construct validity of a measurement device. The extent to which experts' individual conclusions about what the measurement device appears to be measuring agree with each other is believed to provide an indication of the construct validity of the device. Another common face validity procedure does not involve any systematic process at all. Researchers simply accept the instrument as logically related to the construct. However, as noted before, face validity, regardless of how it is established, is an unacceptable form of validity (AERA, 1999).

Acceptable approaches to establishing the construct validity of a measurement device include intervention studies, differential population studies, and related measures studies.

Intervention studies demonstrate that participants respond differently to the measure after receiving some sort of experimental intervention (Graziano & Raulin, 2010). For example, to validate a new measurement device measuring an individual's test anxiety, we might sample 50 college students majoring in science, with students randomly assigned to two groups of 25 each. One group (experimental group) is told that the science test is necessary to continue pursuing a degree in science, whereas the other (control group) is told that the science test is only to provide professors information with which to guide the development of their courses. At that point, all of the students are given the test anxiety inventory. If the experimental students display significantly greater test anxiety on the inventory than the control students, then this finding would provide evidence to support the construct validity of the inventory.

The differential population approach to establishing the construct validity of a measurement device involves demonstrating that individuals representing distinct populations score differently on the measure. For example, to validate a new self-report social adjustment scale, we would administer the scale to students identified as having behavioral disorders and to those without behavior disorders. If the students with behavioral disorders display significantly lower levels of social adjustment than the students without behavior disorders, this finding would provide evidence of the construct validity of the scale.

The related measures approach to establishing the construct validity of a measurement device involves demonstrating a correlation (either positive or negative depending on the measurement device) between participants' scores on the measurement device and their scores on another measure. For example, to validate a new measure of collaboration skills, a group of individuals would be administered the new measure, along with a measure of individualism. Because one would expect individuals with collaborative skills to display less individualism, and vice versa, one would expect a negative correlation between the measures. This example illustrates that the correlation can be positive or negative depending on the measure involved.

Although there are a number of approaches to establish the construct validity of measurement devices, researchers rarely provide evidence to indicate that they are indeed measuring the constructs (inferences) that they purport to measure. Construct validity is a particularly important factor to consider when there is no clear, widely accepted definition of the construct of interest, such as with intelligence, attitude, and personality measures. In some instances, construct validity is not an important factor to consider. In those cases in which the construct is clear and there is a widely accepted definition (e.g., ability to compute mathematical problems correctly), construct validity may not be important to consider. Additionally, construct validity may not be an issue when the concern is to identify a measurement device that has predictive validity for a particular purpose and there is not an intent to appeal to theory. In this case, researchers are most interested in whether the measurement device predicts some established outcome.

Content Validity

Content validity is important because it is generally impossible for a measurement device to encompass all of the relevant items that would prompt individuals to display the behaviors characteristic of a particular construct. Content validity is primarily of importance in assessing the skills and competencies of individuals, such as in achievement testing. The content validity of a measurement device is ensured when it includes items that represent the entire range of skills and competencies, and emphasizes each particular area of skills and competencies according to its importance in providing evidence of the construct.

Generally one approach is used to establish the content validity of measurement devices.

> **Construct validity** *of a measurement device is the extent to which it can be shown to measure a hypothetical construct.*
>
> **Content validity** *refers to the representativeness of the sample of items included in the measurement device.*

Achieving content validity requires that the construct be translated into a set of distinctive behaviors. These behaviors are then described in terms of how people act, or occasionally in terms of what others say about these people. The measurement device is then constructed, with items that are representative in type and proportion, to prompt people to display these characteristic behaviors. Because most measurement devices measure a number of different subtypes (i.e., behaviors) in a given content area, they must include a proportionate number of items to represent each subtype. Essentially, a *proportionally stratified item development procedure* is employed to ensure that each subtype includes the same number of items as the proportion in the given content area. This procedure helps to ensure that the measurement device includes a balance of items. In contrast, a *nonproportional item development procedure* involves simply selecting a specified number of items to represent each subtype, regardless of its proportion in the content area.

Looking closely at the content validity of the measurement device is especially important when different intervention approaches are being studied. In such cases, the measurement device may favor one intervention over another. For example, if researchers use a mathematics achievement test that emphasizes computational skills to assess the relative intervention effects of a new program emphasizing understanding of mathematical concepts, they may conclude that the new program is not any more effective than the traditional program. The outcomes might have been different if the researchers had employed a mathematics achievement test that emphasized both computational skills and understanding of mathematical concepts. Critical research consumers should carefully consider the content validity of the measurement device in cases that involve the comparison of the effects of different interventions.

Criterion-Related Validity

Two forms of **criterion-related validity**—concurrent and predictive (see Figure 3.7)—are used to infer an individual's probable standing on some criterion variable (e.g., aptitude, intelligence, work-related skills) and differ only in a temporal manner. Statements of concurrent validity

indicate the extent to which the measurement device may be used to estimate an individual's present standing on the criterion variable. On the other hand, statements of predictive validity indicate the extent to which the measurement device may be used to estimate an individual's future level on the criterion variable. Thus, the primary difference between concurrent and predictive validity is the time interval. Predictive validity requires that a substantial time interval occur between administration of the measurement device being validated and gathering the criterion data. With concurrent validity, no such time interval is present. It should be apparent that the legitimacy of the criterion measurement device is critical to both concurrent and predictive validity. The criterion measurement device must be valid if meaningful statements about the concurrent and predictive validity of a measurement device are to be made.

The concurrent or predictive validity of a measurement device is established by collecting both the scores of a group of individuals obtained with a certain measurement device and their scores from other devices administered at approximately the same time (concurrent validity) or a future date (predictive validity). The scores are then correlated to provide an estimate of the concurrent or predictive validity of the measurement device.

Interpretation of the coefficient of concurrent or predictive validity is relatively straightforward. These coefficients, like reliability coefficients, vary between values of –1.00 to +1.00. A 0.00 correlation coefficient between the scores of two measurement devices means that they have no systematic relationship to each other—scores on one measurement device tell us nothing about scores on the other measurement device. The greater the value of the coefficient, the more accurate the prediction of the scores of one measurement device to the other, and vice versa. If the coefficient is either –1.00 or +1.00, a perfect prediction can be made.

Looking closely at the concurrent validity of the measurement device used is critical in those cases in which researchers have used a short, easily administered measurement device in place of one that is long or not easily administered. In such cases, researchers are trying to get an efficient estimate of the construct of interest. This administration is not problematic if they employ a measurement device that has a high degree of concurrent validity with a "valid" criterion measurement device. Looking closely at the predictive validity of the measurement device is critical in those cases in which researchers want to predict future performance. Predictive validity is the most commonly used form of criterion-related validity used by researchers.

Concurrent validity can be illustrated by the following example. Let's say a school district has developed its own curriculum-based measure of academic performance. District representatives need to ask the question, "Does our assessment device actually measure achievement?" At this point, the district needs to find a valid criterion measure. According to Salvia, Ysseldyke, and Bolt (2009), there are two basic choices for this criterion measure: (1) another achievement test that is presumed to be valid, and (2) judgments of academic performance made by teachers, parents, or the students themselves. If the new curriculum-based measurement correlates significantly with the other achievement test, the district can conclude that there is evidence for the new assessment's concurrent validity with another criterion measure.

Predictive validity can be illustrated by the following example noted by Salvia et al. (2009). If a district develops a test of reading readiness, teachers can ask, "Does knowledge of a student's score on the reading readiness assessment allow an accurate estimation of the student's actual readiness for instruction some time in the future?" As noted before for concurrent validity, the district must first find a valid criterion measure, such as a valid reading achievement test. If the district's test of reading readiness corresponds closely with the validated reading achievement test and accurately estimates how the student will perform in subsequent instruction, it has established a measurement device that has predictive validity.

WHAT ARE RELIABILITY AND VALIDITY ISSUES IN QUALITATIVE RESEARCH?

As mentioned before, both quantitative and qualitative researchers are concerned about the reliability and validity of the data collected.

Additionally, many qualitative researchers are concerned with reliability and validity; however, it should be noted that others in the qualitative community do not view reliability and validity as necessarily important (see Chapter 9). It is difficult to establish the reliability and validity of qualitative research using quantitative methods, because the researcher *is* the measurement device. There are several reasons why quantitative methods for establishing reliability and validity are generally not relevant to data collected using qualitative methods. First, qualitative researchers generate a narrative rather than a numerical representation of the target features of the participants and study environment. The traditional methods for estimating the reliability and validity of measurement devices were developed for numerical representations of the target features of the participants and the study environment.

Second, because qualitative researchers use an emerging rather than a predetermined design approach, two researchers are not likely to produce the same results (Denzin & Lincoln, 2005; Maxwell, 2005). In essence, qualitative researchers expect quantitative researchers to collect distinct information, because their backgrounds and interests differ, which is likely to influence the design of the study. Additionally, qualitative researchers also interpret the data differently and reach different conclusions because of their varied backgrounds and interests. Although qualitative researchers are likely to produce differences in findings and interpretations about the same inquiry area, these differences do not necessarily mean that the findings are incomplete or inaccurate.

Third, quantitative methods for establishing reliability are not generally relevant to qualitative studies because of the influence of contextual variables that operate in natural settings (Marshall & Rossman, 2011). Examples of contextual variables in a study of violence prevention efforts in schools might include community demographics and resources, school

> **Criterion-related validity** *refers to the extent to which an individual's score on a measurement device is used to predict his/her score on another measurement device.*

organizational procedures and practices, staff characteristics, and student and family characteristics. The same researcher may obtain different or contradictory data because of these contextual variables rather than attributing them to lack of reliability. In short, differences in the findings by changes in context may be produced rather than being a function of measurement error.

The final reason that quantitative methods for establishing reliability are not generally relevant to qualitative research centers on differences in the underlying theoretical stance of these two research methods (Marshall & Rossman, 2011). Qualitative researchers collect data that are subjective, dynamic, and changeable over time. As mentioned previously, participants' views and perceptions are influenced by changes in the context. In contrast, quantitative researchers collect data that are objective, stable, and static. These researchers use predetermined designs to control or account for changes in the context.

Reliability Issues

Because of these aforementioned issues, qualitative researchers have redefined reliability in a manner more congruent with qualitative theory and methodology. Qualitative researchers view *reliability* as the fit between what actually occurs in the setting under study and what is recorded as data (Denzin & Lincoln, 2005; Marshall & Rossman, 2011). Given this view, qualitative researchers use methodological procedures in which they fully explain their procedures, verify their observations, and cross-check their sources. Qualitative researchers provide the following specific evidence of reliability (Marshall & Rossman, 2011):

1. Description of the method, including the underlying logic.
2. Qualifications of the researcher as participant observer.
3. Assumptions of the researcher.
4. Research questions that are stated and directly connected to the study procedures.
5. Description of the study period, as well as range and cycle of activities observed.
6. Data collected from multiple sources.

Validity Issues

Although quantitative and many qualitative researchers have similar views regarding the validity of their data (i.e., accuracy of the inferences drawn from the data), they differ in the methods used to establish the validity of their data. Validity in qualitative research is relative to the researchers' purpose and the circumstances under which the data were collected. The inferences drawn by qualitative researchers differ depending on their background and interests. In essence, qualitative researchers expect quantitative researchers to interpret the data differently and reach different conclusions because of their varied backgrounds and interests. Although qualitative researchers are likely to produce differences in findings and interpretations about the same inquiry area, these differences do not necessarily mean that the interpretations are invalid. Qualitative researchers provide the following specific evidence of validity (Maxwell, 2005):

1. Description of how an ethical stance toward participants was maintained.
2. Description of fieldwork and analyses, including the logic and theoretical base of the data categorizations.
3. Description of cases or situations that might challenge the emerging hypotheses or conclusions.
4. Data collected from multiple sources.
5. Description of how the quality of the data was checked.
6. Description of the formulation and reformulation of the interpretations of the data.
7. Description of how the impact of value judgments was minimized.
8. Discussion of how the study is linked to a theoretical base.
9. Discussion of the limitations of the study.

Illustrative Example of Reliability and Validity Procedures

The following information obtained from a methods section of a qualitative study provides an example of how qualitative researchers establish the reliability and validity of a study (this is also the illustrative study at the end of Chapter 10). The purpose of the study, to identify variables associated with successful inclusion of students with disabilities in science, appeared to be robust across grade levels and specific categories of disability (Scruggs & Mastropieri, 1994).

Scruggs and Mastropieri (1994) went to great lengths to ensure that their data collection was accurate and systematic, and that their conclusions logically proceeded from the interactions of those data sources with their personal perspectives. They obtained multiple sources of evidence in support of each of their conclusions and had extended interactions with the participants. They addressed the issue of consistency by independently confirming all of their conclusions across the classrooms. A detailed description of the participants section of the article is provided to show the level of detail used.

The participants were from a middle SES school district with about 50,000 students in a western metropolitan area. This district was one of four with whom the project staff collaborated as part of a larger project to study science and disability. District science education administrative personnel, building-level administrators, teachers, and special education personnel were interviewed to identify reputed cases of mainstreaming success in science. Project staff also observed three classrooms in three different schools. During the first and second project years, the project staff worked with district teachers and specialists (along with those of the three other school districts) to develop and refine guidelines for including students with disabilities in science classes. Project staff presented the teachers and specialists with draft versions of project guidelines developed from information from previous literature and previously published guidelines and solicited and received written feedback. Project staff revised the guidelines based on teacher/specialist feedback on two separate occasions throughout the 2-year period. The authors noted that the final product contained information on characteristics of specific disability categories, general inclusion strategies applied to science classes, and strategies for adapting specific science activities (e.g., electricity units) for students

with disabilities. Copies were distributed to all cooperating teachers and administrators. Teachers in the three targeted classrooms were asked to refer to the guidelines in the final product when needed, but they were under no obligation to do so. All teachers reported informally that they had frequently referred to the guidelines.

Scruggs and Mastropieri (1994) fully described each of the three classrooms, including the number of students, as well as other pertinent demographic information (e.g., SES, ethnicity, disability category). They described the teachers in terms of their training and years of experience. The curriculum was described in detail, including what was used, how it was used, and why it was used. The background of the project staff was also described in detail (e.g., staff beliefs and preparation for the project). The description of data collection included how and when data were collected. The researchers indicated that the data were analyzed for consistencies and inconsistencies. Out of the data grew a list of seven variables that seemed to be consistent and robust with respect to all data sources across the three different classrooms. Researchers further indicated that these variables also were supported by previous research literature including both convergent and divergent instances. Importantly, the conclusions made by the project staff were reexamined to ensure that they were directly supported by evidence gathered in this investigation. This reexamination is a feature sometimes missed in qualitative research on learning and behavior, as noted by the authors.

With regard to reliability and validity, Scruggs and Mastropieri (1994) reported the following:

> Although it may have been less appropriate to address concerns of "reliability" and "validity," at least in the more traditional quantitative sense, in this investigation, we nevertheless wished to ensure that our data collection had been accurate and systematic and that our conclusions logically proceeded from the interactions of those data sources with our personal perspectives. We addressed these issues by obtaining multiple sources of evidence in support of each of our conclusions and by planning and implementing extended interactions with the participants. We also addressed the issue of consistency by confirming that all conclusions

were supported by evidence from each classroom, considered independently. (p. 793)

WHAT IS INTEROBSERVER AGREEMENT?

Interobserver agreement is a direct measure of behavior, in which two or more observers independently record the occurrence and nonoccurrence of specific behaviors and compare their findings. A primary approach to measurement in educational and psychological research concerned with the direct measurement of behavior is the use of observers to record the occurrence and nonoccurrence of specific behaviors (Cooper et al., 2007). It is necessary to qualify the conclusions about data that interobserver agreement permits before we describe researchers' procedures to establish interobserver agreement. This qualification is necessary, because the concept of interobserver agreement or reliability of observations is not the same as the concept of reliability used in educational and psychological research, which incorporates indirect measurement of behavior.

Recall that reliability focuses on the precision with which one may generalize behavior from one sample to other samples obtained with measurement devices. The other samples may be obtained at different points in time, as in the case of the coefficient of stability. Alternatively, they may be obtained with other sets of items drawn from the universe of possible items and, in some cases, may involve both different items and a different time (i.e., coefficient of equivalence). Additionally, the other samples may be obtained from sets of items on a single form of the measurement device, as in the case of the coefficient of internal consistency.

In contrast, interobserver agreement says nothing about whether the observations of two independent observers are reliable. Although a high degree of agreement between two independent observers recording responses during a session enhances the believability of the data, it only allows the conclusion that their total values for a session were in agreement. It does not indicate that the observers identified the same responses, because each observer may have failed to identify or mistakenly identified different responses (albeit the same number of responses). In other words, just because two observers say that they saw something does not mean that it really happened. Establishing the degree of interobserver agreement enables the researcher to accept the believability of the data, because independently verified reports often are more accurate than a single report.

Interobserver agreement is used to assess the occurrence and nonoccurrence of not only the dependent variable (Cooper et al., 2007) but also the independent variable (Belfiore et al., 2008). That is, interobserver agreement assesses not only behavior but also integrity of implementation of the treatment procedures. Measures of interobserver agreement help in answering the question "Is that what I would have seen if I had been there?"

In general, interobserver agreement has four primary functions: (1) it provides information on whether the definitional aspects of the response and intervention are replicable; (2) it provides information with which to assess the extent to which the definitional aspects of the response and the intervention plan are employed competently; (3) it provides information with which to assess the believability of the experimental effects; and (4) it provides information with which to assess the believability of the absolute level of responding aside from any experimental effects shown.

The first two functions concern the replicability of the study. Adequate descriptions of the definitional aspects of both the response and the measurement procedures and the intervention are necessary to ensure that the study can be replicated. The remaining two functions focus on the believability of the reported data. Confidence in the reported findings is enhanced when two independent observers achieve a high degree of agreement regarding the occurrence and nonoccurrence of the response and the intervention.

WHAT ARE THE METHODS OF ESTABLISHING INTEROBSERVER AGREEMENT?

Although a small number of studies has used correlation coefficients to establish the level of interobserver agreement (Barlow et al., 2008;

Kazdin, 2003), the percentage of agreement between two independent observers is the most common method for reporting interobserver agreement (Cooper et al., 2007). Thus, we focus on the procedures used by researchers to establish the percentage of agreement between two independent observers.

Five behavioral and procedural issues should be considered when assessing interobserver agreement. First, it is critical that a clear, specific definition be developed to ensure that the observers are able to identify characteristics and the beginning and end of the behavior. Second, the frequency with which observations are conducted should be analyzed. Although there are no set rules, the frequency of interobserver measures used by researchers must fall between the ideal (every recorded response) and the minimum (once per condition; e.g., once before intervention and once during intervention). It is common practice to assess interobserver agreement on at least 20 to 25% of total sessions (Cooper et al., 2007). Third, interobserver agreement should be reported for both the dependent variable and the independent variable. Fourth, agreement data should be reported for each behavior for each participant. Finally, the level of interobserver agreement should meet an acceptable level. Although a minimum criterion for the acceptability of interobserver agreement has not be established, the usual convention is to expect independent observers to achieve an average of at least 80% agreement (Barlow et al., 2008; Cooper et al., 2007).

Of course, the 80% rule is arbitrary and must be interpreted within the context of the study. For example, if the average interobserver agreement for a study using permanent products, such as written answers to mathematics problems, is 80%, one would view the data cautiously, whereas this level of interobserver agreement may be acceptable in cases in which the researcher was measuring more complex behaviors, such as initiating social interaction, using activity schedules to sequence activities, or following instructions.

The specific formulas used by researchers to establish interobserver agreement are dependent upon the observational procedure used and include measures of permanent products, event recording, latency and duration recording,

and interval recording (Cooper et al., 2007). The observational procedures and associated methods for calculating interobserver agreement follow.

Measures of Permanent Products

Researchers sometimes use permanent products (e.g., completed worksheets or puzzles, written examinations or spelling words) to assess the effects of an intervention. With this procedure, the researcher observes the product of a participant's behavior. The actual behavior itself is not observed. For example, a researcher might use the number of mathematics problems completed correctly to assess the effects of a self-management intervention on the on-task behavior of students. Although it may seem unnecessary to assess the level of agreement with permanent products that are easily identified, discrete responses, mistakes do occur in the scoring. The following formula is used to establish the percentage of agreement between independent observers measuring permanent products. The percentage of agreement equals the number of agreements divided by the total number of agreements and disagreements multiplied by 100:

$$\frac{\text{Percentage}}{\text{of agreement}} = \frac{\text{Agreements}}{\text{Agreements} + \text{Disagreements}} \times 100$$

Inspection of the formula reveals that as the number of disagreements goes up, the percentage of agreement goes down. For example, let's say that interobserver agreement was achieved on 90 of 100 math problems. In this scenario, disagreement between observers occurred on 10 problems. By substituting these numbers into the formula, the percentage of interobserver agreement would be 90% (i.e., 90 agreements/[90 agreements + 10 disagreements], with the result of .90 multiplied by 100). In contrast, if interobserver agreement had been achieved on 75 of the math problems (the observers disagreed on

---

Interobserver agreement *is a comparison of recordings of behaviors of two or more observers.*

25 of the problems), the percentage of interobserver agreement would drop to 75%.

Event Recording

Researchers may simply tally the number of times a response (e.g., talk outs) occurs within a defined period of time to assess the effects of an intervention. Event recording establishes the numerical dimension of behavior. This observation procedure is used in cases in which there are discrete behaviors with a clear beginning and end, and the behaviors are roughly equivalent in duration. Examples of behaviors that are amenable to event recording include a tally of the number of correct oral responses a student provides, the number of times a student is tardy or absent, the number of times a student uses profanity, and the number of self-injurious behaviors of a student with autism (e.g., face slapping). Nonexamples of behaviors without a clear beginning and end include on-task behavior, out-of-seat behavior, and social engagement. Event recording is also limited by high-frequency behaviors (e.g., motor movement of a child with attention deficit disorder), because the observer becomes overwhelmed and may lose count when trying to tally behaviors. The following formula is used to establish the percentage of agreement between independent observers measuring events. The percentage of agreement equals the smaller total divided by the larger total multiplied by 100. As the discrepancy between the smaller total and larger total becomes greater, the level of interobserver agreement decreases, and vice versa.

$$\text{Percentage of agreement} = \frac{\text{Smaller total}}{\text{Larger total}} \times 100$$

The percentage of agreement with event recording should be interpreted cautiously, because it does not provide any assurance that the two observers are recording the same behavior. For example, one observer recorded that a child talked out 31 times during a 40-minute observation period, and a second observer recorded 30 times during the sample period. However, the first observer recorded 26 occurrences during the first 20 minutes of the observation period and five occurrences during the last 20 minutes, whereas the second observer recorded only 15 occurrences during the first 20 minutes of the observation period and 15 occurrences during the last 20 minutes. The calculation for this observation is the smaller total of 30 divided by the larger total of 31, resulting in .97, which is then multiplied by 100, for a percentage agreement of 97%. Thus, the percentage of agreement would have been inflated and not accurately reflect their actual level of agreement. A solution to this problem is to shorten the time interval within which interobserver agreement is computed. The 40-minute observation period used in the preceding example could be broken down into twenty 2-minute intervals. Percentage of agreement could then be calculated for each interval. Thus, it is important to examine the length of interval used to compute the percentage of agreement in the case of event recording.

Latency and Duration Recording

Latency and duration recording procedures, like event recording, are used in cases in which there is a discrete behavior with a clear beginning and end; however, in contrast with event recording, the behaviors exhibited are not roughly equivalent in time. For example, say tantrums occur often for a young child with autism but vary in the length of time of their occurrence (e.g., one lasts 10 minutes, the next lasts 15 minutes). Simply counting these behaviors loses large amounts of information. What is worse—one tantrum or two? The answer is that you really do not know, because one tantrum may have lasted 45 minutes, and two tantrums may have lasted a total of 10 minutes.

Latency recording involves recording the time from a specified event (e.g., an instructional cue, such as "What color is this?") to the start of the targeted behavior or completion of the response (e.g., "blue"). As noted before, event recording establishes the numerical dimension of behavior; duration recording provides the temporal dimension.

Duration recording simply involves measuring the length of time a response lasts. For example, latency recording may be used to measure the time between a request from a teacher to begin work on an assignment to the actual initiation of the assignment by the child; duration recording may be used to measure the amount of time a student appropriately interacts with others on the playground. Duration recording is also used in those cases in which the behavior is emitted at high rates. For example, some individuals with severe disabilities emit high rates of self-injurious behaviors, such as head hitting. Although event recording might be used, because head hitting has a distinguishable start and finish, counting each occurrence if it occurs at high rates may make it difficult to achieve adequate interobserver agreement. Thus, recording the total amount of time the individual is engaged in head hitting may not only be easier but also achieve a higher level of interobserver agreement. The percentage of agreement equals the shorter latency or duration divided by the longer latency or duration multiplied by 100.

$$\text{Percentage of agreement} = \frac{\text{Shorter latency/duration}}{\text{Longer latency/duration}} \times 100$$

An example of using this formula to calculate interobserver agreement follows. Let's say that one observer recorded 50 minutes of on-task behavior of a student, and the other recorded 40 minutes of on-task behavior. The interobserver agreement is 40 (short duration) divided by 50 (longer duration), which equals .80. This value would then be multiplied by 100 for a percentage of agreement of 80%.

Two problems experienced by observers must be examined closely when interpreting interobserver agreement using latency and duration recording. First, the procedures for ensuring that both of the observers begin the observation period at the same time must be established. Small variations between observers can distort the percentage of agreement. Second, as with event recording, high agreement does not necessarily ensure that observers reported the same latencies or durations for the same occurrences of behavior. These issues should be examined closely by the researcher when assessing the results of the study.

Interval Recording

Researchers often use interval recording procedures to provide an estimate of the number of occurrences or the duration of a behavior. They are useful for behaviors that do not have a clear beginning and end, that occur over time, and that occur at a relatively high rate (thus preventing use of frequency counting). Interval recording procedures involve dividing observational periods into units of time. There are three basic types of interval recording procedures: whole-interval recording, partial-interval recording, and momentary time sampling.

1. *Whole-interval recording.* The whole-interval procedure requires the observer to record the target behavior only if it occurs throughout the entire specified time interval. This procedure provides a conservative estimate (i.e., underestimates the occurrence) of an observed behavior, because it does not count a behavior unless it occurs for the entire interval.

2. *Partial-interval recording.* The partial-interval procedure requires the observer to record the target behavior if it occurs at any point during the specified time interval. This procedure provides a more liberal estimate (i.e., overestimates the occurrence) of the observed behavior than the whole-interval procedure.

3. *Momentary time sampling.* The momentary time sampling procedure requires the observer to record the target behavior if it occurs immediately after the end of the specified time interval. This procedure provides the most liberal estimate of the observed behavior.

The decision with regard to which of the interval recording procedures should be used is based on three factors: (1) the conditions in which the behavior is being recorded; (2) the type of behavior being recorded; and (3) the direction of the expected intervention effects. First, the whole-interval and partial-interval recording procedures require an independent observer, whereas the momentary time sampling procedures do not necessarily require one. Thus, momentary time sampling is used in cases in which the observer might disrupt the intervention, an independent observer is not available, or the teacher or observer does not have the time to watch the student for the entire interval. Second, the types of behaviors being measured play a role in the type of interval recording procedure used. The general rule is that a more conservative interval recording procedure (e.g., whole-interval) should be used when behaviors are emitted at a high frequency or for extended periods of time; a more liberal recording procedure (e.g., partial-interval) should be used when behaviors are emitted at a lower frequency or for shorter periods of time. Finally, the expected direction of the effects of intervention plays a role in the type of interval recording procedures used. The general rule is that a more conservative interval recording procedure (e.g., whole-interval) should be used in those cases in which the intervention effects are expected to increase the frequency or duration of behavior; a more liberal interval (i.e., partial-interval) should be used in those cases in which the intervention effects are expected to decrease the frequency or duration of behavior.

The following example illustrates why we should use a partial-interval recording system with behaviors we want to decrease, and a whole-interval system for behaviors we want to increase. Let's say we wish to take partial-interval data on in-seat behavior that we would like to increase. We define this behavior as "buttocks flat on chair seat; child facing forward in seat, feet flat on floor." We set up 10-second intervals for 5 minutes. If Jerry, a student who needs to improve his in-seat behavior, stays seated for 2 seconds for each 10-second interval, he receives a "plus" for the interval, because he was in-seat at least part of the time. He could do this for all 30 intervals (six 10-second intervals per minute for 5 minutes) and achieve a percentage of 100% for staying in his seat. This method obviously inflates (overestimates) Jerry's behavior. On the other hand, if we were using whole-interval recording, Jerry would receive 0% of intervals in-seat, because no intervals included a full 10 seconds of sitting in his seat.

This scenario can be changed to illustrate why whole-interval recording is used for increasing behaviors. Let's say we wish to decrease Marybeth's pencil-tapping behavior in the classroom during independent seatwork. We set up 15-second whole intervals for 10 minutes. If Marybeth taps her pencil for 13 of the 15 seconds for each interval, she receives a "negative" or "check" in each interval. She could do this for all of the intervals. In essence, she could be tapping her pencil quite extensively, yet receive 0% of intervals of pencil tapping using whole-interval recording. Partial-interval recording would record this behavior as 100% intervals of pencil tapping.

The following formula is used to establish the percentage of agreement between independent observers for each of the interval recording procedures. The percentage of agreement equals the number of agreement intervals divided by the total number of agreement and disagreement intervals multiplied by 100.

$$\text{Percentage of agreement} = \frac{\text{Agreement intervals}}{\text{Agreement intervals} + \text{Disagreement intervals}} \times 100$$

The basic method for establishing interobserver agreement with interval recording involves computing the level of agreement for all of the intervals (total agreement). To provide a more conservative estimate of interobserver agreement, both the scored interval (i.e., occurrence agreement) and unscored interval (i.e., nonoccurrence) methods for establishing interobserver agreement should be used (Cooper et al., 2007). Both the scored and unscored interval methods use the preceding formula: agreement intervals (scored or unscored) divided by the total agreement and disagreement intervals (scored or unscored) multiplied by 100. An example of scored, unscored, and total interval interobserver agreement follows.

Look at the example of scored intervals provided in Figure 3.8. One minute's worth of 10-second intervals are compared. Now, total interobserver agreement can be computed. Total interobserver agreement relates to how well both observers agree on what they see and do not see. Agreement is noted for Intervals 1, 3, 4, and 5. Therefore, the number of agreements

	Interval						
	1	2	3	4	5	6	
Observer 1	+	+	+	−	+	−	+ = Occurrence
Observer 2	+	−	+	−	+	+	− = Nonoccurrence

FIGURE 3.8. Example of interval recording by Observers 1 and 2.

(4) is divided by the number of agreements (4) plus disagreements (2), then multiplied by 100, for a total agreement percentage of 67%. We now can examine scored interval interobserver agreement. We have agreement on intervals that were scored (i.e., behaviors recorded as a plus) for Intervals 1, 3, and 5. We disagree on when we saw the behavior occur in Intervals 2 and 6. Therefore, the number of agreements on when the behavior was scored as occurring (3) is divided by the number of agreements (3) plus disagreements (2), then multiplied by 100, for an agreement percentage of 60% for scored intervals. Finally, we can examine unscored interval interobserver agreement. We have agreement on intervals that were unscored (i.e., agreement that the behavior did not occur, recorded as a check) for Interval 4. We disagreed on when we saw the behavior occur in Intervals 2 and 6. Therefore, the number of agreements on when the behavior was scored as not occurring (1) is divided by the number of agreements (1) plus disagreements (2), then multiplied by 100, for an agreement percentage of 33% for unscored intervals. Analyzing the data this way gives us important information. We now know that the observers agreed on what they saw and what they did not see. This information is helpful for data collection purposes and study replications.

WHAT ARE THE FACTORS THAT INFLUENCE INTEROBSERVER AGREEMENT?

A number of environmental conditions that have an impact on observers and influence the quality of data collection should be considered by both the researcher and research user. These environmental conditions include reactivity, observer drift, complexity of the measurement system, and observer expectations (Kazdin, 2003).

Reactivity

Reactivity refers to differences in interobserver agreement that result from observers being aware that their observations will be checked. Reactivity typically results in higher levels of interobserver agreement and accuracy of observations (Cooper et al., 2007). Reactivity can be overcome by providing random interobserver checks, audiotaping or videotaping the observations and randomly selecting those that will be scored, or conducting interobserver agreement checks 100% of the time.

Observer Drift

Observer drift occurs when observers change the way they employ the definition of behavior over the course of a study (Kazdin, 2003). In contrast to what one may think, observer drift does not necessarily result in lower levels of interobserver agreement. Observers can develop a similar drift if they work closely together and communicate about how they record the observed behavior. This drift will affect the accuracy of the data. Conversely, observer agreement decreases over the course of the study if observers do not work closely together and communicate about how they record the observed behavior. Observer drift can be prevented, or at least diminished, through booster training on the definitions of the behavior(s) and by having data collected by individuals experienced in conducting observation sessions.

Complexity of the Measurement System

The complexity of the measurement system is influenced by the number of individuals observed, the number of behaviors recorded, the duration of the observations, and the size of the time intervals in interval recording (Gall et al., 2007). Generally, the greater the complexity, the lower the levels of interobserver agreement (Cooper et al., 2007). Thus, researchers must balance the complexity of the measurement system with the need to obtain reasonable levels of interobserver agreement and accuracy. Achieving this balance might involve observing fewer individuals, recording fewer behaviors, or changing the duration of the interval.

Observer Expectations

Observer expectations can influence their observations. Observers who expect the intervention to have a specific effect are more likely to observe the effect if they are aware of the intended effect. Observer expectations appear to be most problematic when the researcher provides them feedback on how the study is progressing, on the intervention, on the condition of the study, and on how individuals are responding (Kazdin, 2003). The impact of observer expectations can be decreased by keeping the observer "blind" to the specifics of the investigation (e.g., intervention, condition, purpose of the investigation) and by using individuals with experience in conducting observations.

WHAT ARE THE FACTORS TO CONSIDER WHEN ASSESSING MEASUREMENT DEVICES IN THE CONTEXT OF A STUDY?

The selection of measurement devices by researchers is one of the most important decisions they make in the design and implementation of a study. Selection of measurement devices is especially difficult for researchers, because the time and resources available to assess the target features of the participants and study environment are almost always limited. Thus, critical research consumers should reflect on such issues as they assess the measurement devices

used by researchers. There are four key issues that critical research consumers should consider when assessing the quality of the measurement devices selected by researchers: (1) description of the measurement device, (2) adjustments to the measurement device, (3) appropriateness of the measurement device, and (4) cooperation of participants.

Description of the Measurement Device

The first issue to consider is the description of the measurement device provided by researchers. The information provided by researchers regarding measurement devices varies depending on whether they are using well-known, less well-known, or unknown measurement devices. When researchers use well-known standardized measurement devices, they usually assume that we are familiar with the devices and do little more than name them, because information on the reliability and validity of such devices is reported extensively elsewhere. Critical research consumers can rely on administration and technical information manuals, and reviews of standardized measurement devices such as the *Mental Measurements Yearbooks* (e.g., Spies & Plake, 2005) when researchers use well-known standardized measurement devices. When measurement devices are less well known, researchers typically describe or give examples of them and evidence of their reliability and validity, or direct the reader to studies establishing the reliability. Researchers commonly provide reliability and validity information in the case of unknown measurement devices. If direct observations are conducted, researchers describe how they were done and how the observers or interviewers were trained.

Adjustments to the Measurement Device

The second issue focuses on any adjustments of the measurement device made by researchers. One of the biggest dilemmas faced by researchers in designing and implementing their research is administering adequate measurement devices of the target features of the participants and study environment. The amount of time available to assess participants is almost always limited. In these situations, researchers might administer a short form of the measurement device. In such cases, it is important for critical research consumers to assess the effects of these options on the results. Reducing the length of measurement devices reduces the reliability and may also bias its content. This reduction requires that researchers provide detailed information on the process used to shorten measurement devices, as well as information regarding the reliability and validity of the devices. The reliability and validity data developed on the original test can be applied to the shortened version only with great caution.

Appropriateness of the Measurement Device

The third issue centers on the appropriateness of the measurement device in terms of administration. On one level, critical research consumers must evaluate whether the readability of the measurement device is appropriate. Assessing the appropriateness of the readability of measurement devices is especially important when participants are young or there are potential language issues, because the responses or scores to some degree depend more on vocabulary and reading ability than on target features of participants for which the test is valid. On a second level, critical research consumers must evaluate the appropriateness of the administration procedures. This evaluation includes not only determining whether the administration procedure is appropriate for the participants but also ensuring that the researcher appropriately

administers the measurement device. Generally, measurement devices can be administered either individually or to groups. The age or behaviors of participants affect whether measurement devices can be administered individually or to groups. Very young children usually cannot be assessed as a group, because their attention span is limited and they do not have the reading skills required by group tests. These findings may also be the case with other groups, such as individuals with disabilities. Delinquents and potentially recalcitrant groups may require individual assessment if there is reason to believe that their performance during group administration is unreliable.

Cooperation of Participants

The final issue focuses on whether participants' cooperation has been secured. Critical research consumers must assess procedures used by researchers to ensure the maximum performance of participants. On one level, researchers need to provide participants with a comfortable physical environment. Such an environment enhances participants' cooperation and performance. On another level, researchers need to be familiar with the administration procedures. The performance of participants is likely to be affected if the researcher does not convey the importance of the research by being conversant with the measurement device and its administration. On still another level, researchers should try to heighten the cooperation of participants by making the administration of the measurement device a reinforcing event.

SUMMARY

❖ The primary goal of measurement is to obtain a complete and accurate record of the targeted features of the participants and study environment. Qualitative researchers view reliability as the fit between what actually occurs in the setting under study and what is recorded as data, whereas quantitative researchers view reliability as the consistency across different observations. Single-case researchers report interobserver agreement, a special case of reliability in

which the degree of agreement between independent observers provides a measure of the trustworthiness of the data. Qualitative, quantitative, and single-case researchers consider their findings valid if the inferences they draw about the matter under study are accurate.

❖ Reliability has traditionally been considered a necessary but insufficient condition in measurement use. In order for a measurement device to be valid (*Note.* it is not the measurement device that is valid, but the inferences made by the researcher based on this measurement device), it must be reliable. Unreliable measurement devices cannot be valid. Yet the reliability of a measurement device does not guarantee that it is valid.

❖ There are three ways of securing evidence regarding the reliability of the measurement device used by quantitative researchers—(1) coefficient of stability, (2) coefficient of equivalence, and (3) coefficient of internal consistency. Reliability coefficients vary between values of 0.00 and 1.00, with 1.00 indicating perfect reliability and 0.00 indicating no reliability. The higher the reliability, the smaller the influence of measurement error due to the following: (1) variations in individuals, (2) variations in the conditions of administration from one administration to the next, (3) biases associated with the measurement device, (4) biases associated with participants, and (5) biases associated with the administrator of the measurement device. The *SEM* can be viewed as an estimate of the variability of an individual's score if the measurement device is administered over and over again.

❖ Validity and reliability refer to different aspects of a measurement device's "believability." There are three types of validity—*construct validity* (the extent to which it can be shown to measure a hypothetical construct), *content validity* (the representativeness of the sample of items included in measurement devices), and *criterion-related validity* (the extent to which an individual's score on a measurement device is used to predict his or her score on another measurement device).

❖ Many qualitative researchers are concerned with reliability and validity; however, it should be noted that others in the qualitative community do not view reliability and validity as necessarily important. Qualitative researchers view reliability as the fit between what actually occurs in the setting under study and what is recorded as data. Validity in qualitative research is relative to the researchers' purpose and the circumstances under which the data were collected.

❖ Interobserver agreement is a direct measure of behavior in which observers record the occurrence and nonoccurrence of specific behaviors and compare their findings. Interobserver agreement serves four primary functions: (1) it provides information on whether the definitional aspects of the response and intervention are replicable; (2) provides information with which to assess the extent to which the definitional aspects of the response and the intervention plan are employed competently; (3) provides information with which to assess the believability of the experimental effects; and (4) provides information with which to assess the believability of the absolute level of responding aside from any experimental effects shown.

❖ Five behavioral and procedural issues should be considered when assessing interobserver agreement: (1) A clear, specific definition should be developed to ensure that the observers are able to identify the characteristics and the beginning and end of the behavior; (2) the frequency with which observations that include interobserver agreement measures should be analyzed; (3) interobserver agreement should be reported for both the dependent variable and the independent variable; (4) agreement data should be reported for each behavior for each participant; and (5) the level of interobserver agreement should meet an acceptable level of at least 80%. The methods of establishing interobserver agreement include the following: (1) permanent products (the number of agreements divided by the total number of agreements and disagreements, multiplied by 100); (2) event recording (the smaller total divided by the larger total multiplied by 100); (3) latency and duration recording (the shorter latency or duration divided by the longer latency or duration multiplied by 100); and (4) interval recording (the number of agreement intervals divided by the total number of agreement and disagreement intervals multiplied by 100).

❖ Four environmental conditions that can have an impact on observers and influence the quality of data collection should be considered by both the researcher and research user—(1) reactivity, (2) observer drift, (3) complexity of the measurement system, and (4) observer expectations.

❖ There are four key issues that critical research consumers should consider when assessing the quality of the measurement devices selected by researchers: (1) description of the measurement device, (2) adjustments to the measurement device, (3) appropriateness of the measurement device, and (4) cooperation of participants.

DISCUSSION QUESTIONS

1. How do the types of validity differ? In your answer, provide an example of each type.

2. What is your recommendation in terms of the most important type of validity for measuring emotional intelligence that must be taken into consideration for the selection process? Why?

3. What type of validity do colleges and universities depend on when using the test scores to make admittance decisions? Explain.

4. What are the three basic reliability categories, and what type of error is each category attempting to control?

5. What type of reliability is most important for a questionnaire assessing students' attitudes toward smoking? Why?

6. How are reliability coefficients and the *SEM* related? Explain the importance of having high reliability estimates and a low *SEM*.

7. Is there a problem with an observational method if a researcher used a partial-interval recording method to measure the on-task behavior of the students? Why or why not? For what type of behavior would a partial-interval observational method be appropriate and why?

8. What is the purpose of reporting total, occurrence, and nonoccurrence agreement percentages? What are the other basic interobserver agreement categories, and what is the advantage of reporting interval agreement for interval measures versus the other categories?

9. Is it possible to have validity without reliability? Explain.

10. How do qualitative researchers' views of reliability and validity differ from those of quantitative researchers?

PRACTICE EXERCISES

Reliability

Decide which reliability approach (stability, equivalence, or internal consistency) is described for the following five exercises.

1. A researcher develops a test to assess the effects of a new science curriculum. She computes a split-half coefficient.

2. A researcher develops a new stress inventory for teachers. He administers the inventory to a group of teachers, then readministers it 3 weeks later and correlates the teachers' scores on the two administrations.

3. A test publisher creates two forms of an academic achievement test and readministers different forms to the same group of students after a 4-week period.

4. A researcher develops a questionnaire assessing students' attitudes toward smoking. She computes Cronbach's coefficient alpha.

5. A test publisher develops a new high school science achievement test and readministers it to a group of high school students after a 2-week period.

Validity

Decide which validity approach (construct, content, and criterion) is described in each of the following exercises.

1. A group of experts in social studies judges the adequacy of coverage of a test of students' social studies knowledge.

2. A researcher administers a mathematics aptitude test to a group of high school students, all of whom will be enrolling in a college algebra class the following year. At the end of the students' first term of college algebra, she computes a correlation coefficient between students' mathematics aptitude scores and their achievement scores in the college algebra class.

3. Scores on a newly developed test of self-esteem are correlated with scores on the widely used Coopersmith Self-Esteem Inventory.

4. A science aptitude test is administered to eighth-grade students 2 days before they take the district-wide test of science skills.

5. Scores on the GRE taken during college students' senior year are correlated with their grade point average (GPAs) in graduate school 2 years later.

PART III

·····

Quantitative Research Methods

CHAPTER 4

■ ■ ■ ■

Basic Statistical Concepts and Sampling Procedures

OBJECTIVES

After studying this chapter, you should be able to . . .

1. Explain how statistics should be thought of in the overall picture of quantitative research.
2. Illustrate the scales of measurement.
3. Clarify what is meant by a univariate frequency distribution.
4. Explain how to describe data sets.
5. Describe the role hypotheses play in research.
6. Outline parametric and nonparametric tests of statistical significance.
7. Clarify what is meant by statistical significance.
8. Explain what is meant by Type I and Type II errors and power.
9. Illustrate the types of statistical significance testing methods.
10. Outline the different sampling methods.
11. Describe the sampling decisions researchers make.
12. Clarify what is meant by sampling error.

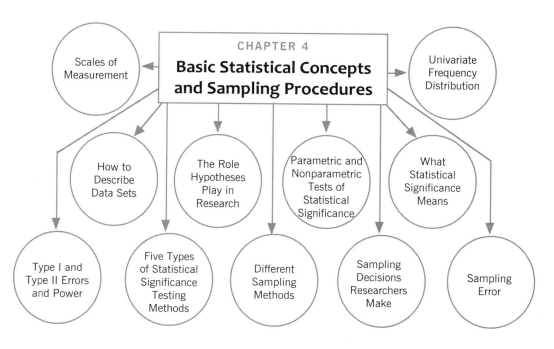

OVERVIEW

When we begin to study research methods, especially quantitative research methods, we may find the statistical aspect of research somewhat daunting. As stated in Chapter 2, statistics is only one of the tools that help us analyze the data we gather. The purpose of this chapter is to introduce basic but important statistical concepts that serve as a foundation for our discussion of experimental designs. After this chapter, specific statistical procedures for particular designs are described in terms of data analysis. Our goal is not to inundate you with statistical concepts and theory. Rather, we want to provide enough detail regarding each of the statistical procedures to ensure that you can adequately interpret the findings of quantitative research.

In this chapter, the following basic statistical concepts are introduced: scales of measurement, univariate frequency distribution, null hypotheses and alternative hypotheses, directional and nondirectional alternative hypotheses, statistical significance, parametric and nonparametric tests of statistical significance, and Type I and Type II errors. In addition, because there is a critical concern about how quantitative research is interpreted for purposes of internal and external validity, a comprehensive description of sampling is included. The method of sampling is a major determinant of the type of research design and the type of statistical analysis required. In this chapter, we describe probability and nonprobability sampling methods. Finally, we discuss sampling error and sampling decisions.

WHAT ARE THE SCALES OF MEASUREMENT?

The process of measurement in quantitative research involves representing in numbers the targeted features of the participants and study environment. Using numbers to describe these targeted features is especially useful, because it permits the targeted features represented by a sample of data to be compared to another sample of data of the same kind. Four distinct scales of measurement enable researchers to measure the targeted features of interest under a range of different conditions and levels of precision (Cicchetti et al., 2006; see Figure 4.1). The level of precision provided by the scales of measurement plays a key role in what tests of statistical significance can be employed (described below). These scales of measurement include the (1) nominal, (2) ordinal, (3) interval, and (4) ratio scales.

Nominal Scale

The nominal scale offers the lowest level of precision, because numbers simply act as identifiers, names, or labels. In other words, the numbers only make identification possible; they serve no other function. For example, by using a nominal scale to specify the gender of participants, each female participant could be represented by a "1" and each male by a "2." Although the nominal scale appears straightforward, it is sometimes misunderstood. The question to ask is whether the numbers represent a measure of any particular quality of the targeted feature of the participants or study environment. If the numbers do not represent a measure, then they represent names or labels. Thus, a nominal variable permits researchers to state only that a participant is the same as, or different from, another participant with respect to the targeted feature in question.

Ordinal Scale

An ordinal scale is one step up in precision from the nominal scale. An ordinal scale preserves the presence or absence of differences in the targeted feature of interest but not the magnitude.

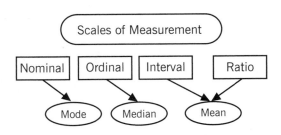

FIGURE 4.1. The four scales of measurement and the appropriate measures of central tendency with each scale.

Data represented on an ordinal scale indicate whether two values are equal or one is greater than the other. Thus, the values can be ordered in relation to each other. For example, if a teacher ranked a group of students in the order of their ability in mathematics, this ranking would be an example of data representing an ordinal scale. Although we could conclude that the student ranked first has greater ability in mathematics than the 10th-ranked student, it cannot be further inferred that he/she has, for example, twice the ability of another student.

Interval Scale

The interval scale is one step up in precision from the ordinal scale. The interval scale, like the ordinal scale, preserves not only the presence or absence of differences in the targeted feature of interest but also the magnitude. The interval scale provides equal intervals between equidistant points on the scale. For example, a 5-point difference between 5 and 10 on a 50-point scale is considered the same as the difference between scores of 45 and 50. Thus, we can infer not only which participant has "more" or "less" of some targeted feature but also "how much more" or "how much less" of it. However, interval scales do not have an absolute-zero point; thus, we cannot state that the difference between a score of 45 and 55 is twice the amount of the difference between a score of 45 and 50.

Ratio Scale

The ratio scale, the most robust of the four scales of measurement, possesses not only all of the attributes of the other three scales but also a true zero point, or the absence of the variable being measured. Possessing a zero point is important because, as the name of the scale indicates, it means that any measure of a variable on a ratio scale can be described in terms of its ratio to other measures. For example, a ruler comprises a ratio scale, because it has a true zero or the absence of length. The ratio scale enables us to say a piece of wood that is 20 inches in length is twice as long as one that is 10 inches in length.

It is important to note that in education and psychology, ratio scales are not used as frequently as other scales of measurement. A problem for social scientists arises, because although a measurement device may represent a ratio scale, it cannot be interpreted as such. An example clarifies this point. In the field of educational assessment, an academic achievement score of zero is clearly possible. However, obtaining a zero cannot be interpreted to mean the complete absence of achievement in the individual being tested. Thus, the scores must be treated as if they are derived from an interval scale.

WHAT IS A UNIVARIATE FREQUENCY DISTRIBUTION?

When we measure certain attributes of participants, we may wish to make certain assumptions about the population to help with interpretation of our data. Thus, one assumption we make is the shape of the population distribution (i.e., how individuals within a population compare to others within that population) on the measured attribute. One type of distribution is called the *univariate distribution* (Johnson, Kemp, & Kotz, 2005). The normal distribution is one of the most common univariate distributions. It is used extensively by researchers to interpret research findings. (*Note.* This is not the case for qualitative and single-case researchers.)

A distribution is the name given to any set of scores organized in a way that enables the shape of the data to be seen. A univariate frequency distribution entails counting the number of times each different score occurs in a data set. A univariate distribution is obtained by plotting the frequency of each different score along the horizontal (*x*) axis. Figure 4.2 presents a set of scores and the corresponding frequency distribution.

HOW CAN WE DESCRIBE DATA SETS?

The frequency distribution represents how a data set can be represented graphically. Consider how data sets can be described (called *descriptive statistics*). Researchers use descriptive statistics, a very simple and parsimonious system to describe any data set mathematically, including the central tendency, the variation,

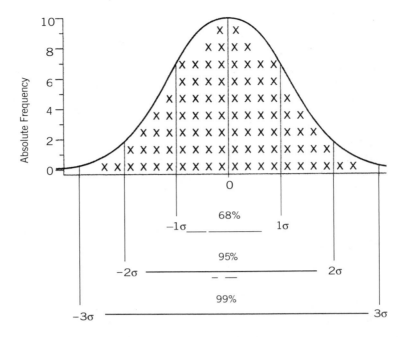

FIGURE 4.2. Frequency distribution of 100 scores depicting 68, 95, and 99% confidence intervals. (σ is the population standard deviation.)

and the shape of the distribution. Researchers typically use three measures of central tendency to describe a central reference value that is usually close to the point of greatest concentration in a set of scores. In many aspects of research, the measure of central tendency is thought to represent best the whole data set.

Measures of Central Tendency

We describe three measures of central tendency: arithmetic mean, median, and mode.

Arithmetic Mean

The most common measure of central tendency is the **arithmetic mean**. The arithmetic mean, or average, is obtained by summing the scores for a data set and dividing by the number of participants or entities in that data set. Consider the following scores on an exam:

80   75   90   95   65   86   97   50

We sum the scores (638) and divide by the number of scores (8) in the data set. The arithmetic mean is 79.8. Although it is beyond the scope of this book to detail the properties of the arithmetic mean and the importance of these properties to many statistical procedures in research, it is important to note that the arithmetic mean provides a better estimate of a population parameter than any other measure of central tendency, because it takes into account *all* scores in the data set.

Median and Mode

Two other commonly used measures of central tendency are the **median** and the mode. The median is the point above and below which half of the scores fall. Consider the following scores arranged in rank order:

2   5   8   8   12   14   15   17   19

In this example, the median is 12. Four scores fall above it, and four scores fall below it. If another observation is added, then the number of scores is an even number. The common convention for dealing with an even number of scores is to take the arithmetic mean of the two middle values. For example, if we were to add the value 20 to the preceding set of scores, the median would be 13 (12 + 14 divided by 2). The median is a measure that is not influenced by extreme scores such as the arithmetic mean. Finally, the most frequently occurring score in a data set is the **mode**. In the previous data set, the mode is 8 (it occurs twice).

When to Use the Different Measures of Central Tendency

The decision of when to use each measure of central tendency depends to a large extent on the scale of measurement used (see Figure 4.1). The arithmetic mean is an appropriate measure of central tendency for interval and ratio scale variables (Graziano & Raulin, 2010). The median is an appropriate measure for central tendency with ordinal variables, whereas the mode is used with nominal variables (Gall et al., 2007). Comparisons can be made using the mean, median, and mode with interval and ratio scale variables. If the frequency distribution is symmetrical, the mean, median, and mode will be relatively the same. If the frequency distribution is skewed, these three measures of central tendency will differ substantially. The shape of the distributions is discussed more fully in what follows.

Measures of Variation

In addition to describing the central distribution of a data set, researchers should describe variation within it. Variation of the characteristic under study is always important to consider. Researchers commonly use three statistics to describe the variation in a data set: the range, the standard deviation, and the variance.

Range

The **range**, the simplest measure of variation, is calculated by subtracting the smallest score from the largest score. Consider the following scores:

12   9   15   24   20   8   11   21   22   14

The range for this set of scores is 24 − 8, or 16. (*Note.* Some statisticians consider the range to be defined as the difference between the largest and smallest numbers plus one; e.g., 24 − 8 + 1 = 17.) The use of the range as an indicator of the variation in a data set is appropriate only in those cases in which the sample is small. When sample sizes increase, the range becomes increasingly unstable as a measure of variation, since it only takes into consideration two scores from the total number of scores.

Standard Deviation and Sample Variance

The **standard deviation** and sample variance are the most commonly used statistics for describing variation in the responses or scores in a data set. The standard deviation can be best understood by considering the meaning of the word *deviation*. In research, a deviation is the distance of a score from the mean for the data set. If the mean of a data set is 10, then the deviation for a score of 12 is 2 (i.e., 12 − 10). The deviation of a score of 6 is −4 (i.e., 6 − 10). Twelve is above the mean, and 6 is below the mean. The standard deviation, symbolized as *SD*, is a statistic that describes how much the scores are spread out around the mean. The larger the standard deviation, the more "spread out" the scores.

The sample variance is simply the square of the standard deviation; that is, the standard deviation is multiplied by itself. For example, if the standard deviation for a set of scores is 3, the variance would be 9. The standard deviation and the sample variance not only indicate the degree of spread in a data set but also provide the basis for many of the statistical procedures used by researchers.

---

*The **arithmetic mean** is obtained by dividing the sum of all scores by the number of scores.*

*The **median** is the point at which 50% of the scores fall above and 50% fall below.*

*The **mode** is the most frequently occurring score.*

*The **range** is the difference between the largest and smallest scores.*

*The **standard deviation** is a statistic that describes how much the scores are spread out around the mean.*

Shape of the Distribution

In addition to describing the central tendency and variation in a data set, researchers often examine the shape of the distribution. Although not commonly described in research studies, it is important to consider the shape of a distribution, because it may affect interpretations of the data and distort the outcomes of some statistical procedures. Distributions of scores can take on three primary shapes: unimodal, bimodal, and skewed.

A *unimodal distribution* is one in which there are several average scores, with fewer high and low scores on each side of the mode. The normal distribution is a unimodal distribution (described in what follows). A *bimodal distribution* is one in which the scores accumulate at two different parts of the scale. Skewed distributions are those in which scores are mainly high or low. A distribution is *positively skewed* when the scores are mainly low (i.e., most scores are low, with a few high scores that stretch out the curve to the right), whereas a distribution is *negatively skewed* when the scores are mainly high (i.e., most scores are high, with a few low scores that stretch out the curve to the left). Although the shape of a set of responses or scores can be examined graphically, a number of available statistics describe the shape of a distribution. It is important to note that researchers rarely report these statistics. Rather, researchers typically examine the shape of the distribution and transform it to approximate the normal distribution prior to conducting more advanced statistical analysis procedures.

The idea of a distribution of frequencies provides the basis for the normal distribution, as well as all other distributions (see Chapter 7). The normal distribution is a purely theoretical distribution obtained by plotting theoretically obtained probabilities across the whole range of possible values, from minus infinity to plus infinity along the horizontal axis. The normal distribution is important in research for several reasons. First, many variables in nature can be shown to approximate the shape of the normal distribution. For example, psychological variables such as intelligence and achievement scores tend to approximate the normal distribution when plotted from an adequately large sample.

Second, the sampling distribution of the mean (i.e., the theoretical frequency distribution of means of an infinitely large number of samples drawn from any given population) approximates a normal distribution as long as researchers have a reasonably large number of sample means. This phenomenon even occurs when the population from which the scores have been drawn is not normally distributed.

Finally, the unique properties of the normal distribution mean that it provides a way of assigning probabilities to scores, so that the association between the sample data and the population can be clearly expressed. This association between sample data and population is especially important, because researchers in education and psychology rarely have access to the entire population, and because researchers can never be certain of what is actually occurring in the population.

The normal distribution, like all distributions, is really a family of distributions that always possesses five key characteristics. First, the normal distribution is perfectly symmetrical about its mean. This distribution allows for the exact division of the area under the curve. Second, the total area under the normal distribution includes all possible values of a given variable. This distribution enables researchers to make precise predictions regarding the probability of a given true score falling within a specified range of scores. Third, the mean, median, and mode of the distribution are the same. That is, the arithmetic average is equal to the central value in the normal distribution, which is equal to the most frequently occurring score. Fourth, the tails of the distribution extend out infinitely in both directions. This phenomenon means that although the tails of the normal distribution continue forever to grow closer and closer to the horizontal, or *x*, axis, they never actually touch the axis (i.e., reach a zero frequency). Finally, there is a consistent relationship between the shape of the normal distribution and the *standard deviation from the mean* (i.e., the statistic that shows how much scores are spread out around the mean). This consistent relationship enables researchers to identify the area in which a given score falls under the normal curve.

Given that there is a consistent relationship between the shape of the normal distribution and the standard deviation from the mean, we examine the types of statements that can be made. Figure 4.2 presents 100 scores distributed normally. By counting the X's, you can confirm the following statements:

1. Approximately 68% of the scores will fall within one standard deviation above and below the mean.

2. Approximately 95% of the scores will fall within two standard deviations above and below the mean (approximately 2.5% of the scores in each tail). (*Note.* We are rounding up from 1.96 standard deviations.)

3. Approximately 99% (again, we are rounding) of the scores will fall three standard deviations above and below the mean (approximately 0.5% in each tail).

4. A percentile score indicates what percentage of the group had scores as low or lower than the given score.

WHAT ROLE DO HYPOTHESES PLAY IN RESEARCH?

Taking into consideration how scores of the population on an attribute are distributed, quantitative researchers make predictions about the outcome of any study before data are collected. These predictions, termed *hypotheses*, represent statements about what findings are expected and used in inferential statistics (Creswell, 2009).

Inferential Statistics

Unlike descriptive statistics that allow researchers to describe their data sets, inferential statistics allow for statistical inference; that is, researchers are able to generalize their results to the larger population or make an "inference" about the population based on the responses of the experimental sample. This ability to generalize to the population is critical, since researchers rarely have the opportunity to study an entire population. Thus, we attempt to learn about the population by studying a representative sample of that population.

The Role of Hypotheses

We now look at the role hypotheses play in assessing whether two groups differ from one another. As we have discussed, most educational and psychological research begins with the development of hypotheses that predict, on the basis of theory and what has already been found, the results of the investigation. Suppose that two sets of collected data represent behavior under two different conditions. The hypotheses constructed before the collection of data assert that a difference is expected between the two conditions. **Statistical significance** refers to a difference between sets of scores that may be so great that there is a likelihood, at some level of probability, that it is the result of one variable influencing another rather than a function of chance due to sampling or measurement error. Recall that the problem addressed by statistical significance testing is whether the difference between the two sets of data can be attributed to the effects of a given variable (systematic variance) rather than chance factors (i.e., sampling and measurement errors). Even in tightly controlled experiments, visual inspection does not allow for a sound decision, because any differences that can be seen in the data may merely reflect chance or random influences rather than the effect of one variable on another. It is clear from our discussion of statistical significance that what is needed is an objective process of determining whether the prediction is, at least at some level, supported by the data. At this point, hypotheses that come into play have a critical role in inferential statistics.

Null and Alternative Hypotheses

The two types of hypotheses developed by researchers are called the *null* (pertaining to

> **Statistical significance** *refers to the probability that the results of a study are likely or unlikely due to chance factors.*

nullifiable) *hypothesis* and the *alternative* or *experimental hypothesis* (Gall et al., 2007). **Null hypotheses** state that there is no difference between two groups of data. **Alternative hypotheses** are statements of statistically significant relationships between variables being studied or differences between values of a population parameter. In this case, an alternative hypothesis would state that there is a statistically significant difference between two groups of data. Null hypotheses and alternative hypotheses are always used in conjunction with one another in tests of statistical significance. For example, the null hypothesis and associated alternative hypothesis illustrated in what follows show how they are used in conjunction with one another. Additionally, hypotheses should be concise statements of the relationship or difference that is expected. Not only are brief and concise hypotheses easier for the researcher to test, but they are also easier for us to understand. The following are examples of null and associated alternative hypotheses:

Null: There will be statistically nonsignificant differences in the achievement scores of students with learning disabilities in skills-grouped classrooms and those in heterogeneous-grouped classrooms.

Alternative: There will be statistically significant differences in the achievement scores of students with learning disabilities in skills-grouped classrooms and those in heterogeneous-grouped classrooms.

The function of null hypotheses and alternative hypotheses is to express statements about differences between parameters of the population from which the samples are taken (Graziano & Raulin, 2010). Why are researchers interested in hypotheses about possible differences between population parameters rather than possible differences between samples? The reason centers on the notion that researchers are generally interested in sample data only to the extent that the data can tell them something about the population from which the sample

was drawn. In other words, differences between the means of two samples are largely trivial, unless they suggest that the same differences would be found in the population.

The use of null and alternative hypotheses and associated statistical significance tests are like "playing devil's advocate." The null hypothesis provides a basis for the argument that there is no systematic difference between the scores of the experimental and control groups. Except for sampling errors and measurement errors, the performance of the two groups is indistinguishable. If, according to a formal statistical test (e.g., the *t* test) the data are consistent with this argument, then an all-chance explanation is justifiable. This explanation is typically described as "accepting the null hypothesis." On the other hand, if the data are inconsistent with the all-chance explanation, the null hypothesis is rejected and the systematic plus-chance explanation is justifiable. Finally, it is important to note that the standard terms of *accept* or *reject* the null hypothesis are too strong. Statistical significance testing should be viewed as an aid to judgment, not as a declaration of "truth." It should be clear that the null hypothesis is virtually never literally true (Cohen et al., 2007), and that critical research consumers should consider the results of tests of statistical significance within the context of the entire study.

Directional and Nondirectional Alternative Hypotheses

One final piece of information is important to understand with regard to the alternative hypothesis. An alternative hypothesis is either directional or nondirectional. A *directional alternative hypothesis* is one in which the population parameter (e.g., mean) is stated to be greater or smaller than the other population parameter. In contrast to the example of the alternative hypothesis provided before, a directional alternative hypothesis goes beyond just stating that there will be a difference. This type of alternative hypothesis is also referred to as a *one-tailed hypothesis*, because it specifies at which end of the sampling distribution the computed value from the test of statistical significance will fall—providing evidence to reject the null hypothesis. In the case of an alpha level of $p <$

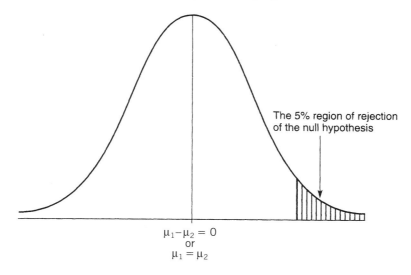

$$\mu_1 - \mu_2 = 0$$
or
$$\mu_1 = \mu_2$$

FIGURE 4.3. Region of rejection for a directional (one-tailed) hypothesis, with $\alpha = .05$, μ_1 = Population 1, μ_2 = Population 2.

.05 (i.e., the probability of obtaining a difference between groups this large or larger is less than 5%), the 5% region of rejection on the distribution is depicted in Figure 4.3. The shaded region depicts the area (5% of either end of the distribution) within which lie those p values obtained from tests of statistical significance that are so low as to require the rejection of the null hypothesis.

A *nondirectional alternative hypothesis* is one in which a difference between two population parameters is stated but no direction is specified. The alternative hypothesis provided earlier is an example of a nondirectional alternative hypothesis. This type of alternative hypothesis is also called a *two-tailed hypothesis*, because it does not specify at which end of the sampling distribution of the test of statistical significance the computed value will fall—providing evidence to reject the null hypothesis. In the case of an alpha level of $p < .05$, the 5% region of rejection on the distribution is depicted in Figure 4.4. The shaded regions depict the area (2.5% of both ends of the sampling distribution) within which lie those p values of the test of statistical significance that are so low as to require the rejection of the null hypothesis.

The choice of a one- rather than two-tailed hypothesis testing strategy can influence

research outcomes. Indeed, this choice is a source of controversy among social scientists (Gall et al., 2007). For example, two different groups of researchers drew different conclusions about the effects of single-sex and coeducational secondary schools using the same data from a national survey. Lee and Bryk (1989) employed one-tailed hypothesis tests to explore whether students attending single-sex schools outperformed students attending coeducational schools. They concluded that single-sex schools produced better outcomes than did coeducational schools. Marsh (1989a) found that some of the differences favoring single-sex schools in the Lee and Bryk (1989) study would have failed to reach statistical significance had two-tailed tests been used. Although Lee and Bryk defended their use of the one-tailed hypothesis tests, Marsh (1989b) stated that a review of previous literature provided no clear basis for the use of a directional hypothesis.

Which type of alternative hypothesis is appropriate? There are two factors one should

> **Null hypotheses** *state that there is no difference between two groups of data, while* **alternative hypotheses** *state that there are differences between two groups of data.*

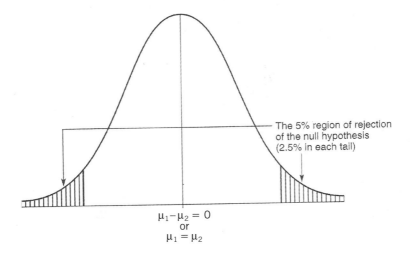

FIGURE 4.4. Region of rejection for a nondirectional (two-tailed) hypothesis, with $\alpha = .05$, μ_1 = Population 1, μ_2 = Population 2.

consider when using a one-tailed alternative hypothesis. First, and most importantly, there should be <u>clear evidence for the prediction</u> <u>made by the researchers</u>. Unfortunately, there is good reason to question whether most educational and psychological theories are powerful enough, empirical generalizations are robust enough, and a priori predictions are accurate enough to warrant the use of such tests (Cohen et al., 2007). Inconsistent and conflicting research outcomes are common in education and psychology (Maxwell, 2004; Wakeley, Rivera, & Langer, 2000). Second, related to the first issue, <u>researchers must make the decision</u> <u>to use a one-tailed alternative hypothesis at the</u> <u>outset of the study</u>. If researchers decide on the type of alternative hypothesis after they have analyzed the data, then there is the possibility that their decision could have been influenced by the data. This decision may introduce bias into the process.

WHAT ARE PARAMETRIC AND NONPARAMETRIC TESTS OF STATISTICAL SIGNIFICANCE?

Researchers must decide which type of test of statistical significance to use in analyzing their data. The type of test we select is from one of two test categories. The decision of which category of test to use is based on several issues (described below).

Parametric Tests

Thus far, we have discussed the assumption that scores in a population are normally distributed. When researchers make this assumption and conduct a test of statistical significance, they are conducting what is called a parametric test. A *parameter* is used to describe some aspect of a set of scores for an entire population. Thus, parametric tests of statistical significance are based on certain assumptions about population parameters (Gall et al., 2007). One assumption is that the scores in the population are normally distributed about the mean. Many complex human behaviors or performance measures (e.g., intelligence scores) are believed to be normally distributed. Another assumption is that the population variances of the comparison groups in a study are equal. This assumption, called *homogeneity of variance*, means that the distribution of scores that "spread out" from the mean in the comparison groups is identical. Yet another assumption involves having at least interval or ratio scale data.

Nonparametric Tests

When there are large deviations from the assumptions of parametric tests of statistical significance in the research data and the data are generated from nominal or ordinal scales, the use of parametric tests of statistical significance may be problematic. That is, the assumptions underlying parametric tests may not be met. Therefore, nonparametric tests of statistical significance are used to test the null hypothesis in such cases. As we might guess, nonparametric tests of statistical significance do not rely on any assumptions about the shape or variance of the population scores. Such tests also do not rely on data derived from a measure that has equal intervals (interval and ratio scales). We discuss the advantage of parametric tests over nonparametric tests later in the chapter.

WHAT IS STATISTICAL SIGNIFICANCE?

Educational research and psychological research are best described as probabilistic rather than truly deterministic endeavors. What this means is that the findings from educational and psychological research do not yet and may never achieve the ability to determine, or to predict, exactly what will happen in any particular situation. Human behavior is far too variable to make perfect predictions of future behavior. We only have to reflect on our own lives to understand the range of events that affect our behavior. Thus, researchers must determine whether a difference (e.g., between the means of two samples) may be so great that there is a likelihood, at some level of probability, that it is the result of one variable influencing another rather than a function of chance due to sampling or measurement error. This is why the significance test of a null hypothesis has become a staple procedure in educational and psychological research. As stated previously, *statistical significance* refers to a difference between sets of scores that may be so great there is a likelihood, at some level of probability, that it is the result of the influence of a systematic variable (independent, extraneous, or some combination of the two) on the dependent variable rather than a function of chance

due to sampling or measurement error. The use of statistical significance dates back about 300 years to studies of birth rates by John Arbuthnot in 1710, and it was popularized in the social sciences by Sir Ronald Fisher and by Jerzy Neyman and Egon Pearson (Huberty, 1987, 1993). Despite some ongoing controversy over its use, statistical significant testing has a relatively long history.

Before looking more closely at what statistical significance means, we should explore the issue of systematic versus chance explanations for findings. Exploring these types of explanations is necessary to understand the nature of statistical significance. As stated in Chapter 2, a *systematic factor* (independent variable or an extraneous variable) is an influence that contributes in an orderly fashion to another factor (dependent variable), for example, the reduction in heart disease (dependent variable) by individuals who watch their diet and stay active (independent variables). A *chance factor* is an influence that contributes haphazardly to another factor, with the amount of influence being unspecifiable. In some cases, researchers may overestimate the influence of systematic factors relative to chance factors. The upshot of this tendency is to jump naturally to systematic conclusions rather than use chance as an explanation. This tendency is why researchers test for statistical significance.

Researchers need a way to protect themselves from favoring systematic conclusions over data that may have occurred due to chance factors. So researchers should understand that although statistical calculations have an aura of being exact, they are always conducted against a background of uncertainty. A major step in making reasonable conclusions for data is to make a judgment about the relative influences of systematic and chance factors.

Statistical significance enables researchers to make such a judgment, because a statistically significant difference is one that is so great as to be unlikely to have occurred by chance factors alone (i.e., occurring because of sampling or measurement error). Consider a simple research study in which the participants are assigned randomly to either an experimental or a control group. Members of the two groups perform the identical experimental task except for the additional manipulation of a single factor of interest in the experimental group, the receipt of training. The researcher wishes to test whether the experimental factor makes a systematic difference in a participant's performance on a specific task.

In this case, performance measures on the task vary from individual to individual. The question is, "Why does performance vary from individual to individual?" The systematic explanatory factor is that the experimental factor, on average, improved the task performance in the experimental group by some unknown amount, over and above the performance of the control group. Calculating the mean difference provides an estimate of the magnitude of this systematic effect. However, there are also chance factors in this situation that influence the performance measures of individuals.

Sampling and measurement errors are two of the primary chance factors about which researchers must be concerned. Sampling errors (e.g., a group's mean may be different each time it is sampled) might arise from the "luck of the draw" in randomly assigning participants to the experimental and control groups. For example, the control group may contain a predominance of participants with somewhat lower (or higher) abilities than members of the experimental group. Thus, the mean difference could be a function of a sampling error rather than a function of an experimental factor. *Measurement errors* refer to unknown and unrepeatable causes of variability in task performance over time and context. (Recall our discussion of reliability in Chapter 3.)

Three possible factors account for performance differences between experimental and control groups. The variability of performance from individual to individual can be completely explained by (1) the experimental factor, (2) chance factors (sampling and measurement errors), or (3) variability that is a function of both the experimental factor and chance factors (i.e., sampling and measurement errors).

Accepting the first account would require that variability in the scores of the experimental group be different from all the scores in the control group. Although such a finding might occur in the physical sciences, where chance variability can be small, this outcome is quite rare in

education and psychology, and does not require statistical inference (Skinner, 1963). Thus, researchers are left with a choice between the all-chance explanation and the systematic-plus-chance explanation. At this point, statistical significance testing comes into play. Statistical significance helps researchers decide whether the observed difference is great enough to reject the null hypothesis (differences due to chance factors alone); it also helps researchers accept the alternative hypothesis (differences due to systematic and chance factors). The systematic and chance factors explanation must be used if chance factors do not adequately account for the findings.

Of course, referring to the statistical significance of any difference in itself is not very revealing unless a specific level of probability is set. This probability enables researchers to interpret how a difference due to sampling or measurement errors is unlikely. The significance level can range from 0.0 to 1.0 and is specified by researchers. This significance level provides to researchers a basis for accepting or rejecting their hypotheses. However, because the aim is always to have the smallest possible risk of rejecting the null hypothesis incorrectly, the probability values always lie close to zero.

The values of $p < .05$, $p < .01$, or $p < .001$ are the most commonly used probability values in educational and psychological research. The significance level sets the maximum acceptable probability of rejecting the null hypothesis, because the difference is great enough to conclude that it did not occur by chance when, in fact, chance caused the results. Thus, the null hypothesis should not have been rejected. We clarify the concept of statistical significance through the following example. Suppose we established a significance level of $p < .05$ to reject the null hypothesis. This level indicates that the maximum desired probability of making the wrong decision about rejecting the null hypothesis when it is true should be less than 5 in 100 (i.e., the probability of getting results or differences between groups by chance is less than 5%). The significance level sets the boundary between what is and what is not an acceptable risk.

However, there is more to the significance level than we have discussed thus far. The significance level in any study is the probability of the obtained results given the sample size and assuming that the sample is derived from a population in which the null hypothesis is true (Graziano & Raulin, 2010). Thus, the significance level must be interpreted in the context of not only population parameters (i.e., what actually exists in the entire population from which the sample was drawn) and size of the research sample but also possible problems with the logic of the significance level. See Daniel (1998) and Johnson (1999) for a discussion of this issue.

Errors Made in Interpretations of the Significance Level

Critical research consumers should understand two common errors in the interpretations of statistical significance. Avoiding these two errors allows us to understand the limited but important role statistical significance plays in interpreting the results of a study.

The first error commonly made by researchers is to view statistical significance as being the same as replicability. It is not unusual for researchers to conclude that smaller significance levels mean that increasingly greater confidence can be vested in a conclusion, and that sample results are replicable (Carver, 1978; Daniel, 1998). The significance level does not tell us anything about the extent to which the findings are replicable. Carver (1978) found numerous examples, even in research textbooks, where researchers mistakenly claimed that the significance level indicated the extent to which the findings of the study could be replicated.

The second error centers on the importance of the findings in a study. Too many researchers believe that statistically significant results are inherently important. In short, significance tells us nothing about the importance or magnitude of the findings (McLean & Ernest, 1998). Some scholars suggest that significance levels are only informative with regard to the magnitude of the results when the findings are counterintuitive (e.g., statistically significant results are obtained with a small sample size). Many scholars (e.g., Rosenthal, 1994a) argue that a more meaningful interpretation of results comes from examining *effect size*, a statistical procedure for determining the magnitude of the difference between two or more groups (see Chapter 15). That is, effect size takes into account the extent, or degree, of difference between two or more groups.

These are critical errors in interpretation of statistical significance. When interpreted correctly, statistical significance informs research consumers whether the observed difference is great enough to reject the null hypothesis (differences occurred due to chance factors alone). Carver (1993) described four ways to minimize the misinterpretation of statistical significance testing:

1. Insist that the word *statistically* be placed in front of significance test results.
2. Maintain that the results always be interpreted with respect to the data first, and statistical significance, second.
3. Require reporting of effect size.
4. Encourage journal editors to publicize their perspectives on statistical significance. (p. 287)

WHAT ARE TYPE I AND TYPE II ERRORS AND POWER?

It is important that critical research consumers understand three concepts related to statistical significance—Type I error, Type II error, and power. If critical research consumers can understand these three related concepts, then they will be well on their way toward understanding the logic behind statistical significance testing. The logic of statistical significance tests requires that researchers establish the level of statistical significance (usually $p < .05$ or $p < .01$) prior to the computation of the test. In other words, researchers should establish the level of statistical significance at which the null hypothesis will not be accepted at the outset of the study. This level of significance is called "alpha" (symbolized as α). The level of significance actually obtained is called the "probability value," and is indicated by the symbol p. A higher level of statistical significance corresponds to a lower p value. For example, $p < .01$ is a lower p value than $p < .05$, but a difference that is statistically significant at the .01 level suggests that chance was less a likely cause of the obtained difference between the groups than a difference that was significant only at the .05 level.

Type I Errors

Given that an alpha (α) level is chosen at the outset of the study and we can never be certain whether to "accept" (i.e., fail to reject) or "reject" the null hypothesis, researchers sometimes unwittingly misinterpret the results of tests of statistical significance. There are two possible misinterpretations. Researchers may reject or fail to accept the null hypothesis when it is true; that is, they incorrectly conclude that any difference between sample groups was due to a systemic variable when the difference was due to chance alone. This type of misinterpretation is called a **Type I error** (a false positive), or α. This type of misinterpretation occurs in tests of statistical significance when the test statistic yields a value that falls in the rejection region by chance alone. Because of the decision-making process associated with tests of statistical significance, the researcher rejects the null hypothesis and consequently accepts the alternative hypothesis. The probability of making a Type I error is set by the significance level (α). For example, a significance level of $p < .05$ means that the probability of making a Type I error is less than 5 in 100. Likewise, a significance level of $p < .01$ means

that the probability of making a Type I error is less than 1 in 100, and so on. The equivalent of a Type I error (α) in criminal law is imprisoning an innocent person. The consequence in educational research is serious as well; for example, it is analogous to concluding that a reading program effectively increases reading scores when in fact it is not effective.

Consider the information presented in Figure 4.5. We assume that our null hypothesis is true. In other words, the differences between the groups are only due to chance factors. We know that if we randomly select from the population and randomly assign participants to one of two groups, then we get differences in the groups' mean scores by chance. For example, Group 1 may have a mean score of 110 and Group 2, a mean score of 105. If we repeat the same process of randomly selecting and assigning participants an infinite number of times, then we would get a sampling distribution of mean differences. The most frequently occurring mean difference is zero (i.e., Group 1 − Group 2 = 0). We would by chance have mean differences that fall nearer and farther from this zero score by chance. Some of these differences would fall outside of the set alpha level. Thus, we would

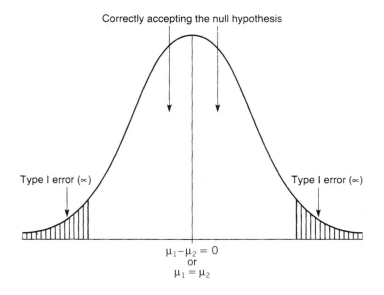

FIGURE 4.5. Normal curve, with $\alpha = .05$, $\mu_1 = \mu_2$ or $\mu_1 - \mu_2 = 0$. The vertical shaded areas represent $\alpha = .05$; a correct decision is represented when the differences between samples are between the α areas for a two-tailed test (when the null hypothesis is true, which is our assumption).

assume that 5% of the scores fall beyond the .05 level. This scenario illustrates the Type I error rate, or α.

Type II Errors

Researchers sometimes accept or fail to reject the null hypothesis when, in fact, there is a difference due to a systematic variable; that is, they are incorrectly concluding the differences between groups were due to chance factors when they were not. This type of misinterpretation is called a **Type II error** (a false negative; symbolized as β). Type II errors occur in tests of statistical significance when the test statistic yields a value that falls outside the rejection region by chance alone. Because of the decision-making process associated with tests of statistical significance, this finding leads researchers to accept the null hypothesis when the experimental factor has a systematic influence on the dependent variable. The probability of making a Type II error (β) is influenced by a number of factors, such as the significance level (i.e., as the p value decreases, the possibility of a Type II error increases), the type of statistical test, and the sample size. To pursue the legal analogy, the equivalent of a Type II error (β) in criminal law is acquitting a guilty individual. In educational research, the equivalent of a Type II error is to conclude that a reading program is ineffective in increasing reading scores when it in fact is effective.

Consider the information contained in Figure 4.6. Suppose we had information that the samples really come from two different populations (e.g., we took a sample of participants from Population 1 and another from Population 2). Realize that we will never fully know this in a research study. In fact, we make the assumption that the samples come from the same population; this assumption is our null hypothesis. However, pretend for the moment that we have this information available. We would take a sample from each population with different means. In this example, Population 1 has a mean of 90 (symbolized μ_1), and Population 2 has a mean of 130 (symbolized μ_2). By chance, we are going to have samples with means that differ from the population means. These sample means fall on either side of the population mean. Most sample means are the same as the population means, but some fall nearer and some farther from the population means.

If we look at Population 1 minus Population 2 ($\mu_1 - \mu_2$), we get a score of 40. However, if we take a sample from each population and subtract one sample mean from the other, we get some mean differences that are more than 40 and others that are less than 40. If a mean difference is sufficiently less than 40, then the mean difference could fall beyond the alpha setting. If we take an infinite number of samples from each population and subtract one from the other, then we get some mean differences that fall close to the null hypothesis (i.e., $\mu_1 - \mu_2 = 0$ or [$\mu_1 = \mu_2$]). If a sample mean difference falls within the alpha level, we are not going to reject the null hypothesis. We are going to conclude that the samples probably came from the same population, and the difference is likely due to chance, not a systematic variable. This scenario illustrates a Type II error, or β.

Relative Seriousness of Type I or Type II Errors

It is important to consider which of these types of errors is most serious. Making a Type I error is more serious, because it leads researchers to believe that the independent variable systematically influenced the dependent variable. This finding is especially problematic, because positive results are much more likely to be reported in the research literature, leading to erroneous conclusions and misdirecting future research. On the other hand, making a Type II error is less serious, because it still leaves open the possibility that a replication of the study will lead to statistically significant findings. Thus, if researchers are going to make an error, they will make a conservative one. Both types of errors point to the importance of replication studies

> **Type I errors** *occur when researchers incorrectly conclude that any difference between sample groups is due to a systematic variable.*
>
> **Type II errors** *occur when researchers incorrectly conclude that the differences between groups are due to chance factors.*

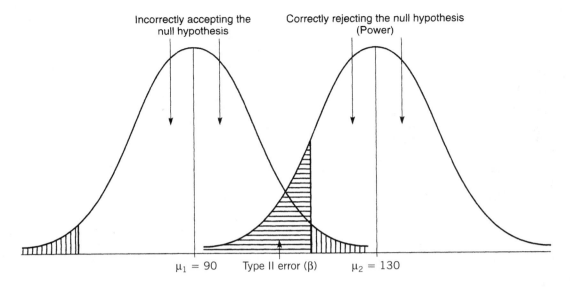

FIGURE 4.6. Normal curves, with $\alpha = .05$ with $\mu_1 \neq \mu_2$. The vertical shaded areas represent $\alpha = .05$; the horizontal shaded area represents a Type II error rate, or β; an incorrect decision is represented on the left curve when the differences between samples are between the α areas for a two-tailed test; a correct decision (power) is made when the sample differences are to the right of β (when the null hypothesis is false).

in education and psychology. It is important for researchers to repeat their own work, as well as the work of others, to explore the possibility that an inaccurate decision was made.

Power

Notice in Figure 4.6 that when the difference falls outside of the alpha level, this is referred to as **power**, defined as correctly detecting a difference when one is actually present, or correctly rejecting the null hypothesis (Faul, Erdfelder, Lang, & Buchner, 2007). Mathematically, power = 1 – Type II error rate, or power = 1 – β. Although the power of a test can be calculated, the procedure for doing so is beyond the scope of this book.

Before discussing power in detail, we must first discuss the four decisions that are made in a statistical significance test. Table 4.1 shows that two of these differences are correct and two are incorrect. If the null hypothesis is correct and we accept it, we will make a correct conclusion. If the null hypothesis is incorrect and we fail to accept it, we will make a Type I error (α). If the null hypothesis is incorrect and we accept it, we

will make a Type II error (β). If the null is incorrect and we fail to accept it, we will make a correct decision (power).

Five Methods of Increasing Power

If power is so desirable, then critical research consumers must understand what affects this probability of detecting differences due to systematic variables when they are present (i.e., rejecting the null hypothesis). There are five basic methods of increasing the power of a test (Cohen et al., 2007; Graziano & Raulin, 2010): (1) Use parametric tests; (2) decrease sources of error variance; (3) relax the alpha level; (4) make a directional alternative hypothesis; and (5) increase sample size. These methods are described below.

Use Parametric Tests

First, researchers can use parametric tests of statistical significance, since they are always more powerful than nonparametric tests. Again, it is beyond the scope of this book to discuss the reasons why this is the case.

TABLE 4.1. Possible Decisions in Statistical Significance Testing

	Accept null hypothesis	Fail to accept null hypothesis (or reject the null hypothesis)
Null hypothesis true (our assumption)	Correct decision	Type I error (α)
Null hypothesis false	Type II error (β)	Correct decision (power)

However, suffice it to say that parametric tests of statistical significance are recommended even when the data do not meet the assumptions of normal distribution or homogeneity of variance (sameness of the fluctuation of scores) but are derived from interval or ratio scores. This recommendation is made because moderate departures from the theoretical assumption about shape and variance have had little effect on parametric tests of statistical significance (Gall et al., 2007). Additionally, because nonparametric tests of statistical significance are less powerful, they require larger sample sizes to yield the same level of statistical significance as parametric tests of statistical significance. That is, they are less likely to provide evidence that the null hypothesis should be rejected. Finally, suitable nonparametric tests of statistical significance are not always available for problems encountered in educational and psychological research.

Decrease Sources of Error Variance

A second method to increase the power of a test is by decreasing sources of error variance from the sampling and measurement process. Recall that scores are going to change from one time to another because, among other things, there is a lack of 100% reliability in the measurement device. If we have a test that is 50% reliable and make an infinite number of sample comparisons, the variability of the mean differences will increase. On the other hand, if we have a test that is 100% reliable, we have lower variability of sample mean differences. Put another way, unsystematic variance makes it more difficult to detect systematic variance. If we can decrease

the unsystematic variance in a study, we are more likely to detect the presence of systematic variance and correctly reject the null hypothesis (power). One source of unsystematic variance is error variance for the sampling and measurement process.

Relax the Alpha Level

The third way to increase the power of a test of statistical significance is by increasing, and thereby relaxing, the significance or alpha level. For example, the power of a given statistical test of significance is greater if a researcher requires an alpha level of $p < .10$ rather than $p < .05$ to reject the null hypothesis. Consider the information in Figure 4.7. If the alpha level is increased, the Type I error rate increases, the Type II error rate decreases, and power increases. We move from having a Type I error rate of 2.5% in each tail to 5% in each tail. The advantage is that researchers are better able to detect systematic variance; the disadvantage is that researchers commit more Type I errors if the differences between the groups occur by chance.

Make a Directional Alternative Hypothesis

The fourth method to increase power is by making a directional alternative hypothesis. Figure 4.8 demonstrates what occurs when a one-tailed versus a two-tailed hypothesis is made. As shown, the Type I error rate for each

> **Power** *is when we correctly conclude that the differences between groups are due to a systematic variable.*

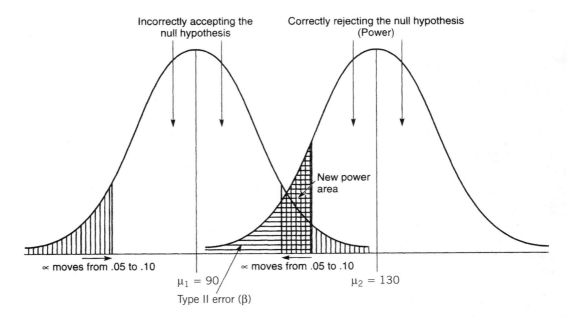

FIGURE 4.7. Normal curves, with α = .10, with $\mu_1 \neq \mu_2$. The vertical shaded areas represent α = .10; the horizontal shaded area represents a Type II error rate, or β; an incorrect decision is represented on the left curve when the differences between samples are between the α areas for a two-tailed test; a correct decision (power) is made when the sample differences are to the right of β (when the null hypothesis is false).

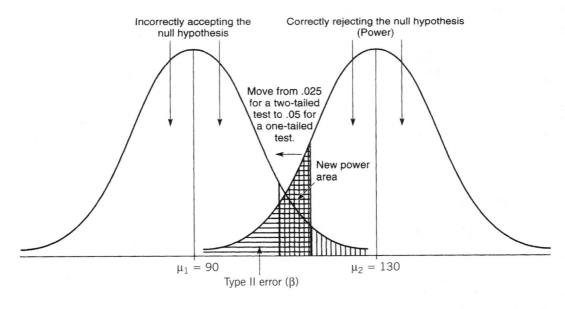

FIGURE 4.8. Normal curves, with α = .05 with $\mu_1 \neq \mu_2$. The vertical shaded areas represent α = .05; the horizontal shaded area represents a Type II error rate, or β; an incorrect decision is represented on the left curve when the differences between samples are to the left of the α area for a one-tailed test; a correct decision (power) is made when the sample differences are to the right of β (when the null hypothesis is false).

tail of a two-tailed test is 2.5%, with alpha set at .05. With a one-tailed hypothesis, the error rate increases to 5% on the single tail. Thus, if the Type I error rate increases, the Type II error rate decreases, thereby increasing power. Additionally, obtaining the evidence needed to accept a two-tailed alternative hypothesis is much harder than accepting a one-tailed alternative hypothesis. The probability of making a Type I error decreases in this case. However, as stated previously, there should be clear evidence for predicting the direction of researchers' findings, and the prediction should be made at the outset of the study. The decision to use a one-tailed test should not be based solely on the wish to increase power.

Increase Sample Size

The final method to increase the power of a test is by increasing sample size. As the sample size increases, so does the probability of a correct rejection of the null hypothesis. Here is the reason why. As the sample size increases, the sample begins to be a better representation of the population. The degree of deviation of the sample mean from the population mean decreases on successive sampling. For example, if we take two samples from two different populations with different means and those samples represent 20% of each population, there will be much smaller deviations in successive comparisons of the groups than if each sample represents only 10% of each population. Figure 4.9 demonstrates this hypothetical example. If we compare Figure 4.9 and Figure 4.6, notice that the variability is smaller. There is also considerably less overlap of the distributions, and power increases. The Type II error rate decreases. The Type I error rate remains at .05.

WHAT ARE THE TYPES OF STATISTICAL SIGNIFICANCE TESTING METHODS?

As stated previously, researchers must choose from one of two categories which type of test of statistical significance to use in analyzing their data: parametric tests or nonparametric tests of statistical significance.

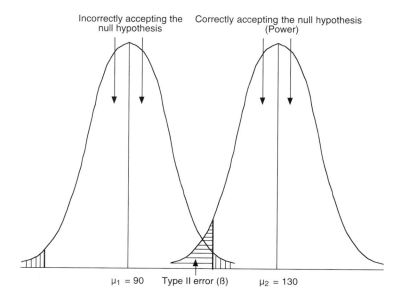

FIGURE 4.9. Normal curves, with $\alpha = .05$, with $\mu_1 \neq \mu_2$. The vertical shaded areas represent $\alpha = .05$; the horizontal shaded area represents a Type II error rate, or β; an incorrect decision is represented on the left curve when the differences between samples are between the α areas for a two-tailed test; a correct decision (power) is made when the sample differences are to the right of β (when the null hypothesis is false).

Parametric Tests of Statistical Significance

Figures 4.10 and 4.11 display flowcharts showing when to use specific inferential statistical analysis procedures. Figure 4.10 shows which procedures to use when there are two means (i.e., one or two groups), and Figure 4.11 shows which procedures to use when there are two or more means (i.e., one, two, three, or more groups). Refer to these figures throughout this section, as well as throughout the analysis of data sections in Chapters 5 and 6.

Comparison of Two Means

The *t*-test, a powerful parametric test of statistical significance, compares the means of two sets of scores to determine whether the difference between them is statistically significant at the chosen alpha level. Recall that in any situation, some degree of difference is always observed.

Thus, the question to ask is not simply whether the two means are different, but whether the difference is so great as to be unlikely to have occurred by chance factors (i.e., sampling and measurement errors). If the result of the *t*-test indicates that the difference is statistically significant, then it provides evidence that enables researchers to conclude that it is unlikely the obtained difference between the means is great enough to have occurred by chance factors alone. Additionally, it is important that the results of the *t*-test be reported along with the summary statistics, such as the mean and standard deviation, to assist the critical research consumers' understanding of what the analysis means. These summary statistics should be reported for any findings from statistical inference testing.

The use of *t*-tests depends on no major violations in the three assumptions about the obtained scores of parametric tests detailed earlier (Erseg-Hurn & Mirosevich, 2008): (1) The

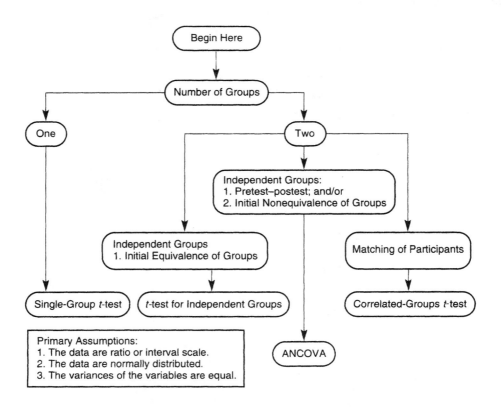

FIGURE 4.10. Selecting inferential statistical analysis procedures: Comparing two means.

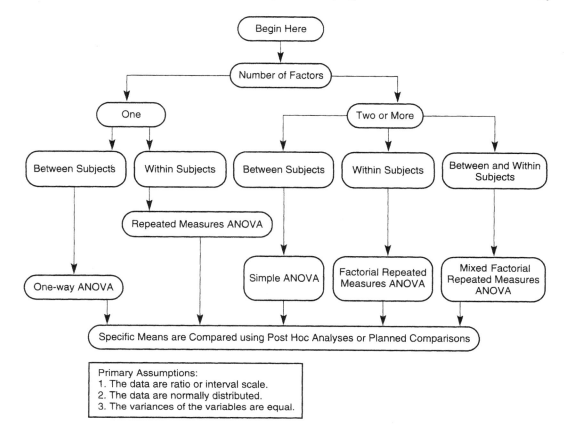

FIGURE 4.11. Selecting inferential statistical analysis procedures: Comparing two or more means.

scores are from an interval or ratio scale of measurement; (2) the scores of the populations under study are normally distributed (normal distribution); and (3) the score variances for the populations under study are equivalent (homogeneity of variance). Of course, if we are concerned about possible violations of these assumptions, one of the nonparametric tests (i.e., the Mann–Whitney U test or the Wilcoxon signed rank test, described later in this chapter) could be computed. If the tests of statistical significance yield different results, the results of the nonparametric test should be reported.

It is not uncommon for researchers to compare two groups or the same group on a number of dependent variables, each requiring a separate t-test. Given the logic of tests of statistical significance, each comparison increases the chances of finding a statistically significant difference between the means of groups on a dependent variable by comparing the groups on many dependent variables. That is, the risk of making a Type I error increases as the number of t-test comparisons increases. For example, a researcher compares two groups on 20 different variables (this requires 20 separate t-tests) and has set alpha at $p < .05$. Even if there are no systematic differences in the groups on any of the variables, we would expect to find at least one statistically significant finding based on chance alone.

The use of multiple t-tests is much less a problem if the predicted direction of the group difference on each variable is based on some theoretical model and/or previous research findings. If the predictions are confirmed, the null hypothesis that the findings are the result of chance factors has low plausibility. On the other hand, if the predictions are not confirmed, the null hypothesis that the findings are the result of chance factors has high plausibility. Of course, it is important to recall our discussion of the problems associated with making predictions in education and psychology.

The three types of *t*-tests commonly used by researchers all are fairly powerful and robust tests of statistical significance. As a result, the *t*-tests can be used with relatively small sample sizes. Although there are no set rules, *t*-tests should not be used with means that comprise fewer than 10 scores, since the assumption of normality may be violated. If there are fewer than 10 scores, nonparametric tests of statistical significance may be used. At least theoretically, larger samples are better. Any increases in the size of the sample have to be balanced against the possibility of increasing sampling and measurement errors due to experimental factors such as fatigue. Thus, for most experiments, a moderate sample size comprising 20 to 25 or more scores for each mean, coupled with careful attention to factors that influence sampling and measurement errors, is appropriate in most cases. The three types of *t*-tests used by researchers are described below.

The t-Test for Independent Means. The *t*-test for independent means is used when the means of two samples are considered *independent* of one another (that is, one sample is not somehow related to another). This type of *t*-test is the most common and typically is used in studies in which researchers are interested in comparing two independent samples on some dependent variable or variables.

The t-Test for Correlated Means. The *t*-test for correlated means is used in cases in which the means of two samples are *related* in some fashion. There are two situations in which the *t*-test for correlated means is used. The first involves an experimental situation in which two groups have been matched on some characteristic, such that their scores on that characteristic vary systematically with their scores on the dependent variable or variables to be compared. The second situation in which the *t*-test for correlated means is appropriate is an experimental situation in which the same group of participants is studied across two different contexts or two points in time.

The t-Test for a Single Mean. Researchers typically compare the mean scores of two samples to determine whether the difference is statistically significant. However, there are times when researchers are interested in whether the difference between a sample mean and a specified population mean is statistically significant. In this case, a *t*-test for a single mean is used. For example, as part of an investigation exploring the intelligence of high school graduates with learning disabilities, the mean score of a group of these graduates on the Wechsler Adult Intelligence Scale–IV (Wechsler, 2008) is compared with the population mean of 100.

Comparison of Two or More Means

Several tests are reviewed that compare two or more means, including (1) analysis of variance, (2) analysis of covariance, (3) repeated measures analysis of variance, (4) multivariate analysis of variance, and (5) tests for differences between variances.

Analysis of Variance. The analysis of variance (**ANOVA**) is a powerful parametric test of statistical significance that compares the means of two or more sets of scores to determine whether the difference between them is statistically significant at the chosen alpha level (Gall et al., 2007; Graziano & Raulin, 2010). Again, the question to be asked is not simply whether the means differ from one another, but whether the difference is so great that it is unlikely to have occurred by chance. If the result of the ANOVA indicates that the difference is statistically significant, then it provides that evidence enables us to conclude there is a statistically significant difference among the means of three or more sets of scores. In other words, the difference is great enough that it is unlikely to have occurred by chance factors alone (sampling and measurement errors). However, the ANOVA does not pinpoint which of the differences between the particular pairs of means are statistically significant.

In most cases, the ANOVA is an initial step in the analysis of the data. Researchers must then pinpoint which differences between the particular pairs of means are statistically significant. A number of multiple-comparison statistical testing procedures (e.g., Neuman–Keuls, Tukey, & Scheffé) can be used to pinpoint such pairs of means (Rafter, Abell, & Braselton, 2002).

Multiple-comparison procedures are special *t*-tests that adjust for the probability that researchers will find a significant difference between any given set of mean scores, simply because many comparisons are made on the same data (Rafter et al., 2002). Although it is beyond the scope of this book to detail each of the multiple-comparison procedures, it is important to note that such procedures are typically conducted in a post hoc fashion. That is, multiple-comparison procedures are most commonly applied only if the *p* value obtained with the ANOVA is statistically significant. In rare cases, the researchers may make a priori comparisons (planned) based on previous findings or some sound theoretical base. In such cases, the researchers may forego the ANOVA and simply use one of the multiple-comparison procedures. This scenario is rarely played out because, as we mentioned earlier, few (if any) theoretical bases in education and psychology would provide researchers with the level of precision necessary to make a priori predictions.

The use of ANOVA depends on no major violations in the same three assumptions about the obtained scores of parametric tests detailed previously. Of course, if we are concerned about possible violations of these assumptions, one of ANOVA's nonparametric counterparts (e.g., chi-square) could be computed. If the tests of statistical significance yield different results, the results of the nonparametric test should be reported. Three variants of ANOVA are described in what follows.

Analysis of Covariance. Analysis of covariance (ANCOVA) is used when researchers need to determine whether a difference between two or more groups on a particular variable can be explained, at least in part, by differences in the groups on another variable (Keselman et al., 1998). ANCOVA is used to control for initial differences between or among groups statistically before a comparison is made. The effect of ANCOVA is to make the groups equivalent with respect to one or more control variables (potential explanatory variables). A statistically significant difference obtained while controlling for the influence of the control variable(s) provides evidence that the control variables do not systematically influence the dependent variable or explain the obtained effect.

Repeated Measures Analysis of Variance. Repeated measures ANOVA is used when researchers need to determine whether two or more groups differ on some dependent variable (Potvin & Schutz, 2000). Determining this difference is common in causal–comparative research when examining developmental changes in children. For example, researchers may measure communication skills in two samples of children (one with autism spectrum disorder and the other with typical development) at ages 3, 6, and 9. Repeated measures would be compared across the two groups.

As in the case of the general ANOVA procedure, the repeated measures ANOVA is an initial step in the analysis of the data. Post hoc multiple-comparison tests must be conducted to pinpoint which of the differences between the particular pairs of means are statistically significant. Additionally, multiple-comparison procedures might be used to answer the following questions:

Do the group means increase significantly in a linear fashion?

Is a straight line a good fit to the group means, or do significant deviations from linearity exist?

Do the group means increase and then decrease in an inverted "U" fashion?

Multiple-comparison procedures can answer such questions.

> The **ANOVA** is a parametric test of statistical significance that compares the means of two or more sets of scores.

Multivariate Analysis of Variance. Multivariate analysis of variance (MANOVA) is used when researchers need to determine whether two or more groups differ on more than one dependent variable (Keselman et al., 1998). In other words, the MANOVA differs from the *t*-test and the ANOVA (which can determine only whether groups differ on one dependent variable) in that it allows researchers to determine whether groups differ on more than one dependent variable. If the result of the MANOVA indicates that the difference is statistically significant, it provides evidence enabling researchers to conclude that there is a statistically significant difference among the groups on one or more of the dependent variables. However, the MANOVA does not pinpoint the dependent variable(s) on which the groups differ.

In most cases, the MANOVA is an initial step in the analysis of data. Researchers must then pinpoint both the dependent measure and the particular pairs of means that are statistically significant. Thus, if the results of the MANOVA are statistically significant, researchers perform an ANOVA on each of the dependent variables to determine which one produces statistically significant differences between or among the mean scores of the groups being studied. If more than two groups are included in the study, researchers then analyze differences in the mean scores of groups using post hoc multiple-comparison procedures (described earlier). It is possible (albeit highly unlikely) to obtain a statistically significant MANOVA without a statistically significant finding with any of the ANOVAs. It is not necessary to include all of the dependent variables in a single MANOVA. Rather, the dependent variables should be grouped into meaningful clusters and analyzed with separate MANOVAs.

Tests for Difference between Variances. Occasions may arise in which researchers want to test the statistical significance of the difference between the variances in scores for two or more samples. A variable may reflect itself in not only a mean difference between two groups but also a variance difference. There are two primary reasons for testing the statistical significance of the difference between variances in scores. Given our discussion of the assumptions underlying parametric tests of statistical significance, the first reason is that most commonly used statistical tests are based on the assumption of homogeneity of variances. Although these tests are not greatly affected by minor violations of this assumption (as well as other assumptions), if there are marked differences in the score variances, one of the nonparametric procedures should be employed.

The second reason for testing the statistical significance of the difference between variances in scores is to test a hypothesis concerning the variability of sample scores. The statistical procedure used to test whether the observed difference between variances of these groups is statistically significant is the *t*-test for independent means.

If two sets of scores are obtained from independent samples, the test for homogeneity of independent variances indicates the statistical significance of the difference between the variance in two sets of scores. In contrast, the test for homogeneity of related variances indicates the statistical significance of the difference between the variance in two sets of scores obtained from matched samples or from repeated measures on a single sample. The *F* maximum test for homogeneity of variance (Wu & Hamada, 2000) is used when researchers need to test the statistical significance of the variance of three or more sets of scores.

Nonparametric Tests of Statistical Significance

Figure 4.12 is a flowchart showing when to use specific nonparametric statistical analysis procedures when there are one, two, three, or more groups and nominal or ordinal scales. Refer to this figure throughout this section, as well as throughout the analysis of data sections in Chapters 5 and 6. We describe (1) the chi-square (χ^2) test comparing relative frequencies, or association between variables; (2) the chi-square goodness-of-fit test; (3) comparisons of two independent medians or means (i.e., Mann–Whitney *U* test); (4) comparisons of two related medians or means (i.e., Wilcoxon signed rank test); and (5) comparisons of three or more medians or means (i.e., Kruskal–Wallis ANOVA).

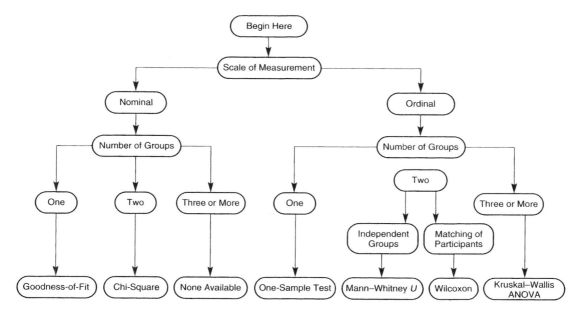

FIGURE 4.12. Selecting nonparametric statistical analysis procedures: Comparing two or more scores.

Comparisons of Relative Frequencies

The chi-square (χ^2) test, a nonparametric test of statistical significance (Zimmerman & Zumbo, 2004), compares the number of participants, objects, or responses that fall into two or more categories, each with two sets of data, to determine whether the difference in the relative frequency of the two sets of data in a given category is statistically significant at the chosen alpha level.

There are two types of chi-square tests: the test for association between variables and the goodness-of-fit test. In essence, chi-square tests compare the data obtained and a set of expected frequencies. If the difference between the observed and expected frequencies is small, the value for chi-square will also be small, and vice versa. The greater the value obtained in the chi-square test, the lower the probability that the difference between observed and expected frequencies could have been due to chance factors alone. Note that the chi-square tests do not allow for the use of directional hypotheses.

Recall that the use of nonparametric tests such as the chi-square test does not rely on any assumptions regarding the population (i.e.,

normal distribution and homogeneity of variance). The chi-square test can be used under the following conditions: (1) The data to be analyzed comprise frequencies organized into the matrix, with each cell of a matrix containing only one specific category of data; (2) the categories used in the chi-square test are defined so that an individual observation qualifies for inclusion in only one of the categories; (3) each data point must be completely independent of every other data point, which means that each individual participant is allowed to contribute once to only one cell; and (4) the purpose of the study is to test for a statistically significant association between two variables or to determine whether an observed frequency distribution differs significantly from the distribution predicted by the null hypothesis. Finally, there are two stipulations to be made concerning the total size of the sample.

1. The sample must contain a minimum of 20 scores when there are only two categories.

2. The sample size must be such that the expected frequency for each cell of the matrix should be at least five observations.

Yates's correction procedure or Fisher's exact test is employed in cases in which the expected frequency is less than five.

The chi-square test is necessary not only when the data comprise frequency counts but also when there are major violations about the assumptions of population parameters underlying a parametric test of statistical significance. For this latter reason, the chi-square test provides a way to deal with imperfect interval scale data by converting the data into frequencies. The two types of chi-square tests used by researchers are described next.

Chi-Square Test for Association between Variables. The chi-square test for association between variables is used to determine whether there is a statistically significant relationship or association between two variables (Gall et al., 2007). Of course, we cannot conclude that one variable has caused the observed pattern of frequencies in the other variable. The association may be due to the existence of some other variable. The establishment of a causal link would be primarily a function of the quality of the research design and procedures. For example, if one of the variables comprises different experimental groups to which participants have been randomly assigned, then it would be valid to infer causality.

Chi-Square Goodness-of-Fit Test. The chi-square test for goodness of fit is used to determine whether there is a statistically significant relationship or association between an observed set of frequencies and a particular hypothetical distribution (Gall et al., 2007). To obtain a significant chi-square value suggests that the obtained frequency differs significantly from what we expect from chance. Again, we cannot conclude that one variable has caused the observed pattern of frequencies in the other.

Comparisons of Two Independent Medians or Means

The Mann–Whitney U test, a nonparametric test of statistical significance, compares the medians or means of two sets of scores to determine whether the difference between them is statistically significant at the chosen alpha level (Oja & Randles, 2004). It is one of the most powerful nonparametric tests available, and it provides an alternative to the parametric t-test when the researcher wants to avoid its assumptions. The Mann–Whitney U test can also be used in those cases with an ordinal scale of measurement. Additionally, the Mann–Whitney U test, like its parametric counterpart, the t-test, allows for both nondirectional and directional hypothesis. Of course, the previously discussed problems associated with making a directional hypothesis in education and psychology apply here.

Although it is beyond the scope of this book to detail the computations underlying the Mann–Whitney U test, a brief explanation of how it works will help critical research consumers to understand it. The Mann–Whitney U test works by first merging the two sets of data to obtain a single rank ordering that is independent of the exact magnitude of the difference between values. Because high values in the rankings indicate higher scores in the data, the set for which the sum is larger will contain the higher relative scores. The Mann–Whitney U test uses these rankings to generate a measure of the difference between the two sets of scores, called a U. The value of U is determined by the number of times that a score from one set of data precedes (i.e., has been given a lower ranking) a score from the other set.

Comparisons of Two Related Medians or Means

The Wilcoxon signed rank test, a nonparametric test of statistical significance, compares the medians or means of two sets of scores that are considered to be related in some fashion (Oja & Randles, 2004). Recall that there are two situations in which the Wilcoxon signed rank test is used. The first involves an experiment in which two groups have been matched on some other characteristic such that their scores on a characteristic vary systematically with their scores on the dependent variable or variables to be compared.

The second situation in which the Wilcoxon signed rank test is appropriate involves an experiment in which the same group of participants is studied across two different contexts or two points in time. The Wilcoxon signed rank test provides an alternative to the parametric *t*-test for correlated means when researchers want to avoid the assumptions of the *t*-test. The Wilcoxon signed rank test can also be used in those cases in which an ordinal scale of measurement has been used. Additionally, like its parametric counterpart, the *t*-test, it allows for both a nondirectional and directional hypothesis. Of course, our discussion of the problems associated with making directional hypotheses in education and psychology applies here.

The Wilcoxon signed rank test works by first determining the magnitude of the difference between the two scores generated by each participant. The differences are then rank-ordered, with the larger differences receiving higher rankings and vice versa. Each ranking is given a "+" or "−" sign to indicate the direction of differences. It is these signed rankings that provide the means for determining whether the differences between two sets of data are statistically significant. If chance factors alone are responsible for the differences between the two sets of data, then we would expect these differences to be equally divided between positive and negative directions. In contrast, if the differences between the two sets of data are the result of the systematic influence of the variable under study, then we would expect these differences to be unequally distributed between positive and negative directions.

Comparisons of Three or More Medians or Means

The Kruskal–Wallis ANOVA, a nonparametric test of statistical significance, compares the medians or means of three or more sets of scores (assuming at least ordinal scale data). It parallels the parametric ANOVA described earlier (Oja & Randles, 2004). The Kruskal–Wallis ANOVA is used when assumptions for a parametric test are violated.

WHAT ARE THE DIFFERENT SAMPLING METHODS?

In Chapter 2, we discussed the importance of *population validity* (i.e., inferring the results of a study from a sample to a population). Sampling provides the basis for experimental research. If everyone in the population cannot be included in the study, then researchers must select a sample. A *sample* is a subset of the population. The quality of the sampling technique in experimental studies enables researchers to maximize the degree to which the selected sample represents the population. Indeed, the quality of the sampling technique employed by researchers plays a large role in all research methods. However, the method of sampling will differ depending on the type of research conducted. For example, qualitative and single-case researchers rely not on probability sampling methods but on nonprobability methods in their selection of participants. (*Note*. Probability and nonprobability sampling methods are discussed later in the chapter.)

A *population* is a group of potential participants, objects, or events to whom or to which researchers want to generalize the results of a study derived from a sample within that population. The generalizability of results is one of the most important aspects of a study if the findings are to have any meaning beyond the limited setting in which the results were obtained. When results are generalizable, they can be applied to groups of individuals with the same characteristics in different settings.

It should be clear that the role of a sample is to represent a much larger, but typically inaccessible, population of individuals. The extent to which researchers can demonstrate that the sample is representative of the population enhances the generalizability of the findings from a study. Regardless of how large a sample is obtained or how carefully the data are collected, researchers' efforts will be wasted if their sampling technique produce a sample that is unrepresentative of the population.

We examine a number of sampling issues before describing some of the most common sampling techniques employed by researchers. The first issue centers on the two types of samples: probability samples and nonprobability samples. A *probability sample* is one in which the likelihood of any one individual, object, or event of the population being selected is known. For example, if 8,000 students are enrolled in a 2-year community college, and there are 3,500 second-year students, the odds of selecting one second-year student as part of a sample is 3,500 divided by 8,000, or .44. A *nonprobability sample* is one in which the likelihood of any individual, object, or event of the population being selected is unknown. For example, if we do not know the total enrollment or the number of second-year students in our community college example, the likelihood of one second-year student being selected cannot be determined.

Probability Sampling

Probability sampling techniques are most commonly used by researchers, because the selection of individuals, objects, or events is determined by random rules or chance. Before describing the different probability sampling techniques, we look at the three meanings of the word *random*, because it is tied directly to probability sampling techniques. First, the word *random* refers to our subjective experiences that certain events occur haphazardly. This meaning has no relevance to sampling techniques in experimental research. Second, *random* is used in an operational way to describe techniques or methods for ensuring that individuals, objects, or events are selected in an unsystematic way. Drawing numbers from a drum after they have been thoroughly mixed is an example of a random technique. Finally, the word *random* refers to the theoretical assumption about the equiprobability of events. Thus, in a random sample, every individual, object, or event has an equiprobability of being included. Of course, the probability sampling techniques we describe later do not truly ensure that every individual, object, or event has an equiprobability of being included in the sample. Rather, probability sampling techniques ensure that who will end up in the sample is determined by nonsystematic means. Now we look at some of the most common probability sampling techniques.

Simple Random Sampling

Of the probability sampling techniques, only simple random sampling ensures that each individual, object, or event has an equiprobability of being included in the sample. Indeed, simple random sampling is the standard against which all other probability and nonprobability sampling techniques can be compared. With simple random sampling, each individual, object, or event is taken from a defined population in such a way to ensure that (1) every individual, object, or event has an unknown chance of being included in the sample; and (2) the inclusion of every individual, object, or event is independent from the inclusion of any of the others (i.e., the choice of one does not influence the choice of another).

The process of simple random sampling comprises three steps. The first step involves listing all members of the population. Simple random sampling requires researchers to have complete access to the population, which means that every individual, object, or event of the defined population is known. For example, suppose a researcher wants to take a random sample from the students enrolled in a high school. The defined population would be the students enrolled at that particular high school. The exact number of students enrolled in the school is known.

The second step in the process of simple random sampling involves assigning each individual, object, or event an identifying number. Researchers typically start with "1" and continue in order, number by number, until all of the individuals, objects, or events have been assigned a number.

The third step in simple random sampling involves using a criterion to choose the sample that ensures every individual, object, or event equiprobability and an independent chance of being selected. To accomplish this, researchers typically use either statistical analysis packages or a table of random numbers. An illustrative example helps us to understand how simple random sampling works.

Table 4.2 lists 60 names and associated assigned numbers (Steps 1 and 2) that represents a population. Let's say we are interested in selecting 10 individuals randomly from this population, using a table of random numbers. A table of random numbers comprises a large number of integers generated by a computer procedure (the same procedure used to select a random sampling in statistical analysis packages), virtually guaranteeing that as every integer is selected, it is entirely independent of

TABLE 4.2. List of 60 Names and Associated Assigned Numbers

1. Jeff P.	21. Meredith L.	41. Jean S.
2. Mary Jean M.	22. Rueben W.	42. Emily B.
3. Tara E.	23. Saul A.	43. Liesel L.
4. Don S.	24. Winston C.	44. Joan M.
5. Terry L.	25. Melia L.	45. Linda M.
6. Melvin J.	26. Wei-Ping L.	46. Olaf H.
7. Fred E.	27. Manuel G.	47. Leisha S.
8. Stacy P.	28. Lindo T.	48. Barbara M.
9. Aaron S.	29. Botheina M.	49. Mario B.
10. Tran W.	30. Elona S.	50. Juan V.
11. Bear R.	31. Hobart C.	51. Bethany S.
12. Lance E.	32. Tamara A.	52. Tom C.
13. Alfred R.	33. Telisha P.	53. Malcolm M.
14. Carolyn E.	34. Bob D.	54. Abraham L.
15. Cory M.	35. Richard N.	55. Raymond H.
16. Elfie M.	36. Mark M.	56. Rigger W.
17. George W.	37. Luke N.	57. Albert S.
18. John C.	38. Shelbee O.	58. Bernard O.
19. Marilyn C.	39. Steven S.	59. Matthew P.
20. Mary Jo B.	40. Eric N.	60. Jamal C.

those that precede it. Therefore, no systematic patterns leading to bias or error are evident when the table of random numbers is used. For example, Table 4.3 contains an equal number of 1's, 2's, 3's, and so on. As a result, the likelihood of selecting a number ending in a 1, a 2, or a 3 is equal. When names are attached to numbers, the likelihood of selecting any particular name is also equal.

Before proceeding with our example, we consider how a table of random numbers is used. Tables of random numbers include integers generated independently from one another that are

then placed into groups of four numbers (see Table 4.3). Tables of random numbers can be used to obtain one-, two-, three-, or four-digit random numbers with equal ease by simply reading across the required number of digits. We can begin to read off numbers at any point on the table, then proceed in any direction we want from that starting point. For example, to pick a starting point somewhere in the middle of a table of random numbers and then continue up the column gives just as random a sample as starting at the top left-hand corner and reading from left to right. Additionally, the number of

TABLE 4.3. Table of Random Numbers

2889	6587	0813	5063	0423	2547	5791	1352	6224	1994	9167	4857
1030	2943	6542	7866	2855	8047	4610	9008	5598	7810	7049	9205
1207	9574	6260	5351	5732	2227	1272	7227	7744	6732	2313	6795
0776	3001	8554	9692	7266	8665	6460	5659	7536	7546	4433	6371
5450	0644	7510	9146	9686	1983	5247	5365	0051	9351	3080	0519
2956	2327	1903	0533	1808	5151	7857	2617	3487	9623	9589	9993
3979	1128	9415	5204	4313	3700	7968	9626	6070	3983	6656	6203
5586	5777	5533	6202	0585	4025	2473	5293	7050	4821	4774	6317
2727	5126	3596	2900	4584	9090	6577	6399	2569	0209	0403	3578
1979	9507	2102	8448	5197	2855	5309	4886	2830	0235	7030	3206
4793	7421	8633	4990	2169	7489	8340	6980	9796	4759	9756	3324
8736	1718	1690	4675	2728	5213	7320	9605	6893	4169	9607	9750
8179	5942	3713	8183	9242	8504	3110	8907	7621	4024	7436	4240

digits considered is dependent on the total number of individuals, objects, or events included in the population. For example, if the population included 1,500 individuals, we would consider four digits at a time, whereas if the population included 50 individuals, we would consider two digits at a time.

Now we select 10 names from Table 4.2 using the partial table of random numbers in Table 4.3. The first step is to pick a starting point. Again, it does not matter where we begin with a table of random numbers. We can begin at the start of a group of integers or anywhere within a group of integers. For this example, our starting point is the first number 2 (4240: bottom right-hand corner of Table 4.3); we read the table from right to left. The first two-digit number considered is 24 (reading right to left). Because the population comprises 60 individuals, and there is a name (Winston C.) associated with the number 24, this individual is the first to be included in the sample. Reading from right to left, the next number considered is 47. Leisha S. becomes the second individual to be included in the sample. We then continue to select two-digit numbers in this manner until 10 values between 01 and 60 are chosen. We now have a sample of 10 names, selected by chance, from our original population of 60 individuals. The 10 individuals are Winston C., Leisha S., Emily B., Don S., Lance E., Jeff P., Alfred R., Eric N., Bernard O., and Botheina M., following numbers 24, 62, 47, 42, 04, 12, 67, 78, 94, 01, 13, 40, 58, 24, and 29.

Systematic Sampling

Systematic sampling is an alternative to simple random sampling as a means to ensure that each individual, object, or event has an equiprobability of being included in the sample. Systematic sampling involves the selection of every kth individual, object, or event on the list chosen. The term kth stands for a number between zero and the size of the sample we want to select. Like simple random sampling, systematic sampling requires a complete listing of every member of the population. Unlike simple random sampling, systematic sampling involves drawing members of the sample at a regular, predetermined interval from the population rather than using a table of random numbers.

The process of systematic sampling comprises three steps: First, list every member of the population; second, assign a number to each member; and third, determine the criterion used to draw members of the sample from the population. The criterion is determined by (1) establishing the kth number by dividing the size of the population by the size of the desired sample, (2) selecting a starting point randomly from which to start drawing members of the sample from the population, and (3) drawing members of the sample from the population using the sampling fraction.

Consider the earlier illustrative sample in which 10 individuals were to be selected randomly from a population containing 60 members. To establish the kth number, we divide 60 by 10. Thus, we select every sixth individual from the list. We then randomly select a starting point. For example, we might close our eyes and point to a name. In this example, the starting point is number 22 (Rueben W.). Once the starting point is determined, every sixth name is then selected (e.g., Lindo T., Bob D.).

Stratified Random Sampling

Simple random sampling and systematic sampling are used when variables of interest (e.g., IQ, SES) are distributed evenly across the population. In other words, using the previous illustrative example, if we selected another set of 10 names, we would assume that because both groups were chosen randomly, they would be equal on the variable of interest. However, researchers often face situations in which they are interested in sampling from a population that is not homogenous on variables that may influence the data. For example, the findings in an experimental study of the effects of an intervention on the reading performance of students that do not take into account that students from different socioeconomic levels have different learning histories may not be representative of the population at large. The problem in such cases is to select a sample that is representative of a heterogeneous population.

Stratified random sampling is used in cases in which the population to be sampled is heterogeneous with respect to one or more variables that may affect the outcomes of the study.

For example, if the population includes 60% European Americans, 30% Hispanics, and 10% African Americans, the sample should have the same ethnic breakdown if ethnicity is an important variable in the first place. A representative ethnic sample is not necessary if ethnicity is not considered an important variable.

The process of systematic sampling comprises three steps. The first step involves listing every member of the subgroups of a population separately. The second step involves assigning a number to each member of the subgroups. The final step involves randomly drawing a proportionate number of members for each of the subgroups, using a statistical analysis package or a table of random numbers.

Going back to our illustrative example, assume that the list of 60 names in Table 4.2 represents a stratified population of males and females, and that their attitudes toward sex education in public schools are of interest. Because gender differences are important, we want a sample that is representative of gender differences in the population. The list of 60 names contains 35 females and 25 males, or approximately 60% female and 40% male. To mirror the population, a stratified random sample of 10 would include six females and four males.

Although simple stratified random samples such as this are relatively common in research in education and psychology, we may encounter situations in which there is a need to stratify a population on more than one variable or characteristic. For example, in a study of the effects of a science curriculum, researchers may stratify the population by gender, grade, and IQ to ensure the representiveness of the sample.

Cluster Sampling

Cluster sampling involves selecting units of individuals, objects, or events rather than individual members themselves. Cluster sampling is often used when an exhaustive list of the population cannot be obtained, or when it is possible to subdivide the population according to some logical structure or principle. Cluster sampling involves subdividing the population into a relatively large number of units, then sampling from these units to obtain a further group of smaller units, and so on, until the members of the final

sample are identified. For example, cluster sampling could be used to conduct a survey of students regarding the quality of library services at a university. In this case, undergraduate and graduate courses representative of each major would be identified. Then one undergraduate and one graduate course would be randomly selected from the identified courses. Students in these courses would constitute the sample. This process may be taken even further by randomly selecting students from these identified courses.

Nonprobability Sampling

Nonprobability sampling techniques involve sample selection in which the probability of selecting a single individual, object, or event is not known. In essence, nonprobability sampling techniques provide researchers a way to select individuals, objects, or events when it is not possible to specify exactly how many members are in the population. Nonprobability sampling techniques are less desirable than probability sampling techniques in quantitative research, because they tend to produce samples that are not representative of the population. Nevertheless, nonprobability sampling techniques are used extensively by researchers in education and psychology. We now look at some of the most common nonprobability sampling techniques.

Quota Sampling

In many respects, quota sampling is similar to the stratified sampling technique previously described. The intent of quota sampling is to derive a sample from a heterogeneous population for which researchers do not have an exhaustive list of the members of the population. Quota sampling can result in a relatively representative sample if the population can be subdivided on one or more variables, if the subdivisions constitute known proportions of the population, and if these relationships are maintained within the sample taken from each subdivision. For example, if a population is known to comprise 75% males and 25% females, then the proportion of males and females in the final samples should also be 75% and 25%, respectively. Of course, the samples derived from quota sampling will be representative of the population only in relation to the variable on which the population is initially divided. Researchers have no way of knowing whether the derived samples are representative of the population in relation to other variables. This situation is not a problem if researchers have subdivided the group on all of the key variables.

The process of quota sampling involves three steps. The first step involves identifying the key variable, or variables, on which the sample is required to be representative of the population and determining what proportion of the population falls into each of the different categories to be used. For example, if a population of at-risk students is to be subdivided on the basis of gender, then the population needs to be subdivided into the proportion of males and females identified as being at risk. The second step is to determine the desired sample size and associated quota for each category. In the final step, researchers select the members of each subdivision using one of the nonprobabilistic sampling procedures described in what follows.

Convenience Sampling

Convenience sampling involves using those individuals, objects, or events that are available to the researcher. Although convenience sampling is an easy way for researchers to generate samples, the samples tend not to be representative of the population. The usual method of putting together a convenience sample is for researchers to use members of a population who are available. For example, a professor in psychology includes all of the students enrolled in an Introduction to Psychology class to explore some psychological phenomenon. Convenience sampling results in a sample that is representative of the population only if the group of individuals, events, or objects available to the researcher are representative of a population. If this is not the case, generalizing beyond the members of the sample would be problematic.

Opportunity Sampling

Opportunity sampling is similar to convenience sampling in that researchers use individuals, objects, or events that are readily available.

However, opportunity sampling means using members of the population who are willing to take part in the research. For example, using our college course example, the professor includes students enrolled in an Introduction to Psychology class who are willing to participate in the research study. In contrast to convenience sampling, opportunity sampling rarely results in representative samples. Thus, any inferences made beyond the members of the sample are problematic.

Volunteer Sampling

Volunteer sampling involves directly advertising for participants in a research study. The distinguishing aspect of volunteer sampling is that participants are self-selected; that is, rather than researchers approaching each member of the population to ask if he/she wants to be included in the sample, the volunteers approach the researchers and ask to participate in the study. It is important to note that members of self-selected samples tend to be different from the population. Thus, any inferences made beyond the members of the sample must be done cautiously.

WHAT ARE THE SAMPLING DECISIONS RESEARCHERS MAKE?

There are a number of decisions that researchers must make with regard to selecting the particular sampling technique they use in a study. The first, and most important, decision that researchers must consider focuses on how important is it that the sample be representative of the population of interest. If it is critical that the results of the study generalize to a particular population, researchers must use a probabilistic sampling technique, such as simple random sampling. A nonprobabilistic sampling technique may be appropriate if it is not critical that the results of the study generalize to a particular population. As we mentioned, it is plausible that samples derived from nonprobabilistic sampling techniques, such as convenience sampling, can be representative of a particular population. The important point to keep in mind is that the use of nonprobabilistic sampling techniques does not render a study useless. Rather, such sampling techniques limit the extent to which inferences regarding the results of the study generalize to a particular population.

The second decision that researchers must consider with regard to selecting a particular sampling technique relates to two basic issues. The first issue is whether researchers have access to an exhaustive list of the members of the population. If not, researchers will not be able to use simple random or systematic sampling techniques. In such cases, quota sampling may be an alternative that results in a reasonably representative sample. The second issue targets the resources (e.g., time, money, and assistance) available to researchers. Probabilistic sampling techniques tend to require more resources than do nonprobabilistic sampling techniques.

The final decision that researchers must make deals with the size of the sample. How many members of the population should researchers select to ensure that the sample is representative of the population? The less representative a sample is of the population, the more sampling error is present, and the less generalizable the results will be to the population. In general, the larger the sample is, the more likely it is representative of the population. However, there is a point of diminishing returns; that is, increasing the amount of resources needed to collect data from large samples does not result in greater precision. The method used by researchers to calculate the sample size needed to be representative of a particular population for an experimental study is as follows:

$$n = \frac{2(SD)^2 \times t^2}{D^2}$$

where n is size of sample, SD is the standard deviation of the dependent variable in the population, t is the critical value needed for rejection of the null hypothesis, and D is the estimate of the average difference between the two groups.

We now examine an illustrative example to see how a researcher can determine the sample size needed to be reasonably representative of a particular population. The goal of this study is to determine the effects of a behavioral intervention on the social adjustment of students with behavioral disorders. The researcher is using a pretest and posttest design with an experimental group and a control group. The standard deviation is estimated by reviewing previous studies. In our example, a social adjustment scale is used, and the standard deviation in the population is 10. The researcher then considers the critical value associated with the particular test of statistical significance that reflects the difference between groups that would be obtained by chance alone (and not any intervention effects). Critical values can be obtained from tables included in statistics textbooks. In our example, the critical value associated with the t-test is 2.00. Finally, the researcher estimates what she expects the magnitude of the difference to be. This estimate is based on previous studies using similar interventions. In our example, say that the researcher expects a 5-point increase. The values for our example are as follows:

$$SD = 10$$
$$t = 2.00$$
$$D = 5$$

Substituting these values into the preceding formula reveals that the researcher would need about 16 members each in the experimental and control groups.

$$n = \frac{(2 \times 10^2) \times 2.00^2}{5^2}$$
$$= 400/25$$
$$= 16$$

Substituting different values into the formula reveals that the expected difference between groups plays the largest role in determining the size of the sample. For example, if the researcher changed the estimated expected difference in her sample to 2, she would need about 100 members in each group. Accordingly, the larger the difference between groups, the less representative the groups have to be of the population to detect the experimental effect, if it exists.

Finally, there are some general issues to keep in mind. The first issue is the size of the sample. Generally, the larger the sample, the smaller the sampling error. Of course, the level of precision achieved with even larger sample sizes decreases dramatically. The second issue is how the sample will eventually be broken down for analysis. The initial selection of participants should be large enough to account for the final breakdown of participant groups. The final issue is choosing an appropriate sample of participants based on the purpose of the research. If a sample is inappropriate for the purpose of the research, then it will not matter how many participants are included in the sample.

WHAT IS SAMPLING ERROR?

We discussed the notion of sampling error in our description of tests of statistical significance. As we might expect, it is virtually impossible for researchers to select samples that are perfectly representative of the population of interest. In other words, regardless of the sampling technique used by the researcher, the characteristics of the sample will differ to some degree from those of the population. The difference between the characteristics of the sample and those of the population is referred to as *sampling error*. For example, the average IQ in the population is 100. If we select 20 samples of 100 individuals randomly and compute the mean IQ scores for each group of individuals, we end up with 20 averages. If all those averages are exactly 100,

there will be no sampling error. Of course, this scenario would never happen. The average IQ scores for the group would vary to some degree from 100. Some would be above 100 (e.g., 100.6, 100.2) and others would be below 100 (e.g., 99.9, 99.4). The amount of variability in these values provides an indicator of the amount of sampling error present.

Although the exact computations of sampling error are beyond the scope of this book, critical research consumers should understand that the researcher's main goal is to minimize this value. The smaller the value, the smaller the sampling error. We already know that the larger the sample, the smaller the sampling error and, consequently, the more representative the sample is of the population. The more representative the sample, the more accurate the tests of statistical significance will be. That is, better sampling leads to more accurate tests of population differences.

Minimizing sampling error requires researchers to focus on two key aspects. The first centers on ensuring the use of sampling techniques that result in samples that are representative of the population. The second aspect focuses on the size of the sample. Remember, in general, the larger the sample, the more likely it is to be representative of the population.

SUMMARY

❖ Statistics should be thought of as only one tool that helps in the analysis of data we gather.

❖ Four distinct scales enable researchers to measure the targeted features of interest under a range of different conditions and levels of precision—(1) nominal scale (identification), (2) ordinal scale (ranking), (3) interval scale (equal distances from point to point on a scale, no absolute zero point), and (4) ratio scale (possesses all attributes of the other scales and has an absolute zero point).

❖ A univariate frequency distribution entails counting the number of times each different score occurs in a data set. The normal distribution is one of the most common univariate distributions.

❖ The frequency distribution represents how a data set can be represented graphically. Researchers typically use three measures of central tendency to describe a central reference value that usually is close to the point of greatest concentration in a set of scores—(1) arithmetic mean (appropriate for interval and ratio scale data), (2) median (appropriate for ordinal scale data), and (3) mode (appropriate for nominal scale data).

❖ Researchers commonly use three statistics to describe the variation in a data set—(1) range, (2) standard deviation, and (3) variance. Distributions of scores can take on three primary shapes: (1) unimodal (normal distribution), (2) bimodal (scores accumulate at two different parts of the scale), and (3) skewed (scores are mainly high or low at the ends of a scale).

❖ Hypotheses represent statements about what findings are expected and are used in inferential statistics. The function of null hypotheses and alternative hypotheses is to express statements about differences between parameters of the population from which the samples are taken. Two types of hypotheses are developed by researchers: (1) null hypothesis (no difference between two groups of data) and (2) alternative or experimental hypothesis (statistically significant relationships between variables being studied or differences between values of a population parameter). An alternative hypothesis is either directional or nondirectional. A nondirectional hypothesis simply states that there are differences between the population means. A directional alternative hypothesis is one in which the population parameter (e.g., mean) is stated to be greater or smaller than the other population parameter.

❖ Parametric tests of statistical significance are based on three primary assumptions about population parameters: (1) The scores in the population are normally distributed about the mean; (2) the population variances of the comparison groups in a study are equal; and (3) there are at least interval or ratio scale data. Nonparametric tests of statistical significance are used to test the null hypothesis when one or more of these assumptions is violated.

❖ Statistical significance occurs when a difference between sets of scores is so great that there is a likelihood, at some level of probability, that it is the result of the influence of a systematic variable (independent, extraneous, or some combination of the two) on the dependent variable rather than a function of chance due to sampling or measurement error. There are two common errors in the interpretations of statistical significance—(1) to view statistical significance as the same as replicability (if we repeat the study again we will get the same results) and (2) the view that statistical significant results are inherently important.

❖ There are two correct decisions a researcher can make about the results of an

investigation: (1) rejecting or failing to accept the null hypothesis when it is false, that is, correctly concluding the differences are due to a systematic variable when in fact they are due to a systematic variable, and (2) accepting or failing to reject the null hypothesis when it is true, that is, correctly concluding that any differences are due to chance factors.

❖ There are two incorrect decisions a researcher can make about the results of an investigation: (1) Type I error, and (2) Type II error. Type I error is rejecting or failing to accept the null hypothesis when it is true; that is, incorrectly concluding that any difference between sample groups is due to a systematic variable when the difference is due to chance alone. Type II error is accepting or failing to reject the null hypothesis when, in fact, there is a difference due to a systematic variable; that is, incorrectly concluding the differences between groups are due to chance factors when they are not.

❖ There are five basic methods to increase the power of a test: (1) use parametric tests; (2) decrease sources of error variance; (3) relax the alpha level; (4) make a directional alternative hypothesis; and (5) increase sample size.

❖ There are eight primary parametric tests: (1) t-test for independent means, (2) t-test for correlated means, (3) t-test for a single mean, (4) analysis of variance, (5) analysis of covariance, (6) repeated measures analysis of variance, (7) multivariate analysis of variance, and (8) tests for differences between variances.

❖ There are five primary nonparametric tests: (1) the chi-square (χ^2) test comparing relative frequencies, or association between variables; (2) the chi-square goodness-of-fit test; (3) the Mann–Whitney U test; (4) the Wilcoxon signed rank test; and (5) the Kruskal–Wallis ANOVA.

❖ The four most common probability sampling methods are: (1) simple random sampling, (2) systemic sampling, (3) stratified random sampling, and (4) cluster sampling.

❖ The four most common nonprobability sampling methods are: (1) quota sampling,

(2) convenience sampling, (3) opportunity sampling, and (4) volunteer sampling.

❖ Researchers must answer three questions before selecting the particular sampling technique they will use: (1) How important is it for the sample to be representative of the population of interest?; (2) how can the sample be selected? (is there an exhaustive list of the members of the population and what is possible with the resources [time, money, assistance] available?); and (3) how many members of the population are needed to ensure that the sample is representative of the population?

❖ The difference between the characteristics of the sample and those of the population is referred to as *sampling error*. Minimizing sampling error requires researchers to focus on two key aspects—(1) ensuring the use of sampling techniques that result in samples that are representative of the population and (2) the size of the sample.

DISCUSSION QUESTIONS

1. Name an original example for each scale of measurement.

2. Suppose that a student took an IQ test and received a score of 130. The standard deviation for the test is 15, and the mean is 100. What proportion of the population scored the same or higher than the student? What proportion of the population scored the same or lower than the student? What score would a student need to be placed at the 84th percentile?

3. What does it mean that the null hypothesis is a straw man to be knocked down? In your answer, describe the purpose of null hypotheses and alternative hypotheses.

4. What is meant by the term *directional hypothesis*, and what information would a researcher need to form such a directional hypothesis?

5. What is a parametric test, and how does a parametric test differ from a nonparametric test? In your response, discuss assumptions of parametric tests.

6. Are the following conclusions warranted? Why or why not? The results were significant at the .05 level. This means that the results proved that the null hypothesis was false and that the independent variable caused the results. If the study were repeated 100 times, these same results would occur 95 times.

7. What is the Type I error rate if the alpha (α) level is .05? What is meant by the term Type I error? Is making a Type I error worse than making a Type II error? Why or why not?

8. What is meant by *power*? How can power be increased? Why is increasing the power of a test worthwhile?

9. What type of parametric test would you use, and why, in the following scenario? The skills of male and female twin pairs in mathematics are assessed, and the average math performances (i.e., scores on a standardized test) of the gender groups are compared. What type of nonparametric test could you use and why (i.e., under what conditions)? What tests (parametric and nonparametric) would you use if the males and females were not related to one another (i.e., separate samples)?

10. What sampling decisions need to be made (i.e., how many students do you need, and should you use probability or nonprobability sampling methods and why?) to study the best method of teaching first-grade students how to spell? Describe how sampling error can be affected by the sampling method you select.

CHAPTER 5

■ ■ ■ ■

Experimental Designs

OBJECTIVES

After studying this chapter, you should be able to . . .

1. State the goal of the experimental researcher and outline the four key features on which experimental designs depend to control for threats to internal and external validity.
2. Explain what is meant by true experimental designs.
3. Illustrate the most common true experimental designs.
4. Describe what is meant by factorial experimental designs.
5. Depict what is meant by quasi-experimental designs.
6. Outline the common quasi-experimental designs.
7. Express what is meant by preexperimental designs.
8. Illustrate the types of preexperimental designs.
9. Describe when researchers should use each experimental research design.

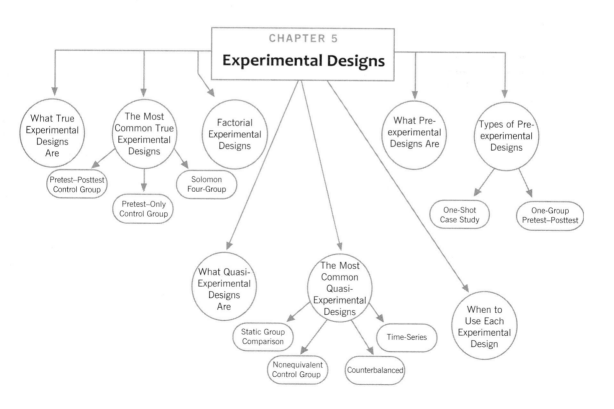

OVERVIEW

Researchers tend to be most interested in why things happen. Establishing cause-and-effect relationships among variables is typically the goal of most research. The experimental research designs described in this chapter test for the presence of a distinct cause-and-effect relationship between variables. In order to achieve this goal, experimental research must control extraneous variables. The results of a study using an experimental design indicate whether an independent variable produces or fails to produce changes in the dependent variable. For example, a simple experimental design would comprise two groups of participants randomly selected from a population in which one group (experimental group) receives the independent variable (intervention), and the other (control group) receives no intervention. Both groups are tested at the conclusion of the study to assess whether there is a difference in their scores. Assuming that the groups are equivalent from the start of the investigation, any observed differences at the conclusion of the investigation may reasonably be attributable to the independent variable, along with measurement and sampling error.

Findings from controlled experiments have led to much of our substantive knowledge in many areas, such as education, learning, memory, perception, and clinical psychology. The control achieved with experimental research designs enables researchers to ensure that the effects of the independent variable on the dependent variable are a direct (causal) consequence of the independent variable and not of other factors (i.e., extraneous variables or threats to internal validity). Of course, the experimental research designs used by researchers to establish cause-and-effect relationships differ widely in their ability to control for threats to internal and external validity (described in Chapter 2).

There are three categories of experimental research designs used by researchers in education and psychology: (1) true experimental, (2) quasi-experimental, and (3) preexperimental designs. These designs differ with regard to the level of experimental control they provide. Researchers must be concerned with the number of extraneous variables (threats to internal validity) that may effect changes in the performance of the experimental or control groups. Researchers must also be concerned with generalizing the results of studies to a broader population and set of conditions (external validity).

The ability of an experimental design to control for threats to internal and external validity is primarily dependent on four key features (Gall et al., 2007). The first key feature centers on the procedures used to select participants from a broader population. The usefulness of any given study is dependent on how well the results of that study can be generalized to a broader population and set of conditions. The second key feature involves the use of a control group or condition. Comparing the performance of an experimental group with that of a control group provides the basis for controlling many of the threats to internal and external validity. The comparison of conditions is critical for establishing whether there is a causal relationship between variables. The third key feature focuses on the initial equivalence of the experimental and control groups. Researchers must ensure this initial equivalence if they are to make relatively definitive conclusions regarding a causal relationship between the independent and dependent variables. The final key feature for experimental research centers on how effectively the investigation is conducted. Although researchers might employ a rigorous design, the results are useless if the investigation is not conducted well.

The three group experimental design categories differ on these design features that account for differences in the levels of experimental control. The final key feature (i.e., quality of implementation) cuts across all three categories of experimental designs. True experimental designs include clear procedures for addressing each of the first three key design features, including (1) the random selection of participants from a population (see Chapter 4), (2) the inclusion of a control group, and (3) the equivalence of the experimental and control groups. Quasi-experimental designs (with the exception of some time-series designs) include procedures for addressing the second key design feature (i.e., the inclusion of a control group). Preexperimental designs include none of these key design features. Table 5.1 summarizes the key design

TABLE 5.1. Key Design Features of True, Quasi-, and Preexperimental Research Designs

	Random selection of participants from a population	Random assignment of participants to conditions	Control group	Equivalence of groups
True	Yes	Yes	Yes	Yes
Quasi-	No	No	Yes	No
Preexperimental	No	No	No	No

features associated with true, quasi-experimental, and preexperimental research designs.

The remainder of this chapter includes a description of each of the true, quasi-experimental, and preexperimental research designs commonly used by researchers in education and psychology. Additionally, methods of analyzing data are described. (Refer to Figures 4.10, 4.11, and 4.12 for information regarding when to use each statistical analysis procedure to analyze data from investigations.) Finally, research examples are provided throughout the chapter to show true experimental and one quasi-experimental design, and an illustrative investigation is included at the end of the chapter for review.

WHAT ARE TRUE EXPERIMENTAL DESIGNS?

True experimental designs are the only experimental designs that can result in relatively definitive statements about causal relationships between variables (Mertler & Charles, 2011). Researchers can argue rather decisively that there is a causal relationship between variables if they have effectively used a true experimental design. The beauty of true experimental designs rests in their simplicity in achieving the three requirements identified by Cook and Campbell (1979) in saying that one variable (independent variable) causes another (dependent variable). That is, true experimental designs ensure that (1) a change in the value of the independent variable is accompanied by a change in the value of the dependent variable, (2) how the independent variable affects the dependent variable is established a priori, and (3) the independent variable precedes the dependent variable.

There are three basic requirements for a research design to be considered a true experimental design. The first requirement is the random selection of participants from a population to form a sample. One of the sampling techniques discussed in Chapter 4 is to ensure that the participants selected are representative of the population. The random selection of participants from a population is a critical issue to the external validity of a study. It is important to note that researchers tend to be much more concerned with random assignment of participants to either experimental or control groups

Research Examples

Beginning with this chapter, we provide examples of research associated with the designs described in the readings. Think about how you would design research to address the questions/hypotheses from these research examples:

- Research Example 1: Do poor early reading skills decrease a child's motivation to read?
- Research Example 2: What are the effects of four first-grade math curricula?
- Research Example 3: What are the effects of pretesting and pedometer use on walking intentions and behavior?
- Research Example 4: What are the effects of sentence length on reading rate and the number of difficult words per paragraph on reading rate? Is there an interaction between the effects of sentence length and number of difficult words per paragraph on reading rates?
- Research Example 5: Do differences exist in dimensions related to quality of life for adults with developmental disabilities compared to adults in the general population?

Research examples appear throughout the chapter.

than with random selection of participants from a population to form a sample. This concern represents the tendency of researchers to be more mindful of a study's internal validity than its external validity.

The second requirement is that research participants must be randomly assigned to the experimental and control conditions. Random assignment helps to ensure that members of the experimental and control groups are equivalent to one another before the implementation of the independent variable. Ensuring that the experimental and control groups are equivalent is critical to the internal validity of the study. However, randomly assigning participants to groups does not necessarily guarantee initial equivalence between groups. Rather, random assignment only ensures the absence of systematic bias in the makeup of the groups. Assigning participants to experimental and control groups is accomplished by using one of the probabilistic sampling techniques discussed previously.

The equal treatment of members of experimental and control groups is the third requirement for a research design to be considered a true experimental design. Research participants in experimental and control groups must be treated equally in every way except in relation to the independent variable. In other words, participants in experimental and control groups are treated differently only with respect to the independent variable. However, note that the comparison of an independent variable (experimental group) with no independent variable (control group) is overly simplistic. The actual comparison in most true experimental studies is what occurs between the independent variable and the activities of the control group during the experimental time frame. Thus, the comparison might be better thought of as being between two *different* independent variables. It is important for critical research consumers to understand the strengths and weaknesses associated with true experimental designs.

WHAT ARE THE MOST COMMON TRUE EXPERIMENTAL DESIGNS?

We now look at three of the most common true experimental designs—pretest–posttest control-group, posttest-only control-group, and Solomon four-group designs. All three of these designs are presented in terms of comparing a single independent variable and dependent variable with a control condition. Designs with more than one independent variable also represent true experimental designs; we discuss these factorial designs separately.

Pretest–Posttest Control-Group Design

The **pretest–posttest control-group design** is one of the most common designs used in education and psychology to demonstrate a causal relationship between an independent variable and a dependent variable. This design begins with random selection of participants from a population to form a sample. Participants from the sample are then randomly assigned to experimental or control groups. Measurement of the dependent variable is taken prior to the introduction of the independent variable. The independent variable is then introduced, followed by postintervention measurement of the independent variable. Figure 5.1 depicts the form of the pretest–posttest control-group design.

The basic assumption of the pretest–posttest control-group design is that participants in the experimental and control groups are equivalent prior to introduction of the independent variable. Any differences observed at the end of the study are assumed to be due to the independent variable. The assumption that the experimental and control groups are equivalent is based on the notion that randomly assigning participants to either group ensures that they are equivalent at the start of the study. The extent to which this assumption is met is based on the technique used to randomly assign participants to groups and the number of participants in each group. Additionally, recall that randomly assigning participants to groups only ensures the absence of systematic bias in the makeup of the groups, not the initial equivalence of the groups.

The goal in a pretest–posttest control-group design is to keep the experiences of the experimental and control groups as identical as possible in all respects except for introduction of the independent variable to the experimental group. Changes in the pretest and posttest scores due to any other extraneous variables (e.g., maturation)

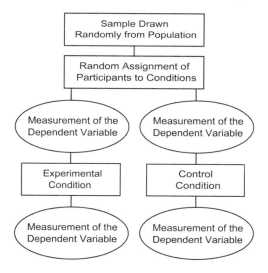

FIGURE 5.1. Pretest–posttest control-group design.

will be reflected in the scores of the control group. In other words, any changes in the posttest scores of the experimental group beyond the changes in the control group can be reasonably attributed to the independent variable.

In some studies using a pretest–posttest control-group design, the control group is administered only in the pretest and the posttest, and receives no specific intervention. In other studies using such a design, the control group is administered an equally desirable but alternative intervention or independent variable. Sometimes researchers refer to the control as a "comparison" group, if the group receives an intervention rather than being in a no-intervention condition. Furthermore, researchers may label the two groups in relation to the interventions the groups receive (e.g., direct instruction group, cooperative learning group).

Analysis of Data

Although the tests of statistical significance discussed in Chapter 4 can be used with the pretest–posttest control-group design, the ANCOVA is preferred. With ANCOVA, the posttest mean score of the experimental group is compared with the posttest mean score of the experimental group, with the pretest scores used as a covariate. Recall from Chapter 4 that ANCOVA

statistically adjusts the posttest scores for initial differences between the experimental and control groups on the pretest. The ANCOVA is the preferred test of statistical significance because it is the most powerful. That is, ANCOVA increases the probability that researchers will detect the effects of the independent variable. Additionally, a nonparametric test, such as the Mann–Whitney U test, should be used if the data violate the assumptions underlying these parametric tests (i.e., homogeneity of variance, normal distribution of data, and interval or ratio scale data).

Internal Validity. The pretest–posttest control-group design in which the control group receives no intervention effectively controls for the eight threats to internal validity that result in changes in the performance of the experimental group. These threats to internal validity include (1) history, (2) maturation, (3) testing, (4) instrumentation, (5) statistical regression, (6) selection, (7) mortality, and (8) selection by maturation interaction. Testing may be a threat to the internal validity of the study if the pretest has a powerful effect on the intervention. The four additional threats to internal validity that cause changes in the performance of the control group are controlled if researchers provide the control group with an equally desirable but alternative intervention. These threats to internal validity include (1) experimental treatment diffusion, (2) compensatory rivalry by the control group, (3) compensatory equalization of treatments, and (4) resentful demoralization of the control group. Table 5.2 summarizes the potential threats to internal validity associated with each of the true experimental research designs.

External Validity. The pretest–posttest control-group design effectively controls for many of the threats to external validity if the study is conducted effectively. Table 5.3 summarizes the potential threats to external validity associated with each of the true experimental research

> The **pretest–posttest control-group design** *includes measurement of the dependent variable before and after implementation of the independent variable.*

designs. The threats to external validity that are controlled for include (1) multiple treatment interference, (2) novelty and disruption effects, (3) the Hawthorne effect, (4) pretest sensitization, and (5) posttest sensitization. It is important to note that novelty and disruption effects, as well as the Hawthorne effect, may be threats to the external validity of a study if the researchers did not provide an equally desirable but alternative intervention. Pretest sensitization also may be a threat to the external validity of the study if the pretest has a powerful effect on the intervention. The remaining threats to the external validity of a study are dependent on the particular characteristics of the study and how well the study was conducted (see Table 5.3). For example, as discussed earlier, if the participants have not been selected randomly from a population to form a sample, then the threats to external validity associated with the population represent potential problems.

> *Recall the research question regarding early reading failure and whether it decreases children's motivation to read? Read on to see how your design compares to how the actual study was designed.*

Research Example 1: Early Reading Failure and Children's Motivation to Read

The pretest–posttest control group design was used to evaluate whether low performance in early reading decreased children's motivation to practice reading, and whether improving word identification skills with a peer tutor would bolster motivation (Morgan, Fuchs, Compton, Cordray, & Fuchs, 2008). Researchers sought to investigate the causal relationship between low performance in early reading and decreased motivation. Thirty classroom teachers were recruited in 15 schools in a large metropolitan area. Within teachers' classrooms, 75

TABLE 5.2. Threats to Internal Validity Associated with True Experimental Designs

Threat	Pretest–posttest control group	Posttest-only control group	Solomon four-group
1. Maturation	Controlled	Controlled	Controlled
2. Selection	Controlled	Controlled[c]	Controlled
3. Selection by maturation interaction	Controlled	Controlled	Controlled
4. Statistical regression	Controlled	Controlled	Controlled
5. Mortality	Controlled	Controlled	Controlled
6. Instrumentation	Controlled	Controlled	Controlled
7. Testing	Controlled[a]	Controlled	Controlled
8. History	Controlled	Controlled	Controlled
9. Resentful demoralization of the control group	Possible concern[b]	Possible concern[b]	Possible concern[b]
10. Diffusion of treatment	Possible concern[b]	Possible concern[b]	Possible concern[b]
11. Compensatory rivalry by the control group	Possible concern[b]	Possible concern[b]	Possible concern[b]
12. Compensatory equalization	Possible concern[b]	Possible concern[b]	Possible concern[b]

Note. This table is meant only as a general guideline. Decisions with regard to threats to internal validity must be made after the specifics of an investigation are known and understood. Thus, interpretations of internal validity threats must be made on a study-by-study basis.

[a]Although testing is generally controlled for, it may be a potential threat to the internal validity of a study if the pretest has a powerful effect on the intervention.

[b]These threats to internal validity are controlled if the control group received an equally desirable but alternative intervention.

[c]Although selection is controlled through the random assignment of participants to groups, the lack of a pretest precludes a statistical test of the equivalence of the groups.

TABLE 5.3. Threats to External Validity Associated with True Experimental Designs

Threat	Pretest–posttest control group	Posttest-only control group	Solomon four-group
		Research design	
1. Generalization across participants	Possible concern[a]	Possible concern[a]	Possible concern[a]
2. Interaction of personological variables and treatment effects	Possible concern[a]	Possible concern[a]	Possible concern[a]
3. Verification of independent variable	Possible concern	Possible concern	Possible concern
4. Multiple treatment interference	Controlled	Controlled	Controlled
5. Novelty and disruption effects	Controlled[b]	Controlled[b]	Controlled[b]
6. Hawthorne effect	Controlled[b]	Controlled[b]	Controlled[b]
7. Experimenter effects	Possible concern	Possible concern	Possible concern
8. Pretest sensitization	Possible concern	Controlled	Controlled
9. Posttest sensitization	Controlled	Possible concern	Controlled
10. Interaction of time of measurement and treatment effects	Possible concern	Possible concern	Possible concern
11. Measurement of the dependent variable	Possible concern	Possible concern	Possible concern
12. Interaction of history and treatment effects	Possible concern	Possible concern	Possible concern

Note. This table is meant only as a general guideline. Decisions with regard to threats to external validity must be made after the specifics of an investigation are known and understood. Thus, interpretations of external validity threats must be made on a study-by-study basis.

[a]Threats to external validity associated with the population are controlled if the sample has been drawn randomly from a population.

[b]These threats to external validity are controlled if the control group received an equally desirable but alternative intervention.

first graders were recruited, including 30 who were high-skilled readers, 15 who were low-skill readers, and 15 additional low-skill readers who received small-group tutoring. Of 30 low-skill participants, 12 were African American, 25 were European American, and 15 participated in Title I schools. Low-skill children were then randomly assigned to a tutoring or nontutoring condition. Tutoring consisted of a mean of 27 hours of small-group tutoring by trained graduate students in phonemic awareness, decoding, and fluency building. Researchers conducted observations measuring the fidelity of tutoring to ensure that tutors adhered to specific teaching steps. Tutoring fidelity was 98%. Tutoring was additive to standard reading instruction. Informal classroom observation confirmed that standard reading instruction was carried out during the study. Eight different measures were used in the pretest and posttest format. Emerging reading skills were measured by administering the Rapid Letter Naming Test from the Comprehensive Test of Phonological Processing (Wagner, Torgesen, & Rashotte, 1999) and three additional tests. Reading skills were measured by the Word Attack and Word Identification subtests of the Woodcock Reading Mastery Test—Revised (Woodcock, 1987) and a first-grade Dolch Sight Word List. Reading motivation was measured by the Reading Self-Concept Scale (Chapman & Tunmer, 1995) and two additional tests. Reading practice was measured by the Reading Frequency Questionnaire (Bast & Reitsma, 1998) and one additional test. Psychometric data were reported on all tests. Results were analyzed using repeated measures ANOVA. Researchers found consistent evidence that reading skill and reading motivation were related. Low-skill readers reported lower reading self-concept than high-skill readers. Teachers rated low-performers as less motivated and more task avoidant during reading. Teachers also rated low-skill readers as less likely to independently practice reading. However, low-skill readers in the tutoring group did not have concomitant changes in reading self-concept, motivation, or task orientation. Although their reading improved, they did not increase their practice of reading. Researchers recommended combining reading tutoring with strategies directly targeting motivation.

Posttest-Only Control-Group Design

The concept of applying a pretest in experimental research is very common in education and psychology. Although it is difficult for researchers to give up the comfort of knowing for sure whether the experimental and control groups are equivalent, applying a pretest is not essential to conducting a true experimental research study. Randomization typically leads to equivalent experimental and control groups (Campbell & Stanley, 1963). The **posttest-only control-group design** is very similar to the pretest–posttest-only control-group design except that pretests of the dependent variable are not administered to the experimental and control groups. The posttest-only control-group design begins with the random selection of participants from a population to form a sample. Participants from the sample are then randomly assigned to the experimental or control groups. The independent variable is then introduced followed by postintervention measurement of the dependent variable. Figure 5.2 depicts the form of the posttest-only control-group design.

The basic assumption of the posttest-only control-group design is the same as the pretest–posttest control-group design. That is, the participants of the experimental and control groups are equivalent prior to the introduction of the independent variable. Any differences observed at the end of the study are assumed to be due to the independent variable. Of course, one of the weaknesses of the posttest-only control-group design is that researchers cannot be certain that random assignment of participants resulted in the initial equivalence of the groups.

The goal of the posttest-only control group design is the same as the pretest–posttest control-group design. This goal is to keep the experiences of the experimental and control groups as identical as possible in all respects except for the introduction of the independent variable to

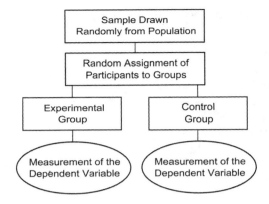

FIGURE 5.2. Posttest-only control-group design.

the experimental group. Changes in the posttest scores due to any other extraneous variables will be reflected in the scores of the control group. Additionally, as with pretest–posttest control-group designs, the control group in a posttest-only control-group design receives no specific intervention in some cases. In other cases, the control group is administered an equally desirable but alternative intervention.

The posttest-only control-group design is used when there is a possibility that the pretest will have an effect on the independent variable, or when researchers are unable to identify a suitable pretest measure (Gall et al., 2007). The posttest-only control-group design is most often used in research exploring the effects of different interventions on the beliefs or attitudes of individuals. For example, say we are interested in studying the effects of a new substance abuse prevention program on high school students' beliefs about alcohol. A pretest in this case might influence participants' responses on the posttest. Thus, participants would be randomly assigned to either the experimental or the control condition. The experimental group would receive the new substance abuse prevention program, and the control group would receive no intervention. At the end of the intervention, a posttest would be administered to both the experimental and the control group. Any differences (statistically significant) in the responses of the experimental and control groups could then be attributed to the effects of the substance abuse prevention program.

Analysis of Data

The data from a posttest-only control-group design are typically analyzed by doing a *t*-test comparing the means of the posttest scores of the experimental and control groups. ANOVA can be used if more than two groups have been studied. If the researcher has collected data on one or more variables unrelated to the purpose of the study, such as gender or IQ, then ANCOVA can be used. Additionally, a nonparametric test such as the Mann–Whitney *U* test should be used if the data violate the assumptions underlying these parametric tests (i.e., homogeneity of variance, normal distribution of data, and interval or ratio scale data).

Internal Validity. The posttest-only control-group design in which the control group receives no intervention effectively controls for the same eight threats to internal validity as the pretest–posttest control-group design (i.e., history, maturation, testing, instrumentation, statistical regression, selection, mortality, and selection by maturation interaction) that result in changes in the performance of the experimental group (see Table 5.2). A disadvantage of the posttest-only control-group design is that it does not enable researchers to check the initial equivalence of the experimental and control groups. Additionally, the posttest-only control-group design effectively controls for the four threats to internal validity (i.e., experimental treatment diffusion, compensatory rivalry by the control group, compensatory equalization of treatments, and resentful demoralization of the control group) that result in changes in the performance of the control group, if that group received an equally desirable but alternative intervention (see Table 5.2).

External Validity. As with the pretest–posttest control-group design, the posttest-only control-group design controls for many of the threats to external validity if the study is conducted effectively (see Table 5.3). A particular advantage is that the posttest-only control group design is able to control for pretest sensitization. That is, because there is no pretest, it is unlikely that participants can gain information allowing them to perform better on the posttest. Novelty and disruption effects and the Hawthorne effect may be threats to the external validity of a study if the researchers did not provide an equally desirable but alternative intervention. Posttest sensitization also may be a threat to the external validity of the study if the posttest has a powerful effect on the intervention. The remaining threats to the external validity of a study are dependent on the particular characteristics of the study and on how well it was conducted (see Table 5.3).

Recall the research question regarding comparison of four different math curricula? Read on to see how your design compares to how the actual study was designed.

Research Example 2: Comparison of Fourth-Grade Math Curricula

A posttest-only control-group design was used to compare four first-grade math curricula (Agodini & Harris, 2010). Over 8,000 first and second graders in 110 schools in 12 districts of 10 states participated. All participants were randomly assigned to one of four curricula. Random assignment was conducted at the school level. A random sample of 10 participants per classroom was included in the analysis. Because of the large number of participants and random assignment, researchers were relatively certain that performance across curriculum groups was equivalent at the outset. Independent variables were the math curricula including (1) Investigations in Number, Data, and Space; (2) Math Expressions; (3) Saxon Math, and (4) Scott Foresman–Addison Wesley Mathematics. Investigations in Number, Data, and Space is a student-centered approach that focuses on student understanding rather than specific problem-solving procedures. Math Expressions is a blend of student-centered and teacher-directed approaches. Saxon Math is a teacher-directed approach, with scripted lessons and daily student practice providing lessons on solving

---

The **posttest-only control-group design** *includes measurement of the dependent variable after implementation of the independent variable.*

only after ind variable

problems. Scott-Foresman–Addison Wesley Mathematics is an approach combining teacher-directed instruction with differentiated student activities, allowing teachers to select relevant and appropriate materials, including manipulatives. Dependent measures were end-of-year test scores on a nationally normed math assessment developed for the Early Childhood Longitudinal Study for first and second graders. For first graders, researchers found that mean math achievement on the posttest was higher for Math Expressions and Saxon Math, although neither was statistically significant. For second graders, researchers found a statistically significant difference with highest performance by the Saxon Math group.

Solomon Four-Group Design

The **Solomon four-group design** offers researchers the greatest amount of experimental control. Like the pretest–posttest control-group and posttest-only control-group designs, the Solomon four-group design assesses the effects of the independent variable relative to a control condition. Unlike these designs, the Solomon four-group design enables researchers to assess the presence of both pretest sensitization and an interaction between the pretest measures and the independent variable. Although the posttest-only control-group design controls for pretest sensitization and for an interaction between the pretest measures and the independent variable, it does not enable researchers to determine their presence. Thus, the Solomon four-group design not only controls for testing (threat to internal validity) and pretest sensitization (threat to external validity), but it also enables researchers to assess their effects on the intervention outcomes.

The Solomon four-group design essentially combines the pretest–posttest control-group design and the posttest-only control-group design (compare Figure 5.3 with Figures 5.1 and 5.2). The Solomon four-group design begins with the random selection of participants from a population to form a sample. Participants from the sample are then randomly assigned to one of four groups. Two groups serve as experimental groups, and two serve as control groups. Measurement of the dependent variable is taken prior to the introduction of the independent variable with one of the experimental groups and one of the control groups. The independent variable is then introduced, followed by postintervention measurement of the dependent variable for all four of the groups. Figure 5.3 depicts the form of the Solomon four-group design.

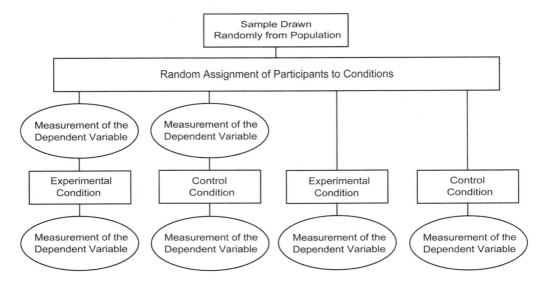

FIGURE 5.3. Solomon four-group design.

The basic assumption of the Solomon four-group design is the same as the pretest–posttest and posttest-only control-group designs, in that the participants of the experimental and control groups are equivalent prior to the introduction of the independent variable. Any differences observed at the end of the study are assumed to be due to the independent variable and, in some cases, the preintervention measures of the dependent variable. As we might expect, the Solomon four-group design requires a great deal more effort and resources to implement than the pretest–posttest and the posttest-only control-group designs. The extra effort and resources needed to implement a Solomon four-group design may be worth it in cases in which it is critical to determine the effects of pretest sensitization and the interaction of the pretest and the independent variable.

The goal of the Solomon four-group design is the same as that of the pretest–posttest and posttest-only control-group designs; that is, the goal is to keep the experiences of the experimental and control groups as identical as possible except for the introduction of the independent variable. Changes in the posttest scores due to any other extraneous variables will be reflected in the scores of the control group.

Analysis of Data

The Solomon four-group design, in its simplest form, is essentially a 2 × 2 factorial design (i.e., two or more independent variables [called factors] affect the dependent variable either independently [main effect] or in combination with each other [interaction effect]), in which the presence or absence of a pretest is one factor (signified by the first "2"), and the presence or absence of the independent variable is the second factor (signified by the second "2"). (*Note.* Factorial designs are discussed below.) Thus, data from a Solomon four-group design is typically analyzed with an ANOVA. Any significant main effects (e.g., differences between the presence and absence of the independent variable) and interaction effects (e.g., the presence or absence of the pretest differentially affects the independent variable such that the independent variable is more or less effective when the pretest is provided) are then explored using post

hoc analysis procedures such as the Scheffé test. Additionally, a nonparametric test, such as the Kruskal–Wallis test, should be used if the data violate the assumptions underlying parametric tests (i.e., homogeneity of variance, normal distribution of data, and interval or ratio scale data).

Internal Validity. The Solomon four-group design controls for all eight of the threats to internal validity (i.e., history, maturation, testing, instrumentation, statistical regression, selection, mortality, and selection by maturation interaction) that result in changes in the performance of the experimental groups (see Table 5.2). As discussed before, an important advantage of the Solomon four-group design over the pretest–posttest and the posttest-only control-group designs is that it enables researchers to determine the effects of the preintervention measurement of the dependent variable on the postintervention measurement of the dependent variable. Additionally, the Solomon four-group design effectively controls for the four threats to internal validity (i.e., experimental treatment diffusion: compensatory rivalry by the control group, compensatory equalization of treatments, and resentful demoralization of the control group). These may result in changes in the performance of the control group if the control group received an equally desirable but alternative intervention (see Table 5.2).

External Validity. The Solomon four-group design controls for many of the threats to external validity if the investigation is conducted effectively (see Table 5.3). Novelty and disruption effects and the Hawthorne effect may be threats to the external validity of a study if researchers do not provide an equally desirable but alternative intervention. Although pretest sensitization is controlled for, posttest sensitization may be a threat to the external validity of the study if the posttest has a powerful effect on the intervention. The remaining threats to the external validity of a study are dependent on the

> The **Solomon four-group design** *is a combination of the pretest–posttest control-group design and the posttest-only control-group design.*

particular characteristics of the study and how well the study was conducted.

Recall the research question regarding the effects of pretesting and pedometers? Read on to see how your design compares to how the actual study was designed.

Research Example 3: Effects of Pretests and Pedometer Use

A Solomon four-group design was used to assess effects of pretesting and pedometers on walking intentions and behavior (Spence, Burgess, Rodgers, & Murray, 2009). The purpose of the study was to determine whether the administration of a pretest questionnaire differentially influenced the posttest self-report of walking behavior of participants as a result of using a pedometer. Participants were 63 female university students randomly assigned to one of four conditions: (1) pedometer and pretest, (2) pedometer and no pretest, (3) no pedometer and pretest, and (4) no pedometer and no pretest. There were 16 participants in all conditions except no pedometer and pretest ($n = 15$). Pretest conditions included questions on walking, intentions to walk, and self-efficacy for walking. The Solomon four-group configuration was used to control for pretest sensitization. Pedometer and pretest participants completed the walking behavior and self-efficacy questionnaires. Pedometer and pretest participants, as well as pedometer-only participants, were then given a pedometer and provided with information about the device. No pedometer and pretest, as well as pedometer and no-pretest participants, were told they would have the opportunity to wear the pedometer later. Posttest conditions were identical to pretest conditions and were administered 1 week later. Data were analyzed using a 2 × 2 (Pedometers × Pretest) ANOVA. The researchers note that significant pretest × pedometer interactions would have indicated the presence of pretest sensitization; however, no such results were obtained. After controlling for pretest reports of walking, wearing pedometers resulted in statistically significant increases in self-reports of walking. About 75% of pedometer users returned log sheets indicating that average number of steps per day was 10,293.

Positive correlations were found between self-reported walking and average number of steps taken per day, and total steps taken per week.

WHAT ARE FACTORIAL EXPERIMENTAL DESIGNS?

Up to now, we have focused on experimental research designs that incorporate one independent variable (i.e., single factor). The goal in such designs is to establish a causal relationship between two variables. However, researchers are often interested in assessing the effects of two or more independent variables (factors) and in identifying which participants benefit most from the independent variable. Researchers use **factorial experimental designs** to assess the effects of two or more independent variables (described in this chapter) or the interaction of participant characteristics with the independent variable (described in Chapter 6, this volume; Graziano & Raulin, 2010). As such, researchers use factorial designs to determine whether the effect of a particular variable studied concurrently with other variables will have the same effect as it would when studied in isolation.

Analysis of Data

The factorial designs and associated statistical analysis procedures used by researchers can be quite complex. For example, a factorial design in a study that compares three methods of teaching reading (i.e., direct instruction, whole language, and language experience) could be extended to include a comparison of short (i.e., periods of intensive instruction) versus massed (i.e., extended period of intensive instruction) learning conditions. The effect on achievement of three methods of teaching and two learning conditions could be investigated with a 3 (direct instruction vs. whole language vs. language experience) × 2 (short vs. massed learning) ANOVA.

It is informative to look more closely at the preceding example to identify the two factors included in factorial designs. The first and second factors are the three methods of reading instruction (i.e., direct instruction, whole language, and language experience) and the type of instruction (short vs. massed learning), respectively. These factors are considered independent variables and are manipulated (termed *stimulus variables*). Additionally, it is important to note that factorial designs may involve repeated measurement of the same participants. The repeated measurement of participants on one or more factors can greatly complicate a factorial design.

A key advantage of factorial designs is that information is obtained about the interaction between factors. Going back to the previous example, one method of teaching reading may interact with a condition of learning and render that combination either better or worse than any other combination. Of course, one of the disadvantages of the factorial design is that the number of combinations may become quite unwieldy to conduct and difficult to interpret. In education and psychology, it is advisable to avoid overly complex factorial experiments. We direct the reader to Ferguson (1989) and McBurney and White (2009) for more information on factorial designs. The particular factorial design used by researchers primarily depends on the following factors:

1. The number of independent variables.

2. The attributes of the independent variable (referred to as a *between-subjects factor* when comparing different groups).

3. Repeated measurement of participants (also referred to as a *within-subjects factor*).

4. Mixing within (repeated measures) and between (comparison of group means) subjects factors.

5. Relative number of participants in each intervention group.

Internal Validity

The threats to internal validity that a factorial design controls for are dependent on the basic underlying true experimental design (see Table 5.2). For example, if the basic, underlying true experimental design is a pretest–posttest control group design, the eight threats to internal validity (i.e., history, maturation, testing, instrumentation, statistical regression, selection,

mortality, and selection by maturation interaction) that result in changes in the performance of the experimental group are controlled. Additionally, the four threats to internal validity that cause changes in the performance of the control group are controlled for in factorial designs, because the different experimental groups are receiving some form of the intervention.

External Validity

One of the greatest strengths of a factorial design is that it enhances the external validity of the study. Analyzing the effects of the intervention on different subsets of the sample increases the extent to which the results can be generalized "across participants" and provides an understanding of the interaction of personological variables and treatment effects. As with all of the true experimental designs, factorial designs control for many of the threats to external validity if the investigation is conducted effectively (see Table 5.3).

Recall the research question regarding the effects of sentence length and number of difficult words per paragraph on reading rates? Read on to see how your design compares to how the actual study was designed.

Research Example 4: Effects of Sentence Length and Number of Difficult Words per Paragraph on Reading Rates

This example was not drawn from experimental literature; it is hypothetical. However, we include it to illustrate important characteristics and processes related to factorial designs. We consider an example comparing a single-factor experimental design and a two-factor design that address the same research question to show how researchers use factorial designs. Suppose we are interested in assessing the effects of sentence length and number of difficult words per paragraph on the reading rates

> **Factorial experimental designs** *assess the effects of two or more independent variables or the interaction of participant characteristics with the independent variable.*

of elementary-school-age students. The two independent variables of interest are sentence length and number of difficult words per paragraph. Suppose we choose two sentence lengths (≤ 20 words and > 20 words) and two levels of the number of difficult words per paragraph (≤ 2 and > 2). We would need to use two separate studies to assess the effects of these two independent variables using single-factor experimental designs. Table 5.4 presents what these two experimental designs might look like. The study on the top (Design 1) is designed to assess the effects of sentence length on reading rate, and the study in the middle (Design 2) is designed to assess the effects of the number of difficult words per paragraph. In both studies, 20 participants would be assigned to each of the experimental conditions, for a total of 40 participants per study (total of 80 participants). Except for students in the sentence length and the number of difficult words per paragraph conditions, all of the participants would be treated the same. At the completion of the study, we would analyze the data and be able to make a statement regarding the influence of sentence length and number of difficult words per paragraph on rate of reading.

Compare these two single-factor studies with the two-factor factorial design (Design 3) at the bottom of Table 5.4. The two independent variables (i.e., sentence length and number of difficult words per paragraph) are manipulated simultaneously. Because both independent variables have two levels, there are four (2 × 2) unique groups. This design would be called a 2 × 2 factorial design. Inspection of Table 5.4 reveals that the sample size in each group is 10. This number was chosen to provide a direct comparison with the single-factor studies (i.e., we start with 40 participants, then randomly assign 10 participants to serve in each of the four groups). At the completion of the study, we would analyze the data and make a statement regarding the influence of sentence length and number of difficult words per paragraph on rate of reading (main effects). We would make a statement regarding the interaction of sentence length and number of difficult words per paragraph (i.e., interaction effects).

Our comparison of two single-factor designs with a two-factor factorial design is only correct up to a point. The factorial design provides the same information as the two single-factor designs only when there is no interaction

TABLE 5.4. Comparison of Single-Factor and Two-Factor Experimental Designs

Design 1

Sentence length	
≤ 20 words	> 20 words
20 participants	20 participants

Design 2

Average number of difficult words per paragraph	
≤ 2 words	> 2 words
20 participants	20 participants

Design 3

Sentence length	Average number of difficult words per paragraph	
	≤ 2 words	> 2 words
≤ 20 words	10 participants	10 participants
> 20 words	10 participants	10 participants

between the two independent variables. There are no interaction effects when the effect of one of the independent variables is the same at each level of the other independent variable. Returning to our example, the effects of sentence length are the same regardless of the number of difficult words per paragraph and vice versa. On the other hand, if the effects of sentence length are different across the different levels of the number of difficult words per paragraph, there is an interaction, and the information provided by the main effect is not the same as that in the single-factor designs. This finding is not problematic, because the researchers would have discovered information that is not available from the single-factor designs—how the two independent variables combine to influence reading rate. Additionally, researchers will not be as interested in the main effects when there is an interaction effect, because anything they say with regard to the effects of one independent variable would have to be qualified by its differential effect across the levels of the other independent variable.

Finally, it is important to address the concepts of main and interaction effects, because they are key concepts associated with factorial designs. We examine an illustrative example in which a 2 × 2 factorial design yields only main effects, and

in which the same 2 × 2 factorial design yields interaction effects. It is important to note that we are presenting a simplified explanation of main and interaction effects here. We direct the reader to Keppel (1973) and Ferguson (1989) for more information on main and interaction effects.

Using the same example noted earlier, Table 5.5 presents Study 1, in which a main effect for sentence length was obtained, and Study 2, in which an interaction effect between sentence length and number of difficult words per paragraph was obtained. Inspection of the results of Study 1 reveals that changes in participants' reading rates for sentences with ≤ 20 words and > 20 words were relatively (statistically similar) consistent across the number of difficult words per paragraph. Participants generally read faster when the sentences contained < 20 words. These results are consistent with only obtaining a main effect. On the other hand, inspection of the results of Study 2 reveals a different pattern. Participants' reading rates differed across the number of difficult words per paragraph. The reading rates of participants were similar regardless of sentence length if there were less than two difficult words per paragraph. However, the reading rates of participants were significantly lower when there were more than two difficult words per paragraph.

TABLE 5.5. Comparison of Main Effects and Interaction Effects

Study 1

Sentence length	Average number of difficult words per paragraph	
	≤ 2 words	> 2 words
	Mean	*Mean*
≤ 20 words	112	114
> 20 words	90	88

Study 2

Sentence length	Average number of difficult words per paragraph	
	≤ 2 words	> 2 words
	Mean	*Mean*
≤ 20 words	110	115
> 20 words	112	85

WHAT ARE QUASI-EXPERIMENTAL DESIGNS?

Quasi-experimental designs differ from true experimental designs in two ways. First, participants are not randomly selected from a specified population. Second, participants are not randomly assigned to experimental and control groups. Participants are intact groups, such as all sophomores in a high school classroom or members of an afterschool study group. Nevertheless, quasi-experimental designs provide a relatively high degree of experimental control in natural settings, and they clearly represent a step up from preexperimental designs (described later), because they enable researchers to compare the performance of the experimental group with that of a control group. In other words, quasi-experimental designs enable researchers to move their experimentation out of the laboratory and into a natural context. It is important for critical research consumers to understand the strengths and weaknesses associated with quasi-experimental designs.

WHAT ARE THE COMMON QUASI-EXPERIMENTAL DESIGNS?

We examine four common quasi-experimental designs—static-group comparison, nonequivalent control-group, counterbalanced, and time-series designs. Note that these four designs are presented in terms of a single independent variable and dependent variable.

Static-Group Comparison Design

The **static-group comparison design** begins with the identification of two naturally assembled experimental and control groups (e.g., students in two classrooms). The naturally assembled experimental and control groups should be as similar as possible, and the assignment to one group or the other is assumed to be random. The independent variable is then introduced to the experimental group, followed by the postintervention measurement of the dependent variable. Figure 5.4 depicts the form of the static-group comparison design.

Analysis of Data

The data from a static-group comparison design can be analyzed with a *t*-test of the difference between the posttest mean scores of the experimental and control groups. Additionally, a nonparametric test such as the Mann–Whitney *U* test should be used if the data violate the assumptions underlying these parametric tests (i.e., homogeneity of variance, normal distribution of data, and interval or ratio scale data).

Internal Validity. The use of a comparison group in the static-group comparison design enhances its experimental control in comparison to preexperimental designs (described later). However, in the absence of random assignment of participants to groups, the lack of a pretest greatly weakens its ability to control for a number of threats to internal validity. Inspection of Table 5.6 reveals that the static-group comparison design controls for four of the threats to internal validity (i.e., statistical regression, instrumentation, testing, and history) that may result in changes in performance of the experimental group. The remaining threats to internal validity (i.e., maturation, selection, selection by maturation interaction, mortality, resentful demoralization of the control group, diffusion of treatment, compensatory rivalry by the control group, and compensatory equalization) represent possible concerns to the internal validity of the static-group comparison design.

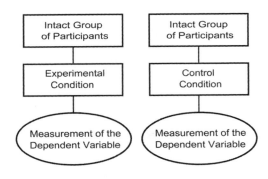

FIGURE 5.4. Static-group comparison design.

TABLE 5.6. Threats to Internal Validity Associated with Quasi-Experimental Designs

Threat	Research design			
	Static group comparison	Nonequivalent control group	Counterbalanced	Time-series
1. Maturation	Possible concern	Controlled	Controlled	Controlled
2. Selection	Possible concern	Controlled	Controlled	Controlled
3. Selection by maturation interaction	Possible concern	Controlled	Possible concern	Controlled
4. Statistical regression	Controlled	Possible concern	Controlled	Controlled
5. Mortality	Possible concern	Controlled	Controlled	Controlled
6. Instrumentation	Controlled	Controlled	Controlled	Controlled
7. Testing	Controlled	Controlled	Controlled	Controlled
8. History	Controlled	Controlled	Controlled	Controlled
9. Resentful demoralization of the control group	Possible concern[a]	Possible concern[a]	Controlled	Not applicable
10. Diffusion of treatment	Possible concern[a]	Possible concern[a]	Controlled	Not applicable
11. Compensatory rivalry by the control group	Possible concern[a]	Possible concern[a]	Controlled	Not applicable
12. Compensatory equalization	Possible concern[a]	Possible concern[a]	Controlled	Not applicable

Note. This table is meant only as a general guideline. Decisions with regard to threats to internal validity must be made after the specifics of an investigation are known and understood. Thus, interpretations of internal validity threats must be made on a study-by-study basis.

[a] These threats to internal validity are controlled if the control group received an equally desirable but alternative intervention.

External Validity. Inspection of Table 5.7 reveals that the threats to external validity associated with the population (i.e., generalization across participants and interaction of personological variables and treatment effects) are a concern, because participants were not randomly selected from a specified population. Novelty and disruption effects, as well as the Hawthorne effect, may be threats to the external validity of the study if the researchers did not provide an equally desirable but alternative intervention. Posttest sensitization also may be a threat to external validity if the posttest has a powerful effect on the independent variable. The remaining threats to the external validity of a study are dependent on the particular characteristics of the study, and on how well the study was conducted.

Recall the research question regarding quality of life for adults with and without disabilities? Read on to see how your design compares to how the actual study was designed.

Research Example 5: Differences in Quality of Life

A static-group comparison design was used to investigate whether differences exist in dimensions related to *quality of life* for adults with developmental disabilities compared to adults in the general population (Sheppard-Jones, Prout, & Kleinart, 2005). *Quality of life* has been defined as "general feelings of well-being, feelings of positive social involvement, and opportunities to

---

Quasi-experimental designs *are similar to true experimental designs except that participants are neither selected from the specified population nor randomly assigned to groups.*

The **static-group comparison design** *is the same as the posttest-only control-group design described earlier, except for the absence of the random selection of participants from a population and random assignment of participants to groups.*

TABLE 5.7. Threats to External Validity Associated with Quasi-Experimental Designs

Threat	Research design			
	Static group comparison	Nonequivalent control group	Counterbalanced	Time-series
1. Generalization across participants	Concern	Concern	Concern[b]	Concern
2. Interaction of personological variables and treatment effects	Concern	Concern	Concern[b]	Concern
3. Verification of independent variable	Possible concern	Possible concern	Possible concern	Possible concern
4. Multiple treatment interference	Controlled	Controlled	Controlled	Controlled
5. Novelty and disruption effects	Controlled[a]	Controlled[a]	Possible concern	Controlled
6. Hawthorne effect	Controlled[a]	Controlled[a]	Possible concern	Controlled
7. Experimenter effects	Possible concern	Possible concern	Possible concern	Controlled
8. Pretest sensitization	Controlled	Possible concern	Controlled	Controlled
9. Posttest sensitization	Possible concern	Controlled	Controlled	Controlled
10. Interaction of time of measurement and treatment effects	Possible concern	Possible concern	Possible concern	Possible concern
11. Measurement of the dependent variable	Possible concern	Possible concern	Possible concern	Possible concern
12. Interaction of history and treatment effects	Possible concern	Possible concern	Possible concern	Possible concern

Note. This table is meant only as a general guideline. Decisions with regard to threats to external validity must be made after the specifics of an investigation are known and understood. Thus, interpretations of external validity threats must be made on a study-by-study basis.
[a]These threats to external validity are controlled if the control group received an equally desirable but alternative intervention.
[b]These threats to external validity are not a concern if the researcher has randomly selected the participants from a specified population.

achieve personal potential" (Shalock et al., 2002, p. 458). Two groups were compared: (1) consumers, that is, individuals with intellectual or other developmental disabilities (e.g., autism spectrum disorder) and (2) the general population. The consumer group comprised 502 randomly selected adults with disabilities receiving state-funded services. Consumers had a mean age of 40 years, were largely single (95%), and lived in varied environments (40% in group homes, 40% with family, 15% in institutions or nursing homes, 5% other). The general population group comprised 576 adults with a mean age of 45, who were largely married (60%) and living on their own (99%). Groups were similar in terms of gender and race. The measurement instrument, called the Core Indicators Consumer Survey (Human Services Research Institute, 2001), was completed in a face-to-face or telephone interview. Items on the survey related to relationships, safety, health, choice-making opportunities, community participation, well-being and

satisfaction, and rights. Individuals responded to survey items using a 3-point Likert-type scale or by responding "yes" or "no." Individuals in the consumer group were interviewed directly, although in 194 cases (38.6%), proxies such as legal guardians responded on behalf of the consumers because of limitations in communication. Individuals in the general population group, interviewed via telephone, were selected randomly in a random-digit dialing procedure. The response rate for the telephone survey was 36.4%. Researchers used MANOVA to analyze survey data. Numerous variables were statistically significant. Results indicated that consumer group members were more lonely, desirous of more work hours, and afraid at home in their neighborhood. Consumers were less likely to have a choice as to where and with whom they lived or to exercise choice in free-time activities. They had fewer options from which to choose in terms of activities, transportation, and place of residence.

Nonequivalent Control-Group Design

The **nonequivalent control-group design** begins with the identification of naturally assembled experimental and control groups. Again, the naturally occurring experimental and control groups should be as similar as possible, and the assignment to one group or the other is assumed to be random. Measurement of the dependent variable is taken prior to the introduction of the independent variable. The independent variable is then introduced, followed by the postintervention measurement of the dependent variable. Figure 5.5 depicts the form of the nonequivalent control-group design.

Analysis of Data

The data from a nonequivalent control-group design are analyzed using ANCOVA, because the primary threat to the internal validity of the nonequivalent control-group design is the possibility that differences on the posttest scores of the experimental and control groups are the result of initial differences rather than the effects of the independent variable. ANCOVA statistically equates initial differences between the experimental and control groups by adjusting the posttest means of the groups.

Internal Validity. Although the nonequivalent control-group design does not provide the same level of experimental control as the pretest–posttest control-group design, it enables researchers to address many of the threats to internal validity adequately. The effectiveness of the nonequivalent control-group design in addressing the threats to internal validity increases with the similarity of the pretest scores of the experimental and control groups. Inspection of Table 5.6 reveals that the nonequivalent control-group design controls for seven of the threats to internal validity (i.e., maturation, selection, selection by maturation interaction, mortality, instrumentation, testing, and history) that result in changes in the performance of the experimental groups. The nonequivalent control-group design does not control for statistical regression that can result in changes in the performance of the experimental group. The four threats to internal validity (i.e., experimental treatment diffusion, compensatory rivalry by the control group, compensatory equalization of treatments, and resentful demoralization of the control group) that result in changes in the performance of the control group are controlled if researchers provide the control group an equally desirable but alternative intervention.

External Validity. As with the static-group comparison design, the threats to external validity associated with the population (i.e., generalization across participants and interaction of personological variables and treatment effects) are a concern, because participants were not randomly selected from a specified population (see Table 5.7). Novelty and disruption effects and the Hawthorne effect may be threats to the external validity of the study if the researchers did not provide an equally desirable but alternative intervention. Pretest and posttest sensitization also may be threats to the external validity if the pretest and posttest have a powerful effect on the intervention. The remaining threats to the external validity of a study are dependent on the particular characteristics of the study.

> *The **nonequivalent control-group design** is similar to the pretest–posttest control-group design described previously, except for the absence of the random selection of participants from a population and the random assignment of participants to groups.*

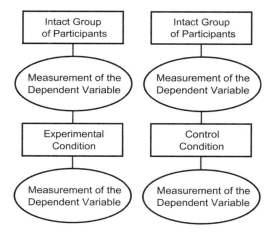

FIGURE 5.5. Nonequivalent control-group design.

Counterbalanced Designs

Counterbalanced designs encompass a wide range of designs in which independent variables are introduced to all participants. Counterbalanced designs are useful when researchers are interested in studying multiple variables. Counterbalanced designs are also useful when it is not possible to assign participants randomly to the experimental and control groups, and when participant attrition may be a problem. The level of experimental control achieved with a counterbalanced design is greater than that of the nonequivalent control-group design, because each participant serves as his/her own control. Counterbalanced designs are also referred to as "rotation experiments," crossover designs, and "switchover designs."

In its simplest form, the counterbalanced design begins with the identification of two naturally assembled groups. Measurement of the dependent variable is taken prior to the introduction of the independent variable. The independent variable is introduced to one of the groups, followed by postintervention measurement of the dependent variable. The independent variable is then introduced to the other group followed by the postintervention measurement of the dependent variable. Figure 5.6 depicts the form of the two-group counterbalanced design using naturally assembled groups. (Researchers may randomly assign participants to groups.)

Analysis of Data

Although data from counterbalanced designs can be analyzed with a number of statistical tests, a repeated measures ANOVA is most commonly used. The advantage of any repeated measurement analysis procedure is that it controls for differences between participants. That is, repeated measurement analyses eliminate differences between participants from the experimental error. Additionally, a nonparametric measure such as the Kruskal–Wallis test should be used if the data violate the assumptions underlying parametric tests (i.e., homogeneity of variance, normal distribution of data, and interval or ratio scale data).

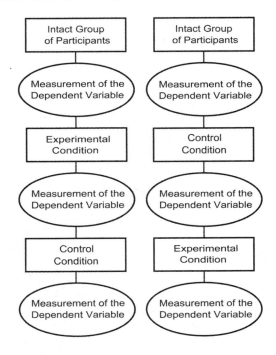

FIGURE 5.6. Two-group counterbalanced design.

Internal Validity. The counterbalanced design provides a higher level of experimental control than does the nonequivalent control-group design. This greater degree of experimental control is achieved because the counterbalancing of the independent variable enables researchers to compare participants' performance in groups rather than in experimental and control groups; thus, counterbalanced designs eliminate the need for groups to be equivalent.

Inspection of Table 5.6 reveals that counterbalanced designs effectively deal with seven of the threats to internal validity (i.e., maturation, selection, statistical regression, mortality, instrumentation, testing, and history) that result in changes in performance of the experimental group. Counterbalanced designs do not effectively control for selection by maturation interaction effects, because there is no nonintervention control group. The four threats to internal validity (i.e., experimental treatment diffusion, compensatory rivalry by the control group, compensatory equalization of treatments, and resentful demoralization by the control group) that result in changes in performance of the control group are controlled for if researchers ensure that there is no treatment diffusion.

External Validity. The threats to external validity associated with the population (i.e., generalization across participants and interaction of personological variables and treatment effects) are not a concern when participants have been randomly selected from a specified population (see Table 5.7). If this is not the case, then these threats to external validity are of concern. Novelty and disruption, the Hawthorne effect, and experimenter effects may be evident because of the ongoing implementation of different independent variables. Pretest and posttest sensitization are unlikely threats to the external validity of a study because of the repeated measurement of the dependent variable. The remaining threats to the external validity of a study are dependent on the particular characteristics of the study and how well it was conducted.

Time-Series Designs

Any effects attributable to the independent variable are indicated by discontinuity in the preintervention and postintervention series of scores. **Time-series designs** differ from single-case designs (see Chapters 11 to 13) in that the unit of analysis is a group of individuals, not single participants. Additionally, time-series designs can be used in an ex post facto or experimental fashion. It is important to note that a variety of time-series designs involve different numbers of groups, independent variables, and so on.

A time-series design begins with the identification of a naturally assembled group. Measurement of the dependent variable occurs a number of times prior to the introduction of the independent variable, which is followed by measurement of the dependent variable a number of more times. Figure 5.7 depicts the form of time-series designs.

Analysis of Data

Data from time-series designs can be analyzed in a variety of ways. Researchers may graph

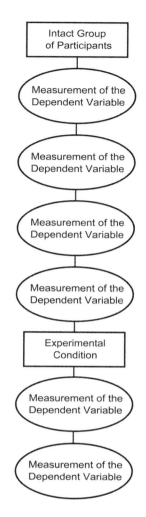

FIGURE 5.7. Time-series design.

In **counterbalanced designs**, *two or more groups get the same independent variables, but the independent variables are introduced in different orders.*

Time-series designs *are quasi-experimental designs involving a series of repeated measurements of a group of research participants.*

the scores and look for changes in the preinter- vention and postintervention pattern of scores. Each score is plotted separately on the graph, and scores are connected by a line. A vertical line is inserted into the series of scores at the point the independent variable is introduced. Researchers then use the graphed data to com- pare the level, slope, and variation in the prein- tervention and postintervention scores. Visual analysis methods for assessing intervention effects are described more completely in our presentation of single-case designs (see Chap- ters 11 to 13). Statistical methods used with data from time-series designs can range from multi- ple regression to log linear analysis procedures. These statistical analysis procedures are all aimed at determining whether the preinterven- tion and postintervention patterns of scores dif- fer statistically from one another. We direct the reader to Box, Hunter, and Hunter (2005) and to Glass, Wilson, and Gottman (2008) for complete descriptions of statistical procedures for analyz- ing data from time-series studies.

Internal Validity. Time-series designs pro- vide a high degree of experimental control even though they do not employ a control group. Inspection of Table 5.6 reveals that time-series designs control for the eight threats to internal validity (i.e., maturation, selection, selection by maturation interaction, statistical regression, mortality, instrumentation, testing, history) that result in changes in performance of the experimental group. Instrumentation might be a concern if the calibration of the measurement device employed by the researcher changed over the course of the study. Of course, it would be unlikely for such a change to occur in direct connection with the introduction of the inde- pendent variable. The four threats to internal validity that result in changes in the perfor- mance of the control group are not applicable with time-series designs.

External Validity. As with all quasi-experi- mental designs, the threats to external validity associated with the population (i.e., generaliza- tion across participants and interaction of per- sonological variables and treatment effects) are a concern, because participants have not been randomly selected from a specified population

(see Table 5.7). Novelty and disruption, the Hawthorne effect, and experimenter effects tend not to be a problem because of the ongo- ing measurement of the dependent variable. Additionally, pretest and posttest sensitization are unlikely threats to the external validity of a study because of the repeated measure- ment of the dependent variable. The remaining threats to the external validity of a study are dependent on the particular characteristics of the study and on how well the study was con- ducted.

WHAT ARE PREEXPERIMENTAL DESIGNS?

Preexperimental designs primarily differ from true experimental designs and two of the quasi-experimental designs (i.e., counterbal- anced and time-series designs) in that they do not include a control group. The lack of a control group essentially eliminates researchers' abil- ity to control for any of the threats to internal validity. The lack of control over possible extra- neous variables that may cause changes in the dependent variable renders preexperimental designs almost useless to furthering knowledge in education and psychology. In short, research- ers cannot ensure that a change in the value of the independent variable is accompanied by a change in the value of the dependent variable, which is one of the three key requirements for asserting that a causal relationship exists between two variables.

Nevertheless, we detail preexperimental designs because they are used extensively in educational and psychological research despite these obvious problems. It is important for critical research consumers to understand the weaknesses associated with preexperimental designs.

WHAT ARE THE TYPES OF PREEXPERIMENTAL DESIGNS?

We consider two preexperimental designs— one-shot case study and one-group pretest– posttest design. Both designs are presented in terms of a single independent variable and dependent variable.

One-Shot Case Study

In the one-shot case study, an independent variable is introduced to a group of participants. The one-shot case study begins with the identification of a naturally assembled group. The independent variable is then administered, followed by the measurement of the dependent variable. Figure 5.8 depicts the form of the one-shot case study.

Analysis of Data

The data from a one-shot case study may be analyzed with the one-sample t-test if there is a specified population mean. In essence, the obtained mean of the study group is compared to the specified population mean. The results of the one-sample t-test indicates whether the obtained mean of the study group differs from that of the specified population mean.

Internal Validity. Researchers utilizing one-shot case studies often collect extensive information or use standardized measures in an effort to document the effects of the independent variable. Although such efforts may seem a reasonable replacement for the experimental control associated with the true experimental designs, they do not lead to any definitive assessment of the potential extraneous variables that may have resulted in changes in the scores of individuals.

Inspection of Table 5.8 reveals that the one-shot case study has low internal validity. Four of the eight threats to internal validity (i.e., history, maturation, selection, mortality) that may result in changes in performance of the experimental group are concerns. The remaining four threats to internal validity (i.e., selection by maturation interaction, instrumentation, testing, and statistical regression) that may result in changes in performance of the experimental group and the four threats to internal validity (i.e., experimental treatment diffusion, compensatory rivalry by the control group, compensatory equalization of treatments, and resentful demoralization of the control group) that result in changes in performance of the control group are not applicable.

External Validity. The one-shot case study does not control for most of the threats to external validity (see Table 5.9). Pretest sensitization is the only threat to external validity that can be controlled. Researchers who are limited to studying one group of participants should include a pretest in their experimental design (this design is described in what follows).

One-Group Pretest–Posttest Design

The one-group pretest–posttest design differs from the one-shot case study in that a pretest measure is administered prior to introduction of the independent variable. Effects of the independent variable are determined by comparing the pretest and posttest scores of the group of participants. The one-group pretest–posttest design begins with the identification of a naturally assembled group. Measurement of the dependent variable occurs prior to the introduction of the independent variable. The independent variable is then introduced followed by measurement of the dependent variable. Figure 5.9 depicts the form of the one-group pretest–posttest design.

Analysis of Data

Data from a one-group pretest–posttest design may be analyzed with a correlated t-test. A paired set of variables is the minimum requirement for a correlated t-test. The pretest scores are compared to the posttest scores. The results of the correlated t-test indicate whether the

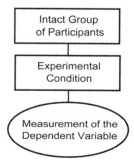

FIGURE 5.8. One-shot case study.

> **Preexperimental designs** *do not include a control group.*

TABLE 5.8. Threats to Internal Validity Associated with Preexperimental Designs

	Research design	
Threat	One-shot case study	One-group pretest–posttest
1. Maturation	Concern	Concern
2. Selection	Concern	Controlled
3. Selection by maturation interaction	Not applicable	Concern
4. Statistical regression	Not applicable	Concern
5. Mortality	Concern	Controlled
6. Instrumentation	Not applicable	Concern
7. Testing	Not applicable	Concern
8. History	Concern	Concern
9. Resentful demoralization of the control group	Not applicable	Not applicable
10. Diffusion of treatment	Not applicable	Not applicable
11. Compensatory rivalry by the control group	Not applicable	Not applicable
12. Compensatory equalization	Not applicable	Not applicable

Note. This table is meant only as a general guideline. Decisions with regard to threats to internal validity must be made after the specifics of an investigation are known and understood. Thus, interpretations of internal validity threats must be made on a study-by-study basis.

TABLE 5.9. Threats to External Validity Associated with Preexperimental Designs

	Research design	
Threat	One-shot case study	One-group pretest–posttest
1. Generalization across participants	Possible concern	Possible concern
2. Interaction of personological variables and treatment effects	Possible concern	Possible concern
3. Verification of independent variable	Possible concern	Possible concern
4. Multiple treatment interference	Not applicable	Not applicable
5. Novelty and disruption effects	Possible concern	Possible concern
6. Hawthorne effect	Possible concern	Possible concern
7. Experimenter effects	Possible concern	Possible concern
8. Pretest sensitization	Not applicable	Possible concern
9. Posttest sensitization	Possible concern	Possible concern
10. Interaction of time of measurement and treatment effects	Possible concern	Possible concern
11. Measurement of the dependent variable	Possible concern	Possible concern
12. Interaction of history and treatment effects	Possible concern	Possible concern

Note. This table is meant only as a general guideline. Decisions with regard to threats to internal validity must be made after the specifics of an investigation are known and understood. Thus, interpretations of internal validity threats must be made on a study-by-study basis.

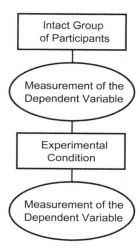

FIGURE 5.9. One-group pretest–posttest design.

pretest and posttest means of the study group differ from one another. Additionally, a nonparametric test such as the Wilcoxon signed rank test should be used if the data violate the assumptions underlying these parametric tests (i.e., homogeneity of variance, normal distribution of data, and interval or ratio scale data).

Internal Validity. Although the use of a pretest in the one-group pretest–posttest design renders it better than the one-shot case study, it still does not provide much experimental control. Inspection of Table 5.8 reveals that the one-group pretest–posttest design does not control for six of the eight threats to internal validity (i.e., history, maturation, testing, instrumentation, statistical regression, and selection by maturation interaction) that may result in changes in performance of the experimental group. The one-group pretest–posttest design does control for selection and mortality that may result in changes in the dependent variable. As with the one-shot case study, the remaining four threats to internal validity (i.e., experimental treatment diffusion, compensatory rivalry by the control group, compensatory equalization of treatments, and resentful demoralization of the control group) that result in changes in performance of the control group are not applicable, because there is no control group.

External Validity. As with the one-shot case study, researchers often provide a great deal of detail in an effort to document the effects of the dependent variable. These efforts should not alleviate concerns regarding the external validity of the one-group pretest–posttest design. Inspection of Table 5.9 shows that the one-group pretest–posttest design does not control for any of the threats to external validity.

WHEN SHOULD RESEARCHERS USE EACH EXPERIMENTAL RESEARCH DESIGN?

Experimental research designs are used to establish causal relationships. It should be clear by now that there is a clear difference in the extent to which true experimental, quasi-experimental, and preexperimental research designs allow researchers to assert with confidence that there is a causal relationship between variables. True experimental research designs provide the highest level of confidence and are the designs of choice to establish a causal relationship between variables. The internal and external validity of true experimental designs are high, because these research designs rely on the random selection of participants from a population and the random assignment of participants to experimental and control groups. The random selection of participants from a population increases the external validity of the study, and the random assignment of participants to experimental and control groups increases internal validity of the study. Establishing the initial equivalence of the experimental and control groups enables the researcher to conclude confidently that any statistically significant differences are due to the independent variables. Thus, researchers who are attempting to demonstrate a cause-and-effect relationship should use a true experimental design if they can randomly select and assign participants.

Although quasi-experimental research designs do not provide the same level of control as true experimental research designs, they control reasonably well for threats to the internal and external validity of studies. Quasi-experimental research designs are extremely useful, because they enable researchers to conduct representative research—that is, research that replicates "real-world" conditions. Quasi-experimental research designs should be employed when it is critical for researchers to conduct a representative study. Quasi-experimental research designs may also be employed when it is impossible for researchers to select participants randomly from a population or randomly assign participants to the experimental and control groups.

The preexperimental research designs have a lack of experimental control that essentially renders them useless for establishing causal relationships between variables. Indeed, we have detailed preexperimental research designs

only because they continue to be used inappropriately by researchers to infer causal relationships between variables. In contrast to true experimental and quasi-experimental research designs, preexperimental research designs do not enable reasonable comparisons to be made. Thus, any causal claims made by researchers are clearly inappropriate. Researchers should use preexperimental designs as a last resort; that is, when they are not able to use true experimental or quasi-experimental designs due to limitations (e.g., limited financial or human resources, teacher, administrative, or parental concerns, scheduling difficulties).

SUMMARY

❖ Establishing cause-and-effect relationships among variables is typically the goal of most research. There are three categories of experimental research designs used by researchers in education and psychology: (1) true experimental, (2) quasi-experimental, and (3) preexperimental designs.

❖ The ability of an experimental design to control for threats to internal and external validity is primarily dependent on four key features: (1) the procedures used to select participants from a broader population; (2) the use of a control group or condition; (3) the initial equivalence of the experimental and control groups; and (4) how effectively the investigation was conducted.

❖ True experimental designs are the only experimental designs that can result in relatively definitive statements about causal relationships between variables. True experimental designs ensure that (1) a change in the value of the independent variable is accompanied by a change in the value of the dependent variable, (2) how the independent variable affects the dependent variable is established a priori, and (3) the independent variable precedes the dependent variable.

❖ There are three basic requirements for a research design to be considered a true experimental design: (1) random selection of

participants from a population to form a sample; (2) random assignment of research participants to the experimental and control conditions; and (3) equal treatment of members of the experimental and control groups.

❖ Three of the most common true experimental designs include (1) pretest–posttest control-group, (2) posttest-only control-group, and (3) Solomon four-group designs.

❖ The pretest–posttest control-group design has the following five attributes: (1) random selection of participants from a population to form a sample; (2) random assignment of selected participants to the experimental or control groups; (3) measurement of the dependent variable prior to the introduction of the independent variable; (4) introduction of the independent variable; and (5) postintervention measurement of the independent variable. Any differences observed at the end of the study are assumed to be due to the independent variable.

❖ A posttest-only control-group design is a true experimental design similar to the pretest–posttest-only control-group design, with the exception that pretests of the dependent variable are not administered to the experimental and control groups. This design has the following four attributes: (1) random selection of participants from a population to form a sample; (2) random assignment of the selected participants to the experimental or control groups; (3) introduction of the independent variable; and (4) postintervention measurement of the dependent variable. Any differences observed at the end of the study are assumed to be due to the independent variable.

❖ The Solomon four-group design is a true experimental design that essentially combines the pretest–posttest control-group design and the posttest-only control-group design; two groups serve as experimental groups and two groups serve as control groups.

Many of the threats to internal validity are controlled in true experimental designs, while many of the threats to external validity remain. The Solomon four-group design not only controls for testing (threat to internal validity) and pretest sensitization (threat to external validity) but also enables researchers to assess their effects on the intervention outcomes.

❖ A factorial experimental design is used to assess the effects of two or more independent variables or the interaction of participant characteristics with the independent variable. It is used to determine whether a particular variable has the same effect when studied concurrently with other variables as it would when studied in isolation. The threats to internal validity controlled for by a factorial design are dependent on the basic underlying true experimental design. One of the greatest strengths of a factorial design is that it enhances the external validity of the study.

❖ In quasi-experimental designs, participants are neither randomly selected from the specified population nor randomly assigned to experimental and control groups. These designs differ from true experimental designs in two ways: (1) Participants are not randomly selected from a specified population, and (b) participants are not randomly assigned to experimental and control groups.

The static-group comparison design is the same as the posttest-only control group design except for the absence of random selection of participants from a population and random assignment of participants to groups.

The nonequivalent control-group design is similar to the pretest–posttest control-group design described previously except for the absence of random selection of participants from a population and random assignment of participants to groups.

Counterbalanced designs encompass a wide range of designs in which independent variables are introduced to all participants. In counterbalanced designs, two or more groups get the same independent variables, but the independent variables are introduced in different orders. Counterbalanced designs are also useful when it is not possible to assign participants randomly to the experimental and control groups, and when participant attrition may be a problem.

Time-series designs are quasi-experimental designs involving a series of repeated measurements of a single group of research participants in the following three steps: (1) Measure the dependent variable a number of times prior to the introduction of the independent variable; (2) introduce the independent variable; and (3) measure the dependent variable a number of more times.

In the absence of random assignment of participants to groups, the possibility of pretreatment differences is present. The lack of a pretest (as in the static group comparison) greatly weakens the ability to control for a number of threats to internal validity. However, the level of experimental control achieved with a counterbalanced design is greater than that achieved with other designs, because each participant serves as his/her own control, and time-series designs provide a high degree of experimental control even though they do not employ a control group. External validity threats are present with these designs, just as they were in the true experimental designs.

❖ Preexperimental designs primarily differ from true experimental designs and two of the quasi-experimental designs (i.e., counterbalanced and time-series designs) in that they do not include a control group. The lack of a control group essentially eliminates researchers' ability to control for any of the threats to internal validity.

The one-shot case study involves the following three steps: (1) identification of a naturally assembled group, (2) administration of the independent variable, and (c) measurement of the dependent variable. The one-group pretest–posttest design differs from the one-shot case study in that a pretest measure is administered prior to the introduction of the independent variable. The effects of the independent variable are determined by comparing the pretest and posttest scores of the group of participants. Preexperimental designs control for threats to neither internal validity nor external validity. Conclusions regarding the results of investigations using these designs must be made with caution.

❖ Researchers who are attempting to demonstrate a cause-and-effect relationship should use a true experimental design if they can randomly select and assign participants. Quasi-experimental research designs should be employed when it is critical for researchers to conduct a representative study, or when it is impossible for researchers to select participants randomly from a population or randomly assign participants to the experimental and control groups. Researchers should use preexperimental designs as a last resort; that is, when researchers are not able to use true experimental or quasi-experimental designs due to limitations.

DISCUSSION QUESTIONS

1. What is meant by a true experimental design? (In your response, discuss the basic design features of true experimental designs.)

2. What are quasi-experimental designs? How are true experimental and quasi-experimental designs similar, and how are they different?

3. Can quasi-experimental designs determine cause-and-effect relationships? Explain.

4. How are threats to the internal validity of the experiment controlled with a quasi-experimental design?

5. How do true experimental designs control for threats to external validity? What are some concerns you might have?

6. Are quasi-experimental designs more or less useful than true experimental designs in determining the external validity of the investigation? Why or why not?

7. What type of design is recommended if you are concerned that males and females have different attitudes toward math and may perform differently in math? Why?

8. What type of design have you used when you pretest a single class, provide the instruction, then posttest the class? What are the problems with this design? What conclusions could you make in terms of internal and external validity?

9. For the example in Question 8, what would be a better design for you to use? How would you do this? How would your conclusions differ?

10. Of the designs discussed in this chapter, which design(s) seem to have the strongest control over threats to internal validity? Which design(s) do you think would be the most difficult to implement in an applied setting? Why?

Note. Beginning in this chapter, we offer an illustrative example of research associated with the designs described in the readings. The example is followed by questions about the research. Finally, there are references to three additional research studies associated with the designs in the readings.

The Effects of Learning Strategy Instruction on the Completion of Job Applications by Students with Learning Disabilities

J. Ron Nelson, Deborah J. Smith, and John M. Dodd

The purpose of this study was to assess the effects of learning strategy instruction on the completion of job applications by students identified as learning disabled. Thirty-three students (average age 15 years 6 months) were randomly assigned by grade and gender to one of two experimental conditions: learning strategy instruction or traditional instruction. The result was 16 students (10 boys and 6 girls) being placed under the learning strategy instruction condition and 17 students (10 boys and 7 girls) being placed under the traditional instruction condition. Results indicated that in addition to statistically significant lower numbers of information omissions and information location errors, holistic ratings of the overall neatness of the job applications were significantly higher for those students under the learning strategy instruction condition. In addition to these positive changes in the performance measures, social validity data suggest that students under the learning strategy condition would be more likely to receive an invitation for a job interview. The findings and future research needs are discussed.

Because employers often receive numerous applications for a single advertised position, the quality of the employment application materials has a direct effect on an individual's ability to secure employment. Employers most often use the employment application form and, when applicable, the personal resume to decide whom to interview for a position. Regardless of otherwise equal qualifications, the content, completeness, and neatness of these employment application materials have an effect on whether an individual is given the opportunity to interview for a specific job (Field & Holley, 1976). Indeed, the skills involved in completing employment application materials may be the foundation upon which other job-finding skills, such as interviewing, are built (Azrin & Philip, 1979; Mathews, Whang, & Fawcett, 1981).

Despite the importance of a complete and accurate employment application, researchers have mostly focused on the effects of training procedures on an individual's job interview performance (e.g., Furman, Geller, Simon, & Kelly, 1979; Hall, Sheldon-Wildgen, & Sherman, 1980; Hollansworth, Dressel, & Stevens, 1977); relatively few studies have been conducted on teaching disadvantaged individuals (Clark, Boyd, & MaCrae, 1975) or those identified as learning disabled (Mathews & Fawcett, 1984) to complete job application forms. Approaches employed in these studies were applied behavioral instruction techniques designed to teach the skills involved in completing employment applications. Mathews and Fawcett, for example, taught three high school seniors identified as having learning disabilities (LD) to complete a job application and write a resume. The training sequence involved the student, with assistance from the experimenter, reading a set of instructional materials containing detailed written specifications for the behaviors, including a rationale and examples for each task. The student then practiced each task with feedback from the experimenter. Following training, each of the three students showed significant changes in the percentage of application items completed accurately.

Although the results of this study demonstrate that students with LD can be taught to more accurately complete job application forms, the students were reported to need assistance with reading the procedural text accompanying the employment application materials. More important, procedures required 2.5 hours of individual instructional time. This would suggest that an effective group training procedure on employment application skills should be designed to facilitate both the acquisition and the expression of information. Students must be taught to understand the procedural text included on job application forms and to provide all of the requested information accurately.

Learning strategy instruction is one instructional approach that might be used to teach students these two related skills that are necessary to independently complete job applications. For the purposes of this article, a learning strategy will be defined as a collection of specific skills that one uses in a particular situation to facilitate the acquisition or expression of knowledge or skills. This type of instruction appears to be especially beneficial for students with LD because these students have been characterized as lacking active task engagement and persistence (Harris, 1986) and as lacking the skills necessary to execute and monitor the cognitive processes central to academic success (Baumann, 1986).

Although, to date, there appears to have been no empirical work conducted with learning strategies designed to facilitate both the understanding of procedural text that is included on a job application and the expression of the requested information, the present study can be placed in the context of recent work on learning strategy instruction in reading (e.g., Borkowski, Weyhing, & Carr, 1988) and writing (e.g., Englert, Raphael, Anderson, Anthony, & Stevens, 1991). Research on reading strategy instruction has focused on how to teach students to (a) determine the main idea (Baumann, 1986; Cunningham & Moore, 1986; Williams, 1986); (b) summarize the information contained in text (Day, 1980; Hare & Borchardt, 1984; Nelson, Smith, & Dodd, 1992; Palincsar & Brown, 1984; Taylor, 1982; Taylor & Beach, 1984; Taylor & Berkowitz, 1980); (c) draw inferences about what they have read (Hansen, 1981; Pearson, 1985; Raphael & McKinney, 1983; Raphael & Pearson, 1985; Raphael & Wonnacott, 1985); (d) generate questions about what they have read (Andre & Anderson, 1978–79; Brown & Palincsar, 1985); and (e) monitor their comprehension of the text (Baker & Anderson, 1982; Vosniadou, Pearson, & Rogers, 1988). In sum, this work has shown that students with LD, as well as other students, can be taught strategies to facilitate their reading and understanding of literary and expository text.

However, following written directions such as those included on job applications differs from other kinds of reading, in that the goal of the reader is to *do* something rather than to *learn about* something. In the case of procedural text or written directions, a partial understanding is insufficient—mastery of the content is required. Reading written directions is further complicated by the fact that writers of directions often overestimate the reader's experience with directions, omit intermediate steps, use technical vocabulary, and employ complex syntax (Henk & Helfeldt, 1987). Furthermore, written directions often contain unclear directional and location cues for entering information in specific places on the application form. In addition, according to Henk and Helfeldt, there is no immediate transfer of academic reading skills to following written directions. Good readers follow written directions well only 80% of the time, and poor readers achieve less than a 50% success rate (Fox & Siedow, 1980).

Paralleling work on reading comprehension, researchers have developed a number of learning strategies designed to facilitate students' abilities to generate expository text (e.g., Englert et al., 1991; Graham & Harris, 1989; Harris & Graham, 1985; Schmidt, Deshler, Schumaker, & Alley, 1988). Schmidt et al., for example, taught high school students with LD four written expression learning strategies: sentence writing, paragraph writing, error monitoring, and theme writing. The results showed improvements both in the quality of themes and in the mechanics of the written text.

Because research and theory suggest that students should be taught to apply different learning strategies to different types of situations (Brandt, 1989), students must possess specific strategies for both understanding and following procedural text or written directions. In other words, the reading and writing strategies demanded by the task requirements of a job application depart from those that students apply elsewhere. The purpose of the present study was to develop a learning strategy and study its effects on completion of job applications by students with LD. This is important because there are significant societal and personal costs associated with the unemployment and underemployment of individuals with disabilities, and, as noted, regardless of otherwise equal qualifications, the content, completeness, and neatness of a job application can determine whether an individual has an opportunity to even interview for a specific job.

METHOD

Subjects

Thirty-three students (20 boys and 13 girls) with LD served as participants in the study. All were receiving special education services in a public high school in a city in the Northwest (population 180,000) and were classified as learning disabled by a school district multidisciplinary evaluation team. Criteria for special education classification include deficits in oral expression (as measured by the Northwestern Syntax Screening Test), listening comprehension (as measured by the Carrow Test for Auditory Comprehension of Language), and/or written expression (as measured by the Comprehensive Tests of Basic Skills). Criteria also included a significant discrepancy (at least 2 years below grade placement) between the student's estimated ability and academic performance.

Students were generally from low-SES families (qualified for free and reduced lunch). Table 1 provides additional descriptions of the participants' sex, age, race, grade level, years in special education, percentage of each school day spent in special education, IQ, and achievement.

TABLE 1. Subject Description

	Learning strategy instruction (n = 16)	Traditional instruction (n = 17)
Gender		
Male	10	10
Female	6	7
Age		
Mean	15.9	16.3
Range	14.5–17.3	14.3–17.5
Race		
White	15	17
African American	1	0
Grade level		
12th	2	3
11th	6	7
10th	6	5
9th	2	2
Years in special education		
Mean	5.9	5.3
Range	4–8	4–9
Percentage of day in special education		
Mode	.50	.50
Range	33–83	33–83
Intelligence[a]		
Mean	98.5	96.2
Range	88–106	84–105
Reading comprehension[b]		
Mean T	35.1	33.4
Range	22–43	25–41

[a]Stanford–Binet Intelligence Scale.
[b]Iowa Test of Basic Skills.

Setting

All participants were enrolled in a pre-vocational education class for students with learning disabilities. The class was taught by a certificated special education teacher with 6 years of teaching experience at the high school level. The classroom aide was a high school graduate with 8 years of classroom assistance experience. The teacher conducted the experimental sessions during two 60-minute instructional periods. The classroom was approximately 10 m by 15 m and had 25 individual desks at which the participating students sat during the experimental sessions.

Dependent Measures

Student Performance Measures

Three mutually exclusive measures were employed to assess the effects of the learning strategy instruction on the completion of job applications by students: information omissions, information location errors, and a holistic rating of overall neatness of the job application. An omission was scored when a required item was not completed. A location error was scored when the correct information was entered in the wrong location (e.g., writing the information on the line directly below where the information was to be placed). A 5-point Likert-type scale (1 = *very messy* to 5 = *very neat*) was used to obtain a holistic rating of the overall neatness of the job application.

Interscorer agreement for omissions and location errors was determined by having two scorers independently score all of the job applications. The scorers' records were compared item by item. For omissions, agreement was noted when both scorers had marked a response as not present. Similarly, an agreement was noted when both the scorers marked the location of the information as correct or if both scorers had marked the location of the information as incorrect. Percentage of agreement for each measure was computed by dividing the number of agreements by the number of agreements plus disagreements. The percentage of agreement was 100% in both cases.

Interscorer agreement was computed for the holistic rating by having two raters independently rate all of the job applications. A Pearson product moment correlation was then calculated to estimate the reliability of the ratings. The correlation was .78, $p < .05$.

Social Validity Measure

To assess the social validity of the effects of the training, the supervisor of classified personnel at a local university employing approximately 1,200 classified staff was asked the following: "Based on this job application, if you had a position open, would you invite this person in for an interview?" The rating was completed on a 5-point Likert-type scale (1 = *very unlikely*, 3 = *undecided*, 5 = *very likely*). The supervisor rated each application and was unaware of whether it was completed under the learning strategy or traditional instruction condition. *External validity*

Design

A pretest–posttest control group design was employed. Students were randomly assigned by age and gender to one of two experimental conditions: learning strategy instruction or traditional instruction. This resulted in 16 students (10 boys and 6 girls) being assigned under the learning strategy instruction condition and 17 students (10 boys and 7 girls) under the traditional instruction condition. The results of a preliminary analysis revealed that there were statistically nonsignificant differences in characteristics (i.e., intelligence, achievement, age, years in special education, and percentage of each school day spent in special education) between the two groups.

Procedure

Job Applications

Job applications for entry-level jobs were obtained from eight local businesses. Two of these job applications were selected for the pretest and posttest; two additional applications were used to conduct the training sessions (demonstration and independent practice). Although these job applications were designed to elicit the same general information, the format (e.g., sequence of information and location cues) differed. The same pretest, posttest, and training job applications were used under the learning strategy instruction and traditional instruction conditions.

Preskill Instructional Module

Students under both conditions (described below) received a prepared instructional module designed to provide the relevant prerequisite vocabulary knowledge necessary to complete a job application. This instruction was conducted, and job application information collected (discussed below), prior to pretesting. The teacher presented the prerequisite vocabulary knowledge module, using a written script, to students under both conditions. The prerequisite information included definitions for the following job application vocabulary words: (a) *birth place*, (b) *nationality*, (c) *previous work experience*, (d) *references*, (e) *maiden name*, (f) *marital status*, (g) *citizenship*, (h) *salary*, and (i) *wage*. Instruction continued until all of the students earned 100% correct on a paper-and-pencil test in which the words were matched with their respective definitions.

Students under both experimental conditions also compiled the information necessary for them to complete a job application, including (a) birth date, (b) social security number, (c) complete address, (d) telephone number, (e) educational experience, (f) previous work experience, (g) references, and (h) felony convictions (if applicable). Students then constructed a job application information card containing this information.

Students under both experimental conditions then completed the pretest job application. The teacher asked them to complete the job application as if they were applying for an actual job. She also explained that typically no one is available to help people complete job applications, and they were to use their job information card for the task. Students were provided as much time as they needed to complete the application. The teacher did not provide the students any assistance during this time. The pretest session was conducted 1 day prior to the training and posttest sessions.

Learning Strategy Instruction Condition

The job application learning strategy taught in this investigation was designed after analyzing the nature of items included on standard job applications for entry-level jobs obtained from a number of local businesses, and after completing a task analysis of the steps involved in completing a job application. The strategy was also designed in accordance with the needs and skill levels of the students. The principle steps were then sequenced and a first-letter mnemonic device was developed to facilitate students' recall of the strategy steps. This resulted in a six-step strategy called "SELECT."

Students first Survey the entire job application and look for the Emphasized words that indicate the type of information requested (e.g., previous experience) and think to themselves, "What information do I have to have to complete the job application?" and "Do I have all of the necessary information to complete the application (check job application information card)?" If not, "What additional information do I need to get?" The students then look closely at the items on the job application for Location cues that indicate where the requested information is to be entered (e.g., line immediately below the request for information) and think to themselves, "Where does the information go?" Next, they think to themselves, "How much space do I need for the information—How big should I print the information?" and then carefully Enter the information requested in the appropriate location. After completing the application, the students then Check to see if the information is accurate (compare with job information card) and that the job application is completed, and think to themselves, "Did I put the right information in the right locations?" If not, "I need to complete another job application." Then, "Did I complete the job application?" If not, "Complete the job application." Finally, the students Turn the completed job application in to the appropriate individual.

The special education teacher used a five-step procedure to teach the students the job application strategy during an approximately 1-hour instructional session. First, the teacher discussed the goal of the job application strategy instruction procedure (i.e., to help students accurately complete a job application) and why it is important to know how to accurately complete a job application. She also explained how they would be able to use the strategy whenever they applied for a job.

Second, an overhead transparency was used to introduce and discuss the six-step job application strategy. The teacher and students discussed the use of the strategy until it was clear that the students fully understood the steps. This was accomplished through choral responding by the students and informal checks by the teacher.

Third, using an overhead transparency, the teacher modeled the job application strategy by completing a standard job application while "thinking out loud." To actively engage the students, the teacher used prompts to encourage an interactive dialogue with the students throughout the demonstration, for example, "What is it I have to do? I need to . . . " and "How am I doing?" The students were encouraged to help the teacher. After modeling, the teacher and students discussed the

importance of using self-questioning statements while completing a job application.

Fourth, students were required to verbally practice the job application strategy steps, including the self-questioning statements, until they were memorized. All of the students were able to do this correctly within a 15- to 20-minute rehearsal period. They were then required to write down the steps and associated self-questioning statements as they worked through a job application. Students were provided only one practice attempt. They were allowed to ask any questions at this time and the teacher provided corrective feedback only upon demand by the students throughout the training session.

Finally, students independently completed the posttest job application. As under the pretest condition, the teacher asked the students to complete the job application as if they were applying for an actual job. She also explained to the students that because there typically is no one there to help them complete job applications, they were to use only their job information card to complete the job application, and that they had as much time as they needed to complete the application. The teacher did not provide the students any assistance during this time. After they completed the posttest job application, the students were asked to independently describe the steps they had used, in an attempt to check whether they had employed the learning strategy. All of the students verbally stated, in sequence, the steps and associated self-questioning statements included in the learning strategy.

Traditional Instruction Condition

The same job application forms used under the learning strategy condition were used for the traditional instruction condition. During an approximately 1-hour instructional session, the special education teacher (same teacher) first discussed the goal of the job application instruction (i.e., to help students accurately complete a job application) and why it is important to know how to accurately complete a job application. She also explained how they would be able to use the things they learned whenever they applied for a job.

Next, the teacher used an overhead transparency to model how to complete a standard job application. Throughout the demonstration, the teacher explained why it was important to accurately complete job applications and instructed the students to be careful to complete all of the information and to be sure that they put the information in the correct place. To actively engage the students, the teacher used prompts throughout the demonstration, such as "What is it I have to do? I need to . . ." and "How am I doing?" The students were encouraged to help the teacher complete the job application. Students were then required to practice completing a job application. They were allowed only one practice attempt, and they were allowed to ask any questions during this time. The teacher provided corrective feedback only upon request throughout the session.

Finally, the students independently completed the posttest job application. The teacher did not provide the students any assistance during this time. Once again, these conditions (job application, instructions, and amount of time) were the same as those employed under the pretest and learning strategy instruction conditions.

Fidelity of Implementation

Fidelity of implementation was assessed under both experimental conditions by observing the teacher on the day of instruction to ensure that she followed the teaching steps associated with each of the experimental conditions. The primary researcher used a checklist to track whether the teacher fully completed the teaching functions described above under each condition.

RESULTS

Preliminary analyses indicated that there were nonsignificant differences between the groups on the pretest measures. Posttest measures were analyzed in condition (traditional, strategy) by gender (male, female) analyses of variance (ANOVAs). For every dependent measure, only a significant main effect for condition was obtained. The F values for these effects, along with the means and standard deviations for each of the dependent measures, are presented in Table 2.

The findings indicate that students who received instruction in the learning strategy condition made statistically significant lower numbers of information omission errors and location errors than students under the job application instruction condition. Additionally, these students received statistically significant higher holistic ratings on their job applications than their counterparts.

TABLE 2. Mean Number of Information Omissions and Location Errors, and Mean Holistic Rating of Overall Application Neatness

Dependent measure	Group A	Group B	$F(1, 31)$ (Condition)
Omissions	5.35 (2.55)	0.63 (0.63)	15.29*
Location errors	1.35 (0.99)	0.25 (0.25)	5.29**
Neatness rating	3.37 (1.05)	4.46 (0.51)	7.25***

Note. Group A refers to the traditional instruction condition and Group B refers to the strategy instruction condition. Numbers in parentheses are standard deviations.
*$p < .001$. **$p < .05$. ***$p < .01$.

There were statistically nonsignificant main effects for gender and nonsignificant condition by gender interactions for all of the dependent measures.

Confidence in these results is strengthened by the results of the checks for fidelity of implementation conducted under both experimental conditions. These findings showed that the teacher fully completed the teaching functions described above under each condition.

The social validity measure was analyzed in a condition (traditional, strategy) by gender (male, female) ANOVA. A significant main effect for condition was obtained, $F(1,31) = 6.12$, $p < .05$. There were statistically nonsignificant main effects for gender and condition by gender interactions for the social validity measure. The effects of the job application training on the ratings (1 = *very unlikely* to 5 = *very likely*) by the supervisor of classified personnel suggest that students under the learning strategy condition (mean = 4.21; SD = 0.46) would be more likely to receive invitations for job interviews after training than those under the traditional condition (mean = 2.88; SD = 1.02).

DISCUSSION

Past research on learning strategies has focused on skills that were general in nature and that apply across subject matters (Brandt, 1989). Recent work on learning strategies, however, has focused on studying how people learn particular things in particular environments. The present study was designed to develop and assess the effects of a learning strategy designed specifically to help students with LD understand the procedural text or written directions included on a job application and provide the requested information.

The results of this study suggest that a sample of students identified as learning disabled according to the state of Washington and federal guidelines were capable of mastering a six-step job application learning strategy in a relatively short time. Because the accurate completion of job applications constitutes an important component in the job search process, these procedures may be very beneficial in facilitating successful job acquisition by students with learning disabilities.

The findings of this study support those of other researchers (e.g., Clark et al., 1975; Mathews & Fawcett, 1984), demonstrating the beneficial effects of teaching students employment application skills. In addition to statistically significant lower numbers of information omissions and information location errors, holistic ratings of the overall neatness of the job applications were much higher for those students under the learning strategy instruction condition. Confidence in the findings of this study are strengthened by the fidelity of implementation data that indicate that the experimental conditions were fully implemented under both conditions.

Most important, in addition to statistically significant positive changes in the three performance measures, the social validity data suggest that the learning strategy instruction resulted in job application forms that would be more likely to elicit invitations for job interviews. The supervisor of classified personnel at the local university indicated that he would be likely to give the students under the learning strategy condition an invitation for a job interview. In contrast, he was significantly less likely to grant a job interview to students under the traditional instruction condition.

It is important to note several limitations of the study. First, the present study provides only one comparison of many potential instructional approaches. Thus, conclusions regarding the efficacy of the learning strategy instruction over any other instructional practices must be made cautiously. Second, because maintenance was not assessed, the long-term impact of the training is uncertain. Third, although students under the learning strategy condition verbally stated that they had employed and articulated the six-steps included in the learning strategy to complete the job applications, the subjective nature of this self-report data does not fully substantiate their claim.

Fourth, the relatively small number of subjects limits conclusions regarding the effectiveness of this strategy with students from other areas of the country or, more important, students with other types of disabilities and abilities. Finally, the limited nature of the task also limits conclusions regarding the effectiveness of this type of instruction for other procedural types of texts. The skills required to understand procedural text and perform the required functions accompanying technological devices, such as videocassette recorders, personal computers, programmable microwave ovens, and so forth, differ from those required to complete a standard job application. Procedural text for these devices, with accompanying illustrations, require an individual to fully understand sequence and direction and location concepts. Readers, for example, must be sensitive to sequence cues such as "then," "next," and "finally," and complex direction and location concepts, such as "down," "outside," "against," "inside," and "up." These complex directions, when combined with manual operations and the need to monitor progress, pose an instructional dilemma.

In summary, the skills addressed in the present study, although important, are relatively simple compared to demands that students may encounter regarding the understanding of procedural text. Further research is needed not only to clarify the results of the present study, but also to address the instructional requirements for preparing students with disabilities and others to effectively manage procedural text. Given our rapidly expanding technological society, the complexity of procedural text is only going to increase. Thus, researchers and teachers must continue to develop instructional procedures to facilitate students' understanding of procedural text.

REFERENCES

Andre, M. E., & Anderson, T. H. (1978–79). The development and evaluation of a self-questioning study technique. *Reading Research Quarterly, 14,* 605–623.

Azrin, N. H., & Philip, R. A. (1979). The Job Club methods vs. a lecture–discussion-role play method of obtaining employment for clients with job-finding handicaps. *Rehabilitation Counseling Bulletin, 23,* 144–155.

Baker, L., & Anderson, R. L. (1982). Effects of inconsistent information on text processing: Evidence for comprehension monitoring. *Reading Research Quarterly, 17,* 281–294.

Baumann, J. F. (1986). The direct instruction of main idea comprehension ability. In J. F. Bauman (Ed.), *Teaching main idea comprehension* (pp. 133–178). Newark, DE: International Reading Association.

Borkowski, J. G., Weyhing, R. S., & Carr, M. (1988). Effects of attributional retraining on strategy-based reading comprehension in learning-disabled students. *Journal of Educational Psychology, 80,* 46–53.

Brandt, R. (1989). On learning research: A conversation with Lauren Resnick. *Educational Leadership, 46*(4), 12–16.

Brown, A. L., & Palincsar, A. S. (1985). *Reciprocal teaching of comprehension strategies: A natural history of one program to enhance learning* (Tech. Rep. No. 334). Urbana: University of Illinois, Center for the Study of Reading.

Clark, H. B., Boyd, S. B., & MaCrae, J. W. (1975). A classroom program teaching disadvantaged youths to write biographical information. *Journal of Applied Behavior Analysis, 8,* 67–75.

Cunningham, J. W., & Moore, D. W. (1986). The confused world of main idea. In J. B. Baumann (Ed.), *Teaching main idea comprehension* (pp. 1–17). Newark, DE: International Reading Association.

Day, J. D. (1980). *Teaching summarization skills: A comparison of training methods.* Unpublished doctoral dissertation, University of Illinois, Urbana–Champaign.

Englert, C. S., Raphael, T. E., Anderson, L. M., Anthony, H. M., & Stevens, D. D. (1991). Making strategies and self-talk visible: Writing instruction in regular and special education classrooms. *American Educational Research Journal, 28,* 337–372.

Field, H. S., & Holley, W. H. (1976). Resume preparation: An empirical study of personnel managers' perceptions. *Vocational Guidance Quarterly, 25,* 229–237.

Fox, B. J., & Siedow, M. D. (1980). Written directions for content area classrooms—Do students understand the teacher? *The Clearing House, 54,* 101–104.

Furman, W., Geller, M., Simon, S. J., & Kelly, J. A. (1979). The use of a behavior rehearsal procedure for teaching job-interview skills to psychiatric patients. *Behavior Therapy, 10,* 157–167.

Graham, S., & Harris, K. R. (1989). Component analysis of cognitive strategy instruction: Effects on learning disabled students' skills at composing essays: Self-instructional strategy training. *Exceptional Children, 56,* 201–214.

Hall, C., Sheldon-Wildgen, J., & Sherman, J. A. (1980). Teaching job interview skills to retarded clients. *Journal of Applied Behavior Analysis, 13,* 433–442.

Hansen, J. (1981). The effects of inference training and practice on young children's reading comprehension. *Reading Research Quarterly, 16,* 391–417.

Hare, V. C., & Borchardt, K. M. (1984). Direct instruction of summarization skills. *Reading Research Quarterly, 20,* 62–78.

Harris, K. R., & Graham, S. (1985). Improving learning disabled students' composition skills: Self-control strategy training. *Learning Disability Quarterly, 8,* 27–36.

Henk, W. A., & Helfeldt, J. P. (1987). How to develop independence in following written directions. *Journal of Reading, 30,* 602–607.

Hollansworth, J. G., Dressel, M. E., & Stevens, J. (1977). Use of behavioral versus traditional procedures for increasing job interview skills. *Journal of Counseling Psychology, 24,* 503–510.

Mathews, R. M., & Fawcett, S. B. (1984). Building the capacities of job candidates through behavioral instruction. *Journal of Community Psychology, 12,* 123–129.

Mathews, R. M., Whang, P. L., & Fawcett, S. B. (1981). Behavioral assessment of job-related skills. *Journal of Employment Counseling, 18,* 3–11.

Nelson, J. R., Smith, D. J., & Dodd, J. M. (1992). *The effects of a summary skills intervention on students' comprehension of science text.* Manuscript submitted for publication.

Palincsar, A. M., & Brown, A. L. (1984). Reciprocal teaching of comprehension-fostering and comprehension-monitoring activities. *Cognition and Instruction, 1,* 117–175.

Pearson, P. D. (1985). Changing the face of reading comprehension instruction. *The Reading Teacher, 38,* 724–738.

Raphael, T. E., & McKinney, J. (1983). An examination of 5th and 8th grade children's question answering behavior: An instructional study in metacognition. *Journal of Reading Behavior, 15*(5), 67–86.

Raphael, T. E., & Pearson, P. D. (1985). Increasing students' awareness of sources of information for answering questions. *American Educational Research Journal, 22,* 217–235.

Raphael, T. E., & Wonnacott, C. A. (1985). Heightening fourth-grade students' sensitivity to sources of information for answering questions. *Reading Research Quarterly, 20,* 282–296.

Schmidt, J., Deshler, D., Schumaker, J., & Alley, G. (1988). The effects of generalization instruction on the written performance of adolescents with learning disabilities in the mainstream classroom. *Reading, Writing, and Learning Disabilities, 4,* 291–309.

Taylor, B. M. (1982). Text structure and children's comprehension and memory for expository materials. *Journal of Educational Psychology, 15,* 401–405.

Taylor, B. M., & Beach, R. W. (1984). The effects of text structure instruction on middle-grade students' comprehension and production of expository text. *Reading Research Quarterly, 19,* 134–146.

Taylor, B. M., & Berkowitz, B. S. (1980). Facilitating childrens' comprehension of content material. In M. L. Kamil & A. J. Moe (Eds.), *Perspectives in reading research and instruction* (pp. 64–68). Clemson, SC: National Reading Conference.

Vosniadou, S., Pearson, P. D., & Rogers, T. (1988). What causes children's failures to detect inconsistencies in text? Representation vs. comparison difficulties. *Journal of Educational Psychology, 80,* 27–39.

Williams, J. P. (1986). Extracting important information from text. In J. A. Niles & R. V. Lalik (Eds.), *Solving problems in literacy: Learners, teachers, and researchers* (pp. 11–29). Rochester, NY: National Reading Conference.

ABOUT THE AUTHORS

J. Ron Nelson, PhD, is an assistant professor in the Department of Applied Psychology at Eastern Washington University. He received his doctoral degree in special education from Utah State University. His major research interests include teaching methods for exceptional students and students at risk for school failure, as well as students' social and intellectual reasoning. **Deborah J. Smith, PhD,** is project director in Disabled Student Services and adjunct professor in the Department of Applied Psychology at Eastern Washington University. She received her doctoral degree in special education from Utah State University. Her major research interests include self-management strategies for classroom deportment and academic performance, as well as cognitive instructional strategies. **John M. Dodd, EdD,** is a professor in the Department of Reading and Special Education at Eastern Montana College. He received his doctoral degree in human development at the University of Kansas. His major research interests include culturally sensitive identification and programming for linguistically and culturally diverse students. Address: J. Ron Nelson, Department of Applied Psychology, MS/92, Eastern Washington University, Cheney, WA 99004.

Source: From Nelson, J. R., Smith, D. J., & Dodd, J. M. (1994). The effects of learning strategy instruction on the completion of job applications by students with learning disabilities. *Journal of Learning Disabilities, 27,* 104–110. Copyright 1994 by the Hammill Institute on Disabilities. Reprinted by permission of SAGE.

ILLUSTRATIVE EXAMPLE QUESTIONS

1. Are there any problems with the way participants were selected and assigned to the two conditions?

2. What type of experimental design was used in the study?

3. Why was fidelity of implementation assessed? Does it increase your confidence in the findings? Why?

4. Why do you think it was important for the authors to use a variety of dependent measures?

5. Are there any problems with treatment diffusion, compensatory rivalry, or resentful demoralization of the traditional instruction group? Why?

6. Was it necessary for the authors to assess the initial equivalence of the two groups?

7. What other statistical analysis procedure could the authors have used to ensure the initial equivalence of the experimental and control groups?

8. What was the purpose of providing the preskill lesson to both of the groups?

9. What could the authors have done to improve the internal validity of the study?

10. What could the authors have done to improve the external validity of the study?

ADDITIONAL RESEARCH EXAMPLES

1. Cheng, C., Wang, F., & Golden, D. L. (2011). Unpacking cultural differences in interpersonal flexibility: Role of culture-related personality and situational factors. *Journal of Cross-Cultural Psychology, 42,* 425–444.

2. Horrey, W. J., Lesch, M. F., Kramer, A. F., & Melton, D. F. (2009). Effects of a computer-based training module on drivers' willingness to engage in distracting activities. *Human Factors: The Journal of the Human Factors and Ergonomics Society, 51,* 571–581.

3. Kellow, J. T., & Jones, B. D. (2008). The effects of stereotypes on the achievement gap: Reexamining the academic performance of African American high school students. *Journal of Black Psychology, 34,* 94–120.

THREATS TO INTERNAL VALIDITY

Circle the number corresponding to the likelihood of each threat to internal validity being present in the investigation and provide a justification.

1 = definitely not a threat   2 = not a likely threat   3 = somewhat likely threat

4 = likely threat   5 = definite threat   NA = not applicable for this design

Results in Differences within or between Individuals

1. Maturation   1   2   3   4   5   NA

   Justification _____

_____

2. Selection   1   2   3   4   5   NA

   Justification _____

_____

3. Selection by Maturation Interaction   1   2   3   4   5   NA

   Justification _____

_____

4. Statistical Regression   1   2   3   4   5   NA

   Justification _____

_____

5. Morality   1   2   3   4   5   NA

   Justification _____

_____

6. Instrumentation   1   2   3   4   5   NA

   Justification _____

_____

7. Testing   1   2   3   4   5   NA

   Justification _____

_____

(continued)

8. History   1   2   3   4   5   NA

     Justification _____

     _____

9. Resentful Demoralization of the Control Group   1   2   3   4   5   NA

     Justification _____

     _____

Results in Similarities within or between Individuals

10. Diffusion of Treatment   1   2   3   4   5   NA

     Justification _____

     _____

11. Compensatory Rivalry by the Control Group   1   2   3   4   5   NA

     Justification _____

     _____

12. Compensatory Equalization of Treatments   1   2   3   4   5   NA

     Justification _____

     _____

Abstract: Write a one-page abstract summarizing the overall conclusions of the authors and whether or not you feel the authors' conclusions are valid based on the internal validity of the investigation.

THREATS TO EXTERNAL VALIDITY

Circle the number corresponding to the likelihood of each threat to external validity being present in the investigation according to the following scale:

1 = definitely not a threat   2 = not a likely threat   3 = somewhat likely threat

4 = likely threat   5 = definite threat   NA = not applicable for this design

Also, provide a justification for each rating.

Population

1. Generalization across Subjects   1   2   3   4   5   NA

 Justification _____

 _____

2. Interaction of Personological Variables and Treatment   1   2   3   4   5   NA

 Justification _____

 _____

Ecological

3. Verification of the Independent Variable   1   2   3   4   5   NA

 Justification _____

 _____

4. Multiple Treatment Interference   1   2   3   4   5   NA

 Justification _____

 _____

5. Hawthorne Effect   1   2   3   4   5   NA

 Justification _____

 _____

6. Novelty and Disruption Effects   1   2   3   4   5   NA

 Justification _____

 _____

7. Experimental Effects   1   2   3   4   5   NA

 Justification _____

 _____

(continued)

8. Pretest Sensitization   1   2   3   4   5   NA

Justification _____

_____

9. Posttest Sensitization   1   2   3   4   5   NA

Justification _____

_____

10. Interaction of Time of Measurement and Treatment Effects   1   2   3   4   5   NA

Justification _____

_____

11. Measurement of the Dependent Variable   1   2   3   4   5   NA

Justification _____

_____

12. Interaction of History and Treatment Effects   1   2   3   4   5   NA

Justification _____

_____

Abstract: Write a one-page abstract summarizing the overall conclusions of the authors and whether or not you feel the authors' conclusions are valid based on the external validity of the investigation.

CHAPTER 6

■ ■ ■ ■

Causal–Comparative Research

OBJECTIVES

After studying this chapter, you should be able to . . .

1. Illustrate the two purposes of causal–comparative research.
2. Outline the causal–comparative research method.
3. Explain when researchers should consider designing a causal–comparative research study.
4. Describe how the causal–comparative approach can be combined with factorial experimental designs.
5. Define when researchers should use the causal–comparative research design.

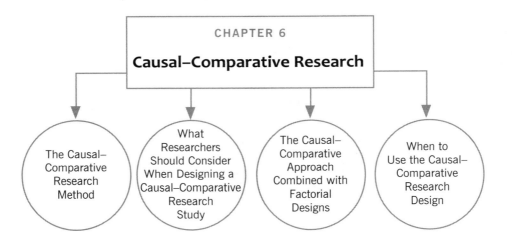

OVERVIEW

As previously noted, one of the primary features of science is that it possesses a set of goals, principles, and procedures that provides a way to construct knowledge that is common to both quantitative and qualitative researchers. The goals, principles, and procedures used by experimental researchers were presented in Chapter 5. This chapter focuses on the causal–comparative research method.

Although all research may share the goal of providing evidence about causal relationships (i.e., about what leads to what), a great deal of research in education and psychology leads only to descriptions of the relationships among variables. Research aimed at studying relationships between and among variables can be used both to rule out causal hypotheses and to provide support for others (Johnston & Pennypacker, 1993). For example, if a "no relationship" finding is obtained, the credibility of a hypothesis is lessened. If a "high relationship" finding is obtained, the credibility of the hypothesis is strengthened in that it has survived disconfirmation. (The link between heavy smoking and lung cancer is a case in point.) These hypotheses can then be checked through experimental manipulation when appropriate.

Two general approaches are used by researchers to explore the relationships among variables (Graziano & Raulin, 2010; see Figure 6.1). The first approach is the causal–comparative method. One purpose of this method is to compare two or more samples or groups of participants that are different on a critical variable but otherwise comparable. For example, juvenile delinquents have been compared to non-delinquents to identify whether levels of moral reasoning are related to delinquency. Another purpose of this method is to compare two or more equivalent samples on a critical variable to identify changes over time. For example, young children's understanding of knowledge has been compared with that of older children to identify developmental changes in children's understanding of knowledge.

The second approach, the correlational method, reduced to its barest essentials, involves collecting two sets of data and determining the extent to which these data sets covary using a correlation statistic. For example, researchers have explored the extent to which scholastic aptitude and grade point average (GPA) are related in an effort to determine if students' scores on a measure of scholastic aptitude can predict their GPAs.

This chapter begins with a general description of the causal–comparative research method, followed by a discussion of how the data in the causal–comparative design are interpreted and an illustrative example of how to interpret the findings of causal–comparative research. Next, a description of how the causal–comparative

---

Research Examples

Consider these issues. Think about how you would design research to address the questions/hypotheses from these research examples:

- Research Example 1: What are the perceptions of future teachers on providing educational service to students with disabilities in general education classrooms?
- Research Example 2: Do opportunities to learn vary as a function of number of students in a classroom identified as English language learners?
- Research Example 3: Does the education level (middle school, high school, or college) of a musician or the musician's primary instrument (brass vs. non-brass) influence one's evaluation of a musical passage?

Research examples appear throughout the chapter.

---

research method can be combined with factorial experiments is provided. Finally, an illustrative example of how to interpret the findings of causal–comparative research is provided for critique.

WHAT IS THE CAUSAL–COMPARATIVE RESEARCH METHOD?

The **causal–comparative research method** involves comparing two groups of individuals drawn from the same population that differ on a critical variable but are otherwise comparable. For example, we could compare students with and without emotional disturbance, drawn from the same population, to identify possible causes of emotional disturbance. In essence, the causal–comparative method is a particular way to collect and analyze data to discover possible causes for a pattern of behavior by comparing participants with this pattern and participants

> The **causal–comparative research method** *involves the comparison of two groups that differ on a critical variable.*

Causal–Comparative	Correlational
Comparing Two or More Samples	Comparing Two or More Sets of Data

FIGURE 6.1. Key differences between approaches used to study relationships among variables.

in whom it is absent (or present to a lesser degree). This method is sometimes referred to as *ex post facto research*, because the causes are studied after they have presumably influenced another variable.

Causal–comparative research is similar to experimental research methods, in that each compares group scores (averages) to determine relationships between the independent and dependent variables. Both experimental and causal–comparative designs use group memberships as a categorical variable. Finally, with the exception of counterbalanced and time-series designs, both compare separate groups of participants.

In essence, the causal–comparative design tends to look like experimental designs. However, there are several differences (Schenker & Rumrill, 2004; see Figure 6.2). First, in experimental designs, the independent variable is manipulated, whereas in the causal–comparative design, the independent variable is not manipulated, because it is either not possible to manipulate the independent variable, as is the case with gender, or it is prohibitive to do so, as in a study on smoking.

For example, it is not possible to take a sample of individuals without sexual identity, then randomly assign half to a female group and the other half to a male group to see the effects of gender on the relative effectiveness of a mathematics curriculum. Likewise, it would be unethical in a sample of nonsmokers to assign half to a nonsmoking group and the other half to a smoking group that would have to smoke two packs of cigarettes a day for a year to determine the effects of smoking. The independent variables (e.g., gender, smoking status) in causal–comparative research are called *classification, subject,* or *organismic variables,* and the

independent variables in experimental research are called *stimulus variables.* Note that a stimulus variable may be manipulated in a causal–comparative design, but for both groups the variable is manipulated with the intention of seeing how the classification, subject, or organismic variable affects the participants' responses.

Another difference between the causal–comparative design and experimental designs involves the issue of cause-and-effect relationships. Despite its name, the causal–comparative design demonstrates a relatively weak indication of a cause-and-effect relationship. The experimental design demonstrates a much stronger causal relationship.

A final difference is that in experimental research the participants may be assigned to groups, whereas in the causal–comparative design participants are already in preformed groups (e.g., males and females).

WHAT SHOULD RESEARCHERS CONSIDER WHEN DESIGNING A CAUSAL–COMPARATIVE STUDY?

There are three critical issues that researchers must consider when designing a causal–comparative study: (1) development of hypotheses, (2) selection of groups, and (3) analysis of data (see Figure 6.3). Critical research consumers should look closely at causal–comparative studies to ensure that these issues have been adequately considered.

Development of Hypotheses

The initial issue centers on the development of hypotheses about the causes or effects of the phenomenon under study. Although the

---

Experimental

- Independent variable is manipulated
- Strong indication of cause-and-effect relationships
- Participants assigned to groups

Causal–Comparative

- Independent variable is not manipulated
- Weak indication of cause-and-effect relationships
- Participants are in preformed groups

FIGURE 6.2. Key differences between experimental and causal–comparative designs.

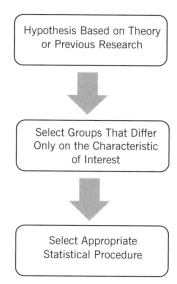

Hypothesis Based on Theory or Previous Research

⬇

Select Groups That Differ Only on the Characteristic of Interest

⬇

Select Appropriate Statistical Procedure

FIGURE 6.3. Key critical issues for designing causal–comparative studies.

hypotheses can initially be based on pure speculation and informal observations, it is critical that researchers look closely at theory and previous research findings to ensure that there is a basis for the hypotheses. Doing so is also critical to ensure that other possible explanatory factors that might influence the phenomenon or characteristic under study can be considered in the research design. As will become clear in our discussion of the data analysis procedures used with causal–comparative research, there are ways of determining the influence of potential explanatory factors other than those of particular interest. Indeed, it is important that researchers explore plausible alternative hypotheses about factors that might explain differences in the characteristic of interest.

Selection of Groups

The second critical issue in designing a causal–comparative study is to select the group that possesses the characteristic under study (experimental group) and a comparison group that does not have the characteristic. Selecting the group that possesses the characteristic requires a precise definition so that not only can a comparison group be selected, but also the results of the study can be interpreted meaningfully. For

example, in a study of the effects of teacher attitudes on the academic performance of students at risk for school failure, it would not be precise enough to say simply that the experimental group includes at-risk students. A more precise definition would be needed, for example, students who are in the lower quartile in academic achievement, who average 10 or more absences (excused and unexcused) a year, and average five detentions or more a year for disruptive behavior. This definition not only enables researchers to identify a meaningful comparison group but also allows the results of the study to be interpreted meaningfully.

A potential problem can arise when selecting a comparison group. In the preceding example, selecting a comparison group would appear to be rather straightforward. Researchers would select students who do not meet the specified criteria. Unfortunately, things are often not so straightforward in selecting a comparison group. In the preceding case, differences in academic performance might be due to other, extraneous factors, such as the type and amount of instruction they receive, intelligence level, and level of parental involvement. There are three ways to solve this problem—matching of participants, equating groups statistically, and selecting extreme groups.

Matching of Participants

Researchers might equate groups on the extraneous factors through a matching procedure to ensure that the variables do not confound the results of the study. They might match the experimental students with regard to the amount and type of instruction they receive (e.g., experimental and control students enrolled in the same class), intelligence (e.g., experimental students matched with control students having an IQ within ± 8 points), and level of parental involvement (e.g., experimental students with high and low parental involvement matched with equivalent control group students).

Equating Groups Statistically

Related to the matching approach, researchers can use a statistical procedure to equate groups on the extraneous variables. This procedure called ANCOVA is described in detail later. Although some researchers question the validity of using ANCOVA to equate groups statistically because it essentially creates an artificial or unnatural comparison group (e.g., Ferguson, 1989; McBurney & White, 2009), it is the preferred procedure of most researchers. The use of ANCOVA to equate groups statistically is preferred for two reasons. First, there simply may not be suitable matches available for some members of the experimental group. Second, matching experimental and comparison participants on all of the extraneous factors is a time-consuming job. In most cases, it is much more efficient to measure the participants on the extraneous factors and equate them statistically using ANCOVA.

Selecting Extreme Groups

The final approach to handling the problem of extraneous variables is called the extreme groups method. As its name implies, this method requires researchers to select experimental and comparison groups at two extremes of a score distribution on the characteristic of interest. The assumption underlying the extreme groups methods is that the comparison group is more likely to differ on other measured factors, but less dramatically than on the variable of interest (Gall et al., 2007). In the earlier study of the influence of teacher attitudes on the academic performance of students at risk for school failure, researchers might select the sample by administering a survey to 100 teachers. Then they might select the top 20 teachers who reported positive attitudes and the bottom 20 teachers who reported more negative attitudes. The remaining 60 teachers might be dropped from the study. The resulting sample of 40 teachers would most likely include a greater number of teachers with very positive and very negative attitudes than would a sample of teachers randomly selected from the population. Selecting these extreme groups is more likely to reveal an effect on the academic performance of students at risk for school failure than selecting groups that do not demonstrate extreme differences on the characteristic of interest.

Analysis of Data

The final issue focuses on collection and analysis of the data. Researchers use a wide range of measurement devices in causal–comparative research. Standardized and criterion-referenced tests, surveys, questionnaires, interviews, and observations are all used by researchers in causal–comparative research. Thus, they must carefully consider the reliability and validity of the measurement device being used. Additionally, because inferential statistics play a key role in interpreting the findings of causal–comparative research studies, it is critical that researchers employ the appropriate tests of statistical significance. Statistical significance testing and the statistical procedures commonly used in causal–comparative research follow.

Determining whether two or more groups differ on some critical variable is accomplished by using various statistical procedures. Use of these statistical procedures depends on a number of issues, including the number of groups, the types of data, and the question(s) being asked. (Refer to Figures 4.10, 4.11, and 4.12 for information regarding when to use each statistical analysis procedure to analyze data from investigations.)

Recall from Chapter 4 that there are parametric and nonparametric tests of statistical significance. Parametric tests are most commonly used in causal–comparative research studies. A t-test is used when researchers are interested in determining whether there is a statistical significant difference between the means of two sets of scores. A t-test for independent means is used when the means of two samples are considered independent from one another. The t-test for correlated means is used when the samples are related to one another, whereas the t-test for a single mean is used in cases in which the researcher is interested in determining whether there is a statistically significant difference between a sample mean and a specified population mean. See Chapter 4 for a description of the nonparametric tests of statistical significance that parallel these t-tests.

ANOVA is used to compare the means of three or more sets of scores to determine whether the difference between them is statistically significant. Recall that the ANOVA does not pinpoint which of the differences is statistically significant. Thus, the ANOVA is an initial step in the analysis of data from a causal-comparative study designed to compare the means for three or more sets of scores. Researchers use multiple-comparison procedures such as the Neuman–Keuls, Tukey, and Scheffé test to pinpoint which pairs of means differ from one another. See Chapter 4 for a description of the nonparametric test of statistical significance that parallels the ANOVA.

Internal Validity

Although some of the threats to internal validity discussed in Chapter 2 typically do not directly apply to causal–comparative research (e.g., maturation, testing, resentful demoralization of the control group, diffusion of treatment, compensatory rivalry by the control group, compensatory equalization; see Table 6.1), researchers should look closely at the design of causal–comparative research studies to assess the potential threats to internal validity.

There are three critical issues to consider in not only designing but also in analyzing and evaluating causal–comparative research. First, as in all research, researchers should rely heavily on theory and previous research. The basis for exploring possible causal relationships should not be based on speculation alone. Second, the selection of experimental

and comparison groups should be done with a high degree of precision, which is necessary for meaningful interpretations of the findings. Table 6.1 indicates that selection is the major threat to the internal validity of a causal–comparative design. Third, as with all research, the data collection and analysis procedures must be appropriate for the given focus of the study, because tests of statistical significance provide the framework for interpreting the findings. This is not to say that tests of statistical significance provide the complete story; rather, they are critical for determining whether, at some established probability level, the results were a function of chance factors alone.

It should be clear that interpretations of causal–comparative findings are limited because researchers do not know whether a particular variable (i.e., classification) is a cause or a result of the pattern of behavior being studied. For example, in a study on whether students with behavioral disorders (BD) understand the cause-and-effect relationship between social interactions and educational and life outcomes (Nelson, Drummond, Martella, & Marchand-Martella, 1997), we found that students with BD did not fully understand the outcomes of

TABLE 6.1. Threats to Internal Validity Associated with the Causal–Comparative Design

Threat	Causal–comparative research design
1. Maturation	Not applicable
2. Selection	Concern
3. Selection by maturation interaction	Not applicable
4. Statistical regression	Not applicable
5. Mortality	Not applicable
6. Instrumentation	Not applicable
7. Testing	Not applicable
8. History	Not applicable
9. Resentful demoralization of the control group	Not applicable
10. Diffusion of treatment	Not applicable
11. Compensatory rivalry by the control group	Not applicable
12. Compensatory equalization	Not applicable

Note. This table is meant only as a general guideline. Decisions with regard to threats to internal validity must be made after the specifics of an investigation are known and understood. Thus, interpretations of internal validity threats must be made on a study-by-study basis.

negative interpersonal social interactions. We did not know the types of interpersonal social interactions patterns that were present before any of the students developed BD. Thus, it was difficult to interpret the findings.

Questions such as the following would have to be addressed in additional studies to clarify the potential cause-and-effect relationships: Do students with more serious BD have a more limited understanding of the cause-and-effect relationship between social interactions and educational and life outcomes? Does the understanding of students with BD regarding the cause-and-effect relationship between social interactions and educational and life outcomes become more limited in the process of becoming BD? Or do other factors such as level of social development or intelligence result in a limited understanding of the cause-and-effect relationship between social interactions and educational and life outcomes?

Nevertheless, the causal–comparative method is useful for identifying possible causal relationships. These tentative relationships can be explored in subsequent experimental or longitudinal studies when possible. Additionally, replications of the study that confirm the causal relationship and disconfirm other potential causal relationships can also increase confidence in the existence of a causal relationship in cases in which it is impossible to conduct experimental studies.

External Validity

As with internal validity, some of the threats to external validity do not typically apply to causal–comparative research (e.g., interaction of personological variables and treatment effects, novelty and disruption effects, pretest sensitization). However, critical research consumers should look closely at the design of causal–comparative studies to assess threats to external validity (see Table 6.2). One of the primary threats to the external validity to consider is "generalization across participants." The procedure for selecting participants is one of the most important factors to consider. It is not uncommon for researchers to use convenience sampling techniques (i.e., readily available participants) rather than random selection procedures. If this is the case, the results of the study are unlikely to generalize across participants.

TABLE 6.2. Threats to External Validity Associated with the Causal–Comparative Design

Threat	Causal–comparative research design
1. Generalization across participants	Possible concern
2. Interaction of personological variables and treatment effects	Not applicable
3. Verification of independent variable	Possible concern
4. Multiple treatment interference	Not applicable
5. Novelty and disruption effects	Not applicable
6. Hawthorne effect	Not applicable
7. Experimenter effects	Not applicable
8. Pretest sensitization	Not applicable
9. Posttest sensitization	Possible concern
10. Interaction of time of measurement and treatment effects	Possible concern
11. Measurement of the dependent variable	Possible concern
12. Interaction of history and treatment effects	Possible concern

Note. This table is meant only as a general guideline. Decisions with regard to threats to external validity must be made after the specifics of an investigation are known and understood. Thus, interpretations of external validity threats must be made on a study-by-study basis.

Additional threats to the external validity of causal–comparative studies to examine closely are those associated with the dependent measure and experimenter effects. For example, the "measurement of the dependent variable" is a potential threat to the external validity of causal–comparative studies, because indirect measurement techniques are typically used by the researchers. Thus, critical research consumers must look closely at the dependent variable to determine whether the results would generalize beyond the dependent measure used in the study.

Finally, an interesting threat may be verification of the independent variable. Consider the study discussed previously about whether students with BD understand the cause-and-effect relationship between social interactions and educational and life outcomes. In order to be part of the investigation, students had to have a BD diagnosis (the independent variable of concern). Thus, we had to rely on the BD label; more importantly, we had to rely on the validity of the assessments that aided in diagnosing students as having BD. If these assessments were not valid (i.e., students without BD were labeled or students with BD were not labeled), the validity of our independent variable would be in question. It is critical to consider the methods used in categorizing participants on a classification variable. Of course, on a variable such as gender, there would be little or no concern. With other variables, especially those that leave room for error in categorization, the verification of the independent variable is important.

Recall the research question regarding the perceptions of future teachers on providing educational service to students with disabilities in general education classrooms? Read on to see how your design compares to how the actual study was designed.

Research Example 1: Not Possible to Manipulate the Independent Variable

A 2×2 within-subject factorial design was used to investigate perceptions of future teachers on providing educational service to students with disabilities in general education classrooms (Shippen, Crites, Houchins, Ramsey, &

Simon, 2005). Factors were time (pretest and posttest) and teacher type (general and special education trainees). A total of 326 graduate and undergraduate preservice teachers (i.e., students working towards teaching licensure) from three universities first took a pretest. The pretest called the Preservice Inclusion Survey (PSIS; adapted from Soodak, Podell, & Lehman, 1998) describes hypothetical students with disabilities in an inclusive class. Following presentation of a paragraph describing students with hearing impairments, LDs, intellectual disability, BDs, or physical disabilities, preservice teachers were presented a list of 17 adjective combinations (e.g., *fearless/scared, uncomfortable/comfortable*). For each adjective combination, teachers rated their perceptions on a 5-point Likert-type scale ranging from *negative feelings* to *positive feelings*. Following the pretest, preservice teachers participated in a semester-length introductory course in special education at one of three universities. According to the researchers:

> By the end of the course, the participants would have been familiar with the characteristics, causation, and interventions for students with hearing impairments, learning disabilities, [intellectual disability], behavioral disorders, or physical disabilities requiring use of a wheelchair. (p. 94)

The purpose of the study was to compare perceptions of preservice teachers on two dichotomous scales (Hostility/Receptivity and Anxiety/Calmness) before and after completion of the course. The same PSIS was administered following the course. Preservice teachers included special educators (29%), general educators (46%), and dually certified educators (21%). Four percent did not respond. Fifty-one percent of preservice teachers were postbaccalaureate or graduate-level educators, and 75% were female. A MANOVA was used to analyze the data. The statistical analysis set time (pre- and posttest) as the factor, with dependent measures including dichotomous scales (Hostility/Receptivity, Anxiety/Calmness). Results indicated significant main effects for time (pretest, posttest) and dichotomous scales. Post-PSIS scores revealed that future teachers were less hostile and anxious about serving students with disabilities in inclusive settings. There were no statistically significant differences for teacher type, gender, or class rank.

Recall the research question regarding whether opportunities to learn vary as a function of number of students in a classroom identified as English language learners? Read on to see how your design compares to how the actual study was designed.

Research Example 2: Prohibitive to Assess Changes in Variable over Time

A causal–comparative design involved a study of the relationship between English language learners (ELLs) and level of opportunity to learn (OTL; Abedi & Herman, 2010). A total of nine teachers and 602 students from urban schools participated in the study. Teachers taught Algebra I to 24 classes of students. To explore whether the concentration of ELL students related to OTL, the sample of classrooms was divided into three groups: (1) classrooms in which ELLs were the majority of students (more than 75% of total students), (2) classrooms in which proportions of ELL and non-ELL students were evenly mixed, and (3) classrooms in which non-ELLs were the majority of students (more than 75% of total students). The researchers' hypothesis was that ELL students achieved less due to decreased levels of OTL. Four OTL measures were used. First, researchers developed an OTL survey addressing content coverage, or actual coverage of core curriculum; content exposure, the amount of time teachers allocate to covering content; content emphasis, the time and attention to certain topics that are part of the core curriculum; and quality of instructional delivery, or how effectively teachers engage students, so that students acquire skills taught. Teachers' and students' OTL surveys were based on self-report. A key component of the OTL survey involved comparison of teacher and student perceptions. Teachers checked whether 28 topics related to algebra had been addressed. Students responded to the same 28 topics. Percentage of agreement between teachers' and students' responses was computed. For ELL students and their teachers, agreement was 54.1%. For non-ELL students and their teachers, agreement was 73.4%. A second measure was a 20-item algebra test specifically

developed for this study. A third measure was a student background questionnaire with self-assessment questions pertaining to comprehension of teacher instructional activities (directions, instruction, tests, etc.). A fourth measure was the Fluency subscale of the Language Assessment Scale (Medina & Escamilia, 1992). Researchers used MANOVA to analyze results from multiple variables. Results indicated that (1) measures of classroom OTL were associated with student performance on the algebra test, (2) ELL students reported lower levels of OTL compared to non-ELL students, (3) classrooms with higher concentrations of ELL students were associated with lower levels of OTL, and (4) English proficiency and self-reported ability to understand teachers' instruction influenced OTL. OTL was related to student performance even after researchers controlled for student math grades. Those students who reported low OTL indicated they did not understand teacher instructions.

CAN THE CAUSAL–COMPARATIVE APPROACH BE COMBINED WITH FACTORIAL DESIGNS?

In Chapter 5, we introduced factorial experimental designs to assess the effects of two or more independent variables and/or the interactions among variables that can be manipulated (Graziano & Raulin, 2010). However, factorial designs also are very flexible and allow use of causal–comparative designs (i.e., using classification variables) when researchers are interested in the effects of classification variables. Factorial designs also allow researchers to combine experimental methodologies (i.e., using stimulus variables) with others, such as a causal–comparative one (i.e., using classification variables). In fact, most factorial designs use a combination or mixture of experimental and causal–comparative methodologies. For example, researchers typically use basic classification variables, such as gender, when analyzing the results of all experimental research designs. We consider two types of these factorial designs—those that include classification variables only, and those that mix stimulus and classification variables (mixed factors).

Classification Variables

There may be times when researchers are interested in the differences between groups based on a classification variable versus a stimulus variable. For example, consider exposing two groups of participants (male and females) and two types of schools (private and public) to a word fluency program and assessing the reading rates of students after the completion of the program (see Figure 6.4). We would have a 2 × 2 factorial design, with each factor being a classification variable. Note that there is a stimulus variable present (i.e., fluency program); however, the stimulus variable is applied equally to both groups. We could determine whether there were differences between males and females with regard to reading, and between students who go to private versus public schools. We could also determine whether there was an interaction effect between gender and type of school attended.

Mixed Factors

In the social sciences factorial designs commonly use an experimental design strategy for one factor and a causal–comparative design for another. These studies involve at least one factor that is a stimulus or manipulated variable and a classification variable such as gender, age, ethnicity, or baseline performance levels. For example, a researcher may want to explore whether a reading intervention has the same effect on students with lower baseline levels of reading skills as on those with higher levels, or whether the effects vary as a function of the gender. In our example of sentence length in Chapter 5, we might have the configuration shown in Figure 6.5. We would have two groups exposed to either sentence length less than or equal to 20

words or greater than 20 words, and less than or equal to two difficult words per paragraph or greater than two difficult words per paragraph, just as we saw in the example in Chapter 5. However, we are also interested in whether gender plays a role in performance. Thus, we can include gender as a third factor to make a 2 × 2 × 2 factorial design in which first two factors are stimulus variables and the third factor is a classification variable (i.e., male and female).

Analysis of Data

As we noted in Chapter 5, the factorial designs and associated statistical analysis procedures used by researchers can be quite complex. For example, a factorial design used in a study comparing two methods of vocabulary instruction (i.e., interactive storybook reading, explicit instruction of word meanings) might be extended to include a comparison of home language (i.e., Spanish, English) and the performance of boys and girls. The effect on vocabulary learning of three methods of teaching, two language conditions, and gender could be investigated with a 2 (interactive storybook reading vs. explicit instruction of word meanings) × 2 (Spanish vs. English) × 2 (male vs. female) ANOVA.

It is informative to look more closely at the preceding example to identify the two primary types of factors included in factorial designs. The first factor (stimulus), the two methods of vocabulary instruction (i.e., interactive storybook reading, explicit instruction of word meanings) is an independent variable being manipulated as a part of the experimental methodology. The other two factors, home language and gender, are classification factors included in the analysis as a part of the causal–comparative methodology. They were present prior to the start of the study and were not manipulated by researchers.

As noted earlier, an advantage of factorial designs is that they allow researchers to combine experimental and other methods, such as causal–comparative methods. Going back to the previous example, one method of teaching vocabulary may interact with the participants' home language and/or gender, and render that combination either better or worse than any

Gender	Type of School	
	Private	Public
Male	10 Participants	10 Participants
Female	10 Participants	10 Participants

FIGURE 6.4. 2 × 2 factorial design with classification variables.

Sentence Length	Average Number of Difficult Words per Paragraph	
	≤ 2 Words	> 2 Words
≤ 20 Words	Male: 5 Participants	Male: 5 Participants
	Female: 5 Participants	Female: 5 Participants
> 20 Words	Male: 5 Participants	Male: 5 Participants
	Female: 5 Participants	Female: 5 Participants

FIGURE 6.5. 2 × 2 × 2 factorial design with mixed factors.

other combination. Internal and external validity issues that pertain to the type of methods used (i.e., experimental, causal–comparative) are present in factorial designs, as explained in Chapter 5.

Recall the research question about whether education level and primary instrument influence one's evaluation of a musical passage? Read on to see how your design compares to the way the actual study was designed.

Research Example 3: Causal–Comparative Design Combined with Factorial Design

A causal–comparative design with classification variables was used to investigate influence of primary musical instrument performance and education level on the evaluation of musical performance (Hewitt, 2007). The factorial design involved 2 (brass instrument as primary musical instrument vs. non-brass instrument) × 3 (education level of student evaluator: middle school, high school, or college) classification variables. In this study, musicians with different educational levels and primary experience in brass or non-brass instruments evaluated six junior high school-age students as they performed the same musical passage using a trumpet. The study examined whether different musicians evaluated a musical passage in similar or different ways using the Woodwind Brass Solo Evaluation Form (WBSEF; Saunders & Holahan, 1997). The WBSEF, which reportedly had high levels of interrater reliability among professional musicians in previous research, requires that the evaluator rate the musician's performance in seven subareas, including tone, melodic accuracy, intonation, rhythmic accuracy, tempo, interpretation, and technique/

articulation. There were 423 participants, including 187 middle school, 113 high school, and 123 college students. Researchers and participants first discussed the content of each subarea of the WBSEF, then participants listened to a "model" recording of Bach's *Gigue from French Suite* on two occasions. Finally, participants evaluated individual, audiotaped performances of junior high students who played the *Gigue*. A general linear model with repeated measures analysis was used to determine relationships between two instrument conditions (brass or non-brass as primary instrument of the participant evaluators) and among three educational levels (education level of student evaluator: middle school, high school, or college) to WBSEF ratings. Generally, results showed that high school and middle school participants rated junior high musicians' performance lower than that of college participants. Statistically significant differences in ratings were found on all subareas of the WBSEF except interpretation. The researcher commented that "results suggest that differences do exist between educational levels on the evaluation of trumpet performances" (Hewitt, 2007, p. 24). The primary performance instrument had no influence on the evaluation of junior high trumpet performances. Researchers recommended that musicians of all education levels receive training in reliable evaluation of musical passages.

WHEN SHOULD RESEARCHERS USE THE CAUSAL–COMPARATIVE RESEARCH DESIGN?

Causal–comparative research is used to explore potential causal relationships between two or more variables. The causal–comparative research method is used under two primary conditions (Schenker & Rumrill, 2004): (1) when it is not possible to manipulate the variables experimentally, such as presenting or taking away BD or mental illnesses; and (2) when it would be prohibitive to assess changes in a variable, such as when ethical concerns about requiring a group to smoke when there are not enough resources to conduct a study over time using a longitudinal research. Much work in developmental psychology is based on the causal–comparative research method, in which the goal is to explore developmental changes over time.

Despite the intent of causal–comparative research to establish causal relationships between or among variables, such interpretations must be made with caution. Causal interpretations of causal–comparative findings are limited for two reasons. First, it is never totally clear whether a particular variable is a cause or a result of the pattern of behavior being studied or the result of some other variable. Second, the logic of statistical significance testing never results in a definitive causal statement; there is always a chance of making a Type I error. Nevertheless, causal–comparative research is useful for identifying possible causal relationships. These tentative relationships can be explored in subsequent experimental or longitudinal studies when possible. Additionally, replications of a study that confirm the causal relationship and disconfirm other potential causal relationships can be used to increase our confidence in the findings when it is not possible to conduct experimental studies. Our acceptance of the link between smoking and lung cancer is a case in point.

SUMMARY

❖ One of the two approaches used by researchers to explore the relationships among variables is the causal–comparative method. This method has two purposes—(1) to compare two or more samples or groups of participants that differ on a critical variable but are otherwise comparable, and (2) to compare two or more equivalent samples on a critical variable to identify changes over time.

❖ The causal–comparative research method compares two groups of individuals drawn from the same population that differ on a critical variable but are otherwise comparable. Causal–comparative research is similar to experimental research methods in three ways: (1) Each compares group scores (averages) to determine relationships between the independent and dependent variables; (2) both use group memberships as a categorical variable; and (3) with the exception of counterbalanced and time-series designs, both compare separate groups of participants. Causal–comparative research is different in three important ways: (1) In experimental designs, the independent variable is manipulated, whereas in the causal–comparative design, the independent variable is not manipulated; (2) the causal–comparative design cannot determine cause-and-effect relationships

the way experimental designs can; and (3) in experimental research, participants may be assigned to groups, whereas participants in the causal–comparative design are already in preformed groups (e.g., males and females).

❖ There are three critical issues that researchers must consider when designing a causal–comparative study: (1) development of hypotheses about the causes or effects of the phenomenon under study, (2) selection of a group that possesses the characteristic under study (experimental group) and a comparison group that does not have the characteristic, and (3) analysis of data using a wide range of measurement devices in causal–comparative research. Selection is a serious threat to internal validity, and generalization across participants is a potential threat to external validity.

❖ Factorial designs allow researchers to use causal–comparative designs (i.e., using classification variables) when the point of interest is the effects of classification variables. Factorial designs also allow researchers to combine experimental methodologies (i.e., using stimulus variables) and others, such as a causal-comparative methodology (i.e., using classification variables). In fact, most factorial designs use a combination or mixture of experimental and causal–comparative methodologies. Internal and external validity issues that pertain to the types of methods used (i.e., experimental, causal–comparative) are present in factorial designs.

❖ The causal–comparative research method is used under two primary conditions—(1) when it is not possible to manipulate the variables experimentally, and (2) when it would be prohibitive to assess changes in a variable.

DISCUSSION QUESTIONS

1. What is causal–comparative research, that is, how is it done?

2. Does the term *causal–comparative* mean that these designs can determine cause-and-effect relationships? Why or why not? (*Note.* In your response, indicate the internal validity threats to the causal–comparative research method.)

3. How are causal–comparative research designs similar to true experimental designs? How are they different?

4. When is it appropriate to use causal–comparative research designs?

5. What are the considerations one must make when designing causal–comparative research studies?

6. Why are the threats to internal validity that result in changes in the performance of the control group not applicable to causal–comparative research studies?

7. How are independent variables in causal–comparative research designs different from those used in experimental designs?

8. How can causal–comparative designs be combined in a factorial design? In your response, include examples of classification variables only and mixed factors.

9. If it were possible to use an experimental design to study the subject matter in a causal–comparative design, what factors would have to be in place for such a study to progress?

10. What kinds of factors should a researcher consider when selecting statistical analysis procedures to analyze data from a causal–comparative research study?

---------------------------------- ILLUSTRATIVE EXAMPLE ----------------------------------

Literate Language Features in Spoken Narratives of Children with Typical Language and Children with Language Impairments

Kellie S. Greenhalgh   *Carol J. Strong*
Utah State University, Logan

ABSTRACT: **Purpose:** *This study focused on literate language features in spoken narratives of school-age children with typical language development and school-age children with language impairments (LI).*

Method: *The spoken narrative retellings from male and female children aged 7 to 10 years were analyzed. The samples yielded scores for the literate language features of conjunctions, elaborated noun phrases, mental and linguistic verbs, and adverbs. A general language*

performance measure (number of different words) also was studied.

Results: *Group membership main effects were statistically significant for conjunctions and elaborated noun phrases, with effect sizes ranging from small to moderate. No statistically significant differences were obtained for age level or gender. Correlations between scores for number of different words and scores for the literate language features were low to moderate.*

Clinical implications: *The measures of conjunctions and elaborated noun phrases differentiated children with LI from those with typical language. When the number of different words was normalized for sample length, support for its use as a general language performance measure was not obtained.*

KEY WORDS: language impairment, literate language, language assessment, narration

What is a literate language style? Language development has been characterized in terms of an oral–literate continuum (Westby, 1985). An oral language style may be broadly defined as "learning to talk"—that is, learning phonology, morphology, syntax, semantics, and pragmatics—whereas a literate language style may be defined as "talking to learn"—that is, using language "to monitor and reflect on experience, and reason about, plan, and predict experiences" (Westby, 1985, p. 181). Clearly, development of a literate language style contributes to the academic success of children. Wallach and Butler (1994) noted that children "who *talk like books*—that is, students who use literate styles of communicating in oral language—tend to match teacher expectations more often than children who do not . . . and tend to be rewarded in school" (pp. 5–6, italics in original).

In contrasting oral and literate language, Paul (2001) pointed to differences in contextualization. Generally, oral language is highly contextualized, with the immediate environment offering abundant cues such as objects, gestures, facial expressions, and intonation. Literate language, by contrast, is highly decontextualized, with "virtually all the information needed for comprehension . . . present within the linguistic signal itself, and little support . . . available outside it" (Paul, 2001, p. 391). Drawing on the work of Westby (1991), Paul (2001, p. 391) enumerated many specific differences between oral and literate language with respect to function, topic, and structure.

Literate language is not a "skill" independent of children's literacy achievement or experiences. Generally, children who are illiterate or semiliterate have had limited opportunity to experience literate language and internalize its functions, topics, and structures (Wallach & Butler, 1994). By contrast, children who can read, who are read to, and who discuss text experiences with adult caregivers have significant advantages in terms of exposure to literate language. "*The most natural and common way of acquiring literate language is*

through print" (Wallach & Butler, 1994, p. 6, italics in original). However, oral experiences—such as hearing planned speeches or sermons—also may enable children to internalize highly literate aspects of language (e.g., conditional and causal conjunctions). Theoretically, literate language may be linked to children's development of meaningful abstract thinking or the ability to recontextualize a previously experienced event or activity (van Oers, 1998) so that a listener also can construct meaning.

Literate language deficits limit a child's ability to convey specific meanings (Paul, 1995). Moreover, they can detrimentally affect literacy acquisition (Lyon, 1999; Snow, Scarborough, & Burns, 1999). Investigators have documented the semantic and syntactic weaknesses of children with language impairments (LI) (Gerber, 1993; Klee, 1992; Paul & Smith, 1993; Watkins, Kelly, Harbers, & Hollis, 1995), and clinicians frequently report these deficits as well. For example, school-age children with LI tend to have (a) small vocabularies characterized by short words that occur frequently (Paul, 1995), (b) high frequencies of nonspecific words (Wiig & Semel, 1984), and (c) fewer complex sentences and less elaboration of noun phrases (Paul, 1995). Research findings indicate that "good readers bring strong vocabularies and good syntactic and grammatical skills to the reading comprehension process" (Lyon, 1999, p. 10).

The assessment of literate language is essential for identifying children whose language limitations may hinder their academic and communication success. In fact, a number of researchers (Gillam, Pena, & Miller, 1999; Nippold, 1988, 1993; and Peterson & McCabe, 1983) have urged clinicians to assess children's literate language. However, clinicians often rely on standardized tests (e.g., Test of Language Development—Intermediate, Newcomer & Hammill, 1991; Comprehensive Receptive and Expressive Vocabulary Test, Wallace & Hammill, 1994; The Word Test—Revised, Zachman, Barrett, Huisingh, & Jorgensen, 1990) for diagnosing semantic and syntactic deficits, even though such tests have limitations. Standardized tests, for example, tap a limited number of words/concepts, require very specific responses, do not gauge learner potential, and do not reflect children's performance in conversation, narration, or classroom discourse (e.g., Nelson, 1994; Palincsar, Brown, & Campione, 1994). One alternative to standardized measures is the use of a general language performance measure for assessing semantic diversity.

GENERAL LANGUAGE PERFORMANCE MEASURE

When estimating semantic diversity in discourse for clinical or research purposes, speech-language pathologists and researchers have calculated the number of different words [NDW] (Klee, 1992; Miller, 1991; Paul & Smith, 1993; Watkins et al., 1995). The NDW measure typically is computed from the first 50 child-initiated utterances in a transcript (Klee, 1992). Each unique word is counted once, with regular forms of nouns and verbs recognized as belonging to the same word root, irregular forms recognized as unique words, and contractions counted as two different words.

Recent findings support the use of NDW for identifying children with LI. For example, Klee (1992) reported that NDW scores moderately correlated with age in groups of children with normal and impaired language ($r = 0.76$), and that mean NDW scores statistically differentiated the groups. Watkins et al. (1995) also reported that mean NDW scores differentiated children with normal language from children with specific LI. Miller (1991) contributed further support for the validity of NDW in the finding that these scores were highly correlated with age in samples of narration ($r = .80$) and moderately correlated in samples of conversation ($r = .75$). Although the NDW measure appears useful for identifying children whose semantic diversity is below expectations, it is a measure of general language performance rather than a fine-grained measure of literate language skills.

This study's purpose was to examine differences in literate language use in spoken narratives for children with LI and for children with typical language across four age levels and for males and females. The correlations between scores for NDW and scores for the literate language features studied here also were examined to estimate the extent to which NDW (a measure of semantic diversity) reflected literate language usage.

LITERATE LANGUAGE MEASURES

The elementary school-age years are critical for literate language development and the acquisition of words and structures "needed to understand and produce language near the literate end of the oral-literate continuum" (Paul, 1995, p. 486). In samples of narrative discourse, a literate language style often is reflected in the richness of the vocabulary used—what Peterson and McCabe (1983) called "sparkle" or Gillam et al. (1999) referred to as the elaborateness of children's vocabulary.

Based on the work of Pellegrini (1985), who documented literate language style in children's narratives produced during play, Westby (1999) described four features as contributors to a literate language style: conjunctions, elaborated noun phrases (ENP), mental and linguistic verbs, and adverbs. The frequency of their use provides an estimate of a child's literate language ability. The rationale for using these features is threefold.

- These linguistic features enhance the quality (effectiveness) of children's narratives so that listeners can build a mental model for the story (Segal & Duchan, 1997).

- The features allow children to recontextualize information more effectively, enabling them to meet the literacy demands of the curriculum (van Oers, 1998).

- Features such as these that occur with low frequency are likely sensitive to linguistic growth (Perera, 1986).

Descriptions of the four features follow.

Conjunctions

Scott (1988) identified adverbial markers and conjunctions that occur with low frequency in the language of school-age children. Although these inter- and intrasentential connectives occur infrequently, children use such structures to organize narratives, clarify event and object relationships in the story, and make meanings explicit (Pellegrini, 1985; Segal & Duchan, 1997; Wallach, 1990).

Segal and Duchan (1997) contended that connectives guide the listener in constructing meaning for a text and help listeners "build a mental model of the narrative" (p. 99). For example, (a) temporal conjunctions, such as *when, while,* and *after,* in subordinate clauses provide background for narrative events (Pellegrini, 1985); (b) causal conjunctions, such as *because* and *so that,* in subordinate clauses provide psychological motivation or physical reasons for narrative events (Scarlett & Wolf, 1979); and (c) coordinating conjunctions, such as *so, but,* and *however,* signal semantic opposition between elements of a text (McClure & Steffensen, 1985; Segal & Duchan, 1997; Westby, 1999). Children organize information and clarify relationships, then, by using both subordinating and coordinating conjunctions. Because these structures signal a literate language style, Nippold (1993) encouraged clinicians to analyze samples for their occurrence.

ENPs

ENPs contribute to the explicitness of character and object descriptions in narration (Pellegrini, 1985). For example, when children use noun modifiers (e.g., *the old, dead log*), qualifiers (e.g., *a hole in the ground*), appositives (e.g., *this boy, Tom,* had a dog), and relative clauses (e.g., *the boy took the baby that liked him home*), they graphically describe and add information about the nouns or pronouns (Westby, 1994). Such elaboration clarifies children's meanings and helps listeners build a mental model of the story's characters and objects.

Nippold (1988) reported that noun phrase postmodification is a "particularly active growth area" (p. 63) during the school-age years. In spoken language, most instances of ENPs follow the verb (e.g., Tom ran toward *the big old frog*); in written language, a higher percentage of ENPs function as subjects (e.g., *The boy who was crying* went home). Nippold recommended tracking children's use of ENPs (both their type and their grammatical role) as evidence of literate language development.

Mental and Linguistic Verbs

The literate language construct includes mental verbs (e.g., *decided, forgot, knew, thought, remembered*) that refer to various acts of thinking and linguistic verbs (e.g., *said, called, told*) that refer to various acts of speaking. As children engage in discussions of spoken and written language in curricular subjects, they develop an understanding and use of more advanced mental verb forms (e.g., *assume, infer, doubt*) and linguistic verb forms (e.g., *interpret, confirm, assert*) (Nippold, 1988).

When children use mental and linguistic verbs in telling or retelling a story, rather than general verbs, they communicate the story's events in a more explicit (or literate) manner (e.g., he *decided* to look for the frog versus he *went* and looked for the frog; he *shouted*, "stay away" versus he *goes*, "stay away"). Analyzing discourse for the presence of mental and linguistic verbs informs language intervention as well because their occurrence indicates children's awareness of characters' mental states and their verbal abilities.

Adverbs

In narration, the elaboration of events through adverbs (e.g., the dog *accidentally* knocked the beehive down) is evidence that children understand subtle differences in meaning. Such subtleties are gradually learned as children participate in the language of the curriculum (Nippold, 1988). Adverbs often indicate time (e.g., *suddenly*), manner (e.g., *angrily*) and degree (e.g., *extremely*) (Nippold, 1988; Westby, 1999).

Summary and Research Questions

In summary, researchers suggest that these four features contribute to a literate language style and are likely sensitive to developmental growth. Consequently, researchers advise clinicians to analyze language samples for their occurrence, along with calculating a measure of general language performance, such as NDW. Although prior researchers have established that the general language performance measure of NDW enables clinicians to document semantic diversity deficits, calculating this measure does not inform or guide language intervention. In contrast, analyzing samples for literate language features can specifically inform intervention planning, and the scores from such measures also may be useful for documenting a language impairment. The problem is that, in the context of spoken narration, it is not known whether mean scores for literate language features differ between children with typical language and those with language impairments, whether the mean scores increase with increases in age, or whether the mean scores differ between males and females.

To investigate this problem, spoken narratives that had been elicited previously using materials and procedures developed by Strong (1998) were analyzed. The independent variables were group membership (children with typical language [TL] and children with language impairments [LI]), age (7 to 10 years), and gender. The dependent measures were NDW and scores for each of the four literate language features. Five research questions guided this study:

1. Will differences be obtained between the mean scores for children with TL and children with LI?

2. Will differences be obtained among the mean scores for age level (7, 8, 9, and 10 years)?

3. Will differences be obtained between the mean scores for males and females?

4. Will there be interactions between or among the independent variables?

5. Will there be a relationship between NDW scores and scores for the literate language features?

METHODS

A causal–comparative design (Gall, Borg, & Gall, 1996) was used, allowing the researcher to study cause–effect relationships under conditions where experimental manipulation is difficult or impossible. In this study, the scores for NDW and the literate language features of children with LI were compared with those of children with TL. The two groups were matched for age and gender to control for potential additional sources of score variability.

Participants

All children attended northern Utah schools from 30 small towns and farms within Cache County. The total county population for 1997 was estimated at 87,900. Utah State University employs approximately 20% of the labor force; the rest of the labor force is employed in local service businesses and light industries or travel out of the area to work in defense-related industries. In 1997, the median family income was $32,474 and the average per capita income was $16,900. Minorities made up 7.7% of the labor force (Cache Chamber of Commerce, 2000).

The school district has 11 elementary schools, 4 middle schools, 2 senior high schools, 2 freshmen centers, and 1 alternative high school. The district has a total enrollment of approximately 13,200 children.

The children with LI had been classified as having mild, moderate, and severe language impairments, according to Utah State Office of Education (1993) criteria. That is, a child was considered as having LI if he or she performed at least one standard deviation below the mean on two or more measures of oral expression or listening comprehension in one or more of three areas—morphology, syntax, and semantics. The tests that had been most commonly administered to diagnose and assess language impairment were the Test of Language Development—Intermediate (Newcomer & Hammill, 1991) and the Clinical Evaluation of Language Fundamentals—Revised (Semel, Wiig, & Secord, 1987). The children with LI had no history or evidence of other disorders and were not classified as having an intellectual handicap (IQ score of 85 or greater on either the Wechsler Intelligence Scale for Children—Revised [Wechsler, 1974], the Leiter International Performance Scale [Leiter, 1979], the Slosson Intelligence Test [Slosson, 1981], or the Kaufman Assessment Battery for Children [Kaufman & Kaufman, 1983]).

The 52 participants with LI were randomly selected from the accessible population of children (ages 7 through 10) with documented LI within the district; the 52 participants with TL were then randomly selected from the same classrooms (36 different classrooms) as those in which the participants with LI were enrolled. All of the 52 children with LI were being educated in regular education classrooms. All participants were Caucasian and their native language was English.

The sample stories were obtained from 104 children—52 with LI and 52 with TL, with 26 at each of the four age levels. These children had retold stories for studies conducted by Strong and Shaver (1991) and Davis (1999), and their existing stories were used for the analyses in this study.

Independent t-tests revealed that, at each age level, the difference between the mean ages for the two groups (see Table 1) was not statistically significant ($p > .05$). Overall, males and females were equally represented; however, as Table 1 indicates, the proportion of males to females at each age level varied.

The Peabody Picture Vocabulary Test—Revised [PPVT-R] (Dunn & Dunn, 1981) was administered as an estimate of each child's vocabulary comprehension. The difference between the mean PPVT-R standard scores was statistically significant, $F(1, 103) = 55.05$, $p < .01$. The mean score of children with TL was higher than the mean score of children with LI at each age level (see Table 1).

PROCEDURE

The researchers met with each of the 104 children four times (Davis, 1999; Strong & Shaver, 1991). During the first session, the researchers administered the PPVT-R and familiarized children with the data collection procedures by eliciting a practice narrative retelling. The remaining three data collection sessions occurred at 1-to-2-week

TABLE 1. Means and Standard Deviations (in Parentheses) for Age, Number of Males and Females by Group, and Peabody Picture Vocabulary Test, Revised (PPVT-R) Standard Scores

Age level	Language impaired	Typical language
Age in years:months		
7	7:4 (0:3)	7:4 (0:4)
8	8:5 (0:3)	8:4 (0:4)
9	9:4 (0:3)	9:3 (0:3)
10	10:6 (0:3)	10:5 (0:5)
Gender		
7	7 (M); 6 (F)	7 (M); 6 (F)
8	10 (M); 3 (F)	10 (M); 3 (F)
9	5 (M); 8 (F)	5 (M); 8 (F)
10	4 (M); 9 (F)	4 (M); 9 (F)
PPVT-R (standard scores)		
7	91.5 (14.9)	107.2 (10.0)
8	79.8 (16.3)	104.2 (8.6)
9	80.7 (14.9)	101.3 (10.0)
10	86.1 (12.4)	97.5 (9.6)

Note: n = 26 at every age level (13 with language impairment and 13 with typical language); M = male; F = female.

intervals and required approximately 15 minutes each. A total of 416 narrative samples were collected, four from each of the 104 children.

Collection of Narrative Language Samples

Several authors have indicated that the construction of stories is a more difficult communication task for children than retelling a story (Martin, 1983; Milosky, 1987; Ripich & Griffith, 1985; Roth, 1986). Ripich and Griffith specifically investigated the effect of narrative task by comparing narrative skills in three retelling tasks versus a task in which the children (ages 7 through 12) were asked to look at a five-picture sequence and generate a story. The authors concluded that "all children performed more poorly on some aspects of generating well-formed stories, indicating that overall this task is more difficult" (p. 4), as compared to retelling tasks. For this study, the spoken language samples were collected by having the children retell a story rather than generate a story. Therefore, the story retelling task should have resulted in a more complete and longer sample of spoken discourse.

The narrative language samples were elicited using procedures and stimulus materials from the Strong Narrative Assessment Procedure (SNAP; Strong, 1998). The examiners used four different stories written for four wordless picture books: *A Boy, a Dog, and a Frog* (Mayer, 1967), *Frog, Where Are You?* (Mayer, 1969), *Frog Goes to Dinner* (Mayer, 1974), and *One Frog Too Many* (Mayer & Mayer, 1975). The stories were written to be similar in length, syntax, content, and cohesion. *Frog Goes to Dinner* was used to familiarize the children with the collection procedures. To control for a possible order effect, the remaining three stories were presented to the children in randomized order.

To create a condition in which the child would tell the story to an uninformed listener, the examiner left the child alone to look at the pictures and listen to the story. The examiner instructed each child to "Look at this book and listen to the story. I have to leave for a few minutes. When I come back, I'd like you to tell me the story. You won't have the pictures to look at when you retell the story." The examiner returned when the story was over and asked the child to retell the story by saying, "I didn't get to hear that story. Please tell it to me as completely as you can."

All narratives were audiotaped. After eliciting all of the narrative samples, an identifying number was randomly assigned to each child's audiotape to control for possible coder-expectancy effects and to ensure confidentiality. A cross-referenced list was filed separately so that the producer of each narrative could be identified. The tape recordings were then transcribed in random order using Strong's (1998) transcription guidelines and conventions. A second researcher, trained to follow the same procedures, listened to the tapes for accuracy of transcribing.

Following transcription, utterances were segmented into C-units (Loban, 1976) using Strong's (1998) procedures. A C-unit includes one main clause with all of its subordinate clauses attached to it. The number of C-units ranged from 5 to 43 for the children with LI and from 5 to 47 for the children with TL. The second researcher then independently segmented all of the transcripts. Intercoder agreement for segmentation was calculated using a point-to-point agreement check (McReynolds & Kearns, 1983), and the percentage of agreement was 98%.

Coding NDW and Literate Language Features

The dependent measures were scored using Systematic Analysis of Language Transcripts (SALT; Miller & Chapman, 1998). Although the four stimulus stories include similar numbers of literate language features, only the 104 retellings for *Frog, Where Are You?* (Appendix A) were analyzed. These were chosen for analysis because mean length scores were greater for this story (Strong, 1998) than for the other three stimulus stories, allowing for more occurrences of the literate language features. (See Appendix B for the literate language coding conventions.)

Reliability of the Scores

The productive use of the literate language features for assessment depends on the reliability of the scores—a necessary, although not sufficient, prerequisite for the validity of the scores (see, e.g., Hopkins & Stanley, 1981; Lord & Novick, 1968; and Nunnally, 1978). Also, when scores lack reliability, true differences between means are obscured and correlation coefficients are attenuated (Strong & Shaver, 1991).

The reliability of the scores was estimated by checking for coder inconsistency. After coding every 10th transcript, the second researcher, previously trained in coding and SALT program use, independently coded 1 randomly selected transcript from among the 10. For 10 of the 104 transcripts, point-to-point intercoder agreement was 95%; disagreements were resolved. The criterion was 90% agreement before resolution of disagreements.

DATA ANALYSIS

The independent variables were (a) group membership—LI or TL; (b) age level—7, 8, 9, and 10 years; and (c) gender—males or females. To adjust for varying sample lengths, proportions were calculated. That is, the raw scores for NDW and each of the literate language features were divided by the number of C-units in the sample (see Table 2).

Given the large number of dependent variables, research questions 1 through 4 were addressed using a multivariate analysis of variance (MANOVA, $p \leq .05$). Univariate follow-up tests were conducted only if the omnibus test was significant. So that readers can examine sample length, means and standard deviations for number of C-units were calculated for both groups of participants at each age level (Table 2) and a MANOVA was conducted as well.

The practical significance (Thompson, 1999) of the results was estimated by calculating effect sizes. The effect size used was Cohen's *d* (Cohen,

TABLE 2. Means and Standard Deviations (in Parentheses) by Age Level and Group for Number of C-Units

Age	LI	TL	Pooled	*d*
7	13.9 (103)	199 (11.9)	16.9 (11.3)	.52
8	18.4 (8.9)	27.6 (11.1)	23.0 (10.9)	.80
9	18.3 (9.5)	28.0 (7.7)	23.2 (9.8)	.85
10	25.2 (10.6)	32.7 (10.4)	28.9 (11.0)	.66
Pooled	18.9 (10.4)	27.1 (11.1)	23.0 (11.4)	.72*

Note. LI = language impaired, TL = typical language, *n* = 26 at every age level (13 with LI and 13 with TL), and *d* = effect size. * = statistically significant group main effect, $p \leq .05$.

1988), the standardized effect size, using the formula $d = M_{TL} - M_{LI}/SD_{pooled}$. Cohen's (1988) guidelines for practical significance were used as arbitrary, but reasonable, criteria to judge the magnitude of *d*s: .2 as a small effect size, .5 as a moderate effect size, and .8 as a large effect size.

The *d* expresses the difference between means in standard deviation units. For example, if the mean score of the TL group for conjunctions per C-unit was .50, with a standard deviation of .10, and the mean score for the LI group was .40, with a standard deviation of .10, the effect size for these data would be 1.0 (.5 – .4/.1 = 1). That is, the mean score for the TL group would be one standard deviation above that for the LI group. Reference to a table or normal curve values (e.g., Ferguson, 1981, p. 519) indicates that 34% of a normal distribution lies in the area from the mean to 1 standard deviation above the mean; consequently, 84% of the distribution lies below that point (fifty percent of the distribution is below the mean.) Assuming that the scores were normally distributed, the effect size of 1.0 indicates that 84% of the TL group scored at or above the mean of the LI group on that measure or, conversely, that 84% of the LI group scored at or below the mean for the TL group (Shaver, 1985).

For research question 5, which concerned relationships between NDW scores and the literate language features, Pearson product–moment correlation coefficients (*r*) were calculated. The coefficient of determination (r^2) was calculated to estimate the amount of variance explained by scores on the two variables.

RESULTS

The scores for the five dependent measures were entered into a MANOVA with group (LI and TL), age level (7, 8, 9, and 10 years), and gender as the independent variables. When analyzed together, this analysis revealed a significant multivariate main effect for group, favoring the TL group [Hotellings F (5, 84) = 3.4, p = .008, η^2 = .17]. No other significant multivariate main effects or interactions were obtained. The follow-up univariate analyses revealed statistically significant group differences, favoring the TL group, for only two of the five measures: conjunctions per C-unit [F (1, 88) = 5.81, p = .018, η^2 = .06] and ENP per C-unit [F (1, 88) = 13.58, p < .000, η^2 = .13].

The correlation ratio, η^2, was calculated by dividing the between-group sum of squares by the total sum of squares. For these calculations, the resulting proportions indicate the degree to which variation in the dependent measurements was associated with group membership. For conjunctions per C-unit, 6% of the variability in the scores was associated with group membership; for ENP per C-unit, the value was 13%.

Post hoc power analyses used to determine the probability of rejecting the null hypothesis, assuming that the effect size obtained is the population value, revealed values ranging from low to high, primarily as a function of the magnitude of the effect sizes (see Table 3). For example, for two variables (ENP per C-unit and conjunctions per C-unit), power was .95 and .66, respectively. For

TABLE 3. Group Means, Standard Deviations (in Parentheses), and Standardized Effect Sizes by Age Level for All Measures Adjusted for Number of C-Units

Age	Means LI		TL		d	SEMD
NDW per C-unit						
7	4.1	(1.1)	3.8	(.8)	−.37	
8	3.3	(.6)	3.6	(1.0)	.37	
9	3.6	(.8)	3.4	(.4)	−.24	
10	3.3	(.8)	3.3	(.7)	.00	
Pooled	3.6	(.9)	3.5	(.8)	−12	.17
Conjunctions per C-unit						
7	.19	(.1)	.22	(.2)	.21	
8	.19	(.1)	.28	(.2)	.64	
9	.24	(.2)	.20	(.1)	−.28	
10	.19	(.1)	.28	(.1)	.64	
Pooled	.20	(.1)	.24	(.2)	.28*	.03
ENP per C-unit						
7	.11	(.1)	.15	(.1)	.40	
8	.09	(.1)	.18	(.1)	.91	
9	.12	(.1)	.19	(.1)	.71	
10	.12	(.1)	.15	(.1)	.30	
Pooled	.11	(.1)	.17	(.1)	.61*	.02
Mental and linguistic verbs per C-unit						
7	.09	(.1)	.09	(.10)	.00	
8	.09	(.1)	.11	(.04)	.30	
9	.07	(.1)	.13	(.05)	.89	
10	.09	(.1)	.11	(.10)	.30	
Pooled	.09	(.1)	.11	(.10)	.30	.01
Adverbs per C-unit						
7	.000	.004 (0.1)	.30			
8	.005 (.01)	.010 (.02)	.32			
9	.008 (.01)	.008 (.02)	.00			
10	.006 (.01)	.008 (.01)	.13			
Pooled	.005 (.01)	.008 (.02)	.19			.003

Note: LI = language impaired, TL = typical language, n = 13 per cell, n = 26 for each, d = effect size, SEMD = standard error of the mean difference, NDW = number of different words, and ENP = elaborated noun phrases.

* = statistically significant, p < .05.

the remaining three variables that lacked statistical significance, power was low and ranged from .11 to .32.

Means, standard deviations, and *ds* for the groups for all five measures appear in Table 3. The *d* for ENP per C-unit was moderate (.61) by Cohen's (1988) guidelines, suggesting a difference that can be considered clinically important. The *d* for conjunctions per C-unit was low (.28). Given the low power for the three remaining measures, the effect sizes reported in Table 3 should be interpreted with caution.

Table 3 also provides a standard error of the mean difference (SEMD) for each dependent measure for calculating: confidence intervals. For this study, with 102 degrees of freedom, the *t* ratio at the .05 level is equal to ±1.98. To calculate the 95% confidence interval for NDW per C-unit, the formula is $[(\pm 1.98) (SEMD) + M_{Diff}]$ or $[(\pm 1.98)(.17) + .1]$. Using this formula, one can estimate that 95% of the time, the true mean difference for NDW per C-unit falls within an interval bounded by –.24 and .44.

The multivariate main effect for age level was not statistically significant [Hotellings F (15, 248) = 1.34, p = .18, η^2 = .08]. Post hoc power analyses revealed that the observed power ranged from low (.09 for verbs per C-unit) to moderate (.66 for NDW per C-unit).

The multivariate main effect for gender was not statistically significant [Hotellings F (5, 84) = 1.24, p = .30, η^2 = .07]. Post hoc power analyses revealed that the observed power was low (ranging from .16 for NDW per C-unit to .48 for conjunctions per C-unit).

With all scores pooled, the correlations between scores for NDW per C-unit and the scores for the literate language features ranged from moderate to negligible, and the coefficients of determination were small: ENP per C-unit, r = .51, r^2 = .26; conjunctions per C-unit, r = .36, r^2 = .13; mental and linguistic verbs per C-unit, r = .15, r^2 = .02; and adverbs per C-unit, r = –.11, r^2 = .01. The correlation between age and scores for NDW per C-unit was small and negative (r = –.26, r^2 = .07). All coefficients were statistically significant, except those for mental and linguistic verbs and adverbs.

In summary, with raw scores converted to proportions in order to control for varying sample lengths, four primary findings were obtained.

1. The mean scores for conjunctions per C-unit and ENP per C-unit differentiated the two groups of children.

2. The differences between the groups' mean scores for adverbs per C-unit, mental and linguistic verbs per C-unit, and NDW per C-unit were not statistically significant.

3. The main effects for age level and gender were not statistically significant.

4. Only negligible to moderate coefficients were obtained between the scores for NDW per C-unit and the scores for the literate language features, and the correlation between age and NDW per C-unit was small and negative.

DISCUSSION

Group Differences

Inspection of the group means for all measures of literate language revealed that means for the TL group were consistently greater than means for the LI group, and the effect sizes ranged from small to moderate. However, only the mean differences for conjunctions per C-unit and ENP per C-unit were statistically significant.

The finding that the group means did not differ statistically for mental and linguistic verbs per C-unit and adverbs per C-unit was not surprising given that few instances of these features occurred in the stories of either group. Inspection of the individual scores revealed that the largest adverb score was 2 (one child with TL), and the largest mental and linguistic verb score was 8 (two children with TL). One explanation for their infrequent occurrence is that the stimulus story did not model these literate language features adequately. However, this explanation seems unlikely because the stimulus story contains 3 adverbs and 11 mental and linguistic verbs. Another possible explanation may be grounded in the instructions, which were not necessarily designed to focus children's attention on the characters' needs, perceptions, and feelings—what Bruner (1986) referred to as the "landscape of consciousness" (p. 14). Rather, children were given general instructions to "retell the story as completely as possible."

The finding that group means did not differ for NDW per C-unit conflicts with those from prior research (Klee, 1992; Watkins et al., 1995). This finding may be associated with (a) the fact that authors of prior studies did not conduct the kind of power analyses that were conducted for this study (power was low for NDW per C-unit in this study); (b) the fact that the children's samples did not meet the 50 C-unit standard that is now considered the research standard for computing NDW (Klee, 1992); or (c) the procedure used to control for sample length (dividing each NDW value by the number of C-units).

With respect to the latter issue, inspection of the individual normalized NDW values revealed values for children with LI that were two standard deviations above the mean for the children with TL. Further inspection revealed that these high NDW per C-unit scores were from children who produced fewer than 10 C-units. As indicated previously, the NDW value usually is calculated from a sample of at least 50 utterances (Klee, 1992). This procedure allows for closed-class words that occur frequently (e.g., articles, auxiliaries, prepositions) to be excluded from the NDW count after their first occurrence and for open-class words that occur less frequently (e.g., nouns, verbs, adverbs, adjectives) to be reflected in the overall vocabulary diversity score. Given the small number of C-units for some children, there were few opportunities for the closed-class words to be repeated. Consequently, those children who produced few C-units received spuriously high NDW per C-unit scores. In contrast, small NDW per C-unit values were obtained from some children with TL, who produced large numbers of C-units. These small NDW values reflect the fact that, as sample length increased, words tended to be repeated and the NDW per C-unit values subsequently decreased.

Age-Level Differences

Prior investigations have yielded findings that NDW scores correlated with age (Klee, 1992; Miller, 1991). Also, researchers have suggested that the literate language features are sensitive to developmental growth (Nippold, 1988, 1993; Perera, 1986). Although the finding of no statistically significant age-level effects conflicts with prior findings and predictions, the finding is not surprising given the low to moderate power associated with this factor for these measures.

Another possibility for the lack of an age effect is that the type of samples in this study (e.g., narrative discourse, short samples, and constrained content) imposed ceiling effects that applied generally to both groups. If this is the explanation, then the fact that there were group membership differences in spite of ceiling effects could be taken to indicate that the findings are a conservative estimate of true differences. Finally, the lack of a significant age effect for NDW per C-unit may reflect the manner in which the scores were normalized.

Male–Female Differences

No investigations were located in which researchers had studied differences between males and females for NDW or for the literate language features. This variable was included in this study to control for potential additional sources of score variability.

Again, power was low for this factor. Consequently, it was not surprising that statistically significant differences were not obtained for any of the dependent variables.

Relationships between the Dependent Measures

Findings from prior research have indicated that NDW is a useful general language performance measure because mean scores differentiate children with LI from children with TL and because scores tend to increase with increases in age (Klee, 1992; Miller, 1991; Watkins et al., 1995). In this study, with NDW raw scores adjusted for sample length, the individual scores did not tend to increase with increases in age.

Only moderate and small correlations were obtained in this study between NDW per C-unit scores and scores for ENP per C-unit and conjunctions per C-unit, respectively, indicating that the NDW scores, when normalized for sample length, shared little variability with the scores for the literate language features. This finding suggests that the measures of literate language would provide assessment information not furnished by the general language performance measure of NDW.

CLINICAL IMPLICATIONS AND LIMITATIONS

Literate language means and standard deviations for narrations obtained for one stimulus story are reported here. Although based on a small sample size for each group ($n = 52$), these statistics enable speech-language pathologists to estimate the adequacy of literate language skills of children ages 7 through 10 for samples of narration collected in the same manner. Speech-language pathologists can obtain important assessment and intervention information for the four literate language features simply by scanning a sample for their occurrence and counting their frequency. In this study, conjunctions and ENP were critical features for assessment.

Because children with LI tend to use the literate language features infrequently in their narrative samples, speech-language pathologists are advised also to analyze samples for the type and grammatical role of the literate language features used. For example, conjunctions can be classified as coordinating, subordinating, or intersentential conjunctions (see Appendix B) and whether they signal a temporal, causal, or adversative relationship (see introduction for examples). ENPs can be classified as modifiers, qualifiers, appositives, and relative clauses (see introduction for examples) and whether they follow the verb or function as subjects of the verb. Mental and linguistic verbs can be distinguished. Finally, -ly adverbs can be analyzed as to whether they indicate time, manner, or degree. Such detailed information will not only serve as benchmarks for ongoing assessment, but also will provide guidance for planning intervention targets.

Potential threats to the internal validity of any assessment study include selection and instrumentation. With respect to selection, the question in a causal–comparative design is whether the groups were equivalent on relevant variables, except on the comparison variable (in this case, language level). No IQ scores were available for either group. The only sources that could be relied on were the judgments of classroom teachers, speech-language pathologists, and reports that IQ scores (filed in the school records) for the children with LI were within normal limits. In future studies, researchers are advised to report cognitive scores for participants to improve the generalizability of their findings. Because measures of cognitive level were not obtainable here, results from this study must be interpreted with caution. With respect to instrumentation (score reliability), high intercoder agreement was established for all scores, and transcription and data entry were checked for accuracy.

An additional concern for future studies is that the narrative retellings analyzed were less than 50 C-units in length. In prior studies, investigators have used 50 utterances or more for assessment (Klee, 1992; Miller, 1991; Watkins et al., 1995). Longer samples would better represent a child's literate language capability by providing more opportunities for using the literate language features. Also, the narrative samples studied here varied in length; therefore, actual comparisons of word and literate language counts across age levels and language groups, based on a specific sample length, could not be obtained. These measures should be studied in longer story samples.

Although not typically considered aspects of a literate language style, Westby (1999) noted that, in addition to mental and linguistic verbs that often encode internal states, it may be useful to code other emotional words. Such words as *delighted* or *distraught* may reflect a child's developing "awareness of the landscape of consciousness" (p. 166) and should be considered when designing future studies of literate language.

Finally, it is possible that the number of literate language features in the stimulus story affected children's use of these features when retelling the story. The effects of using a stimulus story, controlled for literate language occurrences, on literate language scores warrants investigation.

CONCLUSION

From this investigation, two fine-grained measures (conjunctions and ENPs) were found to be useful for differentiating children with LI from those with TL. However, future investigators might conduct a discriminant function analysis to strengthen the "diagnostic accuracy" of the group membership categories. A further benefit of the literate language measures is that their scores inform language intervention. The study did not provide further support for using NDW, when normalized for sample length, as a general language performance measure in discourse samples. As in all studies, only replication can establish the reliability and generalizability of the findings reported here.

REFERENCES

Bruner, J. (1986). *Actual minds, possible worlds.* Cambridge, MA: Harvard University Press.

Cache Chamber of Commerce. (2000). [Website: *http://www.cachechamber.com*].

Cohen, J. (1988). *Statistical power analysis far the behavioral sciences* (2nd ed.). Hillsdale, NJ: Erlbaum.

Davis, S. (1999). *Reference cohesion skill in the spoken narratives of seven-year-old children.* Unpublished master's thesis, Utah State University, Logan.

Dunn, L. M., & Dunn, L. M. (1981). *Peabody Picture Vocabulary Test* (rev. ed.). Circle Pines, MN: American Guidance Service.

Ferguson, G. A. (1981). *Statistical analysis in psychology and education* (5th ed.). New York: McGraw-Hill.

Gall, M. D., Borg, W. R., & Gall, J. P. (1996). *Educational research* (6th ed.). White Plains, NY: Longman.

Gerber, A. (1993). *Language-related learning disabilities: Their nature and treatment.* Baltimore, MD: Paul H. Brookes.

Gillam, R. B., Pena, E. D., & Miller, L. (1999). Dynamic assessment of narrative and expository discourse. *Topics in Language Disorders, 20*(1), 33–47.

Hopkins, K. D., & Stanley, J. C. (1981). *Educational and psychological measurement and evaluation* (6th ed.). Englewood Cliffs, NJ: Prentice-Hall.

Kaufman, A. S., & Kaufman, N. L. (1983). *Kaufman Assessment Battery for Children.* Circle Pines, MN: American Guidance.

Klee, T. (1992). Developmental and diagnostic characteristics of quantitative measures of children's language production. *Topics in Language Disorders, 12*(2), 28–41.

Leiter, R. (1979). *Leiter International Performance Scale.* Chicago, IL: Stoelting.

Loban, W. (1976). *Language development: Kindergarten through grade 12.* Urbana, IL: National Council of Teachers of English.

Lord, F. M., & Novick, M. R. (1968). *Statistical theories of mental test scores.* Reading, MA: Addison-Wesley.

Lyon, G. R. (1999). Reading development, reading disorders, and reading instruction: Research-based findings. *ASHA Special Interest Division I Newsletter: Language Learning and Education, 6*(1), 8–16.

Martin, J. R. (1983). The development of register. In J. Fine & R. O. Freedle (Eds.), *Developmental issues in discourse* (pp. 1–39). Norwood, NJ: Ablex.

Mayer, M. (1967). *A boy, a dog, and a frog.* New York: Dial Books for Young Readers.

Mayer, M. (1969). *Frog, where are you?* New York: Dial Books for Young Readers.

Mayer, M. (1974). *Frog goes to dinner.* New York: Dial Books for Young Readers.

Mayer, M., & Mayer, M. (1975). *One frog too many.* New York: Dial Books for Young Readers.

McClure, E. F., & Steffensen, M. S. (1985). A study of the use of conjunctions across grades and ethnic groups. *Research in the Teaching of English, 19,* 217–236.

McReynolds, L. V., & Kearns, K. P. (1983). *Single-subject experimental designs in communicative disorders.* Baltimore, MD: University Park Press.

Miller, J. F. (1991). Quantifying productive language disorders. In J. F. Miller (Ed.), *Research on child language disorders* (pp. 211–220). Austin, TX: PRO-ED.

Miller, J. F., & Chapman, R. S. (1998). *Systematic Analysis of Language Transcripts.* Madison, WI: University of Wisconsin.

Milosky, L. M. (1987). Narratives in the classroom. *Seminars in Speech and Language, 8,* 329–343.

Nelson, N. W. (1994). Curriculum-based language assessment and intervention across the grades. In G. P. Wallach & K. G. Butler (Eds.), *Language learning disabilities in school-age children and adolescents* (pp. 104–131). New York: Macmillan.

Newcomer, P. L., & Hammill, D. D. (1991). *Test of Language Development—Intermediate.* Austin, TX: Pro-Ed.

Nippold, M. A. (1988). The literate lexicon. In M. A. Nippold (Ed.), *Later language development* (pp. 29–47). Austin, TX: Pro-Ed.

Nippold, M. (1993). Developmental markers in adolescent language: Syntax, semantics, and pragmatics. *Language, Speech, and Hearing Services in Schools, 24,* 21–28.

Nunnally, J. C. (1978). *Psychometric theory* (2nd ed.), New York: McGraw-Hill.

Palincsar, A. S., Brown, A. L., & Campione, J. C. (1994). Models and practices of dynamic assessment. In G. P. Wallach & K. G. Butler (Eds.), *Language learning disabilities in school-age children and adolescents* (pp. 132–144). New York: Macmillan.

Paul, R. (1995). *Language disorders from infancy through adolescence.* St. Louis, MO: Mosby.

Paul, R. (2001). *Language disorders from infancy through adolescence* (2nd ed.). St. Louis, MO: Mosby.

Paul, R., & Smith, R. L. (1993). Narrative skills in 4-year-olds with normal, impaired, and late-developing language. *Journal of Speech and Hearing Research, 36,* 592–598.

Pellegrini, A. D. (1985). Relations between preschool children's symbolic play and literate behavior. In L. Gaida & A. D. Pellegrini (Eds.), *Play, language, and stories* (pp. 79–97). Norwood, NJ: Ablex.

Perera, K. (1986). Language acquisition and writing. In P. Fletcher & M. Garman (Eds.), *Language acquisition* (2nd ed., pp. 494–533). Cambridge, England: Cambridge University Press.

Peterson, C., & McCabe, A. (1983). *Developmental psycholinguistics: Three ways of looking at a child's narrative.* New York: Plenum.

Ripich, D. N., & Griffith, P. L. (1985, November). *Story structure, cohesion, and propositions in learning disabled children.* Paper presented at the meeting of the American Speech-Language-Hearing Association, Washington, DC.

Roth, F. P. (1986). Oral narrative abilities of learning-disabled students. *Topics in Language Disorders, 7,* 21–30.

Scarlett, W., & Wolf, D. (1979). When it's only make-believe: The construction of a boundary between fantasy and reality in storytelling. In E. Winner & H. Gardner (Eds.), *Fact, fiction, and fantasy in childhood* (pp. 29–40). San Francisco, CA: Jossey-Bass.

Scott, C. (1988). Spoken and written syntax. In M. Nippold (Ed.), *Later language development* (pp. 49–96). Boston, MA: College-Hill.

Segal, E. M., & Duchan, J. F. (1997). Interclausal connectives as indicators of structuring in narrative. In J. Costermans & M. Fayol (Eds.), *Processing interclausal relationships* (pp. 95–119). Mahwah, NJ: Lawrence Erlbaum.

Semel, E., Wiig, E., & Secord, W. (1987). *Clinical Evaluation of Language Fundamentals—Revised.* San Antonio, TX: Psychological.

Shaver, J. P. (1985, October). Chance and nonsense: A conversation about interpreting tests of statistical significance, part 2. *Phi Delta Kappan, 67,* 138–141.

Slosson, R. L. (1981). *Slosson Intelligence Test.* East Aurora, NY: Slosson Educational Publications.

Snow, C. E., Scarborough, H. S., & Burns, M. S. (1999).

What speech–language pathologists need to know about early reading. *Topics in Language Disorders, 20*(1), 48–58.

Strong, C. J. (1998). *The Strong Narrative Assessment Procedure.* Eau Claire, WI: Thinking Publications.

Strong, C. J., & Shaver, J. P. (1991). Stability of cohesion in the spoken narratives of language-impaired and normally developing school-aged children. *Journal of Speech and Hearing Disorders, 34,* 95–111.

Thompson, B. (1999). Improving research clarity and usefulness with effect size indices as supplements to statistical significance tests. *Exceptional Children, 65,* 329–337.

Utah State Office of Education. (1993). *Rules and regulations for education programs for the handicapped.* Salt Lake City, UT: Author.

van Oers, B. (1998). The fallacy of decontextualization. *Mind, culture, and activity, 5,* 135–142.

Wallace, G., & Hammill, D. (1994). *Comprehensive Receptive and Expressive Vocabulary Test.* Austin, TX: Pro-Ed.

Wallach, G. P. (1990). "Magic buries Celtics": Looking for broader interpretations of language learning and literacy. *Topics in Language Disorders, 10*(2), 63–80.

Wallach, G. P., & Butler, K. G. (1994). Creating communication, literacy, and academic success. In G. P. Wallach & K. G. Butler (Eds.), *Language learning disabilities in school-age children and adolescents* (pp. 2–26). New York: Macmillan.

Watkins, R. V., Kelly, D. J., Harbers, H. M., & Hollis, W. (1995). Measuring children's lexical diversity: Differentiating typical and impaired language learners. *Journal of Speech and Hearing Research, 38,* 1349–1355.

Wechsler, D. (1974). *Wechsler Intelligence Scale for Children—Revised.* San Antonio, TX: Psychological.

Westby, C. E. (1985). Learning to talk—talking to learn: Oral literate language differences. In C. Simon (Ed.), *Communication skills and classroom success: Therapy methodologies for language-learning disabled students* (pp. 181–213). San Diego, CA: College-Hill.

Westby, C. E. (1991). Learning to talk—talking to learn: Oral-literate language differences. In C. Simon (Ed.), *Communication skills and classroom success: Assessment and therapy methodologies for language and learning disabled students* (rev. ed., pp. 181–218). San Diego, CA: College-Hill.

Westby, C. E. (1994). The effects of culture on genre, structure, and style of oral and written narratives. In G. P. Wallach & K. G. Butler (Eds.), *Language learning disabilities in school-age children and adolescents* (pp. 180–218). New York: Macmillan.

Westby, C. E. (1999). Assessing and facilitating text comprehension problems. In H. W. Catts & A. G. Kamhi (Eds.), *Language and reading disabilities* (pp. 154–221). Boston, MA: Allyn & Bacon.

Wiig, E. H., & Semel, E. M. (1984). *Language assessment and intervention for the learning disabled.* Columbus, OH: Merrill.

Zachman, L., Barrett, M., Huisingh, R., & Jorgensen, C. (1990). *The Word Test—Revised.* East Moline, IL: LinguiSystems.

Contact author: Carol J. Strong, Communicative Disorders and Deaf Education, Utah State University, 2800 Old Main Hill, Logan, UT 84322. Email: *carols@coe.usu.edu*

APPENDIX A. STIMULUS STORY, *FROG, WHERE ARE YOU?*

(Numbers = utterances which have been segmented into C-units)

1. There once was a boy named Tom who had a pet frog/
2. He kept it in a large jar/
3. One night, while he and his dog were sleeping, the frog climbed out of the jar/
4. He left through an open window/
5. When Tom woke up, he leaned over his bed to say good morning to the frog/
6. But the frog was gone/
7. Tom looked everywhere for the frog/
8. And the dog looked for him too/
9. Tom called out the window/
10. When the dog looked in the jar, he got his head caught/
11. And so when he leaned out the window, the heavy jar made him fall/
12. And the jar broke/
13. Tom picked him up to see if he was okay/
14. And the dog licked him for being so nice/
15. All day long Tom called for the frog/
16. He called down holes/
17. A gopher got angry at Tom for disturbing him/
18. And while Tom was calling for the frog in a tree hole, the dog was getting into more trouble/
19. He barked at some bees and jumped at a tree where their bees' nest was hanging/
20. And the bees' nest fell down/
21. The angry bees chased the dog/
22. And an angry owl came out of the tree hole to scold Tom/
23. It scared him/
24. The owl screeched at him to stay away from his home/
25. Next Tom climbed a big rock and called again/
26. He leaned on some branches to see better/
27. But the branches began to move and carry him into the air/
28. They weren't branches/
29. They were a deer's antlers/
30. And the deer ran with Tom on his head/
31. The dog ran along too barking at the deer/
32. The deer stopped quickly at the edge of a cliff and threw Tom over the edge/
33. And he and the dog fell into a pond/

34. Suddenly they both heard something/
35. It was a croaking sound/
36. And they smiled/
37. Tom told the dog to be quiet/
38. And they both crept up and looked behind a dead tree/
39. There was his frog sitting proudly with a mother frog/
40. And they had eight babies/
41. One of the frogs leaped forward to greet him/
42. He liked Tom/
43. And Tom liked him/
44. So Tom took the baby frog home to be his new pet/
45. And he waved good-bye to his old frog who now had a family to take care of/

From *The Strong Narrative Assessment Procedure* (pp. 135–136), by C. J. Strong, 1998, Eau Claire, WI: Thinking Publications. © 1998 by Thinking Publications. Reprinted with permission.

APPENDIX B. CODING CONVENTIONS FOR LITERATE LANGUAGE FEATURES*

CONJUNCTIONS

Count coordinating, subordinating, and intersentential conjunctions; exclude *and* and *then*. Count conjunctions that start a story because they join the examiner's prior instructions with the child's narration. Literate conjunctions include, but are not limited to:

when	since	before	after	while
because	so	if	until	whether
but	therefore	however	although	as

Examples of coordinating conjunctions:

- "The branches got up *but* they weren't really branches." (2 C-units)
- "The boy liked him *so* the boy took the baby home." (2 C-units)
- "The bees got angry at him *so* they chased him." (2 C-units)

Examples of subordinating conjunctions:

- "*While* he was sleeping, the frog slipped out of the jar."
- "*When* he woke up, he looked everywhere for the frog."
- "It started out *when* this boy got a new frog."

Examples of intersentential conjunctions:

- "*Next*, Tom got up with his dog."
- "*Instead*, it was a deer's antlers."

ELABORATED NOUN PHRASES (ENPs)

Count a noun phrase as one ENP when it has more than two modifiers preceding the noun (*the two big dogs*) or has qualifiers such as prepositional phrases and relative clauses following the noun (*the big dog in the pet store; the boy who has a fishnet*). Consider determiners (e.g., *the, a, an, this*) as modifiers. Count appositives as noun phrase elaboration (e.g., "This boy, *Tom*, had a dog and a frog").

Examples of modifiers:

- "He peeked over *the old, dead log.*" (1 ENP)
- "And *one little baby frog* liked Tom." (1 ENP)
- "And then *an angry old owl* came out of the tree." (1 ENP)

Examples of qualifiers:

- "He had a jar *with a frog in it.*" (1 ENP)
- "One *of the babies* jumped to meet him." (1 ENP)
- "The bees *in the hive* fell." (1 ENP)
- "The boy took the baby *that liked him* home." (1 ENP)
- "Tom was looking in a hole *in a tree.*" (1 ENP)

MENTAL/LINGUISTIC VERBS

Count verbs that denote cognitive and linguistic processes of humans, animals, or fictitious characters. In the context of narrating past events, count active, not passive, voice and only verb tenses other than present and present progressive. Count all occurrences of a mental or linguistic verb when it is repeated for emphasis (i.e., "They were *calling* and *calling*").

thought	said	know	promised	forgot
wished	greeted	barked	called	screeched
scolded	told	yelled	asked	decided

Examples of mental verbs:

- "He *decided* to go look for him."
- "The boy's dog *thought*, 'Oh thanks.'"
- "He didn't *know* they were antlers."

Examples of linguistic verbs:

- "Tom *told* his dog to be quiet."
- "An owl came after the boy and *screeched* at him to go away."
- "He *called* down holes."

ADVERBS

Count only *-ly* adverbs that convey tone, attitude, time, or manner, including those that are structurally in error but are used to modify a verb.

Examples of adverbs:

- "It *accidentally* knocked a beehive down."
- "The deer *quickly* stopped."
- "It stopped *quick.*"

*Adapted from Paul, 1995 and Westby, 1999.

Source. From Greenhalgh, K. S., & Strong, C. J. (2001). Literate language features in spoken narratives of children with typical language and children with language impairments. *Language, Speech, and Hearing Services in Schools, 32,* 114–125. Copyright 2001 by the American Speech–Language–Hearing Association. Reprinted by permission.

ILLUSTRATIVE EXAMPLE QUESTIONS

1. How were participants selected? Describe characteristics of the two samples of participants.

2. What primary statistical analysis procedure was used to analyze participants' responses?

3. Were effect sizes reasonable?

4. According to the authors, what general conclusions can be made about the results?

5. What limitations did the authors discuss?

6. Do you see any potential problems with the Number of Different Words (NDW) measure? If so, describe.

7. Did intercoder reliability of transcripts involve an adequate sample of data? Why or why not?

8. What problem was produced when a participant had few C-units?

9. What are some potential threats to the internal validity of this study? Provide a justification for each threat.

10. What are some potential threats to the external validity of this study? Provide a justification for each threat.

ADDITIONAL RESEARCH EXAMPLES

1. Gallo, M. A., & Odu, M. (2009). Examining the relationship between class scheduling and student achievement in college algebra. *Community College Review, 36,* 299–325.

2. Gentry, M., Rizza, M. G., & Owen, S. V. (2002). Examining perceptions of challenge and choice in classrooms: The relationship between teachers and their students and comparisons between gifted students and other students. *Gifted Child Quarterly, 46,* 145–155.

3. Porfeli, E., Wang, C., Audette, R., McColl, A., & Algozzine, B. (2009). Influence of social and community capital on student achievement in a large urban school district. *Education and Urban Society, 42,* 72–95.

THREATS TO INTERNAL VALIDITY

Circle the number corresponding to the likelihood of each threat to internal validity being present in the investigation and provide a justification.

1 = definitely not a threat 2 = not a likely threat 3 = somewhat likely threat
4 = likely threat 5 = definite threat NA = not applicable for this design

Results in Differences within or between Individuals

1. Maturation   1   2   3   4   5   NA

   Justification _____

   _____

2. Selection   1   2   3   4   5   NA

   Justification _____

   _____

3. Selection by Maturation Interaction   1   2   3   4   5   NA

   Justification _____

   _____

4. Statistical Regression   1   2   3   4   5   NA

   Justification _____

   _____

5. Morality   1   2   3   4   5   NA

   Justification _____

   _____

6. Instrumentation   1   2   3   4   5   NA

   Justification _____

   _____

7. Testing   1   2   3   4   5   NA

   Justification _____

   _____

(continued)

8. History   1   2   3   4   5   NA

Justification _____

_____

9. Resentful Demoralization of the Control Group   1   2   3   4   5   NA

Justification _____

_____

Results in Similarities within or between Individuals

10. Diffusion of Treatment   1   2   3   4   5   NA

Justification _____

_____

11. Compensatory Rivalry by the Control Group   1   2   3   4   5   NA

Justification _____

_____

12. Compensatory Equalization of Treatments   1   2   3   4   5   NA

Justification _____

_____

Abstract: Write a one-page abstract summarizing the overall conclusions of the authors and whether or not you feel the authors' conclusions are valid based on the internal validity of the investigation.

THREATS TO EXTERNAL VALIDITY

Circle the number corresponding to the likelihood of each threat to external validity being present in the investigation according to the following scale:

1 = definitely not a threat   2 = not a likely threat   3 = somewhat likely threat
4 = likely threat   5 = definite threat   NA = not applicable for this design

Also, provide a justification for each rating.

Population

1. Generalization across Subjects   1   2   3   4   5   NA

   Justification _____

   _____

2. Interaction of Personological Variables and Treatment   1   2   3   4   5   NA

   Justification _____

   _____

Ecological

3. Verification of the Independent Variable   1   2   3   4   5   NA

   Justification _____

   _____

4. Multiple Treatment Interference   1   2   3   4   5   NA

   Justification _____

   _____

5. Hawthorne Effect   1   2   3   4   5   NA

   Justification _____

   _____

6. Novelty and Disruption Effects   1   2   3   4   5   NA

   Justification _____

   _____

7. Experimental Effects   1   2   3   4   5   NA

   Justification _____

   _____

(continued)

8. Pretest Sensitization   1   2   3   4   5   NA

Justification _____

_____

9. Posttest Sensitization   1   2   3   4   5   NA

Justification _____

_____

10. Interaction of Time of Measurement and Treatment Effects   1   2   3   4   5   NA

Justification _____

_____

11. Measurement of the Dependent Variable   1   2   3   4   5   NA

Justification _____

_____

12. Interaction of History and Treatment Effects   1   2   3   4   5   NA

Justification _____

_____

Abstract: Write a one-page abstract summarizing the overall conclusions of the authors and whether or not you feel the authors' conclusions are valid based on the external validity of the investigation.

CHAPTER 7

■ ■ ■ ■

Correlational Research

OBJECTIVES

After studying this chapter, you should be able to . . .

1. Compare and contrast the correlational research method with causal–comparative research.
2. Describe the correlational research method.
3. Outline the issues in designing a correlational study.
4. Illustrate the statistical procedures used in correlational research.
5. Explain when researchers should use the correlational research method.

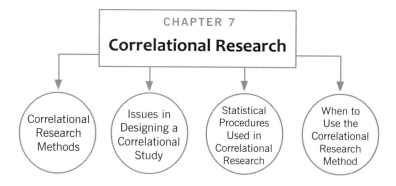

OVERVIEW

The controlled experiment achieves control through precise manipulation of the independent variable by isolating the experiment from extraneous influences via randomization of participants to treatments. The random assignment of participants to treatments helps to ensure that all extraneous influences are equal. The integrity of the controlled experiment lies in the simplicity of its causal model; that is, randomization increases the likelihood that the effects of the independent variable are a direct causal consequence of the independent variable and not due to other causes (e.g., SES or gender residing in initial differences between groups). Despite the simplicity of the controlled experiment for establishing causality, practical considerations (e.g., randomly select participants from the target population, randomly assign participants to groups, and actively manipulate the independent variable) have limited its use. Because of these limitations, researchers employ research methods aimed at identifying the relationships among variables such as the causal–comparative and correlational research methods.

The correlational research method is closely related to the causal–comparative research method in that the primary goal is to explore relationships among variables. Causal–comparative and correlational research also attempt to explain the subject matter of interest and to identify variables that can be tested through experimental research. Neither causal–comparative nor correlational research methods allow for the manipulation of the independent variable that experimental research methods allow. One major difference is that whereas the causal–comparative method takes into consideration scores from two groups of participants, the correlational research method takes into consideration two or more sets of scores from each participant. Thus, the comparison is between groups of participants in causal–comparative research and between scores for each participant in correlational research.

This chapter begins with a general description of the correlational research method, including the analysis of data. It concludes with an illustrative example of how to interpret the findings of correlational research for critique.

WHAT IS THE CORRELATIONAL RESEARCH METHOD?

Correlational research involves collecting two sets of data and determining the extent to which they covary (or vary together). The sets of data can be obtained from the same group at the same point in time or at two or more points in time. The sets of data also can be obtained from two or more groups. In essence, the correlational method is a particular way of collecting and analyzing data to discover relationships

between or among variables and, depending on the data analysis procedures used, the causes for a pattern of behavior.

The correlational research method can be relational or predictive in nature. Relational correlational research explores relationships between or among variables. Predictive correlational research predicts scores on one or more variables from a participant's scores on one or more other variables. In prediction research, the variable(s) used for prediction must be measured prior to the measurement of the variable(s) to be predicted.

WHAT ARE THE ISSUES IN DESIGNING A CORRELATIONAL STUDY?

Before discussing some of the issues that researchers must consider in designing a correlational research study, we should examine the two primary types of variables used in correlational research: predictor variables and criterion variables. In *predictor variables*, participants' scores enable prediction of their scores on some criterion variable. A *criterion variable* is the object of the research, the variable about which researchers seek to discover more information. For example, scores on an IQ test should generally predict scores on a school achievement test. Because experimental research relies primarily on distinctions between independent and dependent variables, we refer to predictor variables as independent variables and criterion variables as dependent variables throughout the remainder of this chapter.

Critical Issues in Correlational Research

The critical issues that researchers must consider in designing a relationship or prediction correlational study parallel those used to design a causal–comparative study. These issues are (1) development of a hypothesis, (2) selection of a homogeneous group, and (3) collection and analysis of data.

Development of a Hypothesis

The first critical issue centers on the development of a hypothesis about the causes or effects

---

Research Examples

Consider these issues. Think about how you would design research to address the questions/hypotheses from these research examples:

- Research Example 1: What is the predictive validity of kindergarten early literacy indicators with regard to later reading performance?
- Research Example 2: Is there a relationship between experience as a peer victim of bullying and compromised academic performance of middle school students?

Research examples appear near the end of the chapter.

of the phenomenon under study. The basis for the study should be grounded on a theoretical framework and previous research. Researchers may explore a large number of variables in those areas in which there is no viable theoretical framework or previous research. However, such a "shotgun" approach must be used cautiously, because variables can be related to one another even if the relationship is not meaningful. For example, there is a high positive correlation between shoe size and earned income, because as people reach adulthood, they are more likely to earn more money than children or adolescents. Although there is a high degree of relationship between shoe size and earned income, the relationship is not a particularly meaningful one.

In addition, when two or more variables are strongly related to one another, they may not reasonably discriminate between or among the variables under study. In correlational research, it is standard practice for researchers to explore the interrelationships among the variables initially to ensure that they reasonably discriminate the variables of interest. Again, if variables are highly related to one another, then the measurement devices may not adequately discriminate between or among the variables of interest. Furthermore, the use of a theoretical framework and previous research is critical to ensure that all variables thought to influence the variable(s) of interest can be considered in the research design. As will become clear with our description of the statistical procedures used in correlational research, there are a number of ways of studying the overall and relative influences between or among a wide range of variables.

Selection of a Homogeneous Group

The second critical issue when designing a correlational research study is to select a homogenous group that possesses the variables under study. As with a causal–comparative study, selecting a homogenous group requires a precise definition of membership. For example, a precise definition of dysfluent speech (Logan, Byrd, Mazzocchi, & Gillam, 2011) was used to determine the relationship between speech rate and speech characteristics of elementary-age students who stuttered and those who did not.

A precise definition not only helps to ensure that the group(s) under study possesses the variables or characteristics of interest but also aids in the interpretation of the findings. If a heterogeneous group is selected, researchers may form homogeneous subgroups that possess different levels of the characteristic. The formation of homogeneous subgroups is common in correlational research studies.

Collection and Analysis of Data

The final issue focuses on collection and analysis of the data. Researchers use a wide range of measurement devices in correlational research. Standardized measurement devices, criterion-referenced tests, surveys, questionnaires, interviews, and observations are all used by researchers in correlational research. Thus, critical research consumers must carefully consider the reliability and validity of the measurement devices being used. Furthermore, because a wide range of correlational statistical procedures has been devised for various purposes, it is crucial that researchers employ the appropriate statistical procedures to describe the relationship between two or more nominal, ordinal, interval, or ratio variables. Many of the most commonly used statistical procedures in correlational research are described in this chapter. Figure 7.1 depicts the general steps in designing a correlational research study.

WHAT ARE THE STATISTICAL PROCEDURES USED IN CORRELATIONAL RESEARCH?

As mentioned earlier, the correlational research method is commonly used by researchers, because it can be applied to areas in which it is implausible to conduct experimental studies and it offers a number of advantages over other experimental research methods. A wide range of available statistical procedures not only depict the degree of relationship among variables but also explore the causal relationships among variables. Exploring causality is important, because many variables under study in education and psychology are influenced by other variables, making it difficult for researchers to

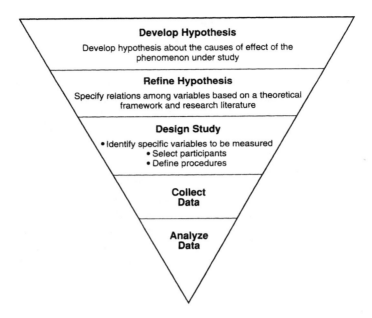

FIGURE 7.1. Steps for designing a correlational research study.

have confidence in what produced the observed effects. True experimental methods tend to limit the number of relationships that can be studied in a given research study.

The reader is directed to Figure 7.2, a flow-chart for the statistical analyses of correlational research data, to achieve additional clarity about the use of each statistic to analyze data.

As with tests of statistical significance, the choice of these procedures depends on a number of issues, including the number of groups and variables being studied, the type of data, and the question(s) being asked. In this section, we describe the common statistical analysis procedures used in correlational research.

Important Concepts

Two primary concepts should be understood before discussing statistical procedures—bivariate frequency distributions and forms of relationships.

Bivariate Frequency Distributions

In Chapter 3, we briefly discussed the use and interpretation of correlation coefficients with regard to the reliability and validity of measurement devices. The correlation coefficient is important, because it has many applications and is the basis for many of the advanced statistical procedures in correlational research. The correlation coefficient is best understood by reference to the bivariate frequency distribution. A bivariate frequency distribution is an extension of the univariate frequency distribution discussed in Chapter 4, in which the scores from *two* variables are plotted in either a table or graph (Holland & Thayer, 2000). Plotting the scores of two variables on a graph (called a *scattergram*) visually depicts the degree of relationship between the two variables or the extent to which they covary. Each set of scores may be displayed separately as univariate frequency distributions. However, such graphs would not show how the variables are related. Thus, the scores for one variable are plotted on the horizontal, or *x* axis, and the scores for the other variable are plotted on the vertical or *y* axis. Displaying two variables graphically is why it is called a bivariate frequency distribution.

A bivariate frequency distribution for a hypothetical set of scores (see Table 7.1) is presented in Figure 7.3. The scores for one variable (*A*)

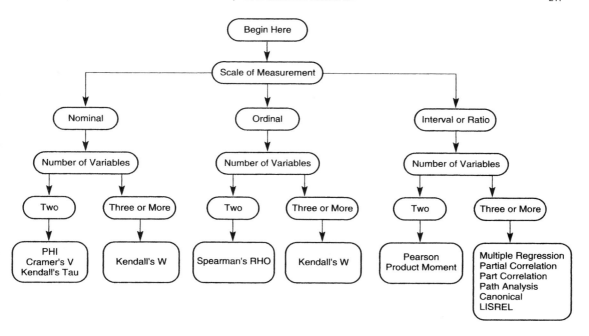

FIGURE 7.2. Selecting statistical analysis procedures: Association between or among two or more variables.

are plotted on the horizontal (x) axis, and the scores for the other variable (B) are plotted on the vertical (y) axis to show they are related to one another. Reading from Table 7.1 we see that Participant 1 scored 6 on Variable A and 13 on Variable B. Follow the horizontal (x) axis (which represents Variable A) until the score of 6 is reached. Draw a vertical line through the score. Next, go up the y axis (which represents Variable B) until the score of 13 is reached. Draw a horizontal line through the score. Place a dot

where these two lines meet. This dot represents the scores for the participant on Variables A and B. Continuing this way with each of the scores yields a bivariate frequency distribution, or scattergram. It is often convenient to draw a line on the scattergram to show the general relationship or trend in the data. This line is called a *regression line*.

Although it is beyond the scope of this book to discuss the computations and theoretical

TABLE 7.1. Scores for Variables A and B

Participant	Variable A	Variable B
1	6	13
2	8	9
3	8	15
4	9	13
5	10	15
6	10	21
7	11	17
8	12	15
9	12	15
10	14	17

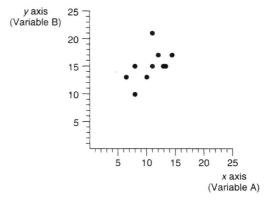

FIGURE 7.3. Scores for variables A or B.

background for the regression line or the line of best fit, it is important to understand that the regression line provides an average statement about how a change in one variable affects another variable. In essence, the regression line describes the trend in the data and is based on all of the observations. For example, each score on Variable *A* has a corresponding score on Variable *B*, and also an estimated score corresponding to a point on the regression line. Thus, this line depicts the average estimate or prediction of scores on one variable to those of another variable.

Forms of Relationships

Relationships between two variables usually take several forms (Gall et al., 2007). We restrict our discussion to linear and curvilinear relationships. *Linear relationships* are those in which a straight line can be visualized in the middle of the values running from one corner to another. *Curvilinear relationships* are those in which the best-fit line is not straight, but may be U-, N-, or W-shaped. An example of a curvilinear relationship that is quadratic is the correlation between age and running speed. From infancy, as we grow older our running speed increases. However, once we reach a certain age, our running speed decreases. Thus, there is a relationship between the two variables, but that relationship is not linear. A variety of statistical procedures can be used to assess the relationship between variables regardless of the form of the relationship.

Correlation Coefficient

Questions such as "Is there a relationship between maternal attachment and children's social adjustment?"; "Is reading achievement related to the amount of time spent reading?"; and "Is quality of child care related to infant development?" are about the relationship between two variables. The **correlation coefficient** is the statistic used to describe the relationship between two variables. Thus, correlational statistics are considered to be descriptive statistics. Correlation coefficients are used extensively in the development and validation

of measurement devices, as we explained in Chapter 3.

Various statistics can be calculated to indicate the degree to which two variables are related to one another depending on the types of variables used. Recall the distinction among nominal, ordinal, interval, and ratio variables. Statistical procedures exist for describing the relationship between two nominal variables, a nominal variable and an interval/ratio variable, two ordinal variables, and two interval or ratio variables. Although we describe each of the correlational procedures used in such cases, we focus on the Pearson product–moment correlation that describes the relationship between two interval or ratio scale variables. We focus on this correlation because it is the most commonly used statistical procedure for deriving a correlation coefficient, and because it provides the basis for many of the more advanced statistical procedures used in correlational research.

General Interpretation of Correlation Coefficients

The correlation coefficient can range from –1.00 to +1.00. Figure 7.4 presents a number of correlation coefficients and associated scattergrams. If the values for the variables plotted on the *x* and *y* axes fall on a straight line, the correlation coefficient has its largest value, +1.00 or –1.00. Graphs in Figure 7.4(a and b) depict a perfect positive and negative correlation between two variables, respectively. The straight diagonal line in both cases, called the *regression line* or *line of best fit*, indicates that each increment in one variable is accompanied by a corresponding increment in the other variable. A perfect correlation between two variables enables a perfect prediction to be made about one variable from the scores on the other variable. Of course, we will probably never encounter a perfect correlation in educational and psychological research due to factors such as measurement error.

If the two variables are not related to one another at all, then the value of the correlation coefficient is zero; see Figure 7.4(g). In such a case, knowing the value for one variable would not enable us to predict the value for the other variable. Between a perfect correlation and zero correlation, the complete range of values can be found. The larger the numbers (e.g., +0.40 vs. +0.20), the more strongly the variables are related to one another. Similarly, the larger the numbers, the better the prediction of the values for one variable from the values of the other variable. Inspection of the scattergrams in Figure 7.4 shows that a strong relationship exists when the points are close to the regression line or the line of best fit; see Figures 7.4(c and d). Predictions can be made with relative confidence when data points are close to the regression line. The actual data points are close to those predicted by the regression line. In contrast, we have relatively little confidence in predictions made when data points are not close to the regression line; see Figures 7.4(e and f).

Figure 7.4 illustrates positive and negative correlation coefficients with the same values. What does it mean when a correlation is positive or negative? In the case of a *positive correlation*, individuals who scored high on one variable tend to score high on the second variable. Conversely, in the case of a *negative correlation*, individuals who scored high on one variable tend to score low on the second variable. In other words, the plus and minus signs determine the direction of the relationship. If the correlation coefficient is positive, then the interpretation is that individuals who had high scores on one variable tended also to have high scores on the second variable and vice versa.

Finally, as we explained in Chapter 3, it is difficult to interpret exactly what a correlation coefficient means. Whether a correlation coefficient of some particular size is important depends on the circumstances or context of the study; that is, whether a correlation coefficient is meaningful depends on the area of research and how it is to be used. Figure 7.5 presents some common interpretations for a range of possible correlations.

Statistical Significance of Correlation Coefficients

We discussed in Chapter 4 the notion that statistical significance enables researchers to draw reasonable conclusions regarding the relative influence of systematic and chance factors on the findings. With regard to correlation coefficients, statistical significance testing allows researchers to draw conclusions (or make inferences) about a relationship in the population from information gained from a sample. Although it is of some interest to describe the relationship between two variables, it is often of greater interest to determine, with some degree of certainty, whether the two variables are associated in the population. For example, if we had drawn representative samples of youth with intellectual disabilities exiting high school, some with part-time or full-time jobs and some without jobs, we would probably find a high positive correlation between having a job and future employment status. That is, completing high school with a job would predict future employment. By testing our correlation coefficient for statistical significance, we would be able to say with some degree of certainty that current employment predicts future employment for the population. Before proceeding with our discussion of statistical significance of correlation coefficients, it is important to know that the obtained correlation coefficient is unique to the sample of participants. In fact, if we were to examine the obtained correlation coefficients based on different samples drawn from the same population, it is highly unlikely that any two correlation coefficients would be identical. Although we would expect them to be similar, there would inevitably be variations in the obtained correlation coefficients.

Testing the statistical significance of a correlation coefficient obtained from a sample enables researchers to speculate about the relationship in the population. The correlation coefficient for a given sample is represented with the letter r and the population value is represented by the Greek letter ρ (rho). Let's consider an example. Suppose you are a curriculum specialist for a school district. You develop a pre-algebra screening test and hypothesize that it will predict how well junior high students perform in a pre-algebra class. You give the test to a random sample of 20 junior high students who have not

> The **correlation coefficient** describes the relationship between two variables.

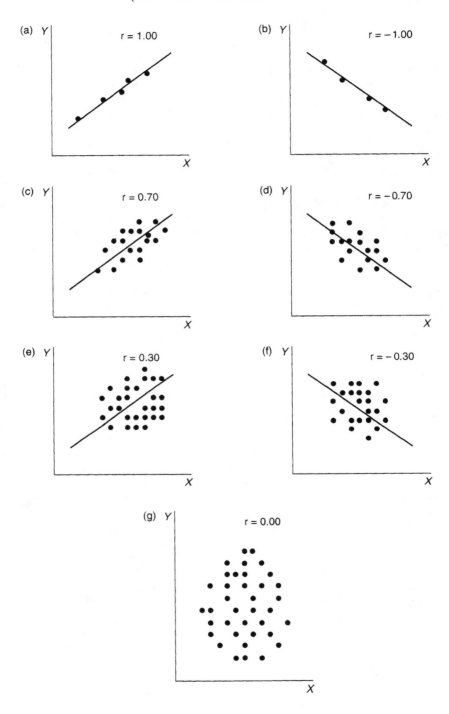

FIGURE 7.4. Positive and negative correlation coefficients.

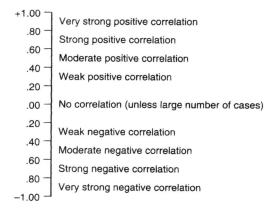

FIGURE 7.5. Rough interpretations for a range of correlations.

TABLE 7.2. Table of Critical Values

Level for a two-tail test	.10	.05	.02	.01	.001
N					
6	.729	.811	.882	.917	.974
7	.669	.754	.833	.874	.951
8	.622	.707	.789	.834	.925
9	.582	.666	.750	.798	.898
10	.549	.632	.716	.765	.872
11	.521	.602	.685	.735	.847
12	.497	.576	.658	.708	.823
13	.476	.553	.634	.684	.801
14	.458	.532	.612	.661	.780
15	.441	.514	.592	.641	.760
16	.426	.497	.574	.623	.742
17	.412	.482	.558	.606	.725
18	.400	.468	.542	.590	.708
19	.389	.456	.528	.575	.693
20	.378	.444	.516	.561	.679
21	.369	.433	.503	.549	.665
22	.360	.423	.492	.537	.652
23	.352	.413	.482	.526	.640
24	.344	.404	.472	.515	.629
25	.337	.396	.462	.505	.618
26	.330	.388	.453	.496	.607
27	.323	.381	.445	.487	.597
28	.317	.374	.437	.479	.588
29	.311	.367	.430	.471	.579
30	.306	.361	.423	.463	.570
35	.282	.333	.391	.428	.531
40	.264	.312	.366	.402	.501
45	.248	.296	.349	.381	.471
50	.235	.276	.328	.361	.451
60	.214	.254	.300	.330	.414
70	.198	.235	.277	.305	.385
80	.185	.220	.260	.286	.361
90	.174	.208	.245	.270	.342
100	.165	.196	.232	.256	.324
150	.135	.161	.190	.210	.267
200	.117	.139	.164	.182	.232
Level for a one-tail test	.05	.025	.01	.005	.0005

yet taken the pre-algebra class. Later, you compare their scores to grades in the pre-algebra class. The correlation is positive (i.e., $r = .561$). Table 7.2 presents the obtained critical values for r. The critical value shown in this table for the .01 two-tailed test for a sample of 20 individuals is $r = .561$. You conclude that the correlation is statistically significant, meaning that the probability of the obtained result, given the sample size and assuming the sample was derived from a population in which the null hypothesis is true, would occur less than 1% of the time.

Finally, it is important to note that whether a correlation coefficient is significant does not provide us any information regarding the magnitude of the relationship between two variables. For example, for a sample of 200, a correlation coefficient of .139 is statistically significant at the .05 alpha level. However, examine the scattergram of a correlation of .139 in Figure 7.6. The figure illustrates a weak correlation even though it is statistically significant. Based on these data, relatively accurate predictions cannot be made.

Variance Interpretation of Correlation Coefficients

The interpretation of the magnitude of a correlation coefficient is problematic, because it is not a proportion. A correlation coefficient of .50 does not represent a degree of relationship twice as great as a correlation coefficient of .25. The difference between correlation coefficients of .80 and .90 is not equal to the difference between the correlation coefficients .30 and .40.

Coefficient of Determination. One of the most informative ways of interpreting the magnitude of correlation coefficients is to consider

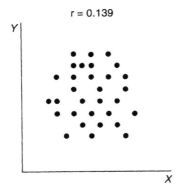

r = 0.139

FIGURE 7.6. Scattergram of correlation of .139.

TABLE 7.3. Values of Coefficient of Determinations and Associated r Values

$R^2 \times 100$	r
1	.10
4	.20
9	.30
16	.40
25	.50
36	.60
49	.70
64	.80
81	.90
100	1.00

the variance or proportion of predictable variance. The proportion of predictable variance, called the **coefficient of determination**, is calculated by squaring the obtained correlation coefficient r^2 and multiplying it by 100. The coefficient of determination is a simple proportion. For example, if $r = .90$, then $r^2 = .81$. Therefore, we can state that 81% of the variance of one variable is predictable from the variance of the other variable. In essence, we know 81% of what we would have to know to make a perfect prediction. In contrast to a correlational coefficient, a .50 coefficient of determination represents a degree of relationship twice as great as a .25 coefficient of determination. The difference between coefficients of determination of .80 and .90 is equal to the difference between coefficients of determination of .30 and .40. Converting the correlation coefficient into a proportion enables us to assess the magnitude of the relationship between two variables. In our preceding example, in which a correlation coefficient of .139 is statistically significant with a sample of 200 individuals, we find that we know less than 2% (i.e., .139 × .139) of what we need to know to make a perfect prediction.

It is generally more meaningful to think in terms of the coefficient of determination than to think of the correlation coefficient itself. Coefficient of determination values of r from .10 to 1.00 are presented in Table 7.3. Note that a correlation of over .80 is needed before we can state that 65% of the variance of one variable is predictable from the variance of another variable.

Coefficient of Alienation. Another way of viewing the magnitude of the correlation coefficient is to consider the lack of association between two variables. The **coefficient of alienation** $(1 - r^2)$ tells us the proportion of variance of one variable that is not predictable from the variance of another variable.

Causality and Correlation

One thing we mentioned before about the correlation coefficient is that it can be applied to any two sets of values from two paired variables. But statistical procedures for obtaining a correlation coefficient do not mean that a meaningful relationship of any kind necessarily exists between the two variables. Thus, the correlational coefficient is only meaningful to the extent that it permits conclusions to be made about the relationship between two variables. Without this connection, the correlation coefficient is simply a value.

On the surface, it might appear that a strong correlation indicates that there must be some kind of causal link between two variables. However, this is not the case. Correlation does not imply causation. Because one variable consistently increases or decreases in unison with another variable does not mean that one causes the other; this is true no matter how strong the correlation coefficient is.

Although correlation does not imply causation, a relationship between variables often provides researchers useful leads to causal relationships.

Of course, if no relationship exists between two variables, a causal relationship may be ruled out. If a relationship does exist between two variables, experimental studies or the use of advanced statistical techniques and the correlational research method are required to confirm whether the variables are causally connected. Cook and Campbell (1979) identified three requirements to say that one variable (independent variable) causes another (dependent variable):

1. A change in the value of the independent value is accompanied by a change in the value of the dependent variable.

2. Some mechanism for asserting beforehand how the independent variable affects the dependent variable.

3. The independent variable must precede the dependent variable. Of course, in correlational research, they may be measured at the same time.

The more advanced statistical procedures used in correlational research, such as multiple regression and structural equation modeling, can be used to meet these three requirements. In contrast to experimental research in which researchers control alternative explanations for changes in the dependent variable through the use of true experimental research designs, researchers using the correlational research method statistically examine the changes in the dependent variable accompanying changes in the independent variable (Graziano & Raulin, 2010). For example, researchers explore the effects of the alternative variables by introducing them into a regression equation and seeing if the relationship between the two variables is affected. If the alternative variables have no effect, this indicates that the relationship may be real. If the relationship between two variables weakens or disappears with the introduction of the alternative variables, then the relationship between the two variables may not be real.

Correlational research typically expresses relationships in diagrams to assert how the causal effect behaves, in contrast to experimental studies, in which the independent variable is directly manipulated to assert how the causal effect behaves. Figure 7.7 presents hypothetical

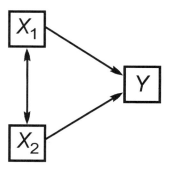

FIGURE 7.7. Reciprocal and causal relationship between variables.

relationships among variables. Researchers represent variables using circles or boxes. Relationships among variables that are not causal in nature are symbolized by curved lines. A single arrow on a line represents a unidirectional relationship. Arrows on both ends represent reciprocal relationships. Relationships between variables can be positive or negative. If a negative sign is not used, it is implied that the relationship is positive. Causal relationships are expressed by straight lines with an arrow on one end. The arrows show the direction of causality (i.e., independent variable to dependent variable) and usually proceed from left to right. Of course, in complex models other arrangements are used to produce a clear diagram.

Inspection of Figure 7.7 reveals that Variables X_1 and X_2 are related to one another in a reciprocal fashion. The relationship between Variables X_1 and X_2 is positive. Variables X_1 and X_2 are causally related to Variable Y. Although this example only includes three variables, it demonstrates how researchers use diagrams to depict relationships under study. We return to

The **coefficient of determination** is calculated by squaring the obtained correlation coefficient r^2 and multiplying it by 100; it tells us the proportion of variance of one variable that is predictable from the variance of another variable.

The **coefficient of alienation** is calculated by subtracting r^2 from 1.00; it tells us the proportion of variance of one variable that is not predictable from the variance of another variable.

these diagrams when we describe the advanced statistical procedures used in correlational research.

Researchers' conceptions of causality differ on this second component (i.e., that the use of some mechanism for asserting beforehand how the independent variable affects the dependent variable). Some researchers believe that a causal relationship can only be established through the direct manipulation of the independent variable, and others believe that such a manipulation is not necessary. It should be clear that researchers who use causal analysis in correlational research do not believe it is necessary to manipulate the independent variable to assert how it affects the dependent variable. Regardless of the position researchers take on this issue, all would assert that the causal relationship between two variables cannot be established given the results of only one study. Replications of the phenomenon under study are necessary for researchers to assert with any confidence that a causal relationship exists between two variables.

Finally, researchers using the correlational research method, like those using true experimental methods, must establish the temporal order of the relationship to make causal statements. In other words, an established relationship between two variables says nothing about which one has a causal effect on the other; researchers must establish the temporal order of the relationship to accomplish this.

Factors Affecting Correlation Coefficients

There are a number of factors that affect the correlation coefficient (Warner, 2007): (1) form of the relationship, (2) outliers in the data, (3) restriction of range, (4) skewed distributions, and (5) attenuation.

Form of the Relationship. One of the primary factors that affects the correlation coefficient is the form of the relationship between two variables. As mentioned earlier, the relationship between variables can take four different forms. The correlation coefficient is only completely satisfactory as an indicator of the relationship if the relationship is linear. The correlation coefficient is not completely satisfactory as an indicator of curvilinear (i.e., quadratic, cubic, and quartic) relationships. Of course, it is important to keep in mind that just because a relationship between two variables is curvilinear does not mean that the variables are unrelated. Rather, the use of the correlation coefficient as an indicator of the degree of relationship between the two variables is inappropriate, and a more appropriate statistical procedure should be used to determine the magnitude of the relationship between the variables.

Many nonlinear relationships can be identified in education and psychology. For example, for most individuals, memory function increases over most of a lifetime, then, depending on age and health, decreases. Thus, a nonlinear relationship exists between memory function and age.

If the relation is nonlinear, low correlations may be obtained even though a systematic relationship may exist between the two variables. Thus, researchers may underestimate the degree of relationship between two variables if the correlation coefficient is used. Although underestimating the degree of relationship between two variables is preferable to overestimating the relationship, researchers are most interested in obtaining an accurate indicator of the degree of relationship between variables. Thus, in interpreting a correlation coefficient, researchers should satisfy themselves that the relationship between two variables is linear. Any gross departure from a linear trend can readily be detected by inspection of the scattergram.

Detecting the particular type of trend through inspection of a scattergram is difficult for small samples (less than 30 to 40 participants). The correlation ratio, also known as the eta coefficient, can be used to detect nonlinear relationships (Mari & Kotz, 2001). The advantage of the correlation ratio is that it provides an indicator of the degree of relationship between two variables when the relationship is considerably nonlinear. The *correlation ratio* is a statistical procedure used to assess the degree of relationship between a nominal scale variable and an interval or ratio scale variable. If the obtained values for the correlation coefficient and correlation ratio substantially depart from one another, then it is likely that the relationship is curvilinear. Conversely, if the obtained values for the correlation coefficient and correlation ratio do not substantially depart from one another, then it is likely that the relationship is linear.

Outliers in the Data. Another factor that affects the correlation coefficient is outliers in the data set. An *outlier* is an individual or other entity (e.g., one or more schools out of a sample of 50) whose score differs considerably from the scores obtained by the other participants or entities of the sample. Outliers can affect the correlation coefficient. Outliers are especially problematic, because they can result in an overestimate or underestimate of the relationship between variables. The scattergram can be used to identify potential outliers. If an outlier is identified, researchers must first determine whether an error occurred in computing or recording the response or score. Some outliers may occur because of simple mistakes on the part of the researcher, such as misplacing the decimal point. If the outlier is not a function of a computation or recording error, researchers should explore other possible explanations. For example, the particular participant may not have been exposed to the independent variable. The decision to eliminate an outlier is difficult. If outliers are left in the sample, then they may distort the obtained correlation coefficient. It may be useful to compare the correlation coefficient obtained with and without the outliers included in the sample before deciding whether to include them in the analysis.

Restriction of Range. Still another factor that influences the correlation coefficient is the homogeneity or heterogeneity of the sample on which the data are collected. Suppose we consider two variables, X and Y, in which the variability (variance) of the X variable is restricted. This restriction reduces the correlation coefficient between the two variables. This restriction is sometimes referred to as *restriction of range* of the correlation coefficient. Researchers should carefully consider the effect discussed here, because some correlational research involves assessing the relationship between variables on highly selected samples. For example, the correlation coefficient between scores on the SAT and GPA in graduate school may be low, because students who gain admission to graduate school

are a highly selected group with little variance in performance.

Researchers can apply a correction for restriction of range when the range of scores for a sample is restricted. This correction procedure enables researchers to estimate what the relationship would be between the two variables if the variability of the responses or scores were not restricted. Use of the correction for restriction of range requires the assumption that the relationship between the two variables is linear throughout their entire range. The correction for restriction of range would not be appropriate in cases in which the relationship is curvilinear.

Skewed Distributions. A skewed distribution is one that deviates substantially from a normal distribution (Graziano & Raulin, 2010). The correlation coefficient will be affected if a variable with a positively skewed distribution (i.e., there are a disproportionate number of high scores) is correlated with a variable with a negatively skewed distribution (i.e., there are a disproportionate number of low scores). In such cases, the variables should be transformed to approximate a normal distribution or, depending on the scale of measurement (e.g., nominal), a nonparametric correlation statistic should be used. The use of the correlation coefficient is based on the assumption that scores are normally distributed. That is, the distributions of the scores for the two variables are normally distributed (see the earlier discussion of the normal distribution). Researchers often explore the relationships between two variables in which their distributions have different shapes.

Attenuation. The obtained correlation coefficient between two variables is always lower than the true correlation. The degree to which the correlation coefficient is lower is dependent on the extent to which the measurement devices are not perfectly reliable. The lowering of the correlation coefficient because of the unreliability of the measure is called *attenuation*. Researchers can apply the correction for attenuation to estimate the relationship between two variables if the measurement devices are perfectly reliable. Applying the correction for attenuation is useful in those cases in which the measurement devices are somewhat unreliable.

Basic Correlational Procedures

Now that we have discussed the correlation coefficient, we examine the wide range of correlational procedures available to researchers conducting correlational research. Several correlational procedures are described, including the Pearson product–moment correlation, part and partial correlation, correlation ratio, Spearman rank correlation coefficient and Kendall rank correlation, Kendall part rank correlation, Kendall coefficient of concordance, phi coefficient, and contingency coefficient. The selection of a particular correlation procedure depends on the scale of measurement involved, the size of the sample, and research questions. Advanced correlational procedures, such as multiple regression, are examined later.

As discussed previously, the Pearson product–moment correlation coefficient is used in those cases in which the scores are interval or ratio scale. The Pearson product–moment correlation coefficient is only appropriate when the two variables of interest are related in a linear fashion and are normally distributed.

A wide range of other correlational procedures can be used to examine the relationship between two variables or among several variables. They can be used to examine the relationship between variables that are related in a linear or curvilinear fashion. They can be used to explore causal relationships among variables.

Part and Partial Correlation

The ability to explore the complex relationships among a wide range of variables is one of the most useful aspects of correlation research. In general, part and partial correlations are used by researchers to explore the influence of an independent variable on the relationship between another independent variable and a dependent variable. The **part correlation** enables researchers to establish the relationship between two variables after the influence or effect of another variable has been removed from one but not both of the variables. The partial correlation coefficient differs from the part correlation in that it enables researchers to establish the relationship between two variables after the influence or effect of a third variable has been removed from both.

We consider a hypothetical study to ensure our understanding of the differences between part and partial correlation coefficients. Figure 7.8 presents a study in which the goal is to explore the relationship between family commitment to education and academic success in high school. In this study, other factors related to academic success include early achievement and socioeconomic level. The influence of these variables on academic success in high school is depicted by straight lines with an arrow. The relationships among family commitment to education, early achievement, and socioeconomic

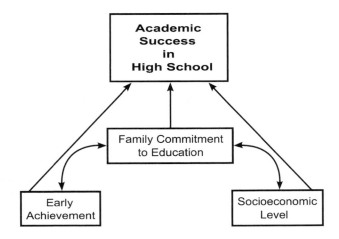

FIGURE 7.8. Determinants of academic success in high school.

level are depicted by curved lines with arrows on both ends.

The **partial correlation** could be used if researchers wanted to establish the relationship between family commitment and academic success in high school, while controlling the influence of early achievement and socioeconomic level. Of course, the partial correlation could also be used to establish the relationship between the other variables (i.e., early achievement and socioeconomic level) and academic success, while controlling the influence of two other variables.

The part correlation could be used if researchers wanted to establish the relationship between family commitment and academic success in high school, while controlling only the influence of early achievement or socioeconomic level. Another use of the part correlation could be to explore the relationship between the other two variables (i.e., early achievement and socioeconomic level) and academic success in high school. The advantage of the partial correlation over the part correlation in this case is its capacity to simplify a potentially complex pattern among family commitment to education, early achievement, socioeconomic level, and academic success in high school, by allowing the researcher to look at only one part of the pattern. Other, more advanced statistical procedures, such as path analysis, multiple regression, and structural equation modeling, enable researchers to examine the complete causal pattern that is hypothesized, with all of the possible influences among variables. We describe each of these statistical procedures later in this chapter.

Correlation Ratio

The **correlation ratio** (η^2) refers to the proportion of the total variability in the dependent variable that can be accounted for by knowing the value of the independent variable. It is appropriate for data in which the dependent variable is measured on an interval or ratio scale, and the independent variable is measured on a nominal or ordinal scale. The correlation ratio does not require a linear relationship or that the dependent variable be normally distributed.

Spearman Rank Correlation Coefficient and Kendall Rank Correlation Coefficient

The Spearman rank correlation and Kendall coefficient are appropriate when both variables are measured on at least ordinal scales.

The Spearman rank correlation is referred to as ρ, and the **Kendall rank correlation coefficient** is referred to as τ, or "tau." The **Spearman rank correlation coefficient** and the Kendall tau provide a measure of the disparity in the rankings between two variables, and involve ranking the scores for each of the variables from smallest to largest and computing the Pearson product–moment correlation coefficient on the ranks. A positive correlation exists as the ranks of one variable increase (or decrease) in conjunction with the ranks of the other variable. Conversely, a negative correlation exists as the ranks of one variable increase (or decrease) in conjunction with the ranks of the other variable. Because a large number of ties affect the Spearman rank correlation coefficient and the Kendall tau, a corrective factor is applied, in which the tied values are replaced with the average rank. If the number of ties is not large, their effect on the Spearman rank correlation coefficient and the Kendall tau is negligible.

---

*The **part correlation** establishes the relationship between two variables after the influence or effect of another variable has been removed from one but not both variables.*

*The **partial correlation coefficient** enables researchers to establish the relationship between two variables after the influence or effect of a third variable has been removed from both.*

*The **correlation ratio** (η^2) refers to the proportion of the total variability in the dependent variable that can be accounted for by the independent variable.*

*The **Spearman rank correlation coefficient** and the **Kendall rank correlation coefficient** involve ranking the scores for each of the variables from smallest to largest and computing the Pearson product–moment correlation coefficient on the ranks.*

Kendall Part Rank Correlation

The Kendall part rank correlation coefficient is used in those cases in which researchers want to control the influence of a third variable on the relationship between two variables. The Kendall part rank correlation coefficient is similar to the part correlation except that it is appropriate when the variables are measured on at least ordinal scales rather than interval or ratio scales. For example, the Kendall part rank correlation coefficient could have been used to explore the relationship between family commitment and academic success in high school, while controlling for the influence of either early achievement or socioeconomic level. Unfortunately, there is no equivalent to the partial correlation coefficient for use when variables are measured in ordinal scales.

Kendall Coefficient of Concordance

The Spearman rank correlation coefficient and the Kendall tau are concerned with measuring the association between the rankings of two variables. The Kendall coefficient of concordance is used when researchers want to establish the relationship among the rankings of several variables, typically in studies of intertest reliability. For example, the Kendall coefficient of concordance might be used in a study whose purpose is to assess the degree of agreement among college professors', principals', and mentors' rankings of the effectiveness of student teachers. A high value for the Kendall coefficient of concordance would indicate that the observers (e.g., professors, principals, and mentors) are applying similar standards in ranking the effectiveness of student teachers. Conversely, a low value for the Kendall coefficient of concordance would indicate that the observers are applying different standards in ranking the effectiveness of student teachers.

Phi Coefficient and Contingency Coefficient

The phi coefficient and contingency coefficient are appropriate when both variables are measured on a nominal scale. The phi coefficient and contingency coefficient are based on chi-square (as discussed in Chapter 4). The phi coefficient and the contingency coefficient are used in place of the chi-square to assess the relationship between nominal variables. The values for the phi coefficient and the contingency coefficient range from 0 to +1. The phi coefficient and the contingency coefficient are useful in cases in which none of the other measures of association we have described are applicable.

Advanced Correlational Procedures

One of the advantages of the correlational research method over experimental methods is that researchers can look at not only the relationships between variables but also the interrelationships among variables. Additionally, researchers are increasingly using the correlational research method to establish causal relationships among variables.

The advanced correlational procedures that follow enable researchers to address a wide range of questions. It is important to note that many of these statistical procedures are used not only in correlational research but also in analyzing data from experimental studies. Thus, it is important for critical research consumers to be familiar with these advanced statistical procedures. We wish to describe each of the statistical procedures in enough detail to enable you to understand them on a basic level. We encourage you to seek more information in case you encounter difficulty interpreting the results of a study (e.g., Allison, 1999; Cohen, Cohen, West, & Aiken, 2003).

Multiple Regression

Multiple regression is an extension of the correlation coefficient in which the overall and relative degree of relationship between a set of independent variables and a dependent variable is obtained. In general, multiple regression is a highly flexible data analysis procedure that may be used whenever a quantitative variable (dependent variable) is to be studied in relationship to, or is a function of, any factors of interest (independent variables). Multiple regression is applicable under the following conditions (Cohen et al., 2003):

1. The form of the relationship under study is not constrained in any way. The relationship may be simple or complex, general or conditional, linear or curvilinear, or combinations of these possibilities.

2. The nature of the factors expressed as independent variables is also not constrained in any way. The factors may be quantitative or qualitative, main effects or interaction effects (as in the ANOVA), or covariates (as in the ANCOVA). The factors may be correlated with each other or uncorrelated. The factors may be naturally occurring properties, such as gender, diagnosis, or IQ, or they may be the result of planned experimental manipulation (treatments). The factors may be single variables or groups of variables. The factors may be nominal, ordinal, interval, or ratio in nature. In short, virtually any information whose bearing on the dependent variable is of interest may be expressed as research factors.

3. The magnitude of the relationship of a factor to the dependent variable is not constrained in any way. The magnitude of the whole relationship or partial relationship of a variable can be determined.

4. The ability to determine the statistical significance of the relationship of a factor to the dependent variable is not constrained in any way. The statistical significance of the whole relationship or partial relationship of a variable can be determined.

Multiple regression is a versatile statistical analysis procedure for analyzing data from correlational research studies, as well as other experimental studies. Remember that the correlation coefficient determines the degree of relationship between two variables: an independent variable and a dependent variable. Multiple regression can be thought of as an extension of the correlation coefficient in which the overall and relative degree of relationship between a set of independent variables (nominal, ordinal, interval, or ratio in nature) and a dependent variable (interval or ratio in nature) is obtained. That is, multiple regression takes the same basic form as the correlation coefficient, but a set of independent variables is involved rather than just one. For example, in a hypothetical study of a set of factors (high school GPA, SAT scores, and absence rate) related to college success (college GPA), multiple regression could be used to determine the overall degree of relationship between the set of factors (high school GPA, SAT scores, and absence rate) and college GPA. Multiple regression would also be used to determine the relative degree of relationship between the set of factors (high school GPA, SAT scores, and absence rate) and college GPA.

Regression Models. A variety of regression models or equations can be constructed from the same set of independent variables to predict the dependent variable. For example, seven different regression models can be constructed from the college example described previously: three models using only one of the independent variables, three with two independent variables, and one with all three of the independent variables. As the number of independent variables increases, so does the number of potential regression models. Although researchers can examine all possible regression models, they typically use forward selection, backward elimination, and stepwise selection procedures to examine the overall and relative relationships between a set of independent variables and a dependent variable. These procedures are all included in standard statistical packages and are described below.

In *forward selection*, the first variable entered into the regression model is the one with the largest positive or negative relationship with the dependent variable. If the first variable selected for entry meets the established criterion (alpha level established by the researcher) for inclusion in the model, forward selection continues. If the independent variable does not meet the criterion for inclusion in the model, the procedure terminates with no variables in the regression model. In this case, none of the independent variables are predictive of the dependent variable. Once

> **Multiple regression** *determines the degree of relationship between a set of independent variables and a dependent variable.*

one independent variable is included in the model, the correlation among the independent variables not in the equation is used to select the next variable. In essence, the partial correlation between the dependent variable and each of the independent variables is computed. The independent variable with the largest partial correlation is the next variable considered in the model. If the established criterion is met, the variable is entered into the regression model. This process continues until there are no other independent variables that meet the established entry criteria.

In contrast to forward selection, which begins with no independent variables in the regression model, *backward elimination* starts with all of the independent variables in the regression model and sequentially removes them. Researchers establish removal criteria rather than entry criteria. The independent variable with the smallest partial correlation with the dependent variable is examined first. If the independent variable meets established criteria for removal, it is removed from the regression model. If the independent variable does not meet the established criteria for removal, it remains in the regression model and the procedure stops. Although backward elimination and forward selection typically result in the same regression model, this is not always the case.

Stepwise selection of independent variables for inclusion in the regression model is a combination of the forward selection and backward elimination procedures. Stepwise selection is the most commonly used procedure. The first independent variable for consideration in the regression model is selected in the same manner as in the forward selection procedure. If the independent variable does not meet the established criteria for inclusion, the procedure is terminated, with no independent variables in the regression model. If the independent variable meets the established criteria for inclusion in the regression model, selection of the second independent variable is based on the highest partial correlation. Stepwise selection differs from forward selection in that the first independent variable is examined to see if it should be removed, based on the established removal criteria, as in backward elimination. Independent variables not in the equation are then examined for

removal. After each step, independent variables already in the regression model are examined for removal. Independent variables are removed until none remain that meet the established removal criteria.

Interpretation of Multiple Regression. In addition to taking the same basic form as the correlation coefficient, interpretation of the results of multiple regression is similar to that of the correlation coefficient. Recall that the correlation coefficient yields r, which provides an index of the degree of relationship between two variables. Similarly, multiple regression yields the coefficient of multiple correlation (R). The coefficient of multiple correlation can be thought of as a simple correlation coefficient between the scores of a set of independent variables and the score on the dependent variable. The R ranges from -1.00 to $+1.00$. Thus, an R value of $+1.00$ indicates that there is a perfect correlation between the independent variables and the dependent variable. In multiple regression, the obtained value for each of the independent variables is called a regression coefficient (R) and its interpretation directly parallels the multiple correlation. Thus, the correlation between a set of independent variables is called the multiple correlation (R), while the correlations between each of the independent variables are called regression coefficients ($R's$).

Furthermore, we indicated that the square of the correlation coefficient (coefficient of determination) tells us the percentage of the variance of the dependent variable that is predicted on the basis of the independent variable. For example, if the correlation of multiple correlation is equal to .70, then one can state that 49% (.7 × .7) of the variance for the dependent variable is predictable on the basis of the set of independent variables.

Because multiple regression can deal effectively with data that are nominal, ordinal, interval, and ratio in nature, it is important to note that the obtained regression coefficients cannot be compared against one another in a meaningful way. In other words, attempts to make direct comparisons of regression coefficients would be like trying to compare apples and oranges. Multiple regression deals with this issue by converting the regression coefficients into comparable units called *beta weights*, which are standardized regression coefficients (i.e., the regression coefficients that would have been obtained if each of the independent variables were equal to one another in terms of means and standard deviations) that enable direct comparisons of the relative relationship of each of the independent variables and the dependent variable. The independent variable that has the largest beta weight (regardless of whether the beta weight is positive or negative) is most strongly related to the dependent variable. Conversely, a small beta weight indicates that the associated independent variable is not strongly related to the dependent variable.

Beta weights are not necessarily favorable regression coefficients. Beta weights and regression coefficients provide different types of information. Beta weights provide information regarding the relative strength of the relationship between the independent variables and the dependent variable, whereas the regression coefficients provide information regarding the overall relationship between a set of independent variables and the dependent variable, or the set of factors that predict the dependent variable. Thus, researchers provide beta weights when they want to show the relative relationship between each set of independent variables and a dependent variable; they provide the regression coefficients when they want to show the overall relationship between a set of independent variables and a dependent variable. Of course, researchers typically provide both the regression coefficients and beta weights, because they want to show both the overall and relative relationship between a set of independent variables and a dependent variable.

When interpreting the magnitude of regression coefficients, our discussion of interpreting correlation coefficients directly applies. As with the correlation coefficient, it might appear that a large regression coefficient would indicate that there is some kind of causal link between independent variables and a dependent variable. Of course, this interpretation is not true. Because a set of independent variables consistently increases or decreases in unison with a dependent variable does not mean that one causes the other. This statement is true no matter how large the regression coefficients are. Additionally,

although it is possible for researchers to use multiple regression to explore causal relationships, they must meet the three requirements identified by Cook and Campbell (1979) to assert that such a relationship exists.

Statistical Significance of Multiple Regression. Before proceeding with our discussion of the statistical significance of multiple regression, it is important to note that the obtained multiple correlation, regression coefficients, and beta weights are unique to the specific sample of participants. Although a wide range of tests of statistical significance can be conducted with multiple regression, three tests of statistical significance are most commonly used by researchers (Cohen et al., 2003).

The first test of statistical significance is commonly used by researchers to establish whether the multiple correlation coefficient or regression coefficients obtained differ significantly from zero. The second test of statistical significance is commonly used by researchers to establish whether the obtained regression coefficients for each of the independent variables differ from one another. Although there will be typically an increase in the multiple correlation coefficient with the addition of each independent variable, it is of interest to determine whether the obtained increase is statistically significant. This type of statistical significance testing can be employed not only to establish the best set of independent variables that can predict the dependent variable but to also explore potential causal relationships between variables. Recall that if an obtained correlation between two variables is unaffected by the addition of other, potentially causal variables, the relationship may be causal in nature. The final test of statistical significance is to establish whether the obtained beta weights differ significantly from zero. The goal of this test of statistical significance is similar to testing the statistical significance of the difference in the obtained regression coefficients. If a particular independent variable is not strongly related to the dependent variable, then the beta weight for this independent variable will be close to zero. On the other hand, if a particular independent variable is strongly related to the dependent variable, then the beta weight for this independent variable will differ significantly from zero. Again, researchers employ this type of statistical significance testing when they are interested in demonstrating, with some degree of certainty, whether the beta weights are significantly different from zero in the population.

Canonical Correlation

Multiple regression is used in those cases when researchers are interested in determining the relationship between a set of independent variables and a dependent variable. Multiple regression can be generalized to cases when researchers are interested in determining the relationship between a set of independent variables and a set of dependent variables. The statistical technique for determining this type of relationship is *canonical correlation*, developed by Hotelling (1935), which is a complex statistical procedure in terms of both calculation and interpretation. Thus, it is used infrequently by researchers. Because it is infrequently used, we will not discuss it further. It is only important that critical research consumers know the canonical correlation procedure is available to researchers in cases in which they are interested in determining the relationship between a set of independent variables and a set of dependent variables.

Discriminant Function Analysis

Multiple regression is applied in situations in which the dependent variable is measured on an interval or ratio scale. **Discriminant function analysis** is employed in those cases in which the dependent variable is nominal in nature (i.e., group membership) rather than ordinal, interval, or ratio. For example, extending from our earlier college example, suppose a particular academic division at a university is interested in determining whether high school GPA and SAT scores predict who will graduate within 4 years rather than students' college GPA. In this case, the dependent variable is dichotomous, because an individual can only fall into one of two groups (those who graduate within 4 years and those who do not). There are two main types of discriminant function analyses. A two-group or *simple discriminant function analysis* is appropriate for nominal dependent variables with two

categories; a *multiple discriminant function analysis* is appropriate with three or more categories.

In contrast to multiple regression, in which the goal is to identify the best set of independent variables that predict a dependent variable, the goal of discriminant function analysis is to identify the best set of independent variables that maximize the correct classification of participants. The coefficients obtained are referred to as *discriminant function* or *structure coefficients*. Now return to our college example in which the goal is to identify students who graduate within 4 years. Using discriminant analysis, high school GPA, SAT scores, and absence rate would be used to predict which students will graduate within 4 years rather than their college GPA.

Interpretation of the discriminant function coefficients directly parallels the interpretation of regression coefficients. Standardized discriminant function coefficients, which have a mean of 0 and a standard deviation of 1, are used by researchers. Additionally, the three types of statistical significance used by researchers with regard to discriminant analysis directly parallel those used with multiple regression. The questions addressed by the tests of statistical significance include the following:

1. Does the obtained overall discriminant function coefficient differ significantly from zero?

2. Do the discriminant function coefficients differ significantly from one another?

3. Do the particular standardized discriminant function coefficients differ significantly from zero?

Factor Analysis

Factor analysis was developed by Spearman in his work on intelligence (Ferguson, 1989). Spearman argued that all functions of intelligence are encompassed within one general function or factor. The general factor was called *g*. Spearman's work led to the extensive use of factor-analytic procedures by researchers in education and psychology. Factor analysis is a multivariate statistical method that is used to identify unobserved or latent variables regarded more commonly as *factors* or *constructs* (Cohen et al.,

2007). Examples of latent variables include self-concept, anxiety, depression, and teacher expectancy. Latent variables represent theoretical constructs that cannot be observed directly and are presumed to underlie particular observed scores on some measurement device.

Factor analysis is used by researchers in an effort to identify factors or latent variables that underlie observed scores. It is most commonly used in the development of measurement devices in which the goal of researchers is either to confirm (confirmatory factor analysis) or identify (exploratory factor analysis) factors included within a measurement device. Factor analysis is also used to identify patterns of relations among a large number of variables in correlational research. In contrast to other correlational statistical procedures in which a distinction is made between independent and dependent variables, factor analysis does not make a distinction between independent and dependent variables. Rather, the concern is with the description and interpretation of interdependencies or interrelationships within a set of variables (Cohen et al., 2007).

Factor analysis, which refers to a variety of methods, can be thought of as a somewhat subjective process in which a large number of items (in the case of a measurement device) or variables (in the case of identifying patterns of interrelationships among variables) is reduced to a smaller set of factors or to a single factor. A single factor (or smaller set of factors) is thought of as more basic, and causal or explanatory explanations may more easily be attributed to them. In other words, the goal of factor analysis is to reduce a large set of variables (or items) describing a complex phenomenon, with the purpose of creating a better understanding of the phenomenon through simplification. For example, an individual's IQ score provides a simplified description of a wide range of extremely complex variables that underlie the construct of IQ.

The goal of factor analysis is to identify a structure or pattern within a set of variables. Consider a bivariate frequency distribution between two variables. The arrangement of the data points for the variables on a scattergram may be haphazard (random). This haphazard arrangement would be considered to be without structure. In contrast, the data points may tend to be arranged along a straight line. This arrangement of the data points with respect to each other would be considered to be a linear structure. Of course, the data points may arrange themselves in any number of structures (e.g., quadratic, cubic). Thus, structure emerges from a set of variables as the arrangement of data points departs from a random state.

Identifying the structure within a set of variables is accomplished through a variety of mathematical methods that underlie factor analysis. In essence, the structures within a set of variables are identified as factors. *Factors* are clusters or variables that are correlated with each other. The first set of variables that cluster together is called the *first factor*, which represents the group of variables that are most interrelated. This factor can then be represented as an individual score for each participant based on the scores from all of the variables included in the factor. The second set of variables that cluster together, called the *second factor*, represents the next group of variables that are most interrelated, and so on. The individual coefficients for each variable are referred to as the loading of each variable on the factor.

Factor Analysis Procedures. There are a variety of factor analyses that yield different solutions or outcomes. The two most common factor-analytic procedures are orthogonal and oblique solutions. An *orthogonal solution* results in factors that are unrelated to one another, and is used when researchers are interested in obtaining a pure set of factors, each measuring a construct that does not overlap with constructs measured by other factors. An *oblique solution* results in factors that are related to one another, and is used when researchers are interested in obtaining a set of factors that measure underlying constructs of some overall general construct. For example, a factor analysis of a stress

Discriminant function analysis *is used when the dependent variable is nominal in nature (i.e., group membership) rather than ordinal, interval, or ratio.*

Factor analysis *is used to identify unobserved or latent variables regarded more commonly as factors or constructs.*

measure might yield such factors as emotional, physical, and social stresses that underlie the general construct of stress.

Interpretation of the Meaning of the Factors. Interpretation of the meaning of the factors is a somewhat subjective process. Researchers need to examine the variables included within each factor and determine the conceptual meaning of the underlying factor. Of course, the same problems regarding the meaningfulness of the variables arise with factor analysis as with any correlational research. Because it is not uncommon for variables to be related to one another, researchers must ensure that the relationship is meaningful.

Path Analysis

Path analysis, which was developed by Wright (1921), is used to determine the amount of variance in a dependent variable that can be accounted for by a set of independent variables. In contrast to multiple regression, path analysis has the additional aim of determining whether the pattern of shared variances among the independent and dependent variables is consistent with particular causal pathways. These causal pathways must be a priori hypotheses by the researcher.

Consider a hypothetical study in which the relationship among home experiences, academic experiences, and college success is of interest. Several causal pathways are plausible. The first step in a path analysis is to diagram the causal pathways among which a choice is to be made. One plausible sequence is that home experiences affect academic experiences, and that academic experiences, in turn, cause college success; see Figure 7.9(a). A second possibility is that both home experiences and academic experiences independently cause college success; see Figure 7.9(b). A third possibility is that home experiences directly affect both academic experiences and college success. In this case, the correlation between academic experiences and college success would be that both are affected by home experiences. Although a number of other possible pathways could explain college success, assume that they have been ruled out on logical grounds by the researcher on the basis

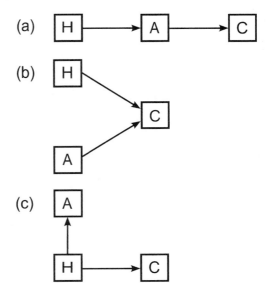

FIGURE 7.9. Three path models of determinants of college success. H, home experience; A, academic experiences; and C, college success.

of previous research and the data collection procedures.

Path coefficients are then computed for the relationships between the dependent variable (college success) and the independent variables (home experiences and academic experiences) in the second step. A *path coefficient* (*P*) is the proportion of variance in the dependent variable for which the independent variable is uniquely responsible, with the effects of the other independent variables partialed out. Path coefficients are regression coefficients obtained by transforming the independent and dependent variables into standard scores that have a mean of 0 and a standard deviation of 1 (beta weight), and computing the regression of the dependent variable on each independent variable in turn, with all of the other independent variables partialed out. The interpretation of path coefficients is the same as regression coefficients. The values for path coefficients can range from –1.00 to +1.00. Additionally, if all of the variance in the dependent variable is accounted for by the independent variables, the path coefficients will add up to 1.00.

Returning to our hypothetical study, suppose we find that the path coefficient for academic experiences is .40, and that the path coefficient for home experiences is .00. This statistic means that, with the effects of home experiences partialed out, academic experiences account for 40% of the variance in college success; with the effect of academic experiences partialed out, home experiences account for none of the variance in college success. The path coefficient for academic experiences and home experiences is then computed to complete the path analysis. We find that the obtained path coefficient is .50.

Figure 7.10 depicts the path diagram showing the coefficients (designated as p) for our hypothetical study. Inspection of the path diagram reveals that of the two independent variables, only academic experiences directly affect college success. Additionally, the diagram shows that home experiences affect college success only by affecting academic experiences.

Limitation on Causal Inferences. There are limitations on causal inferences from path analysis. The first major limitation is that path analysis only enables researchers to choose among several competing causal explanations for a set of coefficients. In our hypothetical study, path analysis made it possible to choose one of the three causal explanations portrayed in Figure 7.9. However, the findings were also compatible with other causal explanations. For example, the coefficient between home experiences and academic learning history might result because children's access to particular academic learning histories results in particular home experiences rather than home experiences resulting in particular academic learning histories. Although such a reversal of the hypothesized causal

relationship would not invalidate the conclusion that academic experiences affect college success, it would invalidate the conclusion that home experiences affect academic experiences.

Another major limitation of path analysis is that other variables may account for more variance in the dependent variable. These other variables might be independent of the variables already identified or they might account for the apparent contribution of the identified variables themselves. For example, if SES were included in our hypothetical study, its presence might reduce the contribution of academic experiences to college success, because the obtained contribution is actually due to the effect of SES. Thus, the effective use of path analysis requires the formulation of clear-cut and comprehensive models based on a sound theoretical base and previous research.

Recall the research question about early literacy predictors posed earlier in this chapter? Read on to see how your design compares to how the actual study was designed.

Research Example 1: Exploratory Relationships Study

An example of correlational research using path analysis is a study conducted to determine the predictability of kindergarten early literacy indicators (Burke, Hagan-Burke, Kwok, & Parker, 2009). The researchers note the increasing focus on moving schools toward formative evaluation of early literacy (National Research Council, 1998) and the importance of accurately predicting reading trajectories. They note that three crucial areas in successful reading development are (1) phonological awareness, (2) phonetic skills related to the alphabet, and (3) automaticity. *Phonological awareness* refers to auditory and oral abilities such as rhyming, alliteration, and breaking apart syllables. *Phonetic skills* related to the alphabet include letter–sound correspondence, unique letter combinations making a common sound, and word blending.

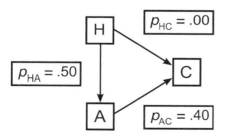

FIGURE 7.10. Diagram of path coefficients relating to college success. H, home experience; A, academic experiences; and C, college success.

> **Path analysis** *is used to determine the amount of variance in a dependent variable that can be accounted for by a set of independent variables.*

Automaticity refers to rapid, fluent, and context-free retrieval of component skills. The purpose of the study was to determine whether early literacy indicators from the kindergarten *Dynamic Indicators of Basic Early Literacy Skills* (DIBELS; Good & Kaminski, 2002) could be used to model reading acquisition. The sample included 218 kindergartners (98 European American, 47 African American, 3 Hispanic, 2 Asian, 9 mixed ethnicities) from one primary school. Four subtests of the DIBELS were administered (Initial Sound Fluency, Phoneme Segmentation Fluency, Letter Naming Fluency, and Nonsense Word Fluency) in middle kindergarten as predictor variables. Four criterion measures were administered in second grade. Data from all assessments were uploaded to a database. Scatterplots were developed between variables and examined for linearity. Correlations were generated to assess strength of associations between predictor variables and criterion variables. Path analysis was used to determine whether the pattern of shared variances among the independent and dependent variables was consistent with particular causal pathways. An initial hypothesized model was developed and evaluated. Results indicated that middle-kindergarten DIBELS scores are valid for predicting complex alphabetic skills. Additionally, results suggested that phonetic decoding efficiency, sight word efficiency, and oral reading fluency can be used to present performance of children who are in the alphabetic phase.

Structural Equation Modeling

Structural equation modeling is part of the linear structural relationship (LISREL) model. It uses one of various computer programs, such as LISREL 8 (Joreskog & Sorborn, 2001), Amos (Arbuckle, 1999), or EQS (EQuation S; Bentler, 2000). This method includes procedures derived from economics, psychometrics, sociometrics, and multivariate statistics (Byrne, 2001). Like some of the other multivariate statistical procedures used by researchers to explore causal relationships, structural equation modeling includes the use of regression models to represent the causal relationships under study. These regression models are similar in nature to the regression models we discussed previously under multiple regression and path analysis.

Structural equation modeling differs in two important ways from other multivariate statistics used by researchers to explore causal relationships (Kline, 2011). The first difference is that it takes an explicit confirmatory rather than an exploratory approach to data analysis. Although other multivariate procedures such as path analysis may be used to explore potential causal relationships, they are typically used in a descriptive or exploratory manner. For example, recall that path analysis only allows researchers to choose from a number of potential explanatory pathways. In contrast, structural equation modeling requires that the nature and pattern of relationship among variables be specified a priori. Structural equation modeling lends itself to inferential data analysis that enables researchers to assess small deviations from an explicit model. Significant deviations from the model would invalidate the hypothesized causal relationships among variables.

The second difference is the ability of structural equation modeling to provide explicit estimates of measurement error. Explicit estimates enable the researcher to obtain a more accurate picture of the relationships among variables than that provided by other multivariate statistical procedures.

Finally, structural equation modeling enables researchers to incorporate both observed and unobserved or latent variables in their models. Recall that latent variables or factors represent theoretical constructs that cannot be observed directly but are presumed to underlie observed measures. The use of latent variables in structural equation modeling enables researchers to combine a number of measures to assess the constructs of interest. Each measure underlying the constructs represents a different aspect of each particular construct, which is the same principle we discussed under factor analysis (i.e., a large number of variables on a measurement device are reduced to a factor or set of factors).

Consider a hypothetical study in which the relationship among several variables is of interest: parental psychological control, parental behavioral control, quality of child care, and child social adjustment. The first step in

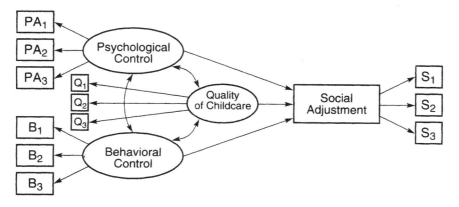

FIGURE 7.11. A figure of the causal relationship among parental psychological control, parental behavioral control, quality child care, and child social adjustment.

structural equation modeling is to specify the causal relationship among each of the latent variables. In our hypothetical study, we use three measures to assess each of the latent variables. Figure 7.11 depicts the causal relationship among parental psychological control, parental behavioral control, quality of child care, and child social adjustment. The model used in the structural equation model is similar to that used in path analysis. The latent variables are depicted by ovals, and the specific measures (referred to as *manifest variables*) used to assess aspects of the latent variables are depicted by rectangles. Inspection of Figure 7.11 reveals that three manifest measures are used to assess each of the latent variables. The straight arrows indicate hypothesized causal relationships. The curved arrows indicate a relationship between variables.

The manifest variables are then combined in the second step through a factor-analytic process. This process identifies the common variance among the manifest variables or the factor they share in common. The factor-analytic process also tests whether each manifest variable correlates at a sufficiently high level with the factor used to represent the particular latent variable.

Path coefficients are then computed for each hypothesized causal relationship between latent variables in the final step of structural equation modeling. Again, a path coefficient is the

proportion of variance in a dependent variable for which the independent variable is uniquely responsible, with the effects of the other independent variables partialed out. Returning to our hypothetical study, let's say that the obtained path coefficients are as follows: .55 for psychological control, .03 for quality of child care, and .70 for behavioral control. We conclude that parental behavioral control and parental psychological control have more influence on child social adjustment than quality of child care, because a larger path coefficient indicates a larger influence.

Structural equation modeling is a statistical procedure commonly used by researchers to explore causal relationships in correlational research. Although structural equation modeling is more sophisticated than path analysis, many of the same limitations we discussed for path analysis apply with structural equation modeling. The strength of structural equation modeling is primarily its ability to measure latent variables with maximal reliability. This

> **Structural equation modeling** is part of the linear structural relationship (LISREL) model and uses one of various computer programs, such as LISREL 8 or EQS. Structural equation modeling is similar to path analysis in that it is used by researchers to test causal relationships among variables.

ability provides a level of precision that is not available with path analysis.

Analysis of Data

Similar to experimental and causal–comparative designs, critical research consumers must determine the extent to which a researcher is able to make cause-and-effect and generalizable statements based on the results of a correlational study.

Internal Validity

As with the causal–comparative research design, the threats to internal validity do not match the correlational design well. There are some obvious threats, but most of the threats discussed previously are not applicable to correlational research, because the correlational research design has not traditionally been used to determine cause-and-effect relationships. However, we can say that interpreting the results of correlational research studies should be done cautiously. Critical research consumers should not assume correlational findings to be proof of cause-and-effect relationships. Researchers must ensure that all of the potential

explanatory variables for the phenomenon under study can be accounted for or included in their analyses. One study cannot account for all of the potential explanatory variables, even when the researcher has employed advanced statistical procedures such as path analysis or structural equation modeling that tend to meet the criteria established by Cook and Campbell (1979) for concluding that a causal relationship exists among variables.

As with experimental studies, causal relationships can only be established through multiple replications. So several threats to internal validity exist for correlational studies. These threats are shown in Table 7.4. As described, the major threats are instrumentation and testing. Instrumentation may be a threat if there is a concern with the reliability of the measurement device. Recall from Chapter 3 that validity is affected by reliability. Therefore, if a researcher is using a test with low reliability, the validity of the results must be in question.

Testing is an obvious problem, because participants are exposed to two assessments. Exposure to the first assessment may affect the performance on the second (usually by increasing scores on the second assessment due to familiarity), increasing the correlation of the two

TABLE 7.4. Threats to Internal Validity Associated with Correlational Research

Threat	Correlational research design
1. Maturation	Not applicable
2. Selection	Not applicable
3. Selection by maturation interaction	Not applicable
4. Statistical regression	Not applicable
5. Mortality	Not applicable
6. Instrumentation	Possible concern
7. Testing	Possible concern
8. History	Not applicable
9. Resentful demoralization of the control group	Not applicable
10. Diffusion of treatment	Not applicable
11. Compensatory rivalry by the control group	Not applicable
12. Compensatory equalization	Not applicable

Note. This table is meant only as a general guideline. Decisions with regard to threats to internal validity must be made after the specifics of an investigation are known and understood. Thus, interpretations of internal validity threats must be made on a study-by-study basis.

assessments. For example, if we test the correlation between teacher attitudes toward students and student success in the classroom, the teacher's exposure to an attitude test may affect the way the teacher interacts with the students (e.g., provides more or less instructional support), which in turn affects students' classroom performance. Thus, the teacher's attitudes toward students may not be the cause of student performance, but the exposure to the first assessment may have led to the change in student performance.

External Validity

As with causal–comparative research, some of the threats to external validity do not typically apply to correlational research (e.g., interaction of personological variables and treatment effects, novelty and disruption effects, pretest sensitization). However, as shown in Table 7.5, several threats are present. A primary threat to the external validity is "generalization across participants." Convenience sampling techniques are frequently used rather than random selection procedures. Therefore, the results of the study are unlikely to generalize across participants.

Other external validity threats include interaction of time of measurement and treatment effects, measurement of the dependent variable, and interaction of history and treatment effects. Interaction of time of measurement and treatment effects is a threat since we would not expect the results to maintain for any length of time unless there was evidence to that effect. The measurement of the dependent variable is also a problem if the measurements are indirect versus direct (e.g., observation). Thus, researchers must look closely at the dependent variable to determine whether the results would generalize beyond the dependent measure used in the study. Finally, there may be an interaction of history and treatment effects if we suspect some event or situation that occurred during the assessments could have affected participants' responses to those assessments. For example, if teachers were undergoing budget cuts when their attitudes toward students were assessed, the responses to the attitude assessment might be different than if they were not going through such cuts in funding. In other words, the concern is whether there would be a similar correlation between attitudes toward students and student classroom performance if teachers in another school district were not faced with similar circumstances.

TABLE 7.5. Threats to External Validity Associated with Correlational Research

Threat	Correlational research design
1. Generalization across participants	Possible concern
2. Interaction of personological variables and treatment effects	Not applicable
3. Verification of independent variable	Not applicable
4. Multiple treatment interference	Not applicable
5. Novelty and disruption effects	Not applicable
6. Hawthorne effect	Not applicable
7. Experimenter effects	Not applicable
8. Pretest sensitization	Not applicable
9. Posttest sensitization	Not applicable
10. Interaction of time of measurement and treatment effects	Possible concern
11. Measurement of the dependent variable	Possible concern
12. Interaction of history and treatment effects	Possible concern

Note. This table is meant only as a general guideline. Decisions with regard to threats to external validity must be made after the specifics of an investigation are known and understood. Thus, interpretations of external validity threats must be made on a study-by-study basis.

Recall the research question about peer victimization posed earlier in this chapter? Read on to see how your design compares to how the actual study was designed.

Research Example 2: Structured Equation Modeling Study

An example of correlational research that explores relationships is a study comparing peer victimization in bullying experiences to compromised academic performance during middle school years (Juvonen, Wang, & Espinoza, 2011). Researchers collected data up to six times across grades 6 through 8 to examine relationships between victimization and decreased school performance. Approximately 2,300 students in 11 urban public schools participated (46% boys, 54% girls; 44% Latino, 26% African American, 10% Asian, 10% European American, 10% Other/Mixed). At the end of eighth grade, the participation rate was 75% of the original sample. Measures included self-perceived victimization, peer nominations of victims, GPA, and teacher reports of academic engagement. Self-perceived victimization assessment included responses to a modified Peer Victimization Scale (Neary & Joseph, 1994). Scale items included statements (e.g., "some kids are often picked on by other kids") followed by responses ("really true for me" or "sort of true for me"). Consistency of scores over time was estimated by computing correlation coefficients. Correlations for self-perceptions of victimization were moderate (i.e., $r = .38$ to $.66$). Peer nominations were high and consistent over time (i.e., $r = .55$ to $.75$). Indicators of academic achievement (GPA, teacher reports) were moderate to high (i.e., $r = .40$ to $.87$). Using structured equation modeling, two multilevel models were developed. Model 1 was designed to examine the overall effects of peer victimization on GPA and academic engagement. Model 2 was similar but captured between-subject differences across all time points and fluctuations in individual mean scores across time points. Results showed that decreased GPA and teacher reports were each predicted by self-perceptions of victimization and peer nominations of victim reputation when controlling for demographic and school-level differences. When controlling for school, gender, and ethnic differences in academic performance indicators, these results were replicated across all 11 urban middle schools. As the authors indicated, "Our findings reveal that students who were generally more bullied (received) lower grades and (engaged in) less academic tasks than did other students" (p. 167). Researchers cautioned that given these results, school administrators and teachers in low-performing schools should not focus exclusively on improving achievement scores, but should also acknowledge socioemotional issues such as bullying.

WHEN SHOULD RESEARCHERS USE THE CORRELATIONAL RESEARCH METHOD?

Researchers commonly use the correlational research method for a number of reasons. First, as with the causal–comparative research method, the correlational research method is used in those cases in which it is difficult or next to impossible to manipulate the variable of interest experimentally, or when researchers are exploring potential causal relationships among variables. Second, although education and psychology rely on an experimental paradigm in which a single presumed causal variable is manipulated while other potential variables are held constant, this paradigm may not adequately address the complexity of matters (e.g., achievement motivation, psychosis, anxiety) studied in education and psychology. The correlational research method enables researchers to manage the multiplicity of factors often associated with any given variable under study. Third, correlational statistical procedures can be used to sort out the effect of relationships among variables, which in some cases may be more important than identifying the overall effect of factors associated with any given variable under study. Fourth, correlational statistical procedures, such as multiple regression, enable researchers to use information from various scales of measurement. Finally, correlational statistical procedures, such as path analysis and structural equation modeling, can be used to establish causal relationships among variables.

SUMMARY

❖ The correlational research method is closely related to the causal–comparative research method in that the primary goal is to explore relationships among variables. Both attempt to explain the subject matter of interest and to identify variables that can be tested through experimental research. Neither research method allows for the manipulation of the independent variable, as do experimental research methods. One major difference is that the causal–comparative method takes into consideration scores from two groups of participants, and the correlational research method takes into consideration two or more sets of scores from each participant.

❖ Correlational research involves collecting two sets of data and determining the relationships between or among variables. The correlational research method can be relational or predictive in nature. Relational correlational research explores relationships between or among variables. Predictive correlational research predicts scores on one or more variables from a participant's scores on one or more other variables.

❖ Exploring causality is important, because many variables under study in education and psychology are influenced by other variables, making it difficult to have confidence in what produced the observed effects. In correlational research, there are two primary types of variables: predictor variables (scores that enable prediction of scores on other [criterion] variables) and criterion variables (the variable about which researchers seek to discover more information).

❖ The three critical issues that researchers must consider in designing a relationship or prediction correlational study are (1) development of a hypothesis, (2) selection of a homogeneous group, and (3) collection and analysis of data.

❖ A wide range of available statistical procedures not only depict the degree of relationship among variables but also explore the causal relationships among variables. As with tests of statistical significance, the choice of these

procedures depends on a number of issues, including the number of groups and variables being studied, the types of data, and the question(s) being asked. The correlation coefficient is important because it has many applications and is the basis for many of the advanced statistical procedures in correlational research. The correlation coefficient is best understood by reference to the bivariate frequency distribution (i.e., the scores from two variables are plotted either in a table or a graph). Relationships between two variables usually take several forms—linear (relationships in which a straight line can be visualized in the middle of the values running from one corner to another) and curvilinear relationships (relationships in which the best-fit line is not straight, but may be U-shaped, N-shaped, or W-shape). The correlation coefficient, the statistic used to describe the relationship between two variables, can range from −1.00 to +1.00. Statistical significance testing of correlation coefficients allows researchers to draw conclusions about a relationship in the population based on information gained from a sample. One of the most informative ways of interpreting the magnitude of correlation coefficients is to consider the variance or proportion of predictable variance or the coefficient of determination. Although correlation does not imply causation, a relationship between variables often provides researchers useful leads to causal relationships. If a relationship does exist between two variables, experimental studies or the use of advanced statistical techniques and the correlational research method is required to confirm whether the variables are causally connected. Five factors affect correlation coefficients: (1) forms of relationship (linear vs. curvilinear), (2) outliers in the data, (3) restriction in range, (4) skewed distributions, and (5) attenuation (unreliable measure). There are nine basic correlational procedures—(1) part correlation, (2) partial correlation, (3) correlation ratio, (4) Spearman rank correlation, (5) Kendall rank correlation coefficient, (6) Kendall part rank correlation, (7) Kendall coefficient of concordance, (8) phi coefficient, and (9) contingency coefficient. There are six advanced correlational procedures—(1) multiple regression, (2) canonical correlation, (3) discriminant function analysis, (4) factor analysis, (5) path analysis, and (6) structural equation modeling. Critical research consumers must determine the extent to which a researcher is able to make cause-and-effect (internal validity) and generalizable (external validity) statements based on the results of a correlational study.

❖ The correlational research method is commonly used by researchers for five reasons. It is difficult or next to impossible (1) to manipulate the variable of interest experimentally or to explore potential causal relationships among variables, (2) to manage the multiplicity of factors often associated with any given variable under study, (3) to sort out the effect of relationships among variables, (4) to use information from various scales of measurement, and (5) to establish causal relationships among variables using correlational statistical procedures such as path analysis and structural equation modeling.

DISCUSSION QUESTIONS

1. What is the purpose of correlational research?

2. What are some of the critical issues that researchers should consider when designing correlational research? Explain.

3. Why is it useful to use a variance interpretation of correlation coefficients in correlational research? Explain.

4. What are beta weights? Why is it more useful to consider beta weights when interpreting multiple correlations?

5. What types of correlational statistical procedures are used to establish cause-and-effect relationships between variables? Explain.

6. What is a bivariate frequency distribution? For the following scores, graph the bivariate distribution and make a statement (i.e., low, moderate, high) about the relationship between the variables by looking at the graph (make an estimate).

Student	Variable A	Variable B
1	20	5
2	15	2

3	25	8
4	10	7
5	18	10
6	12	4
7	14	4
8	10	3
9	23	9
10	22	10

7. What is the logic behind a researcher's decision to use statistical significance testing with correlation coefficients?

8. What is the relationship between the correlation coefficient and causality?

9. According to Cook and Campbell (1979), what are the three conditions researchers must meet in order to infer a causal relationship between two variables?

10. Recall from Chapter 4 that there are several scales of measurement. What correlational statistical procedures are applicable to the different scales of measurement?

Variables That Influence Decoding and Spelling in Beginning Readers

Kathy Strattman and Barbara Williams Hodson
Wichita State University, Kansas, USA

Abstract. *Performances on tasks of phonemic manipulation, working memory, rapid naming, multisyllable word naming, receptive vocabulary and nonverbal intelligence were compared with decoding and spelling scores for 75 beginning readers. Multiple regression analysis revealed that phonemic manipulation accounted for the greatest amount of variance for both decoding and spelling. Working memory and receptive vocabulary added additional unique variance for decoding. Multisyllable word naming and rapid naming contributed significantly to spelling. The major implication of the results is that phonemic manipulation should be included in an assessment battery for beginning readers.*

INTRODUCTION

Literacy is a well-documented educational issue of international concern (UNESCO, retrieved 2003). In addition, the social consequences of literacy failure, the downward spiral that Stanovich (1986) called the 'Matthew effects,' are also acutely known. Those who learn to read with relative ease read and practice more and gain more information; however, those who fail to learn to read efficiently, read less, enjoy reading less, and ultimately, reading becomes a self-defeating task. It is imperative to determine, as early as possible, which children will continue to have difficulty learning to read and spell so that early intervention interrupts or at least diminishes the Matthew effects. Professionals must be guided by scientifically based research to identify and provide efficient and effective instruction for learners along the road to literacy.

There is a sizeable body of scientific research that has provided information about the underlying variables for reading success. Results from three decades of research clearly indicate that problems lie in language coding and processing of phonological information (see Mody, 2003, for review). Although considerable progress has been achieved toward understanding phonological processing, many children are not identified for intervention

until they are already failing. What then are the critical linguistic and cognitive skills necessary for successful development of reading and spelling?

Results of previous studies have identified specific phonological processing abilities contributing to reading success, such as phonological awareness, verbal or working memory, and rapid naming (Bryant et al., 1990; Kamhi et al., 1988; Muter et al., 1997; Wagner et al., 1994). Spelling has only recently been examined as a viable constituent of early literacy (Kamhi & Hinton, 2000). Even fewer studies have focused on both (Muter, 1994; Scarborough, 1998). It is hypothesized that reading and spelling rely on the same cognitive and linguistic underpinnings. Few investigators have studied these together.

Read (1971) called spelling a window to the knowledge children possess about phonology. In contrast to the transitory nature of reading, spelling offers a visible representation of phonological and orthographic understanding. Examining both spelling and reading with the same tasks allows a clearer view of the requisite skills needed for both. There were two objectives for the present study. The first was to investigate relationships among phonological processing variables that have been linked in the literature to decoding and/or spelling, specifically phonemic awareness, working memory, rapid automatized naming (RAN), and production of multisyllable words. The second was to determine which of those variables contributed significantly to the variance of decoding and of spelling independently.

Participants in the present study were in 2nd grade. Ages ranged from 7;2 to 9;2 (years;months). School division levels (e.g., grades) and age of entry generally vary from country to country. In the USA, children typically enter school for formal instruction at 5 years of age (kindergarten). Reading and spelling instruction may begin in kindergarten in some schools; formal instruction, however, begins the following year in 1st grade. In the United Kingdom the 1st year of junior or middle school would likely be the equivalent to 2nd grade in the USA. The 2nd grade is a pivotal time for learning to decode and spell because children have had a solid year of academic instruction in 1st grade (although increasingly more time is being spent on literacy in kindergarten, depending on the school). By 3rd grade, children need to be able to read in order to learn (Chall, 1983) because comprehension then becomes the major focus of reading. Most second graders are still struggling to read novel words (Berninger et al., 2002). Children who have difficulty decoding real and pseudowords in 2nd grade are considered at risk; however, with appropriate intervention severe reading problems can be prevented (Berninger et al., 2003).

PHONOLOGICAL AWARENESS

We know now that phonological awareness is an overarching ability that stretches from a preschooler's tacit sensitivity to word structure outside word meaning (i.e., word play) to the explicit ability to manipulate individual phoneme units in the speech stream (Ball, 1993; Bryant et al., 1990; Chaney, 1998). Numerous correlational and predictive studies have successfully linked phonological awareness to later literacy (see Adams, 1990; Anthony & Lonigan, 2004; Catts & Kamhi, 1999; Ehri, 2000; Mody, 2003; Stanovich, 2000, for reviews). 'Over the last 25 years no variable has proven to be as consistently related to reading (at least word recognition) as phonological awareness . . . explicit awareness of or sensitivity to, the sound structure of speech' (Catts & Kamhi, 1999: 111).

Bryant et al. separated phonological awareness into simpler phonological skills measured by syllabic tasks (rhyme and alliteration) and complex phonological skills measured by sub-syllabic tasks (phonemic segmentation and manipulation). The simpler phonological skills typically develop during preschool years prior to formal reading instruction (Goswami & Bryant, 1990), but the sub-syllabic skills develop reciprocally and for the most part are dependent on explicit instruction (Liberman et al., 1974; Perfetti et al., 1987). Chaney proposed the following sequence of phonological tasks but described them as developmental stages, rather than prerequisite steps for mastery: a) tacit monitoring for correction of speech errors during speaking; b) participation in nursery rhymes and sound play; c) comparing the sounds of words for rhyme and alliteration; d) sound blending/syllable splitting (e.g., recognition of initial sounds); e) phoneme segmentation; and f) phoneme manipulation (adding, deleting, or moving phonemes).

Tasks requiring elision or deletion of phonemes have been strong predictors of later literacy success (Catts et al., 2001; Rosner & Simon, 1971). Phoneme transpositions and manipulations represent more complex phonemic understanding; however, to date there is little information available to demonstrate if these phonemic manipulation skills represent an extension of phonological awareness skills as children progress in school. Lundberg, Olofsson, and Wall (1980) found that Swedish kindergartners' abilities to reverse or transpose phonemes in words was the strongest predictor of reading a year later. Examples of transpositions include moving the beginning phoneme to the end of the word (e.g., *tea* becomes *eat*), moving the ending phoneme to the beginning (e.g., *eat* becomes *tea*), and reversing the beginning and ending phonemes (e.g., *toush* becomes *shout*).

Explicit phonemic awareness required for fluent decoding necessary for comprehension should be assessed through more complex phonological segmentation and manipulation skills (Stackhouse, 1997). Complex skills are required for pig Latin and spoonerisms (Dodd et al., 1996; Perin, 1983; Stackhouse & Wells, 1997). Pig Latin seems to be a slightly more complex task than spoonerisms, requiring not only the ability to segment a word onset and move it to the end of a word but also requiring the addition of the suffix 'ay'. Pig Latin has been used in a few studies for analysing phonological processing with adults (Pennington et al., 1990) and children (Cowan, 1998; Hester & Hodson, 2004). In a study involving sixty-five 3rd graders, Hester and Hodson found that this complex phonological manipulation task was the best predictor of decoding scores, above a working memory task that required concurrent processing, nonverbal intelligence, and receptive vocabulary.

Spoonerisms are naturally occurring, inadvertent exchanges of the initial phonemes or clusters of two words (e.g., *tooth fairy* becomes *footh tairy*) (Fromkin, 1980; van den Broeke & Goldstein, 1980). Stackhouse and Wells (1997) reported use of spoonerisms in treatment with an adolescent boy as a higher level or more complex phonemic awareness task. In a pilot study preceding the current investigation, 2nd graders were not able to learn pig Latin; however, most could produce some spoonerisms and they seemed to enjoy the task.

Simple phonological awareness tasks may have less predictive power as children age, whereas more complex tasks may represent increasingly sophisticated abilities. Some investigators have questioned whether complex tasks of phonological awareness evaluate phonological awareness or working memory (Oakhill & Kyle, 2000; Torgesen et al., 1997).

WORKING MEMORY

Depending on the memory load required by the phonological awareness task, it may be difficult to separate contributions of phonological awareness from working memory (Oakhill & Kyle, 2000; Scarborough, 1998). Working memory required for oddity tasks, in particular, has been studied; however, deletion and manipulation tasks seem to rely on working memory as well. This has not been reported in the literature to date (to the knowledge of the authors).

Working memory has been studied in relation to a variety of language skills, including reading and spelling (Adams & Gathercole, 2000; Baddeley, 1986; Montgomery, 2000). Although working memory is often used as a synonym for short-term memory, others contend that working memory is more complex (Daneman & Carpenter, 1983; Gaulin & Campbell, 1994; Turner & Engel, 1989). Measurement of working memory is confusing, especially when the complexity of tasks is different but reported similarly with respect to reading and spelling skills. One of the sources of confusion is that tasks vary from simple digit span tasks to complex concurrent processing tasks that require temporary storage of a word, while processing some other information (e.g., a cloze task plus word recall) (Leather & Henry, 1994). Historically, in studies of reading, verbal or working memory was measured by memory span of words, nonwords or digits (Gathercole & Baddeley, 1989; Hansen & Bowey, 1994; Mann et al., 1980). A few investigators have explored the contribution of working memory and complex phonological tasks as these relate to decoding, but they typically did not include spelling.

Siegel and Ryan (1989) differentiated between short-term memory and working memory. Although short-term memory tasks require temporary storage and retrieval, working memory tasks require temporary, on-line storage of information, retrieval of information from long-term storage,

and the processing of that information together. Leather and Henry (1994) tested seventy-one 2nd graders using phonological awareness tasks, simple word span tasks and complex working memory tasks. Their results indicated that complex, rather than simple, memory span tasks measure both the storage and the processing capacity of working memory, supporting the earlier findings of Daneman and Carpenter (1983). Most typically, these concurrent processing tasks have been used with comprehension tasks (Daneman & Carpenter, 1983). As children are consciously recoding (sounding out a novel word), they are temporarily storing the sounds for graphemes already decoded, while continuing to process (segmenting and blending) the additional graphemes of the novel word and retrieving phonological information from long-term memory.

RAPID NAMING

In addition to phonological awareness and working memory, the relationship of rapid naming ability and literacy has been investigated. Fluent, efficient reading and spelling require automatized subskills (Fletcher et al., 1997; Meyer et al., 1998b). There has been a recent renewed interest in rapid naming as a measure of automaticity and, therefore, a predictor of reading success (Denckla & Cutting, 1999; Meyer et al., 1998a; Scarborough, 1998; Wolf & Bowers, 2000). Automaticity, which is the 'fast, accurate, and effortless word identification at the single word level' (Hook & Jones, 2002: 9), is measured by both speed and accuracy.

Rapid automatized naming (RAN) has been assessed by a variety of stimuli. Denckla and Cutting (1999) suggested that a continuous format might require more executive functioning, which explains why the continuous formats are better predictors of reading success than discrete trial formats. Meyer et al. (1998b) found that RAN tasks involving colours and objects were better predictors than performance using numbers and letters across all readers in relationship to reading level and vocabulary. These stimuli thus represented a stable factor (i.e., naming speed) not attributable to experience with symbols, as in reading itself.

According to Whitehurst (2001), reading achievement of 1st and 2nd graders is influenced most strongly by letter knowledge and phonological sensitivity. In later elementary grades, once they have cracked the alphabetic code, conceptual and vocabulary skills become more important. In Chall's stage theory of reading (1983), fluency is developing during Stage 2, the period from 2nd to 3rd grade. That fluency includes automatic identification and matching of words and word chunks, as well as rapid graphophonemic correspondence for decoding novel words.

Scarborough (1998) followed 88 children from the end of 2nd grade through 8th grade (68 children). She compared scores of phonological awareness (deletion task), verbal working memory (single process), RAN (object naming), and IQ with reading and spelling scores. The strongest predictors of later literacy were their literacy scores at the end of 2nd grade. Scarborough concluded that the cognitive and linguistic tasks 'had already made their contributions to determining individual differences in reading skill' for typical 2nd graders (Scarborough, 1998: 130). Second grade appears to be a critical school year. The present study was designed to examine similar variables in the first semester of 2nd grade. Children who have failed to learn to decode, critical for the next step in literacy development, and/or spell by the end of the first formal year of instruction could potentially improve with explicit, systematic direct instruction during 2nd grade.

EXPRESSIVE PHONOLOGICAL PRODUCTIONS

Typical 2nd graders have very few, if any, speech sound errors on an articulation test. Stackhouse and Wells (1997) suggested that fuzzy phonological representation might manifest in multisyllable words. Hester and Hodson (2004) investigated multisyllable word naming in relation to decoding. They found a significant relationship, which was subsumed by the variance of the complex phonemic manipulation Pig Latin tasks.

To date only a few investigators have studied relationships of phonological productions of complex speech sound sequences and reading (Kamhi et al., 1988; Larrivee & Catts, 1999; Stackhouse & Wells, 1997) or spelling (Clarke-Klein & Hodson, 1995). Larrivee and Catts determined that the production of complex multisyllable words by kindergarten children, in contrast to one or two syllable words measured by a standard articulation test, were related to reading achievement in 1st and 2nd graders. Assessment of sound productions using multisyllable word productions may be more sensitive for school-age children.

In summary, literacy success has been linked in the literature with phonological processing abilities. Data regarding the relationship among these phonological processes and beginning decoding and spelling are needed. Phonological awareness, particularly phonemic awareness tasks requiring deletion, has been strongly related to early decoding. Less is known about the predictive power of phonemic manipulations after the first year or two of reading and spelling instruction. Information is also needed regarding the relationships among other phonological processing abilities (i.e., working memory, rapid naming, multisyllable word naming) and both decoding and spelling.

PURPOSE

The purpose for the present study was to examine the relationships of cognitive and linguistic variables with decoding and spelling performances of children early in 2nd grade. The variables investigated include: a) phonemic manipulation tasks; b) concurrent working memory; c) multisyllable word production; d) RAN; e) nonverbal intelligence; and f) receptive vocabulary.

METHOD
Participants

Seventy-five 2nd graders (45 females and 30 males) from four regular education classrooms in a midwestern metropolitan public school volunteered (with parents' written consent) for this study. Ages ranged from 86 to 110 months (7;2 to 9;2; $M = 7;10$). They represented a range of ethnic and socioeconomic backgrounds (63% Caucasian, 28% African American and 9% Asian American). Twenty-two per cent of the students in this school qualified for the 'free or reduced lunch' programme, indicating lower socioeconomic status. Participants had passed school-administered hearing and vision screenings during the last academic year or were wearing corrective lenses. None of these participants was receiving speech-language services at the time of this investigation.

Measures
Reading Decoding

Decoding was assessed using the 30-nonword battery of the Word Attack subtest of the *Woodcock–Johnson Revised Test of Achievement (WJ-R)*

(Woodcock & Johnson, 1989). Decoding nonwords requires understanding of grapheme–phoneme correspondence and phonotactic rules. Using nonwords rather than real words to assess decoding reduces the effect of prior sight word knowledge. Presentation of stimuli progressed from easiest to most difficult.

Spelling

Twenty words were selected from the spelling subtest of the *Wide Range Achievement Test–3* (Jastak & Jastak, 1993). The words, which become progressively more complex to spell, require knowledge of specific orthographic and phonotactic rules. Spelling strategies may be revealed when spelling longer, more challenging words (Stackhouse, 1996). A female speaker of Standard American English, using a JVC TDR 462 audiocassette recorder, recorded these words in an IAC booth. During testing, the audiotape was presented free field on a Califone 5230 AV cassette recorder to ensure the same word pronunciations for each group. Small groups of three or four listened to the audio recording of a word, the word in a sentence and the word repeated. The tape was stopped while the participants wrote the word. Spelling performance was scored using the Developmental Scoring for Invented Spellings (Bailet, 1991), a five-point scale ranging from preliterate random strings of letters (0) to some use of spelling strategies to conventional spellings (5).

Phonemic Awareness

Complex phonemic awareness was measured using 10 elision task items and 20 manipulation task items designed by the first author. The elision task included two items requiring syllable deletion (e.g., Say *birthday*. Now say it without *day*) and eight items requiring deletion of an initial or final phoneme (e.g., Say *time*. Now say it without /m/) or a phoneme in a cluster (e.g., Say *desk*. Now say it without /s/). The stimulus words and the answer words were all real words for the elision task.

The four manipulation tasks of five items each required phonemic transpositions of nonwords to real words. Tasks included transpositions of the initial phoneme in CV (e.g., /ko/to *oak*), the final phoneme in VC (e.g., /os/to *so*), and the exchange of initial and final phonemes in CVC (e.g., /saum/ to *mouse*). In addition, there were five spoonerism tasks, requiring the exchange of the onset phonemes of two nonwords to create two real words (e.g., *gall bame* to *ball game*).

Three practice items were provided with corrective feedback prior to each task. Coloured blocks, which were used to demonstrate deletion and transposition visually during the practice items, were available during the assessment. Responses were audio recorded and later scored as correct (1 point) or incorrect (0). A phoneme manipulation composite score was used for statistical analysis.

Working Memory

A concurrent process working memory task, adapted for children by Leather and Henry (1994), was modified for American children. Participants supplied the predictable ending word to complete a sentence read by the investigator (e.g., *I can see with my eyes*). The children were to remember in order the words they had supplied and then were to repeat those words in order at the end of the set of sentences. Two practice sets were provided with corrective feedback. Responses for the three sets of 2, 3 and 4 sentences each were scored. Statistical analysis was based on a possible 54-point working memory composite score of recall accuracy (27) and correct order (27).

Rapid Naming

The ability to name items rapidly was assessed using an array of 30 pictures of four different common objects (*hat, ball, key* and *car*) that were randomly coloured (red, blue, green and yellow). Continuous naming tasks that require shifting between different semantic fields have been used to assess interference with the fluency or automaticity of language retrieval (Wiig et al., 2000). In this nonalphanumeric, continuous naming task developed by the first author, participants were asked to name these coloured pictures 'as fast as you can' (e.g., *red car, blue hat*). A stopwatch was used during testing to encourage rapid naming. The timing scores were actually determined from the audiotape recording of each child's response.

Multisyllable Word Naming

Expressive phonological abilities were assessed using an adapted version of the Multisyllable subtest of the *Assessment of Phonological Processes–Revised* (Hodson, 1986). The 12 words were three to five syllables in length and contained complex phonological sequences (e.g., *stethoscope*). Results of several previous studies have shown that some school-age children made errors on tests of multisyllable words but not on monosyllabic words (Larrivee & Catts, 1999; Lewis & Freebairn, 1992). After the investigator named all 12 pictures randomly and had each child point to the matching pictures, the children then named the pictures. Deviations that were common for the child's age or linguistic community (e.g., lisps, weak syllable deletion, /w/ for /r/) received 1 point, whereas omissions, substitutions and phonological rule deviations (e.g., assimilations, metathesis) were assigned 2 points.

Receptive Vocabulary

The *Peabody Picture Vocabulary Test III (PPVT-III)* (Dunn & Dunn, 1997) was administered to assess receptive semantic and morphosyntactic language abilities. Receptive vocabulary is considered a reliable indicator of a child's general language ability (Gardner, 1985).

Nonverbal Intelligence

The *Test of Nonverbal Intelligence–3 (TONI-3)* (Brown et al., 1997) was used to assess nonverbal problem solving. The *TONI-3* is a nonverbal, language-free assessment of cognitive ability. Results have been found to correlate strongly with other tests of intelligence (Atlas, 1999).

Testing Procedures

All children were tested during two 30-minute sessions in the fourth month of their 2nd grade. Written instructions were read to ensure that each participant received the same directions for a task. In the first session, spelling was assessed in a small group followed by individual administration of the *PPVT-III* and the *TONI-3*. During the second session, the Word Attack subtest of the *WJ-R* was followed by tasks assessing: a) phonological awareness; b) working memory; c) rapid naming; and d) multisyllable word naming. A rotation of 12 different presentation orders was used to counterbalance presentation order effects. Audio recordings of participants' performances were made for later scoring of decoding, phonological manipulations, working memory, RAN, and multisyllable word naming tasks.

Scoring and Reliability

Interscorer reliability was determined for the three tasks that required scorer judgement: a) decoding;

b) spelling; and c) multisyllable word naming. Audio recordings of decoding responses and written invented spelling results for 20 randomly selected participants were scored independently by a graduate student in speech-language pathology and the first author. Pearson product moment reliability coefficients indicated strong interscorer reliability ($r = 0.98$ for decoding and $r = 0.99$ for spelling).

Unit-by-Unit Agreement Index for all items and all participants was used to assess interscorer reliability of speech sound productions of the multisyllable naming task. The first author and a certified speech-language pathologist with research experience transcribing phoneme errors independently scored each word. The percentage of agreement value was 94%. The categorization of phonological errors by both scorers was generally in agreement. Differences in scoring were resolved by consensus before statistical analysis.

RESULTS

Decoding and spelling scores were both compared with performances on tests of six cognitive/linguistic variables: complex phonemic awareness, concurrent processing working memory, RAN, multisyllable word naming, receptive vocabulary, and nonverbal IQ. Means, standard deviations and ranges for these six tasks are in Table 1.

Pearson correlations were computed for criterion and predictor variables (Table 2). Correlation coefficients indicated that all tasks correlated significantly, with the exception of nonverbal intelligence, which did not correlate with phonological awareness and RAN. Correlational analysis indicated strongest correlations between decoding and spelling ($r = 0.77$), and also phonological manipulations and both decoding ($r = 0.79$) and spelling ($r = 0.71$).

Stepwise multiple regression was conducted using SPSS 10.0 (SPSS, 1999). In stepwise regression, complex intercorrelations allow predictor variables that contribute only weakly to the criterion variable to be removed as stronger variables are entered. Criteria for variable entry and removal were as follows: probability of F to enter ≤ 0.05 and probability of F to remove ≤ 0.10 (George & Mallery, 1999). The composite scores of phonological manipulation tasks entered first for both decoding ($R^2 = 0.624$, adjusted $R^2 = 0.619$) and spelling ($R^2 = 0.504$, adjusted $R^2 = 0.497$), accounting for the greatest amount of variance in both decoding and

TABLE 1. Means, Standard Deviations, and Ranges for Beginning Readers (n = 75)

Task	M	SD	Range
Criterion variables			
Reading decoding	12.75	6.90	1–27
Spelling	69.11	12.26	36–89
Predictor variables			
Multisyllable naming	10.17	8.57	0–45
Nonverbal intelligence	98.49	13.02	70–138
Phonemic manipulation	15.68	6.77	4–28
Rapid naming	63.99	11.83	41–98
Receptive vocabulary	103.54	8.57	75–130
Working memory	33.21	6.69	12–45

spelling. (Table 3). In multiple regression analysis, R^2 indicates the proportion of variance and serves as a natural measure of effect size (Cohen & Cohen, 1975). Adjusted R^2 accounts for the number of variables and sample size. Regression analysis yielded significant independent variance for two additional variables for decoding and two different variables for spelling. No variables other than phonemic manipulation accounted for significant variance in both performances.

Decoding tasks were scored correct/incorrect. Scores ranged from 1 to 27 (M = 12.75, SD = 6.9). The total prediction measures accounted for 68% of the variance for decoding. Phonemic awareness accounted for 62% ($F = 118.02$, $p < 0.000$), working memory accounted for an additional 4% ($F = 68.51$, $p = 0.007$), and receptive vocabulary accounted for an additional 2% ($F = 49.79$, $p = 0.031$).

Complex phonemic awareness scores, a composite score of combined elision and transposition tasks, ranged from 4 to 28 (M = 15.68, SD = 6.77). Regression analysis of performance on the

working memory task indicated small but significant independent variance outside of phonemic manipulation for decoding, but not for spelling, although working memory was correlated significantly with both decoding ($r = 0.51$) and spelling ($r = 0.50$).

Spelling performance was scored using a point system for spelling inventions, with higher scores for closer matches to conventional orthography. Scores ranged from 36 to 89 (M = 69.11, SD = 12.26). Three prediction measures accounted for 58% of the variance in spelling. The composite phonemic manipulation score accounted for 50% ($F = 72.15$, $p < 0.000$). Production of multisyllable real words accounted for an additional 5% ($F = 44.04$, $p = 0.005$). Rapid automatized naming (RAN) accounted for an additional 3% ($F = 32.22$, $p = 0.041$). Multisyllable word naming error scores ranged from 0 to 45 (M = 10.17, SD = 8.57). Higher numbers indicated more severe deviations in production, whereas, those with only sound differences typical for their age had lower scores. Only six participants produced all words without any deviations. Multisyllable word naming contributed additional variance outside of phonemic awareness to spelling. The length of time for RAN ranged from 41 to 98 seconds (M = 63.99, SD = 11.83). A higher score indicated a longer time was required for naming. The RAN scores accounted for significant unique variance, after phonemic awareness and multisyllable word naming, for spelling.

DISCUSSION

The first objective was to investigate the relationships among phonological processing variables that have been linked in the literature with

TABLE 2. Correlation Coefficients among Early Literacy Tasks

	1	2	3	4	5	6	7	8
1) Reading decoding	—	0.77*	−0.58*	0.27*	0.79*	−0.50*	0.38*	0.51*
2) Spelling		—	−0.62*	0.30*	0.71*	0.48*	0.34*	0.40*
3) Multisyllable naming			—	−0.24*	−0.62*	−0.38*	−0.45*	−0.23*
4) Nonverbal intelligence				—	0.19	0.17	29*	0.21*
5) Phonemic manipulation					—	−0.43*	0.34*	0.40*
6) RAN						—	−0.34*	0.40*
7) Receptive vocabulary							—	0.28*
8) Working memory								—

*$p < 0.05$.

TABLE 3. Results of Step-Wise Multiple Regression Analysis for Decoding and Spelling

Variables	R^2	Adjusted R^2	β	F	p
Decoding					
Phonemic manipulation	0.624	0.619	0.790	118.02	0.000
Working memory	0.658	0.648	0.811	68.51	0.007
Receptive vocabulary	0.677	0.663	0.823	49.79	0.031
Spelling					
Phonemic manipulation	0.504	0.497	0.710	72.15	0.000
Multisyllable naming	0.557	0.545	0.746	44.04	0.005
RAN	0.584	0.565	0.764	32.22	0.041

decoding and spelling. Results of correlational analyses indicated that in addition to a strong correlation between decoding and spelling, there were significant relationships among all cognitive and linguistic variables, with the exception of nonverbal intelligence and both phonological awareness and RAN.

Decoding and Spelling

In the past, schools have viewed reading and spelling as separate skills; even though both rely on language coding and require processing of phonological information. Ehri (2000) referred to reading and spelling as 'two sides of a coin.' Examining both decoding and spelling within the same study allows a comparison of both 'sides.' Ehri summarized the consistent and significant relationships between reading and spelling ($r = 0.68$ to 0.86) from six previous studies. This same high correlation was found across ages from studies of 1st graders (Griffith, 1991; Juel et al., 1986) and also college students (Greenberg et al., 1997). Results of correlation analyses in the present study support these previous findings (Ehri, 2000; Greenberg et al., 1997; Griffith, 1991). The strength and consistency of correlational analyses support the premise that similar processes are needed for acquisition of both skills. Reading and spelling follow similar development and rely on knowledge of the alphabetic code, graphophonemic correspondence and English phonotactics.

The second objective was to identify which variables contributed uniquely to the variance for decoding and spelling. Although complex phoneme manipulations contributed the greatest amount of variance for both decoding and

spelling, different variables added small, but significant variance for each. Working memory and receptive vocabulary added significantly to decoding. Multisyllable word naming and RAN contributed to spelling. Results of the tasks assessed in this study indicate that there are similarities, but there are also differences in variables that contribute to the successful performance for each.

Phonological Awareness

Results of the current investigation support the findings of numerous studies for decoding and add to knowledge needed relative to spelling. For the participants in this study, tasks of elision and manipulation accounted for the greatest amount of variance in their word attack scores and spelling scores.

Scores on the 10-item elision task ranged from 3 correct to 10 correct; scores on the transposition tasks ranged from 0 to 19. All participants were able to perform the deletion of the second syllable of a compound word; however, nine (12%) could not delete the first syllable of a compound word. Six of those nine scored in the lowest quartile for decoding, spelling and phoneme manipulation. Although 2nd graders had more difficulty with manipulation tasks, strategies were not readily apparent. Some used words that rhymed with the stimulus word rather than a transposition (e.g., *oon* should transpose to *new* but responses were *moon* or *noon*). Some used word or sound associations (e.g., instead of the spoonerism of *one penny* for *pun wenny*, some said *Winnie the Pooh*). Those with higher decoding scores were more successful with these tasks, whereas the poorest readers did not seem to have any understanding, guessed randomly, or reported that the task was 'too hard.' These data demonstrate that phonemic manipulation skills represent an extension of phonological awareness skills as children progress in school.

The ability to manipulate phonemes was the strongest predictor for decoding and spelling. Phonological awareness has been viewed as reciprocal for decoding and for spelling (Masterson & Apel, 2000; Perfetti et al., 1987). Developing skill in one appears to facilitate skill development in the other (Masterson & Apel, 2000). In a six-step developmental model, Frith (1985) proposed an explanation of this reciprocal, facilitative effect. In the logographic stage, reading is an antecedent for spelling; however, spelling as an antecedent for reading is the first step of the alphabetic stage. 'The alphabet is tailor made for writing' (Frith, 1988: 311). At the orthographic stage, reading is again proposed as the antecedent. Because spelling also requires knowledge of English phonotactic rules, participants in the current study demonstrated varying strategies. The spelling by some participants more closely resembled conventional orthography because they applied knowledge of morphology, using prefixes or suffixes (e.g., *decision*) to spell unknown words (Apel et al., 2004). Participants demonstrated a variety of developmental spelling inventions. Only three children used random strings of unrelated graphemes for the longer, more complex words.

Working Memory

As children are learning to read, temporary storage capacity is needed for the on-line phonemic segmentation and blending necessary for conscious decoding. In the current study, working memory was moderately correlated with decoding, spelling and phonemic manipulation scores. After phonological manipulation was partialed out, working memory contributed additional, unique variance for decoding but not for spelling. These results support previous work by Gathercole and Baddeley (1993), who found that working memory, assessed by a simple span task, affected decoding novel words but not sight word reading. Conversely, Gottardo et al. (1996) used a concurrent processing working memory task and found that working memory did not account for significant variance in decoding, but did for word identification (4.5%) and for reading comprehension (12.5%) for students finishing 3rd grade. Perhaps 2nd graders require more working memory

capacity for decoding than 3rd graders, who would be expected to be more fluent decoders. Second graders were still using considerable conscious effort to sound out words, supporting the findings of Berninger et al. (2002).

The relationship between decoding and working memory was expected, based on previous studies; however, the results for spelling are somewhat puzzling. During the act of spelling, the letters children write may actually support working memory. When some students wrote these spelling words, they decoded subvocally and erased. Presumably their decoding did not match the word stored in long-term memory. Storage of an entire word may account for less working memory capacity than separate phonemes.

It also was expected that working memory ability would be related to phonological awareness. The effect of memory load in phonological awareness tasks has been questioned (Oakhill & Kyle, 2000; Wagner et al., 1994), suggesting that working memory performance either compromises or strengthens phonological awareness scores, particularly for oddity tasks. The current findings suggest a similar relationship for deletion or transposition tasks. Brady (1991) proposed that working memory and phonological awareness skills represent the same component of phonological ability because they both rely on the phonological component of language.

Conversely, Hansen and Bowey (1994) suggested that working memory might tap separate processing ability, outside of phonemic manipulations. In a study of sixty-eight 2nd graders, they used an oddity task for assessing phonological awareness and a nonword repetition task for working memory. In the present study, the small, unique contribution of working memory to decoding variance supports Hansen and Bowey's hypothesis.

Phoneme manipulations in this study were demonstrated during practice tasks using coloured blocks to demonstrate the deletion or transposition of phonemes. Participants were each given the opportunity to use blocks as demonstrated by the investigator. This visual representation may have aided working memory and enabled some to be more successful with these tasks, thereby reducing the variance accounted for by working memory. Typically, the children who used the blocks understood the concept of phoneme manipulation and were able to perform the task, but children who did not have this understanding rarely used the blocks.

Receptive Vocabulary

In addition to phoneme manipulation and working memory, receptive vocabulary also contributed small, additional variance for decoding but not for spelling. Correlations for decoding and spelling scores with vocabulary were small, but significant. Stanovich (2000) suggested that vocabulary and reading are reciprocal. Paul (2001) suggested that lower vocabulary may be the result rather than the cause of reading differences.

Multisyllable Word Naming

Although phonemic awareness was most predictive of spelling scores, two other variables contributed small but significant variance for spelling. Multisyllable word naming contributed an additional 5%. Because of the segmental organization underlying phonological awareness, the phonological representations of poor readers may be less differentiated than those of better readers (Fowler, 1991; Stackhouse & Wells, 1997). None of the participants were receiving speech-language services for expressive phonological deviations; yet there were sound production deviations in the multisyllable naming task. Phonological representations for children within this age range may not be firmly developed as they continue to gain experience with words that have multiple syllables. Thirteen of the 20 stimulus spelling words contained multiple syllables ranging from two to five syllables.

Results of a few studies have indicated that children with a history of severe expressive phonological impairment had more difficulties with later reading and spelling (Bird et al., 1995; Clarke-Klein & Hodson, 1995; Gillon, 2000) whereas others did not find a relationship (Bishop & Adams, 1990; Catts, 1993). In the current study, over 60% of the participants demonstrated more than five phonological deviations when naming multisyllable words. These results support Stackhouse's previous work (1997), suggesting that fuzzy phonological representation may continue to affect spelling in the form of weak syllable deletions and assimilations exhibited in multisyllable words. As implied by Larrivee and Catts (1999), assessment of sound productions in more complex words is more sensitive than standard articulation tests for children in 2nd grade. Although no participants were receiving speech-language intervention, the history of such services was not known. The residual effects of a history of severe expressive phonology have been identified (Bird et al., 1995; Clarke-Klein & Hodson, 1995; Lewis & Freebairn, 1995; Webster & Plante, 1992).

Rapid Naming

The RAN contributed small, significant variance for spelling but not decoding, although both correlated significantly with RAN. Scores for RAN were correlated significantly with all other variables, except nonverbal IQ. Some researchers include RAN in the category of phonological processing (Torgesen, 1999), whereas others believe naming speed is a 'second core deficit in dyslexia and largely independent of phonology' (Wolf & Bowers, 2000: 322). Wolf and Obregon (1992) found that naming speed was a predictor of reading achievement. Some children with slower naming speed were poorer readers but did not have deficits in phonological awareness tasks. Others had phonological awareness deficits and slow RAN. They termed this phenomenon 'a double deficit.'

Wagner et al. (1997) cautioned that the influence of RAN might have an age limit because results were nonsignificant in 4th and 5th grades. They suggested that RAN was sensitive in predicting 1st and 2nd grade orthographic skills. Meyer et al. (l998b), who studied the growth curve of rapid naming in an eight-year longitudinal study, reported that the RAN growth curve for all students, regardless of reading skill, was greatest between 1st and 3rd grades. They concluded that RAN can be assessed quickly and those with slower speed may need to be given more intensive help at this stage in literacy development.

Longitudinal studies of 3rd to 8th graders who were poor readers indicated that RAN was predictive only for poor readers but not for average readers (Meyer et al., 1998a). They hypothesized that 'automaticity of retrieval, not knowledge of names itself (as in confrontational naming tasks), gives the predictive power in rapid naming' (p. 106). This hypothesis supports findings of previous studies (Wolf & Bowers, 2000) suggesting RAN may be an independent predictor of literacy skills outside of phonological processing.

IMPLICATIONS

Children who are likely to experience difficulty learning to read and spell need to be identified as early as possible before they 'become discouraged and enter the cycle of failure' (ASHA, 2000: 360). By 2nd grade, most students have been taught basic graphophonemic correspondences. Regardless of differences in their preschool and kindergarten learning experiences, 2nd graders in the USA have had at least a year to learn the elements for decoding and to develop strategies for spelling.

Results of this study support previous research emphasizing the importance of phonemic awareness for decoding and spelling. Complex phonemic manipulation skills contributed significantly to both. Reports of intervention studies have yielded positive results when phonemic awareness is taught (Ball & Blachman, 1991; Lundberg et al., 1980). Those studies that included explicit grapheme-phoneme awareness tasks were linked most successfully with improving literacy skills (Blachman et al., 1994; Bradley & Bryant, 1983; Hatcher et al., 1994; Liberman et al., 1974).

Reading has more frequently been the focus of intervention; however, spelling should be an equally important focus. A child's own spelling is useful for understanding possible language needs (e.g., phonological, morphological). In addition, naming words with multiple syllables was also significantly related to spelling. The integration of phonological rules for production of more complex words was identified by this task but may not be identified through traditional phoneme oriented tests. Higher level phonological processing skills are needed for spelling multisyllabic words. Production of multisyllabic words could also be part of a screening tool for rapid identification of 2nd graders who may be at risk.

Finally, results of this study suggest that RAN speed tapped underlying skill for spelling but not for decoding. Scarborough (1998), in her longitudinal study, found that reading and spelling skills of children with reading disabilities were predicted by RAN speed measured in 2nd grade. Although no child in this study had been identified as reading disabled, some were less skilled readers, and reading levels were differentiated within the 2nd grade level. Indeed, RAN might be another expedient method for identifying those who might need additional support.

In the classroom, utilizing the reading curriculum for spelling and vocabulary enrichment takes advantage of the strong relationship between decoding and spelling identified in this study. In addition, both decoding and spelling could be facilitated through explicit, complex phonemic

manipulation tasks. Phonemic manipulation activities, including spoonerisms, interwoven with literacy experiences increases the awareness of word structures in addition to word meanings.

Information gained from the results of this study could be used for faster identification of children during the 2nd year of formal reading and spelling instruction. The United Nations has declared 2003–2012 as the Literacy Decade (Matsuura, 2003). A major concern of this endeavor by UNESCO is for those persons who lack opportunities to develop literacy. Perhaps this also will be the decade of success for children who have opportunities but who fail because they do not receive early identification and appropriate intervention.

REFERENCES

Adams, A. M., & Gathercole, S. E. (2000). Limitations in working memory: Implications for language development. *International Journal of Language and Communication Disorders, 35*(1), 95–116.

Adams, M. J. (1990). *Beginning to read: Thinking and learning about print.* Cambridge, MA: MIT Press.

American Speech–Language–Hearing Association (ASHA). (2000). *Guidelines for the roles and responsibilities of speech-language pathologists with respect to reading and writing in children and adolescents.* Rockville, MD: ASHA, p. 360.

Anthony, J., & Lonigan, C. (2004). The nature of phonological awareness: Converging evidence from four studies of preschool and early grade school children. *Journal of Educational Psychology, 96*, 43–55.

Apel, K., Masterson, J., & Niessen, N. (2004). Spelling assessment frameworks. In C. A. Stone, E. R. Silliman, B. J. Ehren, & K. Apel (Eds.), *Handbook of language and literacy* (pp. 644–660). New York: Guilford Press.

Atlas, J. A. (1999). Review of the *Test of Nonverbal Intelligence.* In I. B. S. Plake & J. E. Impara (Eds.), *The Supplement to the Thirteenth Mental Measurements Yearbook* (3rd ed., p. 325). Lincoln, NB: Buros Institute.

Baddeley, A. D. (1986). *Working memory.* Oxford: Oxford University Press.

Bailet, L. L. (1991). Development and disorders of spelling in the beginning school years. In A. M. Bain, L. L. Bailet, & L. C. Moats (Eds.), *Written language disorders: Theory into practice* (pp. 1–21). Austin, TX: PRO-ED.

Ball, E. W. (1993). Phonological awareness: What's important and to who? *Reading and Writing: An interdisciplinary Journal, 5*, 141–159.

Ball, E. W., & Blachman, B. A. (1991). Does phoneme awareness training in kindergarten make a difference in early work recognition and developmental spelling? *Reading Research Quarterly, 26*, 49–66.

Berninger, Y., Abbott, R., Vermeulen, K., Ogier, S., Brooksher, R., & Zook, D. (2002). Comparison of faster and slower responders to early intervention in reading:

Differentiating features of their language profiles. *Learning Disability Quarterly, 25*, 59–76.

Berninger, Y., Vermeulen, K., Abbott, R., McCutchen, D., Cotton, S., Cude, J., et al. (2003). Comparison of three approaches to supplementary reading instruction for low-achieving second-grade readers. *Language, Speech, and Hearing Services in Schools, 34*, 101–116.

Bird, J., Bishop, D. Y. M., & Freeman, M. H. (1995). Phonological awareness and literacy development in children with expressive phonological impairments. *Journal of Speech and Hearing Research, 38*, 446–462.

Bishop, D. Y. M., & Adams, C. (1990). A prospective study of the relationship between specific language impairment, phonological disorders, and reading retardation. *Journal of Child Psychology and Psychiatry, 31*, 1027–1050.

Blachman, B. A., Ball, E., Black, R., & Tangle, D. (1994). Kindergarten teachers develop phoneme awareness in low-income, inner-city classrooms. *Reading and Writing: An Interdisciplinary Journal, 6*, 1–18.

Bradley, L., & Bryant, P. (1983). Categorizing sounds and learning to read: A causal connection. *Nature, 30*, 419–421.

Brady, S. (1991). The role of working memory in reading disability. In S. Brady & D. Shankweiler (Eds.), *Phonological processes in literacy: A tribute to Isabelle Liberman* (pp. 129–147). Hillsdale, NJ: Erlbaum.

Bryant, P., MacLean, M., Bradley, L., & Crossland, J. (1990). Rhyme and alliteration, phoneme detection, and learning to read. *Developmental Psychology, 26*, 429–428.

Brown, L., Sherbenou, R. J., & Johnson, S. K. (1997). *The Test of Nonverbal Intelligence (TONI-3)*. Austin, TX: Pro-Ed.

Catts, H. W. (1993). The relationship between speech, language impairments, and reading disabilities. *Journal of Speech and Hearing Research, 36*, 948–958.

Catts, H. W., Fey, M. E., Zhang, X., & Tomblin, J. B. (2001). Estimating the risk of future reading difficulties in kindergarten children: A research based model and its clinical implementation. *Language, Speech, and Hearing Services in Schools, 32*, 38–50.

Catts, H. W., & Kamhi, A. J. (1999). *Language and reading disabilities*. Boston: Allyn & Bacon.

Chall, J. S. (1983). *Stages of reading development*. New York: McGraw-Hill.

Chaney, C. (1998). Preschool language and metalinguistic skills are links to reading success. *Applied Psycholinguistics, 19*, 433–446.

Clarke-Klein, S., & Hodson, B. W. (1995). Phonologically based analysis of misspellings by third graders with disordered-phonology histories. *Journal of Speech and Hearing Research, 38*, 839–849.

Cohen, J., & Cohen, P. (1983). *Applied multiple regression/correlation analysis for the behavioral sciences* (2nd ed.). Hillsdale, NJ: Erlbaum.

Cowan, N. (1998). Short-term memory, working memory, and their importance in language processing. In R. Gillam (Ed.), *Memory and language impairment in children and adults: New perspectives* (pp. 3–27). Gaithersburg, MD: Aspen Press.

Daneman, M., & Carpenter, P. A. (1983). Individual differences in integrating information between and within sentences. *Journal of Experimental Psychology: Learning, Memory, and Cognition, 9*, 561–584.

Denckla, M., & Cutting, L. E. (1999). History and significance of rapid automatized naming. *Annals of Dyslexia, 49*, 29–42.

Dodd, B., Holm, A., Oerlemans, M., & McCormick, M. (1996). *Queensland University Inventory of Literacy*. Brisbane: Department of Speech Pathology and Audiology, The University of Queensland.

Dunn, L., & Dunn, L. (1997). *Peabody Picture Vocabulary Test-3*. Circle Pine, MN: American Guidance Service.

Ehri, L. C. (2000). Learning to read and learning to spell: Two sides of a coin. *Topics in Language Disorders, 20*(3), 19–36.

Fletcher, J. M., Morris, R., Lyon, G. R., Steubing, K. K., Shaywitz, S. E., Shankweiler, D. P., et al. (1997). Subtypes of dyslexia. An old problem revisited. In B. Blachman (Ed.), *Foundations of reading acquisition and dyslexia: Implications for early intervention* (pp. 95–114). Hillsdale, NJ: Erlbaum.

Fowler, A. E. (1991). How early phonological development might set the stage for phoneme awareness. In S. A. Brady & D. P. Shankweiler (Eds.), *Phonological processes in literacy: A tribute to Isabelle Y. Liberman* (pp. 97–113). Hillsdale, NJ: Erlbaum.

Frith, U. (1985). Beneath the surface of developmental dyslexia. In K. Patterson, J. Marshall, & M. Coltheart (Eds.), *Surface dyslexia*. Hove, England: Erlbaum.

Fromkin, V. (1980). *Errors in linguistic performance: Slips of the tongue, ear, pen, and hand*. New York: Academic Press.

Gardner, M. (1985). *Receptive One-Word Picture Vocabulary Test*. Novato, CA: Academic Therapy Publications.

Gathercole, S. E., & Baddeley, A. D. (1989). Evaluation of the role of phonological STM in the development of vocabulary in children: A longitudinal study. *Journal of Memory and Language, 28*, 200–213.

Gathercole, S. E., & Baddeley, A. D. (1993). *Working memory and language*. Hove, UK: Erlbaum.

Gaulin, C., & Campbell, T. (1994). Procedure for assessing verbal working memory in normal school-age children: Some preliminary data. *Perceptual and Motor Skills, 79*, 55–64.

George, D., & Mallery, P. (1999). *SPSS for Windows step by step: A simple guide and reference*. Boston: Allyn & Bacon.

Gillon, G. (2000). The efficacy of phonological awareness intervention for children with spoken language impairment. *Language, Speech, and Hearing Services in Schools, 31*, 126–141.

Goswami, U., & Bryant, P. (1990). *Phonological skills and learning to read*. Hove, UK: Erlbaum.

Gottardo, A., Stanovich, K. E., & Siegel, L. S. (1996). The relationships between phonological sensitivity, syntactic processing, and verbal working memory in the reading performance of third-grade children. *Journal of Experimental Child Psychology, 63*, 563–582.

Greenberg, D., Ehri, L., & Perin, D. (1997). Are word

reading processes the same or different in adult literacy students and 3rd–5th graders matched for reading level? *Journal of Educational Psychology, 89,* 262–275.

Griffith, P. (1991). Phonemic awareness helps first graders invent spellings and third graders remember correct spellings. *Journal of Reading Behavior, 23,* 215–233.

Hansen, J., & Bowey, J. A. (1994). Phonological skills, verbal working memory, and reading ability in second-grade children. *Journal of Child Development, 65,* 938–950.

Hatcher, P. J., Hulme, C., & Ellis, A. W. (1994). Ameliorating early reading failure by integrating the teaching of reading and phonological skills. The phonological linkage hypothesis. *Child Development, 65,* 41–57.

Hester, E., & Hodson, B. W. (2004). The role of phonological representations in decoding skills of young readers. *Child Language Teaching and Therapy, 20,* 115–133.

Hodson, B. W. (1986). *Assessment of Phonological Processes—Revised.* Austin, TX: Pro-Ed.

Hook, P. E., & Jones, S. D. (2002). The importance of automaticity and fluency for efficient reading comprehension. *Perspectives, 9,* 9–14.

Jastak, J. F., & Jastak, S. R. (1993). *Wide Range Achievement Test-3.* Wilmington, DE: Jastak and Associates.

Juel, C., Griffith, P., & Gough, P. (1986). Acquisition of literacy: A longitudinal study of children in first and second grade. *Journal of Educational Psychology, 78,* 243–255.

Kamhi, A. G., Catts, H. W., Mauer, D., Apel, K., & Gentry, B. (1988). Phonological and spatial processing abilities in language- and reading-impaired children. *Journal of Speech and Hearing Disorders, 53,* 316–327.

Kamhi, A. G., & Hinton, L. N. (2000). Explaining individual differences in spelling ability. *Topics in Language Disorders, 20*(3), 37–49.

Larrivee, L., & Catts, H. (1999). Early reading achievement in children with expressive phonological disorders. *American Journal of Speech-Language Pathology, 8,* 118–128.

Leather, C. V., & Henry, L. A. (1994). Working memory span and phonological awareness tasks as predictors of early reading ability. *Journal of Experimental Child Psychology, 58,* 88–111.

Lewis, B. A., & Freebairn, L. (1992). Residual effects of preschool phonology disorders in grade school, adolescence, and adulthood. *Journal of Speech and Hearing Research, 35,* 819–831.

Liberman, I. Y., Shankweiler, D. P., Fischer, M., & Carter, B. (1974). Explicit syllable and phoneme segmentation in the young child. *Journal of Experimental Child Psychology, 18,* 201–212.

Lundberg, I., Olofsson, A., & Wall, S. (1980). Reading and spelling skills in the first school years predicted from phonemic awareness in kindergarten. *Scandinavian Journal of Psychology, 21,* 159–173.

Mann, V. A., Liberman, I. V., & Shankweiler, D. (1980). Children's memory for sentences and word strings in relation to reading ability. *Memory and Cognition, 8,* 320–325.

Masterson, J. J., & Apel, K. (2000). Spelling assessment: Charting a path to optimal intervention. *Topics in Language Disorders, 20,* 50–65.

Matsuura, K. (2003). Message from the director-general of UNESCO: To mark the launch of the United Nations Literacy Decade (203-2012 retrieved 26 August 2003, from *http://portal.unesco.org/education/ev.php?URL_ID=5000%URL_DO=DO_TOPIC&URL_SECTION=201.*

Meyer, M. S. Wood, F. B., Hart, L. A., & Felton, R. H. (1998a). Longitudinal course of rapid naming in disabled and nondisabled readers. *Annals of Dyslexia, 48,* 91–114.

Meyer, M. S., Wood, F. B., Hart, L. A., & Felton, R. H. (1998b). Selective predictive value of rapid automatized naming in poor readers. *Journal of Learning Disabilities, 31*(2), 106–112.

Mody, M. (2003). Phonological basis in reading disability: A review and analysis of the evidence. *Reading and Writing, 16,* 21–39.

Montgomery, J. (2000). Relation of working memory to off-line and real-time sentence processing in children with specific language impairment. *Applied Psycholinguistics, 21,* 117–148.

Muter, V. (1994). Influence of phonological awareness and letter knowledge on beginning reading and spelling development. In C. Hulme & M. Snowling (Eds.), *Reading development and dyslexia.* London: Whurr.

Muter, V., Hulme, C., Snowling, M., & Taylor, S. (1997). Segmentation, not rhyming predicts early progress in learning to read. *Journal of Experimental Child Psychology, 71,* 3–27.

Oakhill, J., & Kyle, F. (2000). The relationship between phonological awareness and working memory. *Journal of Experimental Child Psychology, 75,* 152–164.

Paul, R. (2001). *Language disorders from infancy through adolescence: Assessment and intervention.* St. Louis: Mosby.

Pennington, B. E., Van Orden, G. C., Smith, S. D., Green, P. A., & Haith, M. (1990). Phonological processing skills and deficits in adult dyslexics. *Child Development, 61,* 1753–1778.

Perfetti, C. A., Beck, I., Bell, L. C., & Hughes, C. (1987). Phonemic knowledge and learning to read are reciprocal: A longitudinal study of first grade children. *Merrill–Palmer Quarterly, 33,* 283–319.

Perin, D. (1983). Phonemic segmentation and spelling. *British Journal of Psychology, 74,* 129–144.

Read, C. (1971). Pre-school children's knowledge of English phonology. *Harvard Educational Review, 41,* 1–34.

Rosner, J., & Simon, D. (1971). The auditory analysis test: An initial report. *Journal of Learning Disabilities, 4,* 40–48.

Scarborough, H. S. (1998). Predicting the future achievement of second graders with reading disabilities: Contributions of phonemic awareness, verbal memory, rapid naming, and IQ. *Annals of Dyslexia, 48,* 115–136.

Siegel, L. S., & Ryan, E. B. (1989). The development of working memory in normally achieving and subtypes of learning disabled children. *Child Development, 60,* 973–980.

SPSS 1999: SPSS 10.0. [Computer software]. Chicago, IL: SPSS, Inc.

Stackhouse, J. (1996). Speech, spelling, and reading: Who is at risk and why? In M. Snowling & J. Stackhouse (Eds.), *Dyslexia, Speech and Language: A practitioner's handbook* (pp. 12–30). San Diego, CA: Singular.

Stackhouse, J. (1997). Phonological awareness: Connecting speech and literacy problems. In B. Hodson & M. Edwards (Eds.), *Perspectives in applied phonology* (pp. 157–196). Gaithersburg, MD: Aspen.

Stackhouse, J., & Wells, B. (1997). *Children's speech and literacy difficulties: A psycholinguistic framework*. San Diego: Singular.

Stanovich, K. E. (1986). Matthew effects in reading: Some consequences of individual differences in the acquisition of literacy. *Reading Research Quarterly, 21*, 360–406.

Stanovich, K. E. (2000). *Processes in understanding reading: Scientific foundations and new frontiers*. New York: Guilford Press.

Torgesen, J. K. (1999). Assessment and instruction for phonetic awareness and word recognition skills. In H. Catts & A. Kamhi (Eds.), *Language and reading disabilities* (pp. 128–153). Boston: Allyn & Bacon.

Torgesen, J. K., Wagner, R. K., & Rashotte, C. A. (1997). Approaches to the prevention and remediation of phonologically based reading disabilities. In B. Blachman (Ed.), *Foundations of reading acquisition and dyslexia: Implications for early intervention* (pp. 287–304). Mahwah, NJ: Erlbaum.

Turner, M., & Engel, R. (1989). Is working memory capacity task dependent? *Journal of Memory and Language, 28*, 127–154.

UNESCO (n.d.). United Nations literacy decade: Today, literacy remains a major global challenge. Retrieved August 26, 2003, from *http://portal.unesco.org/education/ev.php?URL_ID=5000%URL_DO=DO_TOPIC &URL_SECTION=201*.

van den Broeke, M. P. R., & Goldstein, L. (1980). Consonant features in speech errors. In V. Fromkin (Ed.), *Errors in linguistic performance: Slips of the tongue, ear, pen, and hand* (pp. 47–66). New York: Academic Press.

Wagner, R. K., Torgesen, J. K., & Rashotte, C. A. (1994). The development of reading-related phonological processing abilities: New evidence of bi-directional causality from a latent variable longitudinal study. *Developmental Psychology, 30*, 73–87.

Wagner, R. K., Torgesen, J. K., Rashotte, C. A., Hecht, S. A., Barker, T. A., Burgess, S. R., et al. (1997). Changing relations between phonological processing abilities and word-level reading as children develop from beginning to skilled readers: A five-year longitudinal study. *Developmental Psychology, 33*, 468–479.

Webster, P., & Plante, A. (1992). Productive phonology and phonology awareness in preschool children. *Applied Psycholinguistics, 16*, 43–57.

Whitehurst, G. J. (2001). Presentation at the White House Summit on Early Childhood Cognitive Development.

Wiig, E. H., Zureich, P., & Hei-Ning, H. C. (2000). A clinical rationale for assessing rapid automatized naming in children with language disorders. *Journal of Learning Disabilities, 33*(4), 359–374.

Wolf, M., & Bowers, P. G. (2000). Naming-speed deficits in developmental reading disabilities: An introduction to the special series on the double deficit hypothesis. *Journal of Learning Disabilities, 33*(4), 322–324.

Wolf, M., & Obregon, M. (1992). Early naming deficits, developmental dyslexia, and a specific hypothesis. *Brain and Language, 42*, 219–247.

Woodcock, R. W., & Johnson, M. B. (1989). *Woodcock–Johnson Tests of Achievement (WJ-R)*. Allen, TX: DLM Teaching Resources.

Address for correspondence: Kathy Strattman, Wichita State University, Department of Communicative Disorders and Sciences, 1845 Fairmount, Wichita, KS 67226-0075, USA. E-mail: *kathy.strattman@* wichita.edu

From Strattman, K., & Williams Hodson, B. (2005). Variables that influence decoding and spelling in beginning readers. *Child Language Teaching and Therapy, 21*, 165–190. Copyright 2005 by Edward Arnold (Publishers) Ltd. Reprinted by permission of SAGE.

ILLUSTRATIVE EXAMPLE QUESTIONS

1. Are there any problems with the population validity of the study? Why or why not?

2. Did the authors base the study on a strong empirical and/or theoretical base? Explain.

3. What dependent measures did the authors use?

4. What primary statistical analysis procedure was used by the authors? In your response, indicate the factors the authors included in their analyses.

5. Did authors' analysis procedures address the stated purpose of the study? Why or why not?

6. According to the authors, how did the results of study relate to previous research findings?

7. According to the authors, what general conclusions can be made about the results?

8. What are some potential threats to the internal validity of the study? Provide a justification for each threat.

9. What are some potential threats to the external validity of this study? Provide a justification for each threat.

10. What limitations did the authors discuss?

ADDITIONAL RESEARCH EXAMPLES

1. Lease, S. H., & Dahlbeck, D. T. (2009). Parental influences, career decision-making attributions, and self-efficacy: Differences for men and women? *Journal of Career Development, 36,* 95–113.

2. Lee, Y., Wehmeyer, M. L., Palmer, S. B., Williams-Diehm, K., Davies, D. K., & Stock, S. E. (2010). Examining individual and instruction-related predictors of the self-determination of students with disabilities: Multiple regression analysis. *Remedial and Special Education, 31*(6), 1–12.

3. Nichols, T. M., Kotchick, B. A., McNamara Barry, C., & Haskins, D. G. (2009). Understanding the educational aspirations of African American adolescents: Child, family, and community factors. *Journal of Black Psychology, 36,* 25–48.

THREATS TO INTERNAL VALIDITY

Circle the number corresponding to the likelihood of each threat to internal validity being present in the investigation and provide a justification.

1 = definitely not a threat   2 = not a likely threat   3 = somewhat likely threat
4 = likely threat   5 = definite threat   NA = not applicable for this design

Results in Differences within or between Individuals

1. Maturation   1   2   3   4   5   NA

   Justification _____

   _____

2. Selection   1   2   3   4   5   NA

   Justification _____

   _____

3. Selection by Maturation Interaction   1   2   3   4   5   NA

   Justification _____

   _____

4. Statistical Regression   1   2   3   4   5   NA

   Justification _____

   _____

5. Morality   1   2   3   4   5   NA

   Justification _____

   _____

6. Instrumentation   1   2   3   4   5   NA

   Justification _____

   _____

7. Testing   1   2   3   4   5   NA

   Justification _____

   _____

(continued)

8. History   1   2   3   4   5   NA

    Justification _____

_____

9. Resentful Demoralization of the Control Group   1   2   3   4   5   NA

    Justification _____

_____

Results in Similarities within or between Individuals

10. Diffusion of Treatment   1   2   3   4   5   NA

    Justification _____

_____

11. Compensatory Rivalry by the Control Group   1   2   3   4   5   NA

    Justification _____

_____

12. Compensatory Equalization of Treatments   1   2   3   4   5   NA

    Justification _____

_____

Abstract: Write a one-page abstract summarizing the overall conclusions of the authors and whether or not you feel the authors' conclusions are valid based on the internal validity of the investigation.

THREATS TO EXTERNAL VALIDITY

Circle the number corresponding to the likelihood of each threat to external validity being present in the investigation according to the following scale:

1 = definitely not a threat   2 = not a likely threat   3 = somewhat likely threat

4 = likely threat   5 = definite threat   NA = not applicable for this design

Also, provide a justification for each rating.

Population

1. Generalization across Subjects   1   2   3   4   5   NA

Justification _____

_____

2. Interaction of Personological Variables and Treatment   1   2   3   4   5   NA

Justification _____

_____

Ecological

3. Verification of the Independent Variable   1   2   3   4   5   NA

Justification _____

_____

4. Multiple Treatment Interference   1   2   3   4   5   NA

Justification _____

_____

5. Hawthorne Effect   1   2   3   4   5   NA

Justification _____

_____

6. Novelty and Disruption Effects   1   2   3   4   5   NA

Justification _____

_____

7. Experimental Effects   1   2   3   4   5   NA

Justification _____

_____

(continued)

8. Pretest Sensitization   1   2   3   4   5   NA

    Justification _____

    _____

9. Posttest Sensitization   1   2   3   4   5   NA

    Justification _____

    _____

10. Interaction of Time of Measurement and Treatment Effects   1   2   3   4   5   NA

    Justification _____

    _____

11. Measurement of the Dependent Variable   1   2   3   4   5   NA

    Justification _____

    _____

12. Interaction of History and Treatment Effects   1   2   3   4   5   NA

    Justification _____

    _____

Abstract: Write a one-page abstract summarizing the overall conclusions of the authors and whether or not you feel the authors' conclusions are valid based on the external validity of the investigation.

CHAPTER 8

■ ■ ■ ■

Survey Research Methods

OBJECTIVES

After studying this chapter, you should be able to . . .

1. Define what is meant by survey research and list three prominent areas where the development and refinement of survey research methods have occurred.
2. Outline the purposes of survey research.
3. Summarize the different types of surveys.
4. Describe the factors in choosing a survey method.
5. Illustrate how survey research is designed.
6. Explain when researchers should use survey research.

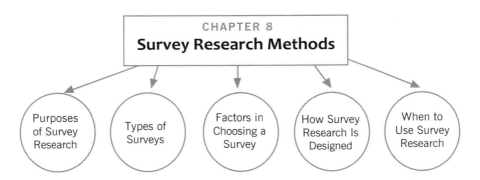

OVERVIEW

A **survey** is a type of quantitative research method that uses questionnaires or interviews to collect data from a sample usually selected to represent a population (Gall et al., 2007). Survey research is the most widely used research method inside and outside of the social sciences. Rarely a day goes by that some survey of opinions, election predictions, or consumer marketing does not receive prominent play in the media. Researchers use a variety of surveys that differ in purpose, length, scope, structure, and content. This survey research can be useful for collecting information from relatively large numbers of dispersed groups of people rather than a small number, as in the case of other research methods (Fowler, 2009; Gall et al., 2007; Graziano & Raulin, 2010).

The use of questions to measure the phenomenon of interest is another essential part of survey research. High-quality survey research requires researchers to construct effective questions and to pose them to respondents in a systematic way. This systematic process is especially important when researchers attempt to measure phenomena that cannot be directly observed, such as attitudes, feelings, and cognitions. Although most surveys have respondents answer self-administered questions, interviewers sometimes ask respondents questions and record their responses. It is critical that interviewers not influence the answers given by respondents, and that questions be posed in a standardized fashion across respondents.

The development and refinement of survey research methods have occurred in three prominent areas. First, the work of the U.S. Census Bureau has played a key role in the sampling and questioning techniques used in survey research (Presser et al., 2004). Although best known for its decennial inventory of the population, the Census Bureau devotes a tremendous effort to ongoing series of sample surveys aimed at providing up-to-date demographic and economic data. Second, commercial polling and marketing firms, such as those organized by Gallup and Harris, have contributed both funds and expertise to the development and refinement of survey research methods. This contribution is particularly reflected in the areas of political polling and consumer marketing. Finally, researchers have played a key role in the development and refinement of survey research methods. Many universities (e.g., University of Massachusetts–Boston, Indiana University, University of Michigan, to name only a few) support centers devoted specifically to the development, refinement, and use of survey research.

Aspects of survey research methods are covered in Chapters 3, 4, 9, and 10. However, whereas these chapters describe basic concepts underlying survey methods, it is important to describe survey research more specifically, so that critical research consumers understand purposes, types, sampling frames, validity issues, and findings. These aspects of survey research are covered here.

We begin the remainder of this section on survey research with a discussion of the varying goals and objectives of survey research, followed by a description of the types of surveys used by researchers. Next, we describe the process used to develop surveys. This section ends with a description of data analysis concerns of survey research and instances when surveys should be used. Research examples highlighting the different designs are presented throughout the chapter, and an illustrative investigation is included at the end of the chapter for critique.

> ### Research Example
>
> Consider this issue. Think about how you would design research to address the question/hypothesis from this research example:
>
> - Research Example: To what extent are young adults with disabilities, who participated in special education, employed in jobs or involved in postsecondary education courses or other learning experiences up to 5 years after high school?
>
> A research example appears near the end of the chapter.

WHAT ARE THE PURPOSES OF SURVEY RESEARCH?

There are as many reasons for conducting surveys as there are surveys. Generally, researchers conduct surveys to explore relationships between and among variables. Business people conduct surveys to determine the demand for their products. Politicians conduct surveys to identify the views of their constituents on key issues that are under consideration. A government agency may conduct surveys to aid in the design of a new set of services. Although the reasons for conducting surveys are numerous, the purpose for conducting surveys can be categorized into three general areas: description, explanation, and exploration. Of course, the purpose of a survey may encompass two or more of these areas.

Description

Surveys are commonly conducted for the purpose of describing some population (Graziano & Raulin, 2010). The primary goal is to identify

> A **survey** is used to identify how people feel, think, act, and vote; it is useful for collecting information from a relatively large number of dispersed groups of people rather than a small number, as in the case of other research methods.

the distribution of characteristics, traits, or attributes of an identified group of people. In other words, researchers are primarily interested in describing the distribution of characteristics rather than why the observed distribution exists. Although researchers often describe subsamples and make comparisons among them, in addition to describing the total sample, the primary purpose of descriptive surveys is to describe the distribution of characteristics, traits, or attributes of interest. The decennial report of the Census Bureau is an example of a survey whose primary purpose is to describe the distribution of demographic characteristics in America.

Explanation

Another purpose of survey research is to explain a phenomenon of interest (Gall et al., 2007). The primary goal is to explain how different variables are related. Survey research that is explanatory in nature typically requires the use of multivariate analysis techniques that enable researchers to examine the relationship between two or more variables. For example, a student's academic performance in elementary school might be explained by variables such as level of parent education, gender, and SES. Researchers would examine the relationship between academic performance and these potential explanatory variables in an attempt to "explain" the academic achievement of students.

Exploration

Researchers also use survey research in an exploratory fashion when they are investigating phenomena not previously studied (Fowler, 2009). For example, researchers wanting to explore the sources of racism on a university campus might survey a group of students with different backgrounds using an in-depth interview or questionnaire to ensure that critical factors are not missed. Researchers could then construct a full-scale probability sample survey, which includes the factors most strongly associated with racism, to identify the sources of racism on the university campus.

WHAT ARE THE DIFFERENT TYPES OF SURVEYS?

One of the most difficult decisions made by researchers conducting survey research is to determine the type of survey or the way the data will be collected. The primary types of surveys include (1) face-to-face interviewing; (2) telephone interviewing; (3) interviewer- and group-administered surveys; (4) self-administered surveys; (5) mail surveys; and (6) online surveys. Although most surveys utilize only one of these data collection methods, a combination of methods may be used. For example, researchers exploring some personal issue, such as drug use, as a part of a larger effort to determine the health and well-being of individuals might have respondents answer a self-administered survey on their past and present use of drugs. Table 8.1 summarizes the advantages and disadvantages associated with each type of survey.

WHAT ARE THE FACTORS IN CHOOSING A SURVEY METHOD?

There are a number of primary factors that researchers should consider when choosing a survey method (see Figure 8.1). These factors include (1) sampling procedures, (2) sampling population, (3) question format, (4) content of questions, (5) response rate, and (6) time and money (Fowler, 2009; Gall et al., 2007; Graziano & Raulin, 2010).

Sampling Procedures

One factor that researchers should consider is on their sampling procedures, which can make it easy or difficult to use a particular type of survey method. For example, the type and the accuracy of information gathered are important if the sampling procedures used by researchers depend on a list. If the list lacks mailing addresses, using a self-administered mail survey is not an option. Another issue focuses on whether there is a designated respondent. If the sampling procedures are based on a list of individuals, any survey method is possible. In contrast, if respondents are not specifically

TABLE 8.1. Advantages and Disadvantages Associated with Each Type of Survey

Method	Advantages	Disadvantages
Face-to-face interviewing	• Enhanced cooperation for completing current interview • Enhanced cooperation for follow-up interview • Address respondent questions • Probe for fuller understanding of responses from respondents • Facilitate the use of more complex instructions or question sequences • Sustain longer interviews • Address personal or sensitive issues • Quality control on responses	• More costly • Requires trained interviewers • Limited supervision of interviewers • Extended data collection period
Telephone interviewing	• Cost-efficient • Supervision of interviewers • Easy to access sample • Short data collection period • Quality control on responses	• Limited to those with telephones • Lower response rate • Limited question formats
Self-administered survey	• Cost-efficient • Use of multiple questions for an area • Address personal or sensitive issues • Efficient data collection, management, and analysis	• Extensive time needed to develop survey • Limited to closed questions • Limited to relatively well-educated and motivated sample • Lack of quality control on responses • Limited to easily accessible sample
Mail survey	• Cost-efficient • Use of multiple questions for an area • Address personal or sensitive issues • Efficient data collection, management, and analysis • Use of widely dispersed sample • More time to complete	• Extensive time needed to develop survey • Limited to closed questions • Limited to relatively well-educated and motivated sample • Lack of quality control on responses

designated and the survey is sent to a household or organization, researchers have little control over who actually completes the survey. In such cases, researchers may want to consider using a telephone survey or personal interview to ensure that respondents possess the specific characteristics of interest. If sampling procedures are based on an e-mail list and online presentation, researchers are dependent on respondents completing the survey without direct interaction between researcher and respondent. Additionally, online surveys sent to large numbers of respondents are based on the assumption that the survey actually gets to the respondent's computer monitor and is not eliminated for computer security reasons as "spam."

Sampling Population

A second factor that researchers should consider when selecting a survey method is the **sampling population**, or the population to which the survey results will be generalized. The reading and writing skills of the sampling population, as well as its motivation to participate, are key considerations when selecting a survey method. Self-administered surveys require more from respondents than do those that rely

> A **sampling population** *is the population to which the sample survey results will be generalized.*

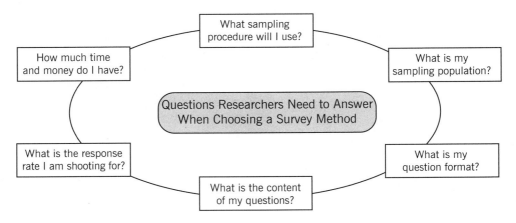

FIGURE 8.1. Primary factors researchers need to consider when choosing a survey method.

on interviewers. Self-administered surveys also require respondents to be more interested in the subject matter under study than do those that rely on interviewers. Thus, researchers should use self-administered surveys only when the sample population is relatively well educated and interested in the subject matter under study.

Question Format

A third factor that researchers should consider when selecting a survey method centers on the question format. Self-administered surveys rely on closed-ended questions in which the respondent checks a box or circles a response from a set of options. Self-administered surveys might include some open-ended questions as well. However, researchers usually treat such information as anecdotal material, because such questions tend to produce data that are incomplete and not comparable across respondents. Additionally, in contrast to open-ended questions, closed-ended question formats enable researchers to collect information on a large number of items or to break down complex questions into a set of simpler questions.

Content of Questions

A fourth factor that researchers should consider is on the content of the questions. Although generally the answers of respondents have

been found to be unaffected by the type of survey (Chandon, Morwitz, & Reinartz, 2005), some sensitive or embarrassing issues may be affected by the survey method researchers use. In the case of such issues (e.g., drug use, sexual preferences), self-administered forms of data collection are preferable, because interviewer-based methods tend to produce socially desirable responses. Additionally, researchers should consider the difficulty of the reporting task. In cases in which researchers are interested in events or behaviors that extend over a period of time (e.g., physical symptoms of stress), self-administered surveys allow the respondent more time for thought and consultation with family, friends, or records.

Response Rate

The fifth factor that researchers should consider centers on the importance of the **response rate**. The response rate is the number of people surveyed (or interviewed) divided by the total number of individuals sampled multiplied by 100. The numerator includes all individuals who were selected and did respond; the denominator includes all the individuals who were sampled regardless of whether they responded. Naturally, researchers prefer that response rates be relatively high. The problem of nonresponse is central to survey research, because researchers have no substantive way to assess fully the extent to which the characteristics of nonrespondents differ from those of respondents. Survey methods that rely on group administration produce the highest response rates. Additionally, telephone surveys and interviewer-administered surveys tend to produce higher response rates than do self-administered surveys.

Time and Money

The final factor that researchers should consider when selecting a survey method is on costs in terms of time and money. Some issues that should be considered by researchers include the amount of time required to develop the survey, the length of the survey, the geographic diffusion of the sample, the education level and interest of the sample, and the availability of trained staff to administer the survey. Survey methods that rely on face-to-face interviews with respondents are more costly than those that do not, such as telephone or self-administered surveys.

HOW IS SURVEY RESEARCH DESIGNED?

Although survey research involves all of the different aspects (e.g., articulating a clear and concise research question) associated with any research method, sampling and question construction are key elements underlying the design of surveys. Before discussing issues associated with sampling and question construction, there are two important points that researchers should consider. First, researchers should thoroughly explore the literature or other sources about the potential for gathering the information they want. Although surveys appear to be a simple solution to learning about some phenomenon of interest, researchers should only undertake surveys when they are certain the information cannot be obtained in other ways. As mentioned earlier, a plethora of survey research is conducted in a variety of areas. It would not be surprising to find that several studies address the phenomenon of interest.

Second, researchers should explore whether there are previously developed, reliable, valid measures to address the phenomenon they are studying. Reference materials such as *The Sixteenth Mental Measurements Yearbook* (Spies

& Plake, 2005) and *Tests in Print VII* (Murphy, Spies, & Plake, 2006) provide information on all of the measures, including surveys used in the social sciences.

Sampling

When conducting survey research, readers are encouraged to review Chapter 4 on sampling techniques. In this section, we present a brief review of some key sampling principles with which to judge the sample or respondents surveyed by researchers.

Although survey researchers use the same research methods as all researchers (i.e., research conceptualization, ethical treatment of participants, sampling, measurement, data collection and analysis, and interpretation), high-quality sampling techniques are critical to survey research. As with any research study, the key to good survey research is to use sampling procedures that give all population members the same (or known) chance of being sampled. In other words, surveys are rarely done for the purpose of describing the particular sample under study. Rather, surveys are conducted for the purpose of understanding the larger population from which the sample was initially selected. Additionally, analyses of survey research typically aim to develop generalized propositions about the phenomena under study. Thus, researchers must define their *sampling frame.*

Sampling Frames

The **sampling frame** is the set of people that has the chance to be selected given the sampling procedure(s) used by researchers. In other words, the sampling frame is the population or defined list from which the sample will be drawn (National Center for Educational Statistics, 2001). It is important that the sampling frame correspond to the population that researchers want to describe. The sampling

> *The* **response rate** *is the number of people surveyed divided by the total number of individuals sampled multiplied by 100.*
>
> *The* **sampling frame** *is the population or defined list from which the sample will be drawn.*

frame and sample selection procedures, including the size and the specific procedures used for selecting individuals to survey, directly influence the precision of the sample estimates. In other words, researchers must determine how closely the characteristics of the sample approximate those of the population. There are three general classes of sampling frames—exhaustive, convenience, and cluster (Gall et al., 2007).

Exhaustive Sampling Frames. In the first class of sampling frames, sampling is done from a more or less complete list of individuals in the population to be studied. This typically occurs when the population is small or clearly defined, and the list is used by researchers to select a sample. For example, the members of the senior class at a regional university might be used as the sampling frame for selecting a sample to assess student satisfaction with a required capstone experience. Sampling frames such as this, referred to as *exhaustive sampling frames*, contain an exhaustive inventory of members of the population.

Convenience Sampling Frames. In the second class of sampling frames, the sampling is done from a set of individuals who do something or go somewhere that enables researchers to administer a survey to them. This class of sampling frame differs from the preceding class in that there is not an advance list from which researchers can sample. Rather, researchers create the list or inventory of the members of the population and sampling occurs simultaneously. For example, researchers might survey every 10th individual coming through the turnstiles at a professional football home game regarding the need for a new stadium.

Cluster Sampling Frames. In the final class of sampling frames, the sampling is done in two or more stages (i.e., cluster sampling). In the first stage(s), researchers sample something other than the individuals to be surveyed. In one or more stages, these primary units are sampled, and from them a final sample is selected. For example, to assess the public's perception of quality of education provided by the local public school district, researchers might randomly select only houses in a neighborhood that have

school-age children. Researchers might then survey a random sample of the adults living in the identified homes regarding their perception of the quality of education provided by the local public school district.

Evaluating Sampling Frames

In addition to determining the characteristics of the sampling frames, there are three general characteristics to consider when evaluating the sampling frame used in survey research—comprehensiveness of the sample, probability of being selected, and response rate.

Comprehensiveness of Sample. The first general characteristic is the comprehensiveness of the sample. A sample can only be representative of the sampling frame. Few approaches to sampling are based on a truly "exhaustive sampling frame" in which every member of the population is known. Furthermore, seemingly comprehensive lists, such as individuals in telephone directories, omit major segments of some populations (e.g., those without phones, unlisted numbers). Thus, a key part of evaluating the sample surveyed by researchers is to look at the percentage of the study population that had a chance of being selected and the extent to which those excluded are distinctive. For example, if researchers intend to sample from a population included on a list (e.g., members of the American Educational Research Association), it is important that they examine in detail how the list was compiled. This examination should focus on the number and characteristics of people not likely to be included on the list.

Probability of Being Selected. The second characteristic focuses on the probability of being selected by researchers to complete the survey. Ideally, to make reasonably accurate estimates of the relationship between sample statistics and the population from which they were drawn, researchers should know the probability of each individual being selected. Researchers are unable to make reasonably accurate estimates of the relationship between the sample statistics and the population from which they are drawn if they do not know the probability of selection. As noted earlier, calculation of the probability of each individual being selected occurs at sample selection or at the time of data collection, depending on the sampling frame or approach used by researchers.

Response Rate. The final characteristic focuses on the response rate. The response rate is a basic parameter for evaluating data collection efforts in survey research. Although there is no agreed-upon standard for a minimum response rate, generally, the lower the response rate, the higher the potential for bias associated with nonrespondents. A response rate of 50% is adequate for analysis and reporting, 60% is good, and 75% or higher is considered very good. Additionally, ensuring reasonable response rates and avoiding procedures that systematically produce substantial differences between respondents and nonrespondents should play a key role in any survey research.

The nature of bias associated with nonresponse differs somewhat across survey methods that rely on personal contact between researchers and respondents (i.e., face-to-face, interviewer- and group-administered surveys) and those that do not (i.e., telephone, self-administered, mail, and online surveys). In the case of telephone surveys, lack of availability is the most important source of nonresponse (Fowler, 2009). For example, the people available to be surveyed will be distinctive if data collection is conducted during Monday through Friday working hours. Such a survey would likely yield high proportions of parents with small children, in-home child care professionals, unemployed individuals, and retired persons.

Lack of accessibility is the major form of nonresponse associated with personal interview surveys. Accessibility is more common in personal interview surveys conducted in central cities than in suburbs or rural areas because it is difficult to access individuals who live in apartments (Cannell, Marquis, & Laurent, 1977). The omission of groups of individuals is another form of nonresponse associated with personal interview surveys. This omission is common when the interview is conducted in areas in which there are large groups of individuals who do not speak English (Fowler, 2009).

The nature of nonresponse associated with mail surveys differs from those conducted by telephone or through personal interviews. Individuals who have an interest in the subject matter are more likely than those who are less interested to return mail surveys. Thus, the results of mail surveys with low response rates may be biased in ways that are directly related to the purpose of the research (Wright, 2005). Another common form of nonresponse in mail surveys is that better-educated individuals are more likely than those with less education to return mail questionnaires (De Winter et al., 2005). Similarly, higher SES individuals who are more likely to have access to Internet are better able to return online questionnaires than those at lower SES levels (Wright, 2005). These forms of bias are more likely to be evident when the subject matter is related (even tangentially) to the education level of respondents.

Developing the Survey Instrument

Using well-designed questions is critical in survey research, because the answer to a question is valuable only to the extent that it has a predictable relationship to facts or the phenomenon of interest. Good questions maximize the relationship between what researchers are trying to measure and the answers of respondents. One goal of survey research is to ensure question reliability (i.e., respondents answer the question in the same way). Another goal is to ensure question validity (i.e., correspondence between the answers of respondents and what is purportedly being measured). Thus, all of the issues discussed in Chapter 3 regarding reliability and validity play a critical role in the development of surveys. Because these issues have already been discussed, the focus in this section is the process used by researchers to develop questions for surveys, which includes (1) identifying key factors (i.e., attributes, characteristics, or behaviors) associated with the phenomena under study, (2) developing questions or statements, (3) formatting and sequencing questions, and (4) pilot-testing the survey (see Figure 8.2).

Identifying Key Factors

Identifying the key factors associated with the phenomenon under study is critical to developing an effective survey. The aim at this point

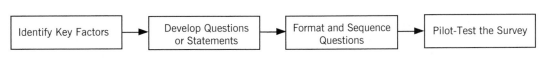

FIGURE 8.2. Process for developing a survey.

in the process of survey design is to identify all of the potential factors associated with this phenomenon. Although researchers might be tempted to rely on brainstorming to identify the factors, they should review the literature and other sources (e.g., experts in the field) to ensure that they identify all of the key factors associated with this phenomenon. Of course, it is important to assess the quality of the questions used by researchers who have done previous work on this phenomenon.

Researchers may begin to prioritize the factors they are interested in exploring, because many possible factors may be associated with the phenomenon under study. Again, researchers should look closely at the literature to identify factors that have been found to be associated most strongly with the phenomenon under study. Identifying factors found to be related to such a phenomenon enable researchers to construct high-quality surveys.

Developing Questions or Statements

Before developing survey questions or statements, researchers must consider response format.

Response Format. Although there are a number of variations, researchers have two categories of options: open- and closed-ended questions. (Although researchers use both questions and statements in survey research, we refer only to questions throughout the remainder of this section.)

Open-Ended Questions. In the case of open-ended questions, respondents are asked to provide their own answers to the questions. For example, respondents who are asked, "What do you think is the most important issue facing public schools today?" might be provided a space to write their answers, or they may report them verbally to interviewers. With open-ended

questions, respondents are free to offer any of a large number of views on a topic. The primary shortcoming of open-ended questions is the lack of uniformity of responses, because respondents can respond in a variety of fashions. This lack of uniformity tends to reduce the reliability and validity of the survey.

Closed-Ended Questions. In the case of closed-ended questions, respondents are asked to select their answers from among those provided by the researchers. Using the preceding example, respondents might be asked to choose the most important issue facing public schools today from a list of possible issues provided by researchers (e.g., funding, violence, substance abuse, availability of well-trained teachers). Additionally, researchers use a variety of scales (e.g., Likert, Thurstone, and Guttman scaling) with closed-ended questions (Tourangeau, Rips, & Rasinski, 2000). Likert-type scales are most commonly used by researchers when respondents are presented a series of questions and asked to indicate "strongly agree," "agree," "undecided," "disagree," or "strongly disagree." Multiple modifications of the wording of the response (e.g., "approve") are used by researchers. The primary shortcoming of closed-ended questions lies in how researchers have chosen and structured the possible responses.

Reviewing Questions Used in Other Surveys. After a response format has been chosen, researchers use the list of key factors to be measured to develop a set of questions to include on the survey. Again, researchers should review questions used by others who have conducted similar surveys. Keep in mind that there is no guarantee that the questions used by researchers conducting similar surveys are good questions or are appropriate for a particular survey. Poorly constructed questions are used in some surveys simply because researchers do not critically evaluate whether question content is appropriate for the population, context, and goals of a particular study.

Ensuring the Reliability and Validity of Questions. All questions should be tested to ensure that they are reliable and valid measures for the population, context, and goals of a particular study. Demographic and background information questions should yield accurate and needed information. These questions are standard to most surveys. Researchers can review other survey instruments to identify common demographic and background questions. General guidelines for constructing reliable and valid questions include (1) use of clear and unambiguous wording; (2) avoidance of double-barreled questions (e.g., "Should America eliminate foreign aid and spend the money on family-friendly programs?"); (3) avoidance of negative items; and (4) avoidance of biased items or terms.

Understanding of Questions. Prior to formatting and sequencing the survey, researchers should explore whether the draft questions are consistently understood and answered by respondents before conducting a more formal pilot test of the survey instrument. To evaluate whether the questions are consistently understood and answered by respondents, researchers typically identify a small group of respondents that is willing to help them understand how the questions work. Researchers ask respondents not only to respond to the draft questions but also to complete an interview regarding the question content and reasons for the responses. The goal is to assess whether respondents' comprehension and responses are consistent with the population, context, and goals of a particular study.

Formatting and Sequencing Questions

Once the questions have been developed and reviewed by a group of respondents for feedback purposes, researchers then format and sequence the questions. Regardless of the type of survey (e.g., interview, self-administered), the primary goal is to format and sequence questions to minimize the work of respondents and, in some cases, to reduce biasing effects associated with

the order of the questions. Six general guidelines for formatting questions follow:

1. The layout of survey instrument should be attractive, clear, and uncluttered. Reduction strategies designed to include more questions on the survey should be avoided.

2. Instructions for completing the survey should be self-explanatory (this is especially critical for self-administered surveys). Enough information should be provided to ensure that respondents can complete the survey as intended.

3. Consistent question forms and response formats should be used. The more the same types of questions and response formats are used, the more reliable the information obtained and the easier the task will be for respondents.

4. The length of time required to complete the survey should be less than 30 minutes. The length of the survey should be adjusted to align with the ability and willingness of respondents to complete the survey.

5. "Skip patterns" should be kept to a minimum (e.g., "Please skip to Question 10 if your answer is NO").

6. The presentation of questions that may affect the answers given by respondents to subsequent questions should be randomized.

Pilot-Testing the Survey

Conducting a pilot test of the survey is the final step in developing a survey instrument. The purpose of a pilot test is to find out how the survey instrument works under realistic conditions. Researchers typically draw 20 to 50 respondents from a population that is the same as, or similar to, the population to be surveyed. The administration procedures should be the same as those used in the actual study. Researchers then use information gained from the pilot test to examine the reliability and validity of the survey. Researchers may also ask questions regarding the survey to ensure that respondents answer the questions as intended. For example, researchers may ask respondents to complete a rating form to evaluate whether

(1) the questions are easy to read and (2) respondents consistently understand and accurately answer the questions.

Analysis of Data

This section considers issues related to internal and external validity of survey research.

Internal Validity

Sampling methods are important in determining the internal validity of a survey (Fowler, 2009). However, the importance has more to do with the sample of items included in the survey than with the sample of the population. How the questions are phrased and the order in which they are placed are critical in determining whether the information received is what the researchers wanted or expected. Thus, critical research consumers should determine whether the questions provided to respondents were adequate in obtaining the information received by the researchers.

Critical research consumers should consider whether the survey was pilot-tested. If it was, two questions should be answered. First, did the authors indicate that modifications were based on the pilot test results? The primary reason for pilot-testing the survey is to determine whether the questions obtain the desired information; researchers usually modify the survey format and/or questions based on the feedback. Second, did the authors indicate who were the pilot test participants? The pilot test participants should be representative of the respondents in the investigation. If they are similar to the respondents, it is likely that the feedback obtained in the pilot test survey was valid in providing feedback on how to modify the survey to obtain important information. If the pilot test participants are not similar to the respondents, there should be a question about the adequacy of any modifications made to the survey.

Once it has been determined that the survey is adequate to obtain the required information, critical research consumers should consider whether cause-and-effect statements can be based on the results. Because an independent variable is not directly manipulated in the same way it would be in an experimental investigation, the determination of a cause-and-effect relationship is not possible. However, through multivariate analysis techniques, it is possible to determine relationships and the strength of those relationships among variables. Thus, the researcher could indicate that a relationship exists. Whether the relationship is causal in nature would then depend on further experimental investigations.

External Validity

The ability to generalize the results of a survey to individuals not included in the survey sample depends on the nature of the sample used (i.e., was it representative?) (Cozby, 2008; Fowler, 2009). Additionally, the description of respondent characteristics is also a critical part of the ability to make generalization claims. Although sampling errors are not the only source of bias in the findings from survey research, they represent a potential source of error.

The sampling process can affect the findings from surveys in several different ways. First, the findings will be biased if the sample frame excludes some individuals from whom we want to collect information. The magnitude of the bias will depend on the extent to which the omitted individuals differ from the respondents. Second, if the sampling approach used by researchers is not probabilistic, the relationship between the sampled population and those sampled is a problem. This is not to say that all nonprobabilistic sampling approaches produce unrepresentative samples. Rather, researchers have no statistical basis for assessing the extent to which a sample is representative of the sampled population. Finally, chance errors will occur if researchers collect data from only a sample of a population.

Recall the first research question about postschool outcomes posed earlier in this chapter? Read on to see how your design compares to how the actual study was designed.

Research Example: Survey

A series of national surveys examined postschool outcomes for young adults with disabilities who had participated in special education (Wagner & Cameto, 2011). The National Longitudinal Transition Study—Second Iteration (NLTS-2), funded by the Office of Special Education Programs in the U.S. Department of Education, sought to provide information on employment, employment training, and postsecondary education of youth with disabilities during their secondary school years and first 5 years after high school. Researchers conducted a national survey with a sample representing youth and young adults with disabilities. They selected a nationally representative sample of 11,276 youth between the ages of 13 and 16 and receiving special education services in 2000–2001. Researchers followed them for 10 years. All types of recognized developmental disabilities (e.g., specific learning disabilities, intellectual disability) and acquired disabilities (e.g., traumatic brain injury) were represented. Researchers conducted surveys in 2003, 2005, 2007, and 2009 with youth or their parents, either over the phone or through a mailed survey format. Wagner and Cameto (2009) reported on results of the final follow-up survey (called *Wave 5*) based on the 2009 telephone interviews. Of the original sample, 6,322 parents or youth responded. Researchers found that up to 8 years after leaving high school, about 60% of young adults with disabilities were engaged in paid employment or preparation for work (i.e., sheltered, supported, or competitive employment). This rate was below the 66% employment rate among out-of-school peers without disabilities. Dropouts were less likely than school completers to be engaged in work, preparation for work, or postschool activities after high school; about 67% of dropouts were engaged in these activities, compared with almost 87% of school

completers. About 34% of the young adults were engaged in a postsecondary educational experience, compared to 51% of young adults without disabilities. Multivariate analyses revealed that disability type and socioeconomic level were associated with an enrollment in 2- or 4-year colleges; those more likely to be involved had a visual impairment or higher cognitive skills, were female, had a relatively well-educated head of household, and/or graduated from high school. More youth were enrolled in 2-year community colleges than in other types of postsecondary schools (44% of the total in postsecondary education).

WHEN SHOULD RESEARCHERS USE SURVEY RESEARCH?

Survey research is appropriate for the study of a wide range of phenomena in education and psychology. However, survey research should be conducted only when other methods are not possible or appropriate to use. If the number of individuals about whom researchers are interested in obtaining information is so large that another methodology is not possible, survey research should be used. Likewise, if the individuals about whom we wish to obtain information are dispersed across a large area, for example, we may not be able to conduct another form of research. In such a case, a survey method would be most appropriate. Finally, some research questions may simply require a survey method, such as asking school psychologists to indicate their support or nonsupport for categorical labeling of special education students (e.g., specific learning disabilities, behavior disorders, intellectual disability).

SUMMARY

❖ A survey is a type of quantitative research method that can identify how people feel, think, act, and vote. A survey is useful for collecting information from a relatively large number of dispersed groups of people. Survey research is the most widely used research method. The development and refinement of survey research methods have occurred in three prominent

areas: Census Bureau, commercial polling and marketing firms, and researchers.

❖ There are three main purposes for conducting survey research: (1) to describe something about a population, (2) to explain some phenomenon of interest, and (3) to explore a phenomenon not previously studied.

❖ There are several different types of surveys: (1) face-to-face interviewing, (2) telephone interviewing, (3) interviewer- and group-administered surveys, (4) self-administered surveys, (5) mail surveys, and (6) online surveys. Each of these types of surveys has advantages and disadvantages.

❖ There are six factors in choosing a survey method: (1) sampling procedures (who receives the survey), (2) sampling population (the population to which results can be generalized), (3) question format (how questions are asked), (4) content of questions (what questions are asked), (5) response rate (the percentage of surveys we would like to get back), and (6) time and money (what we can afford to do).

❖ Two issues should be addressed before designing survey research: (1) whether it is possible to gather the information needed from the literature or from other sources; and (2) whether previously developed measures address the phenomenon being studied. Once these issues are addressed, researchers must decide on a method that samples the population, including the sampling frame. The survey instrument must also be developed. This development includes four steps: (1) identifying key factors (i.e., attributes, characteristics, or behaviors) associated with the phenomenon under study, (2) developing questions or statements, (3) formatting and sequencing questions, and (4) pilot-testing the survey.

❖ Although the survey is the most widely used research method, surveys should be conducted only when other methods are not possible or appropriate to use.

DISCUSSION QUESTIONS

1. In what three prominent areas have development and refinement of survey research methods taken place? Have you or your family been affected directly by one or more of these areas? Explain.

2. In what three areas can the purpose for conducting surveys be categorized? Provide an example of each area you may be interested in studying.

3. In one of the examples you described in question 2, what type of survey would you use? What are the advantages and disadvantages of such a survey?

4. How would your choice of a survey differ if you were studying a culturally sensitive issue (e.g., sexual behavior) rather than an issue that is less sensitive (e.g., preference for presidential candidate)? Explain.

5. What are the factors in choosing a survey method? Provide a description of each.

6. How does the amount of time and money you have affect how you would conduct a survey?

7. What are the two important points researchers should consider when designing a survey?

8. What is a sampling frame? In your answer, describe each of the three classes of sampling frames.

9. What three general characteristics of sampling frames should be considered? What should the researcher be able to report in each of these characteristics?

10. What is the process of developing a survey instrument? In your answer, provide a description of each step in the process.

Teaching Spelling in the Primary Grades: A National Survey of Instructional Practices and Adaptations

Steve Graham
Paul Morphy
Karen R. Harris
Vanderbilt University

Barbara Fink-Chorzempa
State University of New York–New Paltz

Bruce Saddler
University of Albany

Susan Moran
University of Maryland

Linda Mason
Pennsylvania State University

Primary grade teachers randomly selected from across the United States completed a survey (N = 168) that examined their instructional practices in spelling and the types of adaptations they made for struggling spellers. Almost every single teacher surveyed reported teaching spelling, and the vast majority of respondents implemented a complex and multifaceted instructional program that applied a variety of research-supported procedures. Although some teachers were sensitive to the instructional needs of weaker spellers and reported making many different adaptations for these students, a sizable minority of teachers (42%) indicated they made few or no adaptations. In addition, the teachers indicated that 27% of their students experienced difficulty with spelling, calling into question the effectiveness of their instruction with these children.

Keywords: *elementary schools, survey research, instructional practices, spelling, spelling instruction*

Mastering spelling is important to both writing and reading. Spelling errors make text more difficult to read. They can also cause the reader to devalue the quality of the writer's message (Marshall, 1967; Marshall & Powers, 1969). Spelling difficulties can interfere with the execution of other composing processes (Berninger, 1999). Having to consciously think about how to spell a word while writing, for example, may tax a writer's processing memory, leading him or her to forget ideas or plans he or she is trying to retain in working memory (S. Graham, Harris, & Fink-Chorzempa, 2002).

Spelling difficulties can even influence the words writers use when writing, as they are less likely to choose words they cannot spell (S. Graham & Harris, 2005).

McCutchen (1988) and others (Berninger, 1999) have further argued that transcriptions skills, such as spelling, shape young children's approach to writing, as they are so cognitively demanding that children minimize the use of other composing processes, such as planning and revising, that exert considerable processing demands, too. The resulting approach to writing, which persists well beyond the primary grades, mainly involves telling what one knows, with little attention directed to rhetorical goals, whole-text organization, or the needs of the reader (Scardamalia & Bereiter, 1986). Likewise, Berninger (Berninger, Mizokawa, & Bragg, 1991) found that primary-grade children who have difficulty with spelling avoid writing and develop a mindset that they cannot write, leading to arrested writing development. In contrast, learning about spelling can enhance early reading development by shaping children's knowledge of phonemic awareness, strengthening their grasp of the alphabetic principle, and making sight words easier to remember (Adams, 1990; Ehri, 1987; Moats, 2005/2006; Treiman, 1993).

Because spelling is so important to young children's literacy development, it is critical that spelling is taught effectively during the primary grades. This should help minimize spelling's constraints on writing as well as facilitate the acquisition of foundational reading skills, such as word attack and word recognition (see Berninger et al., 1998, and S. Graham et al., 2002, for examples of these effects). The success of such efforts depends, in part, on providing spelling instruction that is responsive to children's individual needs (S. Graham & Harris, 2002). As Corno and Snow (1986) noted, improved educational outcomes depend on adjusting instruction to individual differences among children. This has become increasingly important in recent years, as schools have become more academically diverse (Fuchs & Fuchs, 1998), and most students with disabilities now receive all or part of their education in regular classrooms. In addition, more children come from families living below the poverty line, placing them at greater risk for academic difficulties (Stallings, 1995).

Although educational theorists, teachers, and students agree that instructional adaptations are desirable (Randi & Corno, 2005; Schumm & Vaughn, 1991; Tobias, 1995), there is very little information on how teachers adapt their instruction to meet students' needs. Pressley and colleagues (e.g., Pressley, Rankin, & Yokoi, 1996; Wharton-McDonald, Pressley, & Hampston, 1998) reported that outstanding literacy teachers deliver a common curriculum to all students but adjust their teaching within this framework to meet students' individual needs, especially for those experiencing difficulty. These teachers provide considerable individualized instruction to children. This stands in contrast to other studies that found that typical teachers make few adaptations (e.g., Baker & Zigmond, 1990; Fuchs & Fuchs, 1998) and that their students continue to struggle when adaptations are not made (e.g., Phillips, Fuchs, Fuchs, & Hamlett, 1996).

The study reported here examined primary-grade teachers' instructional adaptations for children experiencing difficulty with spelling. We concentrated specifically on these students because their spelling difficulties put them at greater risk for writing problems and because they are less likely to benefit from the potential positive impact of spelling on reading due to their slow rate of spelling growth. In contrast to Pressley and his colleagues (e.g., Pressley et al., 1996; Wharton-McDonald et al., 1998), who examined the teaching and adaptations of outstanding primary-grade literacy teachers, we focused our investigation on more typical teachers. A national sample of randomly selected primary-grade teachers was surveyed about their instructional practices in spelling and the types of adaptations they made for struggling spellers.

Relatively few studies have examined the spelling practices of contemporary primary-grade teachers or the adaptations they make for struggling spellers. Two recent national surveys of writing instruction (Cutler & Graham, in press; S. Graham, Harris, Fink-Chorzempa, & MacArthur, 2003) found that most primary-grade teachers reported teaching spelling, frequently encouraged the use of invented spelling, and taught spelling words, phonics for spelling, and strategies for spelling unknown words on at least a weekly basis. The only study we were able to locate that examined the adaptations teachers typically make for struggling students was the above survey by S. Graham et al. (2003), but only four of the questions asked focused specifically on spelling. These teachers reported that they more frequently taught phonics for spelling and strategies for spelling unknown words to weaker writers than stronger ones. They further encouraged weaker writers to use invented spellings more often. It is important to note that a sizable minority of teachers (42%) reported making few adaptations (zero to two) for any part of their writing program for weaker writers, with 75% of all adaptations made by just one third of the teachers.

To obtain information on adaptations for weaker spellers in this study, we asked teachers to indicate how often specific spelling activities and procedures were used with weaker and stronger spellers in their class. If a spelling activity or procedure occurred more often with weaker spellers than stronger spellers, then it represented a departure from the general teaching routine and was considered an adaptation. The spelling activities and procedures included in our survey were selected because each is a commonly recommended staple of primary-grade spelling instruction, it is reasonable to expect that teachers might adjust each technique when working with weaker spellers, and there is empirical evidence that the technique is effective with these students (this third criteria was true for most, but not all, techniques; see Method). Teachers were also asked to identify any additional adaptations they made for weaker spellers beyond the activities and procedures that they were queried about directly. Our approach was similar to S. Graham et al. (2003), except we focused on just spelling instead of writing in general. In addition to providing information about spelling adaptations, this survey provided needed information on how spelling is typically taught in primary grades, including how much time is devoted to teaching spelling, the study of spelling words, teachers' use of commercial materials, and how frequently teachers use the selected spelling activities and procedures.

We did not anticipate that participating teachers would report making adaptations for weaker spellers on all of the spelling activities and procedures surveyed, as some adaptations are more acceptable to teachers than others (Schumm & Vaughn, 1991). We did expect, however, that teachers would report making some adjustments in how frequently specific spelling skills were taught as well as modifications in how they taught these skills and promoted successful spelling during writing. Similar kinds of adjustments were reported for weaker writers in S. Graham et al. (2003). On the basis of this prior study, we also anticipated that most teachers would report making some adjustment in their instruction but that most of the adaptations would be made by a small percentage of teachers and that there would be a sizable proportion of teachers who reported making few or even no adaptations. On the basis of findings from previous studies (Cutler & Graham, in press; S. Graham et al., 2003; Pressley et al., 1996; Wharton-McDonald et al., 1998), we further predicted that almost all participating teachers would indicate they teach spelling. Although previous research does not provide a strong foundation for predicting what spelling skills teachers would emphasize and how they would be taught, we anticipated that teachers' spelling instruction would be multifaceted, involving the teaching of a variety of skills and using many different activities and procedures. This is consistent with most recommended approaches for teaching spelling (e.g., S. Graham, 1999; Loomer, Fitzsimmons, & Strege, 1990; Schlagel, 2007).

Although the spelling practices surveyed in this study were not selected so that specific theories of spelling instruction were contrasted, they do provide some evidence on primary-grade teachers' theoretical orientations. The two basic theoretical orientations to teaching spelling are spelling-is-"caught" and spelling-is-"taught" approaches (S. Graham, 2000). With the former, it is assumed that spelling can be acquired as naturally and easily as speaking, by immersing children in literacy-rich environments where they have plenty of opportunities to read and write for real purposes. In contrast, with the spelling-is-taught approach, it is assumed that it is necessary to directly and

systematically teach children how to spell. There are three basic approaches to the spelling-is-taught orientation (Schlagel, 2007): memorization (e.g., students memorize the spelling of specific words), generalization (e.g., students are directly taught rules and skills for spelling unknown words), and developmental (i.e., students connect and extend their grasp of the spelling system through the use of word study activities, such as word sorting). By examining the practices applied by the participating teachers, we can draw some inferences about their theoretical approach to teaching spelling. For example, if teachers indicated that they applied the spelling activities and practices surveyed, it is clear that they do not rely solely on a spelling-is-caught approach. Likewise, if they report that they teach students the skills and strategies needed to spell unknown words, they do emphasize the generalization method from the spelling-is-taught orientation. On the basis of a previous study where primary grade teachers emphasized multiple instructional orientations to teaching writing (S. Graham, Harris, Fink, & MacArthur, 2002), we expected a similar pattern for spelling.

METHOD

Participants and Settings

A random sampling procedure, stratified by grade level, was used to identify 248 first- through third-grade teachers from the population of primary-grade teachers in the United States. The names were selected from a comprehensive list of 558,444 primary-grade teachers in 72,000 private and public schools compiled by Market Data Retrieval. A sample size of 248 teachers is adequate for a population of 558,444 teachers under the following conditions (cf. Dillman, 2000): (a) A plus- or minus-5% sampling error is considered tolerable, (b) expected variation in teacher responses is set at .13 and .87, (c) the statistical confidence level is set at 95%, and (d) a return rate of 70% is obtained. We determined expected variation in teacher responses and the expected return rate by using data from S. Graham et al. (2003). This prior study used the same procedures as this investigation to calculate if a teacher made an adaptation and to solicit surveys from teachers. For each item in this previous study, there was a 13% chance that teachers would report making an adaptation and an 87% chance they would not (thus, the .13–.87 ratio). Furthermore, 70% of their sample completed the survey. Using a formula by Dillman (2000) and the first three conditions above (plus- or minus-5% sampling error; .13–.87 variation in responses, and a statistical confidence level of 95%), we needed 174 teachers to complete the survey to have an adequate sample. Assuming a 70% return rate, the survey needed to be sent to 248 teachers.

Of the 248 teachers identified, 68% (n = 169) agreed to participate in the study. Demographic information for the 169 responders as well as the 79 nonresponders is presented in Table 1. Chi-square analyses revealed no statistically significant differences between responders and nonresponders in terms of gender, grade, or location of the school (all ps > .17). Analyses of variance further indicated that there were no statistically significant differences between responders and nonresponders in terms of school size or annual expenditures for materials per pupil. These findings provide evidence that responders were representative of the whole sample.

Similar to previous surveys with primary-grade teachers (Cutler & Graham, in press; S. Graham et al., 2003) almost all of the teachers were females (see Table 1). For the most part, they were evenly distributed across the three grades (but 11% of them taught multiple grades) as well as across urban, suburban, and rural locations. There was considerable variability in the size of the schools that employed the teachers. As a group, the teachers had taught for slightly more than 16 years (range = 1 year to 48 years; SD = 10.6 years). The average size of their class was 20.7 students (SD = 5.0), with approximately 8.7% of students (SD = 7.0%) receiving free or reduced-cost lunch. One tenth of their students (SD = 9.0) were receiving special education services, and the teachers indicated that 27% (SD = 20.5%) of their students experienced difficulty with spelling. In addition, 65% (SD = 35%) of the teachers' students were White, 16% Black (SD = 27%), 13% Hispanic (SD = 25%), 3% Asian (SD = 9%), and 4% Other (SD = 12%).

Survey Instrument

Teachers were asked to complete a questionnaire that included two parts: One part included questions about the teacher, the classroom, and the general spelling program, and the other assessed the types of adaptations that teachers made for struggling spellers (the survey is presented in the appendix).

TABLE 1. Characteristics of Responders and Nonresponders

Variable	Responders		Nonresponders	
	n	%	n	%
Gender of teacher				
Male	8	5	4	5
Female	156	95	75	95
Grade				
First	50	30	23	29
Second	55	33	21	27
Third	46	27	31	39
Multiple grades	18	11	4	5
Location				
Urban	60	36	23	29
Suburban	49	30	29	37
Rural	56	34	27	34
Size of school				
M	412.5	—	396.4	—
SD	222.2	—	203.9	—
Expenditures per pupil				
M	158.8	—	164.3	—
SD	37.3	—	36.5	—

Note. Information on gender (164 responders, 79 nonresponders), grade (169 responders, 79 nonresponders), location (165 responders, 79 nonresponders), size of school (167 responders, 79 nonresponders), or expenditures per pupil (137 responders, 63 nonresponders) was unavailable for some teachers.

Background Information and General Classroom Practices

Teachers were asked to provide information about number of years teaching, education, and composition of their class (i.e., class size, race of students, number of students who experience difficulty with spelling, number of students receiving special education services, and number of students receiving a free or reduced lunch). They were further asked to indicate how much time they spend teaching spelling, if they used a commercial spelling program, and if they expected students to master a list of spelling words each week. If teachers did use such a list, they were asked to indicate the source for the words on the list (i.e., commercial spelling program, basal reading series, children's reading material, students' writing, or student-selected words).

Teacher Adaptations

In the second section of the survey, we first asked teachers to indicate how many words stronger and weaker spellers studied each week. They were then asked to indicate how often they employed 20 specific spelling activities or practices, using a 7-point Likert-type scale. The Likert-type scale, developed by Pressley et al. (1996), included the following markers: 1 = *never*, 2 = *several times a year*, 3 = *monthly*, 4 = *weekly*, 5 = *several times a week*, 6 = *daily*, and 7 = *several times a day*. The higher the score, the more often an activity or procedure occurred. For each item, the respondent first indicated how often a particular activity or procedure was applied with stronger spellers and then how often it was applied with weaker spellers (this was done on separate scales). A difference between the treatment of weaker and stronger spellers was viewed as an adaptation, and such adaptation could involve providing more or less of an activity or instructional procedure to weaker spellers than stronger ones. Finally, respondents were asked to identify any additional adaptations that were provided to weaker spellers in their classroom beyond what they typically did with students. This provided teachers the opportunity to identify adaptations they were making that were not directly queried through the forced-response items.

The development of the second part of the survey involved six steps. First, we created a possible pool of items by identifying instructional practices used by teachers in previous research studying the teaching of spelling in the primary grades (e.g., Bridge, Compton-Hall, & Cantrell, 1997; S. Graham et al., 2003; Wharton-McDonald et al., 1998). Second, this was supplemented by examining current books and articles on the teaching of spelling (e.g., Bear, Invernizzi, Templeton, & Johnston, 2000; Gentry & Gillett, 1993; Moats, 1995) as well as reviews of the empirical literature on effective spelling practices for young children (e.g., S. Graham, 1999; Loomer et al., 1990). Third, a description of each instructional activity or procedure was developed, and we asked five primary-grade teachers to rate each item (using a 5-point Likert-type scale ranging from 1 point for *strongly disagree* to 5 points for *strongly agree*) on two dimensions: (a) primary-grade teachers typically use the activity or procedure and (b) the activity or procedure can be adapted to help weaker spellers. We included all items on our survey that had a mean of 4.0 on both dimensions, yielding 21 items. Fourth, we created an initial version of the survey, where one activity was answered by identifying the number of words stronger and weaker spellers study each week, and the other 20 items were answered via a Likert-type scale (see above). Fifth, we asked 3 primary-grade teachers to take the survey and record how long it took to complete it. They then reexamined the survey to provide suggestions for improving wording on specific items and the layout of the instrument. These suggestions were incorporated into a final version of the scale. Sixth, we examined the internal consistency of the 20 Likert-type items using the data from this study. Coefficient alpha was .83.

Five of the 21 activities or procedures asked teachers about their teaching of specific spelling skills and strategies (phonological awareness, phonics skills for spelling, strategies for determining the spelling of unknown words, spelling rules, and dictionary skills). With the exception of teaching dictionary skills, there is empirical evidence that all of these activities are effective with struggling spellers (see S. Graham, 1999; S. Graham et al., 2003). Twelve items focused on how frequently teachers applied the following instructional procedures: reduce number of words studied each week, reteach spelling skills and strategies, use games to learn spelling skills, have students work together to learn spelling skills, use word-sorting activities to teach knowledge about spelling, apply computer programs to teach spelling, praise students' correct spelling, apply reinforcement and other motivational strategies to foster spelling performance, conference with parents about their child's spelling, teach spelling skills and strategies through minilessons as the need arises, use mnemonics for remembering the spelling of a difficult word, and conference with students about their spelling. There is empirical evidence that the first nine procedures listed above enhance the performance of weaker spellers (S. Graham, 1999; S. Graham et al., 2003). The final four procedures focused on spelling during writing. This included students' use of spell checkers, encouragement to use invented spellings, proofreading to correct spelling errors, and providing students with feedback on words misspelled while writing. Each of these practices was effective with weaker spellers in one or more empirical studies (Gettinger, 1993; S. Graham, 1999).

Procedures

A cover letter, the survey instrument, and a stamped return envelope were mailed to each teacher during the month of March. The cover letter indicated that we were conducting a survey to gather information on the teaching of spelling and types of adaptations made by teachers. Teachers were asked to return materials in the next 2 weeks if possible. To encourage completion and return of the materials, we included a $2 bill in the package as a thank-you for taking the time to fill out and return the surveys.

Forty-nine percent of the teachers ($n = 122$) completed and returned the survey in the first mailing. The second mailing occurred during the 1st week of April and accounted for another 47 surveys (19%), bringing the grand total to 68%.

RESULTS

Missing Data

Examination of the responses of the 169 teachers indicated that 129 of them had some missing data, although actual percentage of data missing across all surveys was small (mode = 1% of data missing). However, preliminary analysis of the missing data indicated patterns within subjects and across items, suggesting that missing data were not random (e.g., some participants had more missing data than others). Due to the number of participants affected and systematic properties of the missing data, neither listwise deletion nor simple regression imputation was considered a proper remedy.

A multiple imputation of the missing values was completed using an expectation-maximization algorithm (see J. W. Graham & Hofer, 2000). After eliminating 1 outlying participant who was missing 81% of all data, the SPSS missing-values module was employed. This procedure uses all information in the data set to impute values for missing data for all remaining participants ($n = 168$). This enhanced our ability to calculate unbiased parameter estimates while preserving statistical power (J. W. Graham, Taylor, & Cumsille, 2001).

Analyses

First, we examined teachers' responses to the classroom practice questions as well as the Likert-type items assessing how often teachers reported applying 20 spelling activities and instructional practices with stronger and weaker spellers in order to draw a general picture of primary-grade spelling instruction. Next, we examined the types of adaptations teachers made for weaker spellers. This second focus took three forms. One, we examined if there was a difference in how often teachers reported using each of the 21 spelling activities or procedures with stronger and weaker spellers. For each spelling activity or procedure, a one-way ANOVA (with type of speller as the independent variable) was conducted. We reasoned that if teachers were making an adaptation for a specific activity or procedure, then the respective F ratio should be statistically significant. Because of the large number of analyses (21), we set the alpha level at .01. A more conservative probability level was not set to help avoid the possibility of committing a Type II error. Skewness was evident for a majority of these items, so we also conducted each analysis using a nonparametric procedure (Mann–Whitney U test). The outcomes for the nonparametric and parametric analyses were identical; thus, we report only the findings from the ANOVAs here.

Although we expected few if any differences in how often first-, second-, and third-grade teachers reported using the activities and procedures surveyed (as most spelling materials apply the same basic formats and activities in the primary grades; see, for example, Gentry, 2007), we did examine if teachers' reported use of a practice was related to grade taught. Practices such as teaching phonemic awareness and teaching phonics for spelling might be more common in the earlier grades as students are just starting to break the code, whereas the use of a dictionary as a spelling aid may be more common once students have acquired initial competence with spelling. We found only three instances where reported use of a practice was statistically related to grade taught (i.e., teaching phonological awareness, teaching phonics skills for spelling, and reteaching skills and strategies, with teachers indicating that they applied each practice more often with younger students). In no instance was there an interaction between grade and type of speller; thus, scores presented in subsequent sections are averaged across grades.

A second way teachers' reported adaptations were examined was by categorizing and tabulating responses to the open-ended question asking them to identify additional adaptations made for weaker spellers (see further discussion of categorization procedures below). We included in this analysis only adaptations not previously identified via the forced-response items.

Finally, we calculated total number of reported adaptations made by a teacher. This score was based on responses to the forced-response and the open-ended questions. Any time a teacher marked a different score for stronger versus weaker spellers on a forced-response item, it was counted as an adaptation. These adaptations were summed with the number of new adaptations identified from the open-ended question. We also examined if there was a relationship between total number of adaptations and grade taught, school location (urban, suburban, and rural), and years spent teaching.

Spelling Instruction in the Primary Grades

Virtually all of the teachers reported teaching spelling, devoting an average of almost 90 minutes a week to this skill (time spent teaching spelling was not related to grade taught; $p = .09$). This is more than the 60 to 75 minutes per week recommended in previous reviews of the experimental literature (see, for example, Loomer et al., 1990). Nevertheless, there was considerable variability in reported teaching time ($SD = 70.64$ minutes). In addition, 4 teachers did not teach spelling at all (scattered across all three grade levels), 1 teacher devoted 2 minutes a week to it, and another 10 teachers spent only 10 to 20 minutes teaching it.

A slight majority of teachers (57%) reported using commercial materials to teach some aspect of spelling. These teachers reported using a wide range of spelling programs, including stand-alone programs as well as ones that were part of a basal reading program. Whether they reported using a spelling program or not, most teachers (90%) indicated students were expected to master a list of spelling words each week. The sources for the words on these lists were varied and overlapped somewhat: 66% of teachers indicated that words came from spelling programs, 37% from basal readers, 30% from the material students read, 26% from students' compositions, and 14% from student self-selection.

Table 2 presents how often teachers applied (ranging from *never* to *several times a day*) each of the 20 spelling activities and practices assessed with a Likert-type scale (tabulated for both stronger and weaker spellers). Five out of the 6 responding teachers reported using all but 2 of these activities and procedures sometime during the school year. The other 2 procedures, computer programs as an aid for learning spelling words or skills and mnemonics as an aid for remembering difficult spellings, were used by 65% and 74% of teachers, respectively, at some point in the academic year. These data provide additional verification that the 20 spelling activities and procedures are common elements of primary-grade spelling instruction.

On at least a weekly basis, a majority of teachers reported applying 16 activities with either stronger or weaker writers. In order of frequency, these were praise for correct spelling (94%), teaching phonics skills for spelling (92%), instruction in phonological awareness (88%), minilessons to teach spelling skills and strategies (86%), teacher feedback on misspellings (84%), using spelling games to teach skills and strategies (83%), spelling rules instruction (83%), encouraging invented spellings (80%), teaching strategies for spelling unknown words (77%), conferencing with students about their spelling (77%), student use of spell checkers (76%), students helping each other with spelling (76%), student proofreading theirs and others' compositions (71%), reteaching spelling skills and strategies (70%), reinforcement and motivational strategies to teach spelling (63%), and using word sorting to teach spelling (55%).

At least monthly, a majority of teachers reported teaching dictionary skills (62%) and using mnemonics as a way to help students remember difficult spelling words (56%). At least several times a year, most teachers indicated conferencing with parents about their child's spelling (92%) and using

TABLE 2. How Often Primary-Grade Teachers Reported Using Specific Spelling Activities and Instructional Procedures

Spelling Activity or Instructional Procedure	Mean	Standard Deviation	Never (%)	Several Times a Year (%)	Monthly (%)	Weekly (%)	Several Times a Week (%)	Daily (%)	Several Times a Day (%)
Teach Specific Skills/Strategies									
Phonological awareness									
Stronger speller	4.83	1.29	1	5	7	22	29	31	5
Weaker speller	4.97	1.25	1	5	7	18	30	33	7
Phonics for spelling									
Stronger speller	4.82	1.35	3	5	4	26	27	30	6
Weaker speller	4.99	1.29	3	3	2	23	29	33	7
Strategies to spell unknown words									
Stronger speller	4.32	1.48	4	12	9	28	23	21	4
Weaker speller	4.45	1.50	4	10	9	26	24	21	6
Spelling rules									
Stronger speller	4.17	1.18	2	7	10	46	23	10	2
Weaker speller	4.21	1.21	3	7	9	45	23	13	2
Dictionary skills									
Stronger speller	3.11	1.35	10	29	20	29	7	4	2
Weaker speller	3.09	1.35	10	29	21	29	6	4	2
Instructional Activities									
Minilessons									
Stronger speller	4.55	1.38	2	8	7	27	27	24	4
Weaker speller	4.88	1.33	2	5	7	20	30	29	7
Reteaching[a]									
Stronger speller	3.71	1.27	2	18	23	29	21	5	1
Weaker speller	4.07	1.25	1	13	16	30	30	8	2
Spelling games									
Stronger speller	3.59	1.41	2	7	10	46	23	10	2
Weaker speller	3.68	1.43	3	7	9	45	23	13	2
Students work together									
Stronger speller	3.94	1.45	9	8	10	42	18	10	3
Weaker speller	4.00	1.48	10	7	9	41	20	11	4
Word sorting									
Stronger speller	3.29	1.49	17	16	17	27	19	5	0
Weaker speller	3.39	1.47	16	13	16	30	20	5	0
Computer to learn spelling									
Stronger speller	2.60	1.50	35	20	13	22	5	5	1
Weaker speller	2.70	1.60	34	18	12	23	8	5	1
Praise students for correct spelling									
Stronger speller	5.26	1.26	0	4	2	21	21	34	16
Weaker speller	5.41	1.26	0	3	2	23	21	31	22
Use mnemonics for hard words									
Stronger speller	2.95	1.62	26	19	14	23	13	4	2
Weaker speller	3.02	1.68	26	19	14	20	14	7	1
Reinforcement or motivation strategies to promote spelling									
Stronger speller	3.70	1.56	13	14	10	36	14	12	2
Weaker speller	3.79	1.58	11	15	8	34	18	12	2
Conferencing with students[a]									
Stronger speller	3.31	1.51	17	16	14	32	15	5	1
Weaker speller	4.18	1.45	6	10	9	32	28	13	4
Parent conferences[a]									
Stronger speller	1.99	0.68	17	72	5	6	0	0	0
Weaker speller	2.29	079	8	68	12	11	1	0	0

(cont.)

TABLE 2. *(cont.)*

Spelling Activity or Instructional Procedure	Mean	Standard Deviation	Never (%)	Several Times a Year (%)	Monthly (%)	Weekly (%)	Several Times a Week (%)	Daily (%)	Several Times a Day (%)
Spelling When Writing									
Students use spell checkers									
Stronger speller	2.11	1.66	4	12	9	28	23	21	4
Weaker speller	2.11	1.66	4	10	9	26	24	21	6
Encourage invented spelling									
Stronger speller	4.74	1.84	11	5	4	19	14	35	13
Weaker speller	4.72	1.85	11	6	4	18	14	36	12
Student proofreading									
Stronger speller	4.20	1.40	5	6	18	30	20	19	2
Weaker speller	4.20	1.38	4	7	17	30	23	18	2
Teacher feedback on misspellings									
Stronger speller	4.80	1.40	3	3	10	25	23	29	8
Weaker speller	4.78	1.41	3	3	10	27	21	26	10

Note. never = score of 1; *several times a year* = score of 2; *monthly* = score of 3; *weekly* = score of 4; *several times a week* = score of 5; *daily* = score of 6; *several times a day* = score of 7.
[a]Statistically significant difference between stronger and weaker writers ($p < .01$).

computer programs to help students learn spelling words and skills (82%).

Spelling Adaptations: From Forced-Choice Items

Table 2 presents means and standard deviations for stronger and weaker spellers for the 20 spelling activities and practices assessed via Likert-type scales. Because weaker spellers, by definition, experience difficulty mastering the task of spelling, we anticipated that teachers would provide more support and instruction to these students than to the stronger spellers in their classrooms. For the most part, this prediction was not supported by our analyses of the forced-response items, as only 3 of the 20 analyses were statistically significant. In contrast to stronger spellers, teachers reported conferencing more often with the parents of weaker spellers, $F(1, 334) = 29.00$; $MSe = 2.18$, $p < .001$ (Cohen's $d = .57$); conferencing more often with weaker spellers, $F(334) = 13.11$; $MSe = 55$, $p < .001$ (Cohen's $d = .40$); and reteaching skills and strategies to these students, $F(334) = 6.70$; $MSe = 1.58$, $p = .009$ (Cohen's $d = .28$).

There was also a statistically significant difference for the item that asked teachers to indicate how many words they assigned to weekly spelling lists for stronger and weaker spellers, $F(1, 334) = 54.05$; $MSe = 31.44$, $p < .001$ (Cohen's $d = .75$). Weaker spellers were assigned fewer words ($M = 10.3$; $SD = 4.3$) than stronger spellers ($M = 14.8$; $SD = 6.7$).

Additional Adaptations Identified Through the Open-Ended Question

Teacher responses to the open-ended question asking them to identify additional adaptations made for weaker spellers were tabulated and categorized by type. Excluded from this tabulation were any responses that named an adaptation already evident from the forced-response items (e.g., if a teacher wrote, "I provide extra time teaching spelling rules," and conjointly marked a different Likert score for stronger and weaker spellers on the question that specifically asked about teaching spelling rules, the open-ended response was not counted as an adaptation).

In total, 109 of the respondents (65%) provided 294 potential adaptations when responding to the open-ended question. Of these, 190 were determined to be unique. These 190 unique adaptations were then sorted into categories. This process involved two steps. First, the first two authors read through all responses and identified 10 categories that captured the range of teacher responses. These categories were tutoring (from the teacher, another adult, or a peer), computer activities, modified spelling lists, modified procedures for teaching spelling words (flash cards, games, modified regular curricula addressing spelling, multiple minitests, brainstorming), spelling aids for writing (memory facilitation, lists of common words, personal lists of misspelled words), phonics or phonological awareness (explicit phonics, sound-based word games), homework or family connection (all activities sent home regardless of person implementing at home), additional materials (general dictionaries, unique materials not specific to phonics), and test modifications (additional time, preparation time, retesting, and test-scoring modifications not including motivational strategies related to test results).

Next, the second author categorized all responses using the categories just described. To establish reliability of the second author's scoring, 31% ($n = 32$) of teacher's responses (selected randomly) was independently rescored by a second rater. Reliability using Cohen's kappa for number of unique adaptations was .87 and .83 for the categorization of these unique adaptations.

The most frequent additional reported adaptation was tutoring or one-to-one help (32% of responses). This was followed by adaptations involving modified teaching procedures (24%). The next three most frequent adaptations focused on teaching phonics and phonological awareness to weaker spellers (11%), modifying the spelling lists (8%), and modifying homework assignments (8%). Less frequent adaptations included using spelling aids for writing (6%), modifying testing procedures (6%), using the computer to aid spelling (3%), and using additional spelling materials (2%). Only 1% of adaptations were classified as other.

Total Number of Adaptations

Total number of reported adaptations made by each teacher was calculated by summing (a) the number of forced-response items where a different score was marked for stronger and weaker spellers and (b) the number of additional adaptations obtained through our analyses of the open-ended question. For all teachers, the average number of adaptations from these two sources was 3.7. Number of reported adaptations was not significantly related to grade taught ($p = .07$) or to whether teachers worked in an urban, suburban, or rural district ($p = .11$). There also was no statistically significant relation between reported total adaptations and number of years spent teaching ($r = -.11$) or teachers' estimates of how many of their students experienced spelling problems ($r = -.05$). It is important to note that there was considerable variability in total reported adaptations, as the standard deviation was large when compared to the mean ($SD = 3.2$). When all adaptations were summed together

(forced response and open-ended), 42% ($n = 70$) of the teachers reported making just 0 to 2 adaptations. Considered differently, a total of 629 adaptations were reported by all teachers, and of these adaptations, 67% ($n = 422$) were accounted for by just 24% of teachers ($n = 41$).

DISCUSSION

Do Primary-Grade Teachers Teach Spelling and How Do They Teach It?

Although this study mainly focused on primary-grade teachers' adaptations for struggling writers, it also yielded important information on how spelling is taught to young children nationwide. There are little data available on contemporary spelling practices with young children. Consistent with two other recent surveys (Cutler & Graham, in press; S. Graham et al., 2003) and our prediction, virtually all of the primary-grade teachers in this study reported teaching spelling. Only 2% of the teachers reported not teaching spelling at all, and slightly more than 90% indicated that they taught spelling for at least 25 minutes per week. Thus, with the exception of a few participants, enough time was devoted to teaching spelling to allow teachers the opportunity to make adaptations for weaker spellers.

As a group, the participating teachers indicated that they spend 90 minutes a week teaching spelling. This exceeds the average of 60 minutes reported by primary-grade teachers in Cutler and Graham (in press) as well as the traditional recommendation, based on studies that manipulated teaching time (see Loomer et al., 1990), that 60 to 75 minutes a week should be devoted to teaching this skill. However, in both this and the Cutler and Graham (in press) investigation, there was considerable variability in reported teaching time. It is important to note that there was a sizable minority of teachers in this study (45%) who spent less than the empirically supported recommendation for teaching spelling, 60 to 75 minutes a week.

Although the present study did not query teachers on all possible aspects of their spelling instruction, the findings from the current study were consistent with our prediction that primary-grade spelling instruction is multifaceted, involving the teaching of a variety of skills as well as the application of many different activities and instructional procedures. In fact, there was considerable consistency in teachers' reports on how they taught spelling, with many activities and instructional procedures applied by 70% or more of the teachers at least weekly. This included students learning a new list of words each week and the teaching of phonological awareness, phonics for spelling, spelling rules, and strategies for spelling unknown words. Likewise, teachers reported providing minilessons, employing peer learning activities, and using games at least weekly to help students acquire new spelling words and skills. Teachers indicated they frequently praised students for correct spelling, provided feedback on the words children misspelled, and held conferences with students about their spellings. They also reported encouraging students to use invented spellings, spell checkers, and proofreading at least weekly. There is experimental research evidence that all but two of these practices enhance the spelling performance of students in general and struggling spellers in particular (see reviews by S. Graham, 1983, 1999; S. Graham & Miller, 1979; Loomer et al., 1990; Wanzek et al., 2006). Such evidence is not available for conferencing with students and teaching minilessons as the need arises (neither of these techniques has been tested empirically).

Three other evidence-based practices (see S. Graham, 1999; Loomer et al., 1990) were applied by 50% of the teachers on a weekly basis. These were reteaching skills and strategies, word sorting, and reinforcement or other motivational strategies. In contrast, teachers reported that they applied the following two research-supported practices (see review by S. Graham, 1999) infrequently: (a) computer programs to teach spelling and (b) conferencing with parents. The primary-grade teachers in S. Graham et al. (2003) also indicated that they rarely used computers during the writing period. This infrequent use of computer technology is troubling and deserves further study.

Even though the majority of teachers reported that they frequently used a variety of research-supported practices to teach spelling, it is important to note that they also indicated that 27% of their students, on average, experienced difficulty with spelling. Thus, according to their estimates, there was a sizable proportion of students for whom their spelling instruction was not effective. One possible reason for why this was the case is that teachers may not apply these research-supported practices effectively—in the same way they were applied in the studies validating their effectiveness. It is also possible that the participating teachers combined these practices together in ways that reduced their

effectiveness or placed too much emphasis on one procedure and not enough on another. We did not assess either of these possibilities, as the available research does not provide enough evidence to establish clear guidelines for how practices should be combined or if the practices we assessed are differentially effective. Because we did not conduct a comprehensive survey of all instructional practices in spelling, including research-validated procedures, such as the test-study-test method or the corrected-test method, for example (see S. Graham, 1983), it is further possible that teachers did not apply a number of important instructional procedures when teaching spelling, reducing the overall effectiveness of their efforts. Last, it is possible that teachers' knowledge of English orthography and spelling was incomplete, and this may have hampered the impact of their instruction (see Moats, 1995). Future research needs to examine a broader array of spelling practices, including additional research-supported procedures as well as the linkage between the use of such practices, teachers' knowledge, and spelling achievement.

Our findings further provide some insight into primary-grade teachers' theoretical orientations to spelling instruction. Very few of them appeared to embrace only a spelling-is-caught orientation, as almost all of them spent some time teaching children how to spell. Moreover, at least 2 out of every 3 teachers reported applying procedures that were consistent with two of the spelling-is-taught approaches: memorization (students learned a list of spelling words each week) and generalization (i.e., teaching phonemic awareness, phonics skills for spelling, spelling rules, and strategies for spelling unknown words). In addition, 50% of them reported applying an activity (i.e., word sorting) that is commonly used as a tool in the third spelling-is-taught approach, developmental (Schlagel, 2007). As predicted, most primary-grade teachers' spelling instruction embraced multiple perspectives. However, additional research is needed to determine how much emphasis teachers also place on the spelling-is-caught approach. None of the items in this study provided data relevant to this orientation.

Do Primary Grade Teachers Adapt Instruction for Weaker Spellers?

On the basis of the S. Graham et al. (2003) investigation with writing, we expected that the primary-grade teachers in this study would report adapting their instruction for weaker spellers, but most of the reported adaptations would be made by a small percentage of teachers, with a sizable minority of teachers reporting few or no adaptations (0 to 2). These expectations were confirmed, as teachers as a group averaged 3.7 reported adaptations, but two thirds of these adaptations were made by just one fourth of the teachers, with 42% of teachers making virtually no adaptations. These figures are almost identical to S. Graham et al. (2003). Thus, only 1 in 4 teachers was highly sensitive to the needs of weaker spellers, whereas close to one half of them reported making few or no adjustments for these children.

Of the 21 spelling activities and procedures that were directly assessed in our survey, teachers reported making adaptations for only four: the number of words studied each week (fewer words with weaker spellers), how frequently teachers held conferences about spelling with both students and their parents (more often for weaker spellers and their parents), and how often they retaught spelling skills and strategies (more often with weaker spellers). With the exception of conferencing with students (which has not been tested experimentally), all three of these adaptations have improved the spelling performance of struggling spellers in one or more research studies (see S. Graham, 1999). It must be noted, however, that there was little practical difference between how often teachers reported reteaching skills and strategies and conferencing with parents of weaker and stronger spellers.

In contrast to S. Graham et al. (2003), primary-grade teachers in this study did not report encouraging the use of invented spelling more often with weaker than stronger students, nor did they report spending more time teaching phonics for spelling or strategies for spelling unknown words to weaker students. These differences did not appear to be related to how often teachers in the two studies emphasized each of these practices in their classroom, as all three were used frequently and at a similar rate in both investigations. The differences may be a consequence of how the items were worded (weaker "writers" in Graham et al., 2003, and weaker "spellers" in this study), reflect differences in who participated in the two studies, or represent a change in practices over time. Additional research is needed to resolve these discrepancies.

As in the S. Graham et al. (2003) investigations, teachers in this study generated a broad list of additional modifications when asked to describe other modifications they made for weaker spellers. On average, the teachers reported making one additional adaptation beyond what was directly assessed (39% of participants, however, did not report any additional adaptations). The most common other adaptation reported by respondents was the use of tutoring by the teacher, another adult, or a peer. This category accounted for one third of all additional adaptations (26% of all additional adaptations in S. Graham et al., 2003, involved tutoring). One fourth of the other reported adaptations involved modifying procedures for teaching spelling words. This was followed by adaptations in the teaching of phonics and phonemic awareness (11%), modifying the weekly spelling list (8%), assigning homework and making family connections (8%), supplying spelling aids for writing (6%), and modifying spelling tests (6%). Unfortunately, teachers rarely provided enough information about these additional adaptations for us to form judgments about their quality or effectiveness.

An important question raised by this study is why a sizable minority of teachers (42%) reported making few or no adaptations for weaker spellers. One possible reason was that they believed that their spelling program was so effective that adaptations were not needed. We think that this is an unlikely explanation, as teachers who provided two or fewer adaptations indicated that 29% of their students had difficulty with spelling.

It is also possible that these teachers did not view adaptations as particularly valuable and, consequently, were not willing to expend the energy needed to adjust their instruction for weaker spellers. A recent study by S. Graham, Papadopoulou, and Santoro (2006) provides some support for this contention. They examined the acceptability of the writing adaptations primary teachers reported employing in the S. Graham et al. (2003) investigation. Teachers were asked to rate each adaptation on five dimensions: effectiveness, suitability for struggling writers, possible negative impacts, their knowledge of how to implement, and time needed to implement. After controlling for teacher experience, class size, teacher efficacy, percentage of students with writing difficulties, and percentage of students with special needs, they found that these five dimensions accounted for 29% of the variability in teachers' reported use of 14 different adaptations. Thus, teachers were more likely to report making adaptations for struggling writers if they viewed writing modifications as acceptable. Future research needs to examine if these same factors influence teachers' reported and observed use of spelling adaptations.

Another possible reason why some teachers reported making few or no adaptations involves their knowledge about English orthography and spelling and how to teach this complex skill. Some teachers may feel that they do not know enough about spelling to risk modifying how they teach it. Unfortunately, we did not ask teachers about their prior preparation to teach spelling, nor did we try to determine the depth of their knowledge about spelling. Several recent national surveys, however, have asked teachers about their preparedness to teach other aspects of writing. Eighty-eight percent of the primary-grade teachers in S. Graham et al. (2008) reported that they did not receive adequate preparation in their teacher preparation programs to teach handwriting. Likewise, 71% of the participating high school teachers in Kiuhara, Graham, and Hawkin (2008) indicated they received minimal to no preparation to teach writing during college, and 44% continued to report the same level of preparation when in-service and personal learning efforts were included too. Clearly, additional research is needed to assess teachers' preparedness to teach spelling and their knowledge about it, as the studies cited above suggest that many teachers are not adequately prepared to teach writing or its component skills.

Limitations and Assumptions

The present study was based on the assumption that primary-grade teachers would be aware of the elements of their teaching and would be able to relate this knowledge to questions about their teaching practices in the area of spelling, just as other professionals can relate what they do when queried about their actions (Diaper, 1989). Although these findings must be supplemented by research where teachers' practices and adaptations are observed and not just reported, it is important to note that other survey studies querying teachers about their literacy practices are corroborated by observations of these same teachers' classroom instruction (see, for instance, Bridge & Hiebert, 1985; DeFord, 1985).

We also assumed that effective instruction for weaker spellers involves adapting instruction. This assumption would be less valid if the instructional programs used by teachers were so powerful that each child developed the spelling skills needed for success at her or his grade level. This is an improbable scenario, however, as there is no documentation that such a spelling program actually exists, and participating teachers indicated that 27% of their students experienced difficulties with spelling.

When we queried teachers about their use of selected activities and procedures with weaker and stronger spellers, it was tacitly assumed that an important dimension in providing instruction to young, struggling spellers involves adjusting the frequency or quantity of specific aspects of instruction. Although this assumption requires additional validation, providing extra spelling instruction to weaker spellers can boost these children's spelling performance (see Berninger et al., 1998; S. Graham et al., 2003).

Although the number of teachers who completed our survey and were included in the data analysis (168) was slightly less than the number (174) we estimated that we needed to have an adequate sample (see Method), this had a minimal impact on the confidence that can be placed in our findings (sampling error is now 5.1% instead of 5%). Although sampling error could have been reduced with a larger sample, the sampling error is well within acceptable ranges for survey research (Dillman, 2000). Moreover, it would have required a large increase in participants to significantly reduce sampling error in this study. For example, a plus- or minus-1% sampling error in this investigation would require a 25-fold increase to 4,317 teachers sampled.

Last, it was possible that the procedures used to query teachers did not capture all of their adaptations. The forced-response questions did not cover all possible adaptations, and although we asked an open-ended question in order to obtain a more complete account, some teachers may still have failed to provide a full record. For instance, some adaptations may not have been identified because the teacher did not remember making them. Future research can address this problem, at least in part, by asking additional questions, applying direct observation, or using a combination of the two.

In summary, the findings from this study indicated that virtually all primary-grade teachers teach spelling, with the vast majority of them implementing a complex and multifaceted instructional program that uses a variety of research-supported procedures. In addition, some teachers are sensitive to the needs of weaker spellers, making a variety of adaptations for these students. A sizable minority of teachers, however, reported making few or no adaptations. Equally troubling was the finding that teachers indicated 27% of their students experienced difficulty with spelling, calling into question the effectiveness of their instruction.

APPENDIX QUESTIONNAIRE

Dear Colleague,

We know very little about how teachers teach spelling and the types of adaptations they make for different children in their classrooms. To find out more about these topics, the Center to Accelerate Student Learning at the University of Maryland is conducting a survey with teachers from across the United States. **I would like to ask you to complete the attached questionnaire, and return it in the enclosed self-addressed stamped envelope. Please return the questionnaire in the next two weeks if at all possible.** You should be able to complete the questionnaire in 15 to 30 minutes. I have attached a $2 dollar bill to the survey, to say thank you for completing the questionnaire. Thank you for taking the time to complete and return the questionnaire.

Section 1: Please complete the following questions

1. How many years have you taught? _____ What grade(s) do you currently teach? _____
2. Please check your highest educational level: _____ Bachelor _____ Masters _____ Doctoral
3. How many children are in your classroom? _____
4. How many children in your classroom receive a free or reduced lunch? _____
5. How many of the children in your classroom are: _____ Asian _____ Black _____ Hispanic _____ White _____ Other
6. How many of the children in your classroom receive special education services? _____
7. How many children in your class experience difficulty with spelling? _____
8. During an average week, how many minutes do you spend **teaching** spelling? _____
9. Do you use a commercial program to teach spelling? _____ Yes _____ No
   What program(s)? _____
10. Do students in your class study lists of spelling words? _____ Yes _____ No
    If **yes**, please answer the following question:
    Please check the source or sources for students' spelling words. _____ Spelling Series _____ Basal Reader _____ Children's Reading Material _____ Students' Writing _____ Student Selected   Other: _____
    _____

Section 2: If you answered yes to question 10 above, please answer the 2 questions below:

1. During an average week, how many words are studied by good spellers? _____
   How many words are studied by weaker spellers? _____

Please place a check on the item that indicates how often you do the following.

2. Check how often you **conference with students** about their spelling.

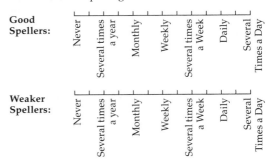

3. Check how often you provide **spelling minilessons** on "things" students need to know right now—skills, words, rules, strategies, or whatever.

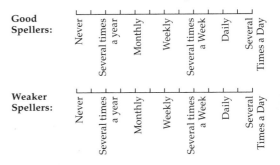

4. Check how often you **reteach** spelling skills or strategies that were previously taught.

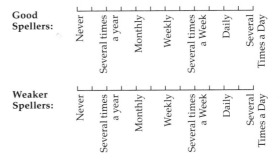

5. Check how often your students use a **spell checker**.

Good Spellers:

Never | Several times a year | Monthly | Weekly | Several times a Week | Daily | Several Times a Day

Weaker Spellers:

Never | Several times a year | Monthly | Weekly | Several times a Week | Daily | Several Times a Day

6. Check how often you teach **strategies for spelling unknown words** (e.g., writing a word out to see if it looks right, sounding it out, using a known word to help spell an unknown one, etc).

Good Spellers:

Never | Several times a year | Monthly | Weekly | Several times a Week | Daily | Several Times a Day

Weaker Spellers:

Never | Several times a year | Monthly | Weekly | Several times a Week | Daily | Several Times a Day

7. Check how often you teach **phonics for spelling**.

Good Spellers:

Never | Several times a year | Monthly | Weekly | Several times a Week | Daily | Several Times a Day

Weaker Spellers:

Never | Several times a year | Monthly | Weekly | Several times a Week | Daily | Several Times a Day

8. Check how often you encourage students to use **invented spellings**.

Good Spellers:

Never | Several times a year | Monthly | Weekly | Several times a Week | Daily | Several Times a Day

Weaker Spellers:

Never | Several times a year | Monthly | Weekly | Several times a Week | Daily | Several Times a Day

9. Check how often you teach **phonological awareness skills** (such as rhyming, identifying the individual sounds in a word, deleting or adding sounds in a word, substituting one sound for another in a word, and so forth).

Good Spellers:

Never | Several times a year | Monthly | Weekly | Several times a Week | Daily | Several Times a Day

Weaker Spellers:

Never | Several times a year | Monthly | Weekly | Several times a Week | Daily | Several Times a Day

10. Check how often your students **use games** to learn spelling words or skills.

Good Spellers:

Never | Several times a year | Monthly | Weekly | Several times a Week | Daily | Several Times a Day

Weaker Spellers:

Never | Several times a year | Monthly | Weekly | Several times a Week | Daily | Several Times a Day

11. Check how often **students work together** to learn spelling words or skills.

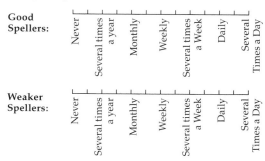

Good Spellers:

Never | Several times a year | Monthly | Weekly | Several times a Week | Daily | Several Times a Day

Weaker Spellers:

Never | Several times a year | Monthly | Weekly | Several times a Week | Daily | Several Times a Day

12. Check how often students in your class do **word sorting** activities (such as sorting words into different piles based on their spelling patterns, the sounds they begin or end with, and so forth).

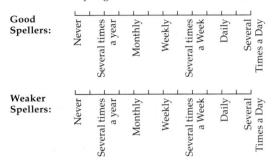

13. Check how often you **conference with parents** about their children's spelling.

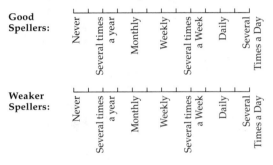

14. Check how often you teach **dictionary skills** for spelling.

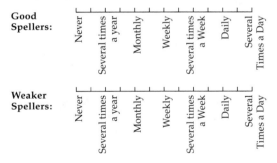

15. Check how often your students use the **computer** to help them learn new words or spelling skills.

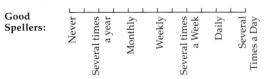

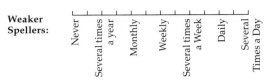

16. Check how often you use **reinforcement or other motivational strategies** to promote spelling.

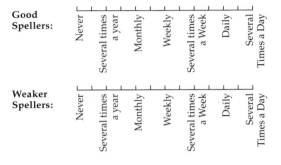

17. Check how often students are taught **spelling rules**.

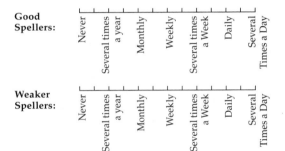

18. Check how often students **proofread** their writing or the writing of others to correct spelling errors.

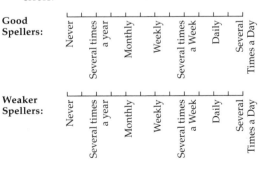

19. Check how often you teach students to use a **mnemonic** for remembering how to spell a difficult word.

Good Spellers:

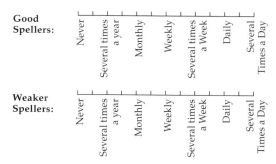

Weaker Spellers:

20. Check how often you **show (circle, underline, etc.)** students the words that are misspelled in their writing.

Good Spellers:

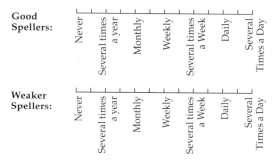

Weaker Spellers:

21. Check how often you **praise** students for correct spelling.

Good Spellers:

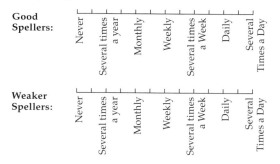

Weaker Spellers:

What types of **additional assistance/instruction** do you provide to students who are weaker spellers? **This is beyond what you typically do with students.** List as many examples as you can.

REFERENCES

Adams, M. (1990). *Beginning to read: Thinking and learning about print*. Cambridge, MA: MIT Press.

Baker, J., & Zigmond, N. (1990). Are regular education classes equipped to accommodate students with learning disabilities. *Exceptional Children, 56*, 515–526.

Bear, D., Invernizzi, M., Templeton, S., & Johnston, F.

(2000). *Words their way: Word study for phonics, vocabulary, and spelling instruction*. Upper Saddle River, NJ: Merrill.

Berninger, V. (1999). Coordinating transcription and text generation in working memory during composing: Automatic and constructive processes. *Learning Disability Quarterly, 22*, 99–112.

Berninger, V., Mizokawa, D., & Bragg, R. (1991). Theory-based diagnosis and remediation of writing disabilities. *Journal of School Psychology, 29*, 57–79.

Berninger, V., Vaughn, K., Abbott, R., Brooks, A., Abbott, S., Rogan, L., et al. (1998). A multiple connections approach to early intervention for spelling problems: Integrating instructional, learner and stimulus variables. *Journal of Educational Psychology, 90*, 587–605.

Bridge, C. A., Compton-Hall, M., & Cantrell, S. C. (1997). Classroom writing practices revisited: The effects of statewide reform on writing instruction. *Elementary School Journal, 98*, 151–170.

Bridge, C. A., & Hiebert, E. H. (1985). A comparison of classroom writing practices, teachers' perceptions of their writing instruction, and textbook recommendations on writing practices. *Elementary School Journal, 86*, 155–172.

Corno, L., & Snow, R. (1986). Adapting teaching to differences among individual learners. In M. Wittrock (Ed.), *Third handbook of research on teaching* (pp. 605–629). New York: Macmillan.

Cutler, L., & Graham, S. (in press). Primary grade writing instruction: A national survey. *Journal of Educational Psychology*.

DeFord, D. (1985). Validating the construct of theoretical orientation in reading. *Reading Research Quarterly, 20*, 351–367.

Diaper, D. (1989). *Knowledge elicitation: Principles, techniques, and application*. New York: Wiley.

Dillman, D. (2000). *Mail and internet surveys*. New York: Wiley.

Ehri, L. (1987). Learning to read and spell words. *Journal of Reading Behavior, 19*, 5–31.

Fuchs, L., & Fuchs, D. (1998). General educators' instructional adaptations for students with learning disabilities. *Learning Disability Quarterly, 21*, 23–33.

Gentry, R. (2007). *Spelling connections*. Columbus, OH: Zaner-Bloser.

Gentry, R., & Gillett, W. (1993). *Teaching kids to spell*. Portsmouth, NH: Heinemann.

Gettinger, M. (1993). The effects of invented spelling and direct instruction on spelling performance of second-grade boys. *Journal of Applied Behavior Analysis, 26*, 281–291.

Graham, J. W., & Hofer, S. M. (2000). Multiple imputation in multivariate research. In T. D. Little, K. U. Schnabel, & J. Baumert (Eds.), *Modeling longitudinal and multilevel data: Practical issues, applied approaches, and specific examples* (pp. 201–218). Mahwah, NJ: Erlbaum.

Graham, J. W., Taylor, B. J., & Cumsille, P. E. (2001). Planned missing-data designs in analysis of change. In L. M. Collins & A. G. Sayer (Eds.), *New methods for the analysis of change* (pp. 335–353). Washington, DC: American Psychological Association.

Graham, S. (1983). Effective spelling instruction. *Elementary School Journal, 83,* 560–567.

Graham, S. (1999). Handwriting and spelling instruction for students with learning disabilities: A review. *Learning Disability Quarterly, 22,* 78–98.

Graham, S. (2000). Should the natural learning approach replace traditional spelling instruction. *Journal of Educational Psychology, 92,* 235–247.

Graham, S., & Harris, K. R. (2002). Prevention and intervention for struggling writers. In M. Shinn, G. Stoner, & H. Walker (Eds.), *Interventions for academic and behavior problems II: Preventive and remedial approaches* (pp. 589–610). Bethesda, MD: National Association of School Psychologists.

Graham, S., & Harris, K. R. (2005, February). *The impact of handwriting and spelling instruction on the writing and reading performance of at-risk first grade writers.* Presentation at Pacific Coast Research Conference, San Diego, CA.

Graham, S., Harris, K. R., & Fink-Chorzempa, B. (2002). Contributions of spelling instruction to the spelling, writing, and reading of poor spellers. *Journal of Educational Psychology, 94,* 669–686.

Graham, S., Harris, K. R., Fink-Chorzempa, B., & MacArthur, C. (2003). Primary grade teachers' instructional adaptations for struggling writers: A national survey. *Journal of Educational Psychology, 95,* 279–292.

Graham, S., Harris, K. R., Mason, L., Fink-Chorzempa, B., Moran, S., & Saddler, B. (2008). How do primary grade teachers teach handwriting: A national survey. *Reading and Writing: An Interdisciplinary Journal, 21,* 49–69.

Graham, S., & Miller, L. (1979). Spelling research and practice: A unified approach. *Focus on Exceptional Children, 12,* 1–16.

Graham, S., Papadopoulou, E., & Santoro, J. (2006, April). *Acceptability of writing adaptations and modifications in writing: A national survey.* Paper presented at the International Conference of the Council for Exceptional Children, Salt Lake City, UT.

Kiuhara, S., Graham, S., & Hawkin, L. (2008). *Teaching writing to high school students: A national survey.* Manuscript submitted for publication.

Loomer, B., Fitzsimmons, R., & Strege, M. (1990). *Spelling research and practice: Teacher's edition.* Iowa City, IA: Useful Learning.

Marshall, J. C. (1967). Writing neatness, composition errors, and essay grades. *American Educational Research Journal, 4,* 375–385.

Marshall, J. C., & Powers, J. M. (1969). Writing neatness, composition errors, and essay grades. *Journal of Educational Measurement, 6*(2), 97–101.

McCutchen, D. (1988). "Functional automaticity" in children's writing: A problem of metacognitive control. *Written Communication, 5,* 306–324.

Moats, L. (1995). *Spelling: Development, disability, and instruction.* Baltimore: York.

Moats, L. (2005/2006). How spelling supports reading: And why it is more regular and predictable than you may think. *American Educator,* Winter, 12–43.

Phillips, N., Fuchs, L., Fuchs, D., & Hamlett, C. (1996).

Instructional variables affecting student achievement: Case studies of two contrasting teachers. *Learning Disabilities Research and Practice, 11,* 24–33.

Pressley, M., Rankin, J., & Yokoi, L. (1996). A survey of instructional practices of primary grade teachers nominated as effective in promoting literacy. *Elementary School Journal, 96,* 363–384.

Randi, J., & Corno, L. (2005). Teaching and learner variation. *British Journal of Educational Psychology, 2,* 47–69.

Scardamalia, M., & Bereiter, C. (1986). Written composition. In M. Wittrock (Ed.), *Handbook of research on teaching* (3rd ed., pp. 778–803). New York: Macmillan.

Schlagel, B. (2007). Best practices in spelling and handwriting. In S. Graham, C. MacArthur, & J. Fitzgerald (Eds.), *Best practices in writing instruction* (pp. 179–201). New York: Guilford Press.

Schumm, J. S., & Vaughn, S. (1991). Making adaptations for mainstreamed students: General classroom teachers' perspectives. *Remedial and Special Education, 12,* 18–27.

Stallings, J. (1995). Ensuring teaching and learning in the 21st century. *Educational Researcher, 24,* 4–8.

Tobias, S. (1995). Interest and metacognitive word knowledge. *Journal of Educational Psychology, 87,* 399–405.

Treiman, R. (1993). *Beginning to spell.* New York: Oxford University Press.

Wanzek, J., Vaughn, S., Wexler, J., Swanson, E. A., Edmonds, M., & Kim, A.-H. (2006). A synthesis of spelling and reading interventions and their effects on the spelling outcomes of students with LD. *Journal of Learning Disabilities, 39,* 528–543.

Wharton-McDonald, R., Pressley, M., & Hampston, J. M. (1998). Literacy instruction in nine first-grade classrooms: Teacher characteristics and student achievement. *Elementary School Journal, 99,* 101–128.

STEVE GRAHAM is Currey Ingram Professor of Special Education and Literacy at Vanderbilt University, Department of Special Education, Peabody #328, 230 Appleton Place, Nashville, TN 37203-5721; e-mail: *steve.graham@vanderbilt.edu.* His research interests are writing, self-regulation, and learning disabilities.

PAUL MORPHY is a doctoral student in special education at Vanderbilt University, Department of Special Education, Peabody #328, 230 Appleton Place, Nashville, TN 37203-5721; e-mail: *paul.morphy@ vanderbilt.edu.* His research interests are statistical analysis, meta-analysis, writing, and reading.

KAREN R. HARRIS is Currey Ingram Professor in Special Education and Literacy at Vanderbilt University, Department of Special Education, Peabody #328, 230 Appleton Place, Nashville, TN 37203-5721; e-mail: *karen.harris@vanderbilt.edu.* Her research interests are strategy instruction, self-regulation, writing, and learning disabilities.

BARBARA FINK-CHORZEMPA is an assistant professor in the Department of Educational Studies, State University of New York-New Paltz, 1 Hawk Drive, New Paltz, NY 12561; e-mail: *chorzembumeuipaltz. edu*. Her research interests are reading, writing, and learning disabilities.

BRUCE SADDLER is an assistant professor of educational psychology and statistics at the University at Albany, Education 226, 1400 Washington Avenue, Albany, NY 12222; e-mail: *bsaddler@uamail.albany. edu*. His research interests are sentence combining instruction, strategy instruction, writing, and learning disabilities.

SUSAN MORAN received her PhD from the University of Maryland; e-mail: *MORANINSEA@aol.com*.

Her research interests are learning disabilities, self-monitoring, and writing.

LINDA MASON is an assistant professor in the Department of Educational and School Psychology and Special Education at Pennsylvania State University, 0210 Cedar Building, University Park, PA 16802; e-mail: *lhm12@psu.edu*. Her research interests are strategy instruction, reading, writing, and learning disabilities.

ILLUSTRATIVE EXAMPLE QUESTIONS

1. What did the survey examine, and what were the sampling procedures?

2. Who were the participants in the survey, and what was the response rate?

3. Describe the development of the second part of the survey.

4. In terms of the use of ANOVA, why did researchers set the alpha level at $p < .01$?

5. How much average time did teachers devote to spelling per week?

6. Summarize the findings with regard to weaker spellers. What are the implications if these results are applied to weaker spellers in general?

7. What findings were consistent with the researchers' predictions (i.e., hypotheses)?

8. Teachers tended to use evidence-based practices, yet 27% of their students, on average, were experiencing difficulty with spelling. How do the researchers account for this finding?

9. In the Discussion, the researchers describe adaptation of instruction for weaker spellers. They reiterate that two-thirds of the adaptations were made by only one-fourth of the teacher respondents, and that 42% of teachers made virtually no adaptations. What future research would you recommend to examine these findings further?

10. What do the findings of this survey mean in terms of teacher preparation programs? What would you recommend?

ADDITIONAL RESEARCH EXAMPLES

1. Boyle-Holmes, T., Grost, L., Russell, L., Laris, B. A., Robin, L., Haller, E., et al. (2010). Promoting elementary physical education: Results of a school-based evaluation study. *Health Education and Behavior, 37*, 377–389.

2. Desimone, L. M., Smith, T. M., & Frisvold, D. E. (2009). Survey measures of classroom instruction: Comparing student and teacher reports. *Educational Policy, 24*, 267–329.

3. Whitted, K. S., & Dupper, D. R. (2008). Do teachers bully students?: Findings from a survey of students in an alternative education setting. *Education and Urban Society, 40*, 329–341.

THREATS TO SURVEY VALIDITY

Internal Validity

1. Were the survey questions adequate in obtaining the information needed   YES   NO   ?
   by the researchers?
   Justification _____

   _____

2. Was the survey pilot-tested?   YES   NO   ?
   Justification _____

   _____

3. Did the authors indicate that modifications were made based   YES   NO   ?
   on the pilot results?
   Justification _____

   _____

4. Did the pilot participants represent the respondents?   YES   NO   ?
   Justification _____

   _____

5. Were there alternative explanations for the results?   YES   NO   ?
   Justification _____

   _____

Abstract: Write a one-page abstract summarizing the overall conclusions of the authors and whether you feel the authors' conclusions are valid based on the internal validity of the investigation.

EXTERNAL VALIDITY

1. What type of sampling frame was used?   Exhaustive?   Convenience?   Cluster?

2. Was the sampling approach used by researchers probabilistic?   YES   NO   ?
   Justification _____
   _____

3. Were the respondents described?   YES   NO   ?
   Justification _____
   _____

4. Was the sample representative of the target population?   YES   NO   ?
   Justification _____
   _____

Abstract: Write a one-page abstract summarizing the overall conclusions of the authors and whether you feel the authors' conclusions are valid based on the external validity of the investigation.

PART IV

····

Qualitative Research Methods

CHAPTER 9

▪ ▪ ▪ ▪

Basic Understandings
in Qualitative Research

OBJECTIVES

After studying this chapter, you should be able to . . .

1. Define what is meant by qualitative research and explain how quantitative and qualitative researchers use their respective methods to answer different questions.
2. Describe the characteristics of qualitative research.
3. Explain the differences between qualitative and quantitative research.
4. Outline qualitative research procedures.
5. Illustrate what is meant by "understanding" in qualitative research.
6. Summarize the evaluative criteria for judging the reliability and validity of qualitative research.
7. Compare and contrast the different types of triangulation methods.
8. Outline how qualitative data are analyzed.

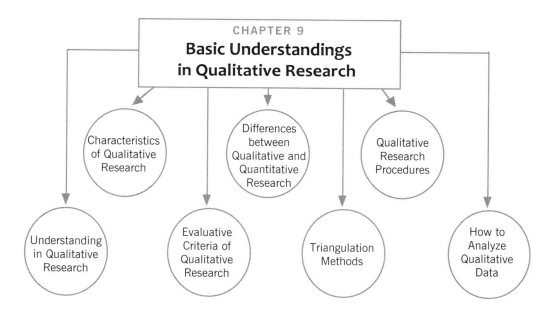

OVERVIEW

Up to this point, we have been primarily discussing quantitative research methods. At this juncture, we turn our attention to the spectrum of qualitative research, which is defined as research whose concern is understanding the context in which behavior occurs, not just the extent to which it occurs; the assessment may be more subjective, in that the dependent variables are not necessarily defined in observable terms; the data are collected in the natural setting; meanings and understandings are reached by studying cases intensively; and inductive logic is used to place the resulting data in a theoretical context. Qualitative research is a flexible but systematic approach to understanding qualities of a phenomenon within a particular context (Brantlinger, Jimenez, Klingner, Pugach, & Richardson, 2005). According to Willig (2001):

> Qualitative researchers tend to be concerned with meaning. That is, they are interested in how people make sense of the world and how they experience events. They aim to understand "what it is like" to experience particular conditions (e.g., what it means and how it feels to live with chronic illness or to be unemployed) and how people manage certain situations (e.g., how people negotiate family life or relations with work colleagues). Qualitative researchers tend, therefore, to be concerned with the quality and texture of experience, rather than with the identification of cause–effect relationships. (p. 9)

As indicated in Chapter 3, qualitative researchers view reliability and validity somewhat differently than do quantitative researchers. Unfortunately, rather than viewing the merits of differing methodologies, we often attempt to discount findings generated from research methods that differ from our own. Many quantitative researchers have tried to discount findings from qualitative methods simply because the data were generated in a qualitative context. Similarly, many qualitative researchers who reject findings from quantitative research say that quantitative researchers do not take into account the process of learning or other critical phenomena occurring outside of the narrowly defined dependent variable. For example, suppose a quantitative researcher generates data to

answer the question of the differential effectiveness of direct instruction and discovery learning on a student group's reading performance and finds one method superior to the other. The qualitative researcher may argue that other, equally important variables were not taken into account—those that cannot be operationally defined before the investigation and directly measured as outcomes, such as self-esteem or student preference.

Unfortunately, often forgotten in the debate between quantitative and qualitative methods are the types of questions answered by the different methodologies. The arguments for or against quantitative and qualitative methodologies seem to assume that both methodologies attempt to answer the same research questions. They do not. Also, we assume that both are based on the same assumptions. They are not. A better way to examine the methodologies is to view the types of questions asked, then to determine whether the methodology used was appropriate to answer the question (Mertens, 2009). This view of matching the methodology to the types of questions is similar to the one expressed in earlier chapters. For example, it is not appropriate to use a preexperimental design to answer a cause-and-effect question (e.g., whether a traumatic event causes anxiety). Similarly, it is not appropriate to use an experimental design to answer questions better addressed through naturalistic inquiry (e.g., understanding social patterns in a teachers' lounge). As noted by Creswell (2009, p. 173), "Qualitative procedures demonstrate a different approach to scholarly inquiry than methods of quantitative research. Qualitative inquiry employs different philosophical assumptions; strategies of inquiry; and methods of data collection, analysis, and interpretation." Therefore, this chapter is concerned with investigating the types of research questions that are appropriate for qualitative research. The best way to think of qualitative and quantitative research is not which is better, but how they can be used to address different issues.

As described in earlier chapters, quantitative research is concerned with the reliable and valid investigation of the impact of independent variables on dependent variables, or the relationships between or among variables. Quantitative researchers are concerned with the outcomes of an intervention and measuring the dependent variable objectively. In contrast, qualitative researchers are concerned with how people feel about classroom procedures, what they believe about certain instructional methods, how they process information, and what meanings they attach to experiences. Qualitative researchers are concerned with understanding the context in which behavior occurs, not just the extent to which it occurs. The assessment may be more subjective, in that the dependent variables are not necessarily defined in observable terms. In fact, qualitative researchers are concerned not with a few narrowly defined variables but with the interaction of multiple variables over a period of time (Mertens, 2009).

For example, let's say we wished to know what makes an outstanding teacher. Quantitatively, we may define specific teaching behaviors that we believe are responsible for positive student outcomes. Once these behaviors are identified, we may randomly assign a sample of teachers to one of two groups. Each group might then be provided an assessment of academic performance. Following the pretest, one group might be taught the instructional behaviors thought to be associated with student achievement, and the other might be provided some form of interaction that lasts an amount of time equal to the instructional training (providing an equal amount of time in interactions with the two groups would control for an alternative explanation of extra attention provided to the "experimental" group). A posttest would then be provided and the groups' mean scores compared. If the students of those who received the instructional training outperformed the other students on an academic performance test, then there would be support for the hypothesis that defined teacher instructional behaviors improve academic performance of students.

Notice how the preceding example answers a particular research question; that is, "Is a set of defined instructional behaviors related to improved student performance?" The example does not answer questions such as "What do the teachers think about the instructional behaviors taught?"; "How do the students feel about the change in how their teachers' approach instruction?"; "Are there other instructional variables

present that could account for improved student performance?"; "Do the assessments that were used measure important learner traits?"; "How do the instructional behaviors taught affect the process of learning rather than just the outcome?"; "Do teachers see the instructional strategies as helpful? If so, which ones are helpful and why? If not, why?"; and "On what do the teachers base their answers or beliefs?" In order to answer these types of questions, other research methodologies must be used. Qualitative methodologies are well suited to answer these questions.

Let's say a qualitative researcher visits a single classroom over time, becomes involved in classroom activities, and examines the nature of the activities in depth. The researcher may set up multiple sources of data gathering, such as interviews with teachers, students, and parents. The investigation may continue for the academic year or even longer. The main attempt here is to get a "real-world" feel for the operations of a classroom, what makes it work, how the teacher and students interact, and what seems to affect student classroom performance. The data generated may come from interviews, narrations, or journal entries by all of the involved parties. Once the investigation is finished, the researcher codes the data in terms of categories and begins to interpret the results. (*Note.* These examples are only meant to be illustrative of possible investigations; the examples are not representative of all possible investigations that can be conducted to answer the aforementioned research questions.)

Notice how the methods, compared to quantitative methods, differ not only in format but also in the nature of questions asked and the types of answers sought. The critical point here is that quantitative research is no better or worse than qualitative research; quantitative research is different than qualitative research in approach and purpose. That said, it does not seem fruitful to argue the superiority of one methodology over the other. A more appropriate discussion should center on when and why each should be used.

> **Qualitative research** *is concerned with understanding the context in which behavior occurs, not just the extent to which it occurs.*

Also, the two methodologies are not mutually exclusive. They can, and in many cases should, be used together. Think of the powerful information that could be gathered if the two methods were combined in the preceding examples. The combination of quantitative and qualitative approaches, called mixed methods, is described in Chapter 10.

Let's return to our classroom example. Suppose there are two groups of teachers in the experimental example. Let's reduce the number of teachers to two and the number of classrooms to two. The instructional behaviors are taught to one class (determined randomly). Qualitative researchers go into both classrooms as described earlier. Since everything is equal in both classrooms except for the instructional training, we still have good experimental control. Granted, the design is not truly experimental but is instead a nonequivalent control-group design (see Chapter 5). We would sacrifice some constraints over the participants but gain a great deal of information from the qualitative data. (*Note.* Many qualitative researchers may be more comfortable using quantitative and qualitative methods in a complementary manner rather than mixing both approaches to develop a "new" research method.)

One way both methodologies can be complementary is by conducting an experimental design and determining the social validity of the outcomes (see Chapter 2). The methodologies can also work together, but not at the same time. For example, if we wanted to determine the effective instructional behaviors necessary for increased academic performance, we could use qualitative research to generate hypotheses. In this case, the qualitative investigation would occur first. Out of the data analysis generated hypotheses would be based on the information gathered. The qualitative research would provide inductive information, and the experimental research would provide deductive information. We would most likely be much more successful in determining when to use certain instructional practices if we first learned about the context under which participants are operating, before we attempt to implement independent variables that may not fit the particular contexts.

This chapter focuses on the characteristics of qualitative research methods. Additionally,

qualitative research procedures are discussed. Finally, methods of understanding the reliability and validity of qualitative research are provided for critique.

WHAT ARE THE CHARACTERISTICS OF QUALITATIVE RESEARCH?

Before we discuss the characteristics of qualitative research, we must point out that there is little agreement among qualitative researchers with regard to what qualitative research is. Patton (1990) provides a detailed discussion of how qualitative research is defined by different scholars (see Table 9.1). The multiple definitions of qualitative research attests to the diversity and breadth of this research spectrum.

Pauly (1991) described a five-step process for conducting qualitative research, including "(a) finding a topic, (b) formulating research questions, (c) gathering the evidence, (d) interpreting the evidence, and (e) telling the researcher's story" (cited in Potter, 1996, p. 7). Silverman (2005) described three distinctive characteristics of qualitative research. Two of the characteristics seem especially relevant for our purposes. First, field research provides a broader perspective on theory than simply a relationship between variables. In other words, a more general version of a theory is one that takes into consideration the mechanisms or processes that generate relationships among the identified variables. For example, rather than simply indicating that there is a strong relationship between social status and academic performance, we may wish to discover how social status affects academic performance, such as the attitudes of parents with high SES backgrounds toward school.

Second, flexibility of field research allows pursuit of theory development in an effective and economical manner. In this way, additional questions are generated that allow researchers to be flexible and possibly move in directions or observe phenomena that they ordinarily would have missed or taken for granted. For example, if we observe a third-grade teacher using direct instruction methods and ours is a narrowly defined observation method (i.e., looking for specific teacher behaviors), we may not see anything remarkable about what is occurring.

TABLE 9.1. Samples of Definitions and Descriptions of Qualitative Research

A. *Formal Definition:* This is a dictionary-type definition in which the essence of the concept is made explicit. This type of definition "centers" readers by telling them what to focus on and where the boundaries are; it provides a foundation for the reader to judge what should and should not be included.

  1. Bogdan and Taylor (1975): "Qualitative methodologies refer to research procedures which produce descriptive data: people's own written or spoken words and observable behavior. [It] directs itself at settings and the individuals within those settings holistically; that is, the subject of the study, be it an organization or an individual, is not reduced to an isolated variable or to an hypothesis, but is viewed instead as part of a whole" (p. 2).

  2. Lindlof (1991): "Qualitative inquiry examines the constitution of meaning in everyday social phenomena. . . . Probably the fundamental touchstone for the term is methodological. Qualitative research *seeks to preserve the form, content, and context of social phenomena and analyze their qualities,* rather than separate them from historical and institutional surroundings" (p. 24, italics in original).

  3. Pauly (1991): "Qualitative studies investigate meaning-making" (p. 2).

B. *Contrasting Definition:* Some scholars define qualitative research in contrast to something else. That something else is usually quantitative research, but the term *quantitative* is usually a synonym for something, such as reductionism, radical empiricism, and so forth.

  1. Bogdan and Taylor (1975), in their book *Introduction to Qualitative Research Methods: A Phenomenological Approach to the Social Sciences,* made a contrast on the philosophical level. They contrasted the positivism of Comte with the phenomenological approach of Weber and Deutscher: "The positivist seeks the facts or causes of social phenomena with little regard for the subjective states of individuals" (p. 2). They stated that "Durkheim advised the social scientist to consider 'social facts,' or social phenomena, as 'things' that exercise an external and coercive influence on human behavior" (p. 2). In contrast, phenomenologists are "concerned with understanding human behavior from the actor's own frame of reference. . . . The important reality is what people imagine it to be" (p. 2). They also defined the phenomenon as "the process of interpretation" (p. 14).

  2. Jensen and Jankowski (1991): In contrasting qualitative with quantitative they asserted that qualitative is concerned with "meaning in phenomenological and contextual terms," not information "in the sense of discrete items transporting significance through mass media" (p. 4). "Qualitative analysis focuses on the *occurrence* of its analytical objects in a particular context, as opposed to the *recurrence* of formally similar elements in different contexts" (p. 4). It also requires an internal approach to looking at indivisible experience through exegesis with a focus on process "which is contextualized and inextricably integrated with wider social and cultural practices" (p. 4). They further stated that "there seems to be no way around the quantitative–qualitative distinction. Although it sometimes serves to confuse rather than clarify research issues, the distinction is a fact of research practice which has major epistemological and political implications that no scholar can afford to ignore" (p. 5).

  3. Lancy (1993) provided a contrast of qualitative with quantitative focusing on the choice of topics, sampling, role of investigator, bias, context, and length of study and report.

  4. Wimmer and Dominick (1991) saw three main differences between qualitative and quantitative. First, they asserted that qualitative believes that there is no single reality, and that each person creates a subjective reality that is holistic and not reducible to component parts. Second, qualitative believes that individuals are fundamentally different and that they cannot be categorized. And third, qualitative strives for unique explanations about particular situations and individuals.

C. *Component Definition:* Some scholars illuminate some components or characteristics. This gives readers a sense of the parts or concerns within the qualitative domain, but it does not provide a sense of the boundaries or limits.

  1. Bogdan and Taylor (1975), who used *phenomenology* as a synonym for qualitative research, argued that phenomenology itself has two components: symbolic interactionism and ethnomethodology. In their view, *ethnomethodology* means qualitative methods, but qualitative methods does not mean ethnomethodology, because there is more to qualitative research than the component of ethnomethodology.

(continued)

TABLE 9.1. *(continued)*

2. Jankowski and Wester (1991) presented two unique elements in their definition. First is the idea of *verstehen*, which "refers to an understanding of the meaning that people ascribe to their social situation and activities. Because people act on the basis of the meanings they attribute to themselves and others, the focus of qualitative social science is on everyday life and its significance as perceived by the participants" (pp. 44–45). The second element is role taking, which expresses the idea that people are active and their roles change across situations.

3. Jensen and Jankowski (1991) examined discourse analysis, textual analysis, reception analysis, ethnography, and history.

4. Lancy (1993) identified ethnography, ethnomethodology, ecological psychology, and history.

D. *Procedural Definition:* Qualitative research can be defined in terms of a list of steps.

1. Lincoln and Cuba (1985) offered two prime tenets: that "first, no manipulation on the part of the inquirer is implied, and, second, the inquirer imposes no a priori units on the outcome" (p. 8).

2. Pauly (1991) attempted to "guide the work of beginners" who want to try qualitative research by providing a "step by step explanation of how one might do qualitative research" (pp. 1–2). He presented five steps: (a) finding a topic, (b) formulating research questions, (c) gathering the evidence, (d) interpreting the evidence, and (e) telling the researcher's story.

E. *Product Definition:* Some theoreticians define qualitative research in terms of the end point of a process.

1. Bogdan and Taylor (1975) asserted that "qualitative methodologies refer to research procedures which produce descriptive data: people's own written or spoken words and observable behavior." It "directs itself at settings and the individuals within those settings holistically; that is, the subject of the study, be it an organization or an individual, is not reduced to an isolated variable or to an hypothesis, but is viewed instead as part of a whole" (p. 2).

Note. Reprinted in abbreviated form from Patton, M. Q. (1990). *Qualitative evaluation and research methods* (2nd ed., pp. 40–41). Newbury Park, CA: Sage. Copyright 1990 by Sage Publications, Inc. Reprinted by permission of SAGE.

This finding may be due to the narrowness of our observational system. If, on the other hand, we visit the same classroom but do not look for predefined behaviors, we may begin to generate a structure through which to organize our observations.

Table 9.2 presents a summary of the characteristics of qualitative research according to Patton (1990). We expand on each of these characteristics throughout the chapter.

WHAT ARE THE DIFFERENCES BETWEEN QUALITATIVE AND QUANTITATIVE RESEARCH?

Qualitative and quantitative research methods are clearly different in many regards (Bogdan & Biklen, 1998). The differences between quantitative and qualitative methods, as seen in Table 9.3, do not make the two methods mutually

exclusive. However, understanding these differences aids critical research consumers in making conclusions about the utility and meaning of the researchers' questions and conclusions.

The obvious difference has to do with how each approaches subject matter. The following is a brief discussion of how quantitative and qualitative methodologies differ.

Contextual Data

First, the direct source of data for qualitative research is the natural setting. Although much quantitative research may be conducted in artificial settings or under artificial contexts, qualitative researchers are concerned with "real-world" or "big picture" questions. There is less concern with isolating variables in high-constraint situations, since those situations, from a qualitative perspective, most likely bear little resemblance to real contexts. Along these lines, the researcher is the key data collection instrument. The assumption is that individuals are affected by their environmental situations or contexts. Therefore, the data collection must occur in those contexts to be understood. If measurement instruments are used out of context, a great deal of information is lost. Additionally, if a researcher uses a measurement device, the variables under study must be narrowly defined. Therefore, interviews, observations, transcripts, historical records, and other methods are used to avoid the narrowness inherent in measurement instruments.

Descriptive Data

Second, qualitative research is descriptive in nature. Although quantitative researchers use numbers to represent the dependent variable, numbers do not represent the whole story.

TABLE 9.2. Major Characteristics of Qualitative Research

1. Naturalistic inquiry	Studying real-world situations as they unfold naturally; nonmanipulative, unobtrusive, and noncontrolling; openness to whatever emerges—lack of predetermined constraints on outcomes
2. Inductive analysis	Immersion in the details and specifics of the data to discover important categories, dimensions, and interrelationships; begin by exploring genuinely open questions rather than testing theoretically derived (deductive) hypotheses
3. Holistic perspective	The whole phenomenon under study is understood as a complex system that is more than the sum of its parts; focus on complex interdependencies not meaningfully reduced to a few discrete variables and linear, cause–effect relationships
4. Qualitative data	Detailed, thick description; inquiry in depth; direct quotations capturing people's personal perspectives and experiences
5. Personal contact and insight	The researcher has direct contact with and gets close to the people, situation, and phenomenon under study; researcher's personal experiences and insights are an important part of the inquiry and critical to understanding the phenomenon
6. Dynamic systems	Attention to process; assumes change is constant and ongoing whether the focus is on an individual or an entire culture
7. Unique case orientation	Assumes each case is special and unique; the first level of inquiry is being true to, respecting, and capturing the details of the individual cases being studied; cross-case analysis follows from and depends on the quality of individual case studies
8. Context sensitivity	Places findings in a social, historical, and temporal context; dubious of the possibility or meaningfulness of generalizations across time and space
9. Empathic neutrality	Complete objectivity is impossible; pure subjectivity undermines credibility; the researcher's passion is understanding the world in all its complexity—not proving something, not advocating, not advancing personal agendas, but understanding; the researcher includes personal experience and empathic insight as part of the relevant data, while taking a neutral nonjudgmental stance toward whatever content may emerge
10. Design flexibility	Open to adapting inquiry as understanding deepens and/or situations change; avoids getting locked into rigid designs that eliminate responsiveness; pursues new paths of discovery as they emerge

Note. Reprinted from Patton, M. Q. (1990). *Qualitative evaluation and research methods* (2nd ed., pp. 40–41). Newbury Park, CA: Sage. Copyright 1990 by Sage Publications, Inc. Reprinted by permission of SAGE.

TABLE 9.3. Differences between Quantitative and Qualitative Research Methods

Quantitative research	Qualitative research
Primary purpose is to determine cause-and-effect relationships.	Primary purpose is to describe ongoing processes.
Precise hypothesis is stated before the start of the investigation; theories govern the purpose of the investigation in a deductive manner.	Hypotheses are developed during the investigation; questions govern the purpose of the investigation; theories are developed inductively.
The independent variable is controlled and manipulated.	There is no specific independent variable; the concern is to study naturally occurring phenomena without interference.
Objective collection of data is a requirement.	Objective collection of data is not a requirement; data collectors may interact with the participants.
Research design is specified before the start of the investigation.	Research design is flexible and develops throughout the investigation.
Data are represented and summarized in numerical form.	Data are represented or summarized in narrative or verbal forms.
Reliability and validity determined through statistical and logical methods.	Reliability and validity determined through multiple sources of information (triangulation).
Samples are selected to represent the population.	Samples are purposefully selected or single cases are studied.
Study of behavior is in the natural or artificial setting.	Study of behavior is in the natural setting.
Use of design or statistical analyses to control for threats to internal validity.	Use of logical analyses to control or account for alternative explanations.
Use of inferential statistical procedures to demonstrate external validity (specifically, population validity).	Use of similar cases to determine the generalizability of findings (logical generalization) if done at all.
Rely on research design and data gathering instruments to control for procedural bias.	Rely on the researcher to come to terms with procedural bias.
Phenomena are broken down or simplified for study.	Phenomena are studied holistically, as a complex system.
Conclusions are stated with a predetermined degree of certainty (i.e., α level).	Conclusions are tentative and subjected to ongoing examination.

(*Note.* Obviously, quantitative researchers also describe events; however, the nature of the descriptions is usually numerical versus narrative.) Numbers summarize what was measured but do not necessarily represent fully what was seen. For example, suppose we wish to determine the extent to which a student improves in a reading class. We could use a standardized measurement device to determine the reading gains the student makes. However, we do not have information on other, possibly important concerns, such as how the student responds each day when reading assignments are required (i.e., happy and feeling excited to become engaged in reading, or moping and depressed about beginning the reading assignment). Information is lacking on whether the student has made connections between what he/she is reading and other subjects, or whether the reading topic is interesting to the student. We do not have information on what the teacher thinks about the program. Does the teacher want to make modifications or drop the program altogether? We do not have information on how others in the classroom or school feel about the program. We do not know whether the school principal or other school personnel are placing pressure on teachers to improve reading scores of students. And we do not have information from parents in terms of their satisfaction with the program. For instance, parents may report their children's excitement about going to school or that they have difficulty motivating their children to go to school. Students may comment about how they love reading class or despise it. Therefore, qualitative researchers attempt to gather as much information as possible to "see the entire movie" rather than "take a few frames from the film." Qualitative researchers insist that because what is missing from the film may be as important as what is captured in the selected frames, descriptive information allows us to see as much of the film as possible to gain more of an appreciation of the larger story.

Process of Change

Third, qualitative researchers consider the process of change as opposed to outcomes. In contrast, whereas quantitative researchers tend to investigate the outcomes (i.e., posttest assessments), qualitative researchers focus on both the process and the outcome. For example, in a quantitative study of reading achievement, we measure the reading performance of students both before and after the reading instruction. We can then determine how much the children have changed in their ability to read. On the other hand, we may wish to investigate why they have changed or how they have improved. The attitudes of the students may have affected the reading performance in some manner. Or the teacher expectations may have had an impact.

The critical questions to be answered are "How are these attitudes or expectations translated into the daily reading activities?"; "How do the interactions of the other students affect the process of reading acquisition?"; and "How does the classroom climate overall affect the process of learning to read?" A more pragmatic difficulty with looking at only outcomes is that once we have a narrowly defined outcome

limited by the variables observed, we have little chance of making a change to improve our instruction, because it is simply too late. If we assess the process of change, we can readily see whether and how the student is being affected. If the student is not progressing, we can make changes before the student fails to achieve. Studying the process of change, then, involves a descriptive and enhanced assessment of the daily changes that occur through interactions, activities, and procedures.

Grounded Theory Development

Fourth, qualitative researchers use a combination of inductive and deductive reasoning in interpreting their research. In contrast, quantitative researchers tend to use a deductive approach. They tend to generate hypotheses from theories and attempt to disprove these hypotheses and/or theories. Qualitative researchers do not generate hypotheses for testing before the investigation. They generate research questions and begin the research without any preconceived notions of possible outcomes. This is not to say that qualitative researchers do not pay attention to existing theory; they do. In fact, they move between inductive and deductive logic in a process called *abduction* or *analytic induction* (Suddaby, 2006). Once findings have been accumulated, theories may be developed.

Such theories are called *grounded theories* (Strauss & Corbin, 1997), because they are based firmly or "grounded" in a solid foundation of research, and because the process that generated the theory cannot be separated from the theory. Our understanding of a phenomenon in grounded theory moves from simple to complex; the amount of previous literature that guides theory development varies from study to study (Hays & Wood, 2011). Thus, **grounded theory** is defined as "a systematic qualitative methodology that emphasizes the generation of theory from data while in the process of conducting research" (Buckley, 2010, p. 116). Thus, a theory is developed while research is being conducted (Chenail, 2011; Mertens, 2009).

> **Grounded theory** *is a theory that is generated from data during the research process.*

As stated by Aldiabat and Le Navenec (2011), "Grounded theory consists of categories that are generated from data analysis and connections about the relationships between categories. These categories represent abstract phenomena at the theoretical level" (p. 1075). The data generated in grounded theory development come from a variety of sources, including observations conducted in the field, interviews, and written accounts (e.g., those from historical records and personal reflections) (Buckley, 2010). A key to the generation of categories in grounded theory development involves the constant comparative approach (Hays & Wood, 2011; Idrees, Vasconcelos, & Cox, 2011). The constant comparative approach uses simultaneous data collection and analysis. In this cyclical process data driven by emerging theory are collected, convergent and divergent categories are developed, additional data are collected, then the categories are revisited, refined, and collapsed. Patterns and sequences are determined, and conclusions regarding causal factors, the way participants respond to these factors, and effects of these factors on participants are determined. This process continues until there are no new data that add to or refute the emerging theory (Hays & Wood, 2011; Idrees et al., 2011).

Constructivist View

Grounded theory traditionally is approached from a constructionist viewpoint. As Buckley (2010) states: "Constructivist grounded theorists assume that data and their analysis are social constructions of reality; that researchers and what they study mutually influence each other; and that *reflexivity* is essential in helping put into perspective researchers' preconceived ideas, personal biases, and values as theory is constructed" (p. 119). According to Suddaby (2006), grounded theory makes statements about how people interpret their realities as opposed to making statements about these realities. Aldiabat and Le Navenec (2011) provide seven main assumptions of grounded theory:

1. The need is to get into the field to discover what is "really going on" in the symbolic world of participants (i.e., to obtain firsthand data taken from its original source).

2. Theory about symbolic world (meanings) is generated from the data.
3. Grounded Theory assumes that persons act on the basis of meanings.
4. Perspectives and social perceptions are defined, developed, negotiated, and contested through interaction.
5. Grounded Theory reflects the complexity and variability of phenomena and of human action.
6. Grounded Theory involves understanding and explaining how participants develop meanings and how those meanings are influenced by other things such as organizational, psychological, social factors, and events.
7. Grounded Theory assumes that persons are actors who take an active role in responding to problematic situations. (p. 1070)

Behavioral View

Grounded theory is frequently defined from a constructivist perspective in which multiple social realities are the main variables, and internal and subjective perspectives are the main concerns. In fact, Suddaby (2006) reported, "It is less appropriate, for example, to use grounded theory when you seek to make knowledge claims about an objective reality, and more appropriate to do so when you want to make knowledge claims about how individuals interpret reality" (p. 634). In essence then, there are two ways to interpret the meaning of grounded theory. First, grounded theory is based on or grounded in the perceptions of the participants with the end goal to develop a theory (Hays & Wood, 2011). The grounding, then, is in the participants' perceptions. Second, grounded theory is based on or grounded in the data collected, not necessarily in subjective and/or constructivist interpretations. According to Glaser (2002), constructivism plays only a small role in grounded theory research. In fact, much of grounded theory development attempts to make the data objective (through methods to correct for bias), and the method used in grounded theory makes the theory as objective as possible (Glaser, 2002). It is this second interpretation of grounded theory that reveals common ground among researchers from different philosophical orientations.

For example, Skinner described theory making in a similar vein. According to Zuriff (1995), Skinner indicated that a theory "evolves as additional empirical relationships are presented in a formal way, and as it develops, it integrates more facts in increasingly more economical formulations" (p. 171). Similarly, Chiesa (1994) stated, "Skinner clearly preferred a Machian approach to explanatory theories; a type of theory that is descriptive, relies on observation, and whose terms integrate relations among basic data" (p. 140). Finally, Skinner himself indicated that "[a theory] has nothing to do with the presence or absence of experimental confirmation. Facts and theories do not stand in opposition to each other. The relation, rather, is this: theories are based upon facts; they are statements about organizations of facts" (1947/1972, p. 302). Thus, it seems that Skinner essentially was saying that theories should be grounded in the data (see Strauss & Corbin, 1997, for a thorough discussion of grounded theory) revealed in observed research findings.

Phenomenology

Fifth, the focus of qualitative research is the meaning that individuals assign to their lives. Qualitative researchers are concerned with phenomena such as values, attitudes, assumptions, and beliefs, and how these phenomena affect the individuals under investigation. Quantitative researchers are more concerned with "hard data" that are objective and narrowly defined. These data usually are not concerned with the meaning or understanding individuals attach to their experiences but with the observable changes enacted upon individuals. Perhaps, more than any of the other four characteristics, this characteristic sets quantitative research apart from qualitative research.

Research that is directed at investigating such phenomena is called **phenomenology**. Researchers "seek to understand the phenomenon through the eyes of those who have direct, immediate experience with it" (Hays & Wood, 2011, p. 291). Thus, phenomenology is the study of "people's experiences in terms of how people make meaning in their lives by examining relationships between what happened and how people have come to understand these events" (Chenail, 2011, p. 1180).

Phenomenological researchers are concerned with cognitive processes (i.e., what and how people think), as well as why participants process information in some manner. These phenomena are not easily defined in operational terms that allow us to observe them directly. Thus, we must use an alternative method of investigation to study these phenomena. Phenomenological research does just that.

Qualitative researchers conducting phenomenological research spend a great deal of time interacting with the participants to assess these difficult-to-measure phenomena. Phenomenology relies on this interaction between the researcher and participants to build relationships. Meaningful data on the participants' inner experiences can be obtained through these relationships (Christensen & Brumfield, 2010). Through extensive interviewing (as well as observations and artifact and document reviews; Christensen & Brumfield, 2010), researchers gather important participant information (Chenail, 2011; Hays & Wood, 2011). Quantitative researchers have a difficult time doing the same thing, since they must attempt to maintain as much objectivity as possible. Their instruments also measure these very complex phenomena by observing their by-products, then summarizing and signifying with numbers what they observed. Qualitative researchers view this practice in isolation as problematic, since large chunks of data are missing; these data include a complex examination of participants' lives.

An important concept in phenomenology research, *bracketing* (Luckerhoff & Guillemette, 2011), involves a process whereby researchers explore their biases and assumptions before their studies begin. Once these biases and expectations are understood, they are set aside so that researchers can reflect on the world of participants. Thus, bracketing is an attempt to "maintain objectivity in its account of subjective experience" (Olivier, 2011, p. 185).

Researchers must follow several steps when conducting phenomenological research (Hays & Wood, 2011). First, researchers bracket their assumptions and approach the phenomenon with a fresh perspective. This step is critical

> **Phenomenology** *is the study of how people come to understand events in their lives.*

given that researchers are the primary data collection instruments and source of data analysis. Second, they conduct interviews to obtain participants' unique perspectives. Participants are selected in a purposeful manner given their experiences with a particular phenomenon and their willingness to share information. Third, researchers look for patterns and variations in participant experiences. In addition, detailed descriptions of each participant and participants as a whole are provided (Christensen & Brumfield, 2010). These descriptions allow analysis of data to be considered within specific demographic information (e.g., educational level, religious views, age, gender, race/ethnicity). Finally, researchers describe the phenomenon, including textural descriptions (meaning and depth of experiences) of individuals and of the group as a whole.

WHAT ARE QUALITATIVE RESEARCH PROCEDURES?

Phases

There are several methods of conducting qualitative research. A major difference between qualitative and quantitative research methodologies is that qualitative methods are more flexible (i.e., they can change during the research). Therefore, no specific steps in designing qualitative methods are the same for all types of designs. However, we can list some phases that researchers typically go through before and during the qualitative research endeavor (shown in Figure 9.1). The reason for pointing out these phases

is to demonstrate how qualitative research is much more flexible than quantitative research. The ways researchers decide to implement each phase form the design. Realize that these phases occur not only before the investigation but also throughout, and not necessarily in the same order as presented here.

Research Question

The first phase is to ask a research question. Obviously, the question can come from several sources, such as observing the world, reading other research, or attempting to solve a problem.

Data Collection

The second phase is to decide how to collect the data. Researchers should decide whether to examine written documents, interview participants, observe participants, or a combination of these. Researchers should decide whether to identify themselves, and, if so, whether to identify themselves as researchers and/or group members. Researchers should also decide whether they will be active or passive observers or active participants. Finally, researchers should decide how long they should collect data to gather enough evidence to make firm assertions about the data.

Sample

The third phase involves deciding on a sample. It is critical to understand that sample size is a concern. However, rather than being concerned

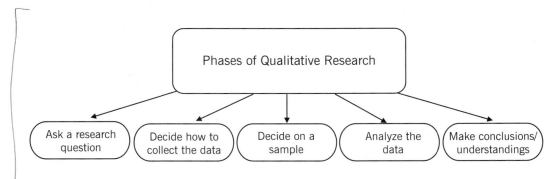

FIGURE 9.1. Phases of the qualitative research process.

about sample size to ensure the representativeness of the sample to the population, qualitative researchers are concerned with access to relevant evidence about a phenomenon (Potter, 1996). Several sampling methods are used in qualitative research and are discussed in more detail later.

Data Analysis

The fourth phase, data analysis, continues throughout the investigation. Researchers must decide on the type of analysis to conduct. This decision is based on the purpose of the investigation. Potter (1996) describes 20 of the most prevalently used techniques placed into four categories: (1) orienting methods, (2) deductive methods of construction, (3) inductive methods of construction, and (4) other methods of construction. A description of each of these methods is beyond the scope of this volume; however, we refer readers to Potter (1996) to gain an appreciation of the complexity of data analysis in qualitative research.

Conclusions or Understandings

The final phase of a qualitative investigation is to reach conclusions or understandings based on the data. These understandings comprise descriptions, interpretations, theories, assertions, generalizations, and evaluations. Understandings are described in more detail later in the chapter.

Sampling

Although sampling procedures were discussed in Chapter 4, a discussion of qualitative sampling procedures seems appropriate, because there are both similarities and distinctions in comparison to quantitative research. Similar to quantitative research, a sample must be chosen, since it is usually not possible to study the entire population. Identifying a sample is one of the first steps in designing a qualitative research study. The setting, population, and phenomena to be studied should also be decided. Under some circumstances, phenomena under study also define the site and the population to be

studied. For example, Gilbride, Stensrud, Vandergoot, and Golden (2003) studied values and beliefs of employers and employees who were open to working with people with disabilities.

Sampling in a qualitative study may or may not be the same as convenience sampling in other methods of research, in which the sample is selected because it is available and relatively easy to integrate into the research. Although the sample may be convenient in many cases, the purpose of selecting the sample is to address the research question specifically. To determine whether the sample is adequate, we must determine the purpose of the research and whether the sample allows generation of answers to the questions posed. Thus, to answer the question of why employers hire employees with disabilities, a business is selected because it has information to answer the question (i.e., employees with disabilities). Thus, although the sample may be convenient in one way, the sample is selected to help answer the research question(s).

The sampling method used most often by qualitative researchers is termed purposeful sampling (Patton, 1987). **Purposeful sampling** (or purposive sampling) is defined as deliberately selecting particular persons, events, or settings for the important information they provide (Maxwell, 1997). Patton (1987) indicated that purposeful sampling is used to select information-rich cases for in-depth study. The samples comprise cases in which a great deal can be learned about issues of central importance for the research. Patton described 10 purposeful sampling methods; however, he indicated that there are other qualitative sampling methods. We should note that these sampling methods are not mutually exclusive. For our purposes, the 10 sampling methods described by Patton suffice (see Figure 9.2; *Note*. Examples used throughout the following descriptions of sampling procedures focus on one topic—reading instruction, due to an attempt to remain consistent throughout).

Purposeful sampling *is selecting particular persons, events, or settings for the important information they provide.*

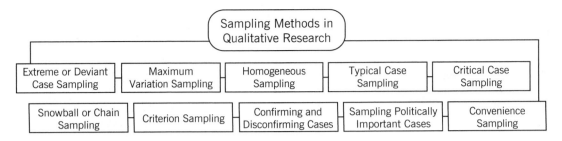

FIGURE 9.2. Ten qualitative sampling methods.

Extreme or Deviant Case Sampling

Extreme or deviant sampling involves selecting those cases that are the most outstanding successes or failures related to some topic of interest because they are expected to yield especially valuable information about the topic of interest (Teddlie & Yu, 2007). For example, if we study reading instruction in a public school, we may choose fourth-grade students with LDs in reading. (*Note.* By the very nature of qualifying for special education services, these students must be generally unresponsive to typical reading instruction; thus, by definition, these students' academic performance deviates from what we expect.) A purpose for doing this might be to obtain valuable information about typical students in reading classes. In other words, if we find that a specific reading method is effective for students with LDs in reading, we may be better able to teach students without LDs how to read, or at least prevent them from being identified as having LDs in the first place.

Maximum Variation Sampling

Maximum variation sampling involves "capturing and describing the central themes or principle outcomes that cut across a great deal of participant or program variation" (Patton, 1987, p. 53). For example, to examine reading instruction, we could select students with LDs in reading, gifted students, and typical students in the fourth grade. The purpose of this sampling method is to obtain high-quality, detailed descriptions of each case to document uniqueness and to determine general patterns that are shared by the heterogeneous sample.

Homogeneous Sampling

Homogeneous sampling is the opposite of maximum variation sampling, in that similar participants are selected to decrease the variation within the sample (Teddlie & Yu, 2007). For example, to assess reading instruction, we could select students in the fourth grade who are at grade level in reading. Note that this sample is homogeneous, not extreme, in that the selected students are all in the same grade and at a similar level in reading skill.

Typical Case Sampling

Typical case sampling involves selecting one or more typical cases (Teddlie & Yu, 2007). What is typical would be decided on by significant others (e.g., parents, teachers, community leaders, administrators) in the setting. For example, if we were to study reading instruction in the fourth grade, we would have the fourth-grade teacher(s) determine the typical reading levels of students and help to select students who meet the definition of *typical*. These students would then comprise the sample involved in the investigation. The purpose of this sampling method is to provide others who are not "familiar with the program . . . a qualitative profile of one or more 'typical' cases" (Patton, 1987, p. 54). Thus, the purpose of typical case sampling is to inform others about the program, not to generalize results to the population, as random sampling procedures in quantitative approaches attempt to do.

Critical Case Sampling

Critical case sampling is used to identify critical cases that are particularly important for some reason (Teddlie & Yu, 2007). For example, say we were studying reading instruction in a fourth-grade class and wished to identify a sample that would allow us to generalize to other cases. We might select students from highly stimulating environments, since we know that a high level of stimulation in the early years (e.g., before entering kindergarten) can have a significant impact on later reading skills (Salvia et al., 2009). We observe our sample and discover that most of the students in a reading class are having difficulty in reading. We then conclude that if these students are having difficulty, others from less stimulating environments placed in similar learning situations probably would also experience difficulties.

Snowball or Chain Sampling

Snowball or chain sampling involves asking others who would be a good choice to include in the sample (Teddlie & Yu, 2007). This sampling method is similar to looking for literature on a chosen topic. For example, suppose we were interested in the research base for whole-language instruction in reading (i.e., a method used to facilitate the development of reading). We could look at the reference section of one article and find other referenced articles (an ancestral search). We could repeat this process across subsequent articles and continue until a large sample of articles is identified. Once the same articles begin to show up in subsequent reference sections, they are considered especially important to the topic. A similar scenario occurs in snowball or chain sampling, in that when we ask who would be particularly adept at teaching reading, several names may be generated, until the same names begin to show up repeatedly. The purpose of this sampling procedure is to identify critical individuals to include in the sample.

Criterion Sampling

Criterion sampling involves setting a criterion of performance; individuals who meet or surpass the criterion are included in the sample. For example, we may want to include teachers with at least 10 years of reading instruction experience in the sample, since these teachers may have particular experiences with success and failure in teaching reading. The purpose of criterion sampling is to provide rich information that improves a program or system.

Confirming and Disconfirming Cases

Confirming and disconfirming cases involve the attempt to confirm what one finds during the exploratory state of the investigation. In other words, some conclusions drawn from the data (in fieldwork or from sources such as stakeholders) should be confirmed or disconfirmed. For example, based on exploratory information, we may want to confirm that students involved in holistic approaches to reading instruction have more positive attitudes toward reading than students involved in teacher-directed reading instruction. Thus, the interpretation is that the type of reading instruction has an impact on student attitudes toward reading. Thus, the researcher could sample students involved in a holistic reading class and students in a teacher-directed reading class, and determine their respective attitudes toward reading. In this manner, the cases involved in the sample either confirm or disconfirm the earlier interpretations. As stated by Patton (1987):

> Thinking about the challenge of finding confirmatory and disconfirming cases emphasizes the relationship between sampling and evaluation conclusions. The sample determines what the evaluator will have something to say about, thus the importance of sampling carefully and thoughtfully. (p. 57)

Sampling Politically Important Cases

Sampling politically important cases is a variation of the critical case strategy. Researchers

---

Extreme or deviant case sampling *involves focusing on cases that have important information because they are unusual or special in some way.*

attempt to select a politically sensitive site or analyze a politically sensitive topic. In some cases, researchers may attempt to avoid the politically sensitive site or topic. For example, in the early to late 1990s, we experienced a political "hot potato" with regard to reading instruction. For various reasons, the use of standardized test scores decreased over a period of several years. (*Note.* Several possible reasons for these decreases are beyond the scope of this example and text.) To better understand this decline, we may purposefully select reading instruction for investigation in an area (e.g., district, school) that has experienced major problems with reading proficiency. The selection of this site for the study could have political consequences but provide critical information about that political climate. One purpose of this sampling method is to increase the usefulness of the gathered information and possibly increase the visibility and impact of the findings.

Convenience Sampling

Convenience sampling was described in Chapter 4. However, although convenience sampling is a common sampling method in both qualitative and quantitative research, it is not viewed as desirable (Patton, 1987). Patton states: "Purposeful, strategic sampling can yield crucial information about critical cases. Convenience sampling is neither purposeful nor strategic" (p. 58).

When reading a qualitative research article, it is important to determine how the sample was selected. Researchers must make certain that the sample was chosen to address the research question directly. The manner in which the sample was chosen addresses directly the credibility of the data. Additionally, according to Patton, there are no rules for sample sizes; the size of the sample must be determined by taking into consideration the needs of interested parties (e.g., stakeholders, decision makers, information seekers). The sample must be large enough to add credibility to the generated data but small enough to allow in-depth analysis of the data. Researchers must be aware that the findings will be critiqued in some manner and anticipate the questions reviewers may raise. They must

make sure that reasons for the selections are stated and explicit (Patton, 1987). An attempt to determine these reasons should add to the credibility of the data.

WHAT IS "UNDERSTANDING" IN QUALITATIVE RESEARCH?

Understanding refers to the way we interpret our data and how that interpretation actually allows us to understand the phenomenon of interest (Mertens, 2009). Maxwell (1992) believed that in qualitative research understanding is more fundamental than validity. Maxwell stated, "I see the types of validity that I present here as derivative from the kinds of understanding gained from qualitative inquiry; my typology of validity categories is also a typology of the kinds of understanding at which qualitative research aims" (p. 281). From a qualitative perspective, *validity* refers to the apparent truthfulness of the collected accounts, not to the data or methods used to gather these data. The inferences drawn from the data may or may not be valid; the item of data itself is neither. This is a critical point. If validity refers to the inferences or conclusions we make about our data, then the validity of our conclusions must be considered. Quantitative researchers many times look at the types of designs or statistical methods used and make a statement of validity or invalidity based on these methods.

For example, if we use a preexperimental design, quantitative researchers might conclude that the validity of the data and any conclusions based on that data are hampered by an inability to control for threats to internal validity. However, qualitative researchers see the conclusions as having paramount importance when compared with the design. For qualitative researchers, a preexperimental design may generate valid or invalid conclusions and inferences; the same can be said about true experimental designs. The design is not the critical aspect in making valid conclusions; however, the data generated with these designs impact the validity of the conclusions. Understanding, then, is concerned with how well we come to learn about a phenomenon. Maxwell (1992) argues that there are five broad categories of understanding in qualitative research and five corresponding types of validity: (1) descriptive, (2) interpretive, (3) theoretical, (4) generalizability, and (5) evaluative. A description of each of the validities follows.

Descriptive Validity

Descriptive validity refers to the factual accuracy of the researcher's or observer's account (Maxwell, 1992). The concern here is whether the gathered data are contrived or distorted. Others should be able to agree that the events or situations occurred. This agreement is similar to interobserver agreement, discussed in Chapter 3. Also, descriptive validity must be viewed in terms of what was included and excluded in the account. For example, if we are interested in studying student reactions to child-centered teaching approaches, leaving out body and facial expressions may be a serious threat to descriptive validity. Descriptive validity, then, refers to the extent to which researchers are able to report accurate data that represent the phenomenon under study. Critical research consumers should take into consideration the extent to which the researcher included and excluded data, or the extent to which others agree on the data gathered.

Interpretive Validity

Interpretive validity refers to the subjective meaning of objects, events, and behaviors to the individuals engaged in and with the objects, events, and behaviors (Dellinger & Leech, 2007). Interpretive validity is specifically relevant to qualitative research. There is no quantitative counterpart to interpretive validity. Rather than being concerned with observed physical aspects, interpretive validity is concerned with those things that cannot be observed, for example, how one believes one is doing is apart from how one is actually doing. Descriptive validity concerns how one is doing in a class; interpretive validity concerns how one believes one is doing in the class. Thus, the participant's perspective is the basis on which a phenomenon is studied and understood.

Interpretive validity relies on not only what people describe to be their beliefs, attitudes, cognitions, intentions, and evaluations but also on the researcher's ability to construct participants' meanings by observing what they say, their body language and past actions, and considering accounts from other sources (e.g., other individuals) also in the situation. Thus, interpretive validity is concerned with the accuracy of the researcher's interpretations with regard to participants' intentions, beliefs, attitudes, evaluations, and cognitions, both consciously and unconsciously. Critical research consumers must be concerned with the researcher's methods to gain the understanding necessary to make valid interpretations, such as asking the participants, asking others, describing nonverbal behaviors (e.g., body position), and gaining information from participants' past.

Theoretical Validity

Theoretical validity is defined as maintaining integrity to ensure accurate interpretation of data (Maxwell, 1997). Maintaining theoretical validity allows the researcher to avoid investigator bias, inattentiveness to discrepant data, or failure to consider alternative understandings. Whereas the first two types of validity refer to the accuracy with which the researcher describes or interprets data, theoretical validity concerns an *explanation*, as well as a description and interpretation of an account (Maxwell, 1992). Theories go beyond the data in that they attempt to provide an explanation for what is observed. Descriptive validity concerns the accuracy of the description; interpretive validity concerns the accuracy of interpretation of the data; and theoretical validity concerns

---

Descriptive validity *refers to the factual accuracy of the researcher's or observer's account.*

Interpretive validity *is concerned with the subjective meanings of objects, events, and behaviors to the individuals engaged in and with the objects, events, and behaviors.*

Theoretical validity *is maintaining integrity to ensure accurate interpretation of data.*

constructing from these descriptions and interpretations a grounded theory to help explain the phenomenon. Maxwell indicates that there are two components to a theory. The first component involves the validity of the concepts that developed the validity, and the second involves relationships among the concepts. For example, as Maxwell (1992) points out,

> One could label the student's throwing of the eraser as an act of resistance, and connect this act to the repressive behavior or values of the teacher, the social structure of the school, and class relationships in U.S. society. The identification of the throwing as "resistance" constitutes the application of a theoretical construct to the descriptive and interpretive understanding of the action; the connection of this to other aspects of the participants, the school, or the community constitutes the postulation of theoretical relationships among these constructs. (p. 291)

Notice that the first aspect of theoretical validity is similar to the construct validity explained in Chapter 3. The second aspect of theoretical validity concerns what we called internal validity in Chapter 2. However, rather than attempting to deal with specific threats to internal validity through a predetermined design, theoretical validity depends more on the community's interpretation and acceptance of the theoretical account. Thus, qualitatively, theoretical or internal validity is a logical and subjective determination rather than an objective one. (*Note.* Many qualitative researchers do not believe that true objectivity exists.) Therefore, even in quantitative research, the determination of internal validity is subjective, since the determination is dependent on the researcher's theoretical framework, beliefs, purposes, and perspective. Critical research consumers should look at how the theory was constructed, whether others agree that the theory is solid, whether the descriptions and interpretations that built the theory are accurate, and how concepts derived from the data were put together. A determination about whether the construction of the theory fits within the overall general framework of what is known about the phenomenon should come from an accumulation of research studies rather than one isolated study.

Generalizability

Generalizability is similar to the external validity described in Chapter 2. (*Note.* Many qualitative researchers reject the concept of generalization. Generalization requires at least some orderliness of phenomena that, according to many qualitative researchers, is not possible when dealing with complex subject matter in human behavior that is context-specific; however, there is a major difference between external validity and generalizability.) As with external validity, *generalizability* refers to the ability to extend the results of an investigation to other persons, settings, or times. The difference lies in the manner in which this extension is accomplished. Recall from earlier chapters that external validity, and specifically population validity, can be enhanced through randomly selecting participants from the population. The assumption is that if the sample mirrors the population, the results found with the sample will most likely hold true for others in the population. However, in qualitative research, random selection of participants is not usually accomplished. As indicated previously, sampling in qualitative research is usually purposeful rather than random. Thus, qualitative researchers must have other ways of generalizing or extending their findings to a broader population.

In one method called *logical generalization*, an inference may be made to others with the same or similar characteristic, such as participants involved in the investigation. A second method is to generate a theory that not only is valid (or seemingly so) for the participants or situations studied (i.e., that makes sense of what they do) but also shows how different results may be obtained in different situations or conditions (Mertens, 2009), and how similar results may be obtained in similar situations or conditions. Generalizability, then, is more a logical or subjective endeavor than an objective or statistical one. Critical research consumers must determine whether the theory makes sense for those in the investigation and whether it is likely to hold up in other situations or conditions, or with other individuals.

Maxwell (1992) discriminates between two types of generalizability: internal and external generalizability. **Internal generalizability** refers to the ability to generalize within the community or group being investigated to those not directly involved in the investigation. For example, Maxwell (2010) describes how studying the interactions of students and teachers in a classroom would be seriously jeopardized if the researcher focused on interviewing only one teacher or one student in the classroom at one particular time of day. A representative sample must be involved in the research to establish internal generalizability.

External generalizability refers to the ability to generalize to other communities or groups. According to Maxwell (1992), internal generalizability is more important to qualitative researchers, who rarely make explicit claims of external generalizability. Some qualitative researchers may in fact insist on a lack of external generalizability in special situations such as studying extreme or ideal cases (Greene & Caracelli, 1997). As Creswell (2009) states, "The value of qualitative research lies in the particular description and themes developed in context of a specific site. Particularity rather than generalizability is the hallmark of qualitative research" (p. 193). Critical research consumers should be aware of the type of generalization being attempted by researchers and determine if the theory makes sense in other situations or conditions. Overall, generalizability is not a central concern of qualitative researchers; descriptive, interpretive, and theoretical validity are more important concerns for qualitative researchers.

Evaluative Validity

Similar to generalizability, evaluative validity is not of central concern to qualitative researchers (Whitemore, Chase, & Mandle, 2001). **Evaluative validity**, or making valid statements, refers to how well a researcher's evaluation of the situation fits with his/her public's evaluation. An example would be the use of corporal punishment in public schools. A researcher's evaluation that corporal punishment is not best practice and should be stopped due to the impact of the punishment on students' self-esteem may be valid for some but not others due to differences in the beliefs about appropriate or inappropriate child management techniques.

WHAT ARE THE EVALUATIVE CRITERIA FOR JUDGING THE RELIABILITY AND VALIDITY OF QUALITATIVE RESEARCH?

Franklin and Jordan (1995) provide several evaluative criteria for judging the reliability and validity of qualitative data or, as qualitative researchers may say, the apparent truthfulness of a study:

> Validity and reliability of qualitative assessment data rest on the credibility, thoroughness, completeness, and consistency of the information interpreted within a narrative assessment report and the logical inferences the clinician uses to draw conclusions from this information about the client. Although accuracy of the clinician's report is difficult to ascertain, the validity and reliability of the interpretations made by the clinician may be evaluated by using the criteria listed below. (p. 291)

The following section describes each of the evaluative criteria for judging qualitative research (i.e., completeness of information; adequacy of interpretation; determination of inconsistencies in data; adequacy of metaphors, pictures, or diagrams; collaboration with participants; and multiple methods to gather data). It is important to note that qualitative researchers such as Howe and Eisenhart (1990) have indicated, "Except at a very high level of abstraction, it is fruitless to try to set standards for qualitative research per se. Even when the focus within qualitative research is significantly restricted, the issues associated with standards are quite complex and extensive" (p. 4). Some qualitative researchers (e.g., Fraenkel & Wallen, 2000; Morse, Barrett, Mayan, Olson, & Spiers, 2002) have called for establishing strong standards of reliability and validity that are interpreted in the same way as quantitative research. Howe

---

Internal generalizability *is the ability to generalize within the community or group being investigated to those not directly involved in the investigation.*

External generalizability *is the ability to generalize to other communities or groups.*

Evaluative validity *refers to making valid statements that fit with the public's evaluation.*

and Eisenhart presented standards for evaluating qualitative research: (1) the fit between research questions and data collection analysis techniques; (2) the effective application of specific data collection and analysis techniques; (3) alertness to and coherence of background assumptions (i.e., existing knowledge); (4) overall warrant (i.e., applying knowledge from outside a particular perspective); and (5) value constraints (i.e., external—worth of research for educators, and internal—research ethics). Thus, standards or criteria should be viewed as general guidelines so as to avoid restrictive interpretations of qualitative research.

Criterion 1: Completeness of Information

The first criterion is concerned with completeness of the information presented. There should be a limited number of gaps in the information, and the data should be coherent enough to make a clear connection with the researcher's conclusions. For example, suppose a researcher wishes to conduct a case study on a particular student in a seventh-grade classroom. The researcher reports complete information for the first semester, but a gap of 2 weeks during the second semester. The student may have been ill during this time; therefore, the researcher should explain this gap.

Criterion 2: Adequacy of Interpretation

The second criterion is concerned with the adequacy of the researcher's interpretations. For example, if the researcher suggests that the student has a developmental disability, missing information about the diagnosis raises a concern.

Criterion 3: Determination of Inconsistencies in Data

The third criterion involves determining whether there are inconsistencies in the data. For example, if a researcher indicates that a student being observed in the classroom is well behaved, then later states that the student had to be disciplined for a class infraction, an apparent inconsistency has occurred and should be explained.

Criterion 4: Adequacy of Metaphors, Pictures, or Diagrams

The fourth criterion is concerned with the adequacy of metaphors, pictures, or diagrams. The use of these techniques should allow for understanding and presenting the information more fully. For example, a picture drawn by the student should allow for more complete understanding of the student and his/her environment.

Criterion 5: Collaboration with Participants

The fifth criterion involves researcher collaboration with the participant(s). The participants' views should be fully reported and integrated throughout the report. These views add credibility to the researcher's conclusions. For example, if the researcher concludes that a student prefers to be placed in an integrated classroom rather than a resource room (where students spend part of the day for extra aid in a subject area), it is beneficial to have statements from the student that back up this conclusion.

Criterion 6: Multiple Methods to Gather Data

The sixth criterion involves the use of multiple methods to gather data. This question is a critical one. Qualitative research methods must have some method of ensuring the reliability and validity of the data collected. One of the most desirable ways to strengthen an investigation's reliability and validity is through triangulation (Silverman, 2005), which is one of the most important methods one can use to document and describe what is going on in the research setting. According to Patton (1990), *triangulation* is the use of "several kinds of methods or data, including using both quantitative and qualitative approaches" (p. 187). The logic behind triangulation is that all data collection methods have strengths and weaknesses. It is to the advantage of researchers to use a combination of data collection methods (e.g., observation, interview, and document analyses) so that the strength of one method can compensate for weakness in another method. (*Note.* Observation, interview, and document analysis methods are discussed in more detail in Chapter 10.)

Observations

According to Patton (1990), observation has several strengths. First, observation provides a picture of what is occurring in the context. What is being observed is occurring at that very point in time in that context. Second, the ability to obtain firsthand experience allows researchers to be more open and discovery-oriented; they can access unexpected information. Finally, observation also allows researchers to view things that may have been missed if observers were not present.

Observational methods have a number of potential weaknesses (Patton, 2002). First, there may be observer bias; that is, what the observer views is not reflected in what he/she documents. Second, there may be reactivity in the observations. Consider your reaction if someone were watching everything you do and taking notes to document your actions. Third, only external behaviors are recorded. Internal behaviors such as beliefs and attitudes are not directly observed. Finally, only a limited sample of the total time period can be observed. Consider observing someone for 4 hours during the day. The concern is whether an observation for 4 hours is an adequate representation of the entire day's activities and behaviors.

Interviews

Interviews can overcome these observational weaknesses in several ways. First, the data are solicited from the participant rather than an observer. Second, there can be a check on the observer's accuracy; that is, if an observer reports something occurring and through an interview a participant also indicated the same thing, the event's likelihood of occurrence is increased. For example, suppose that an observer reports that a participant seemed to have fun with a reading activity. The participant could be asked about his/her reaction to the reading activity. If the participant indicates that he/she had fun or enjoyed the reading activity, our confidence in the accuracy of the observation is increased.

Third, internal behaviors can be measured, albeit indirectly. For example, an observer's report that a teacher used a certain curriculum in her classroom can be documented by watching the teacher's classroom behavior. However, the observer cannot directly report whether the teacher likes the curriculum; the observer would have to make an inference through behaviors such as body position, facial expressions, and tone of voice. An interviewer could ask the teacher to comment on the curriculum. The teacher's attitude toward the curriculum could then be examined in a manner that could not be directly examined through observation. Finally, an interviewer can attempt to sample a much wider range of program activities and situations than could an observer. An interviewer could ask what occurred during the nonobservational period or last year, or even 10 years ago. The point here is that information gained through interviews cannot be gained through observations, because doing so is impossible or impractical.

Although interviews can overcome or compensate for problems with observations, they do have weaknesses. First, there may be distortion in the perceptions or perspectives due to the researcher's state of mind (Seidman, 2006). Statements that reflect anger, bias, or lack of awareness could distort information the researcher provides in an interview. If, for example, we ask about the job performance of someone we do not like, we may be more apt to provide inaccurate information by either downplaying achievements or highlighting failures or weaknesses. Second, there may be a lack of recall during the interview. Based on much memory research, we know that people have a tendency to put in fictitious information where there are gaps in memory. Thus, the reliability and validity of information obtained from interviews may be suspect in certain circumstances, especially when information on obscure events or events that occurred some time ago is needed. Finally, interviews are problematic when there is reactivity to the interviewer. This reactivity may include an interviewee telling the interviewer what he/she thinks the interviewer wants to hear or exaggerating an event to make him-/herself look better, or downplaying an event for the same purposes. Obviously, observation can help to overcome the problems with interviews and verify information provided by interviewees.

Document Analysis

Document analysis involves obtaining data from any number of written or visual sources such as diaries, novels, incident reports, pictures, advertisements, speeches, official documents, files, films, audiotapes, books, newspapers, and so on. Document analyses are popular methods of data collection for qualitative researchers when the data are presented as a permanent product. Document analyses may include incident reports in a school, number and types of arrests on school grounds, newspaper accounts of events, or historical records kept by certain groups.

Document analyses have several advantages over observations and interviews for some types of information. First, document analysis involves permanent products; that is, documents can be studied by several individuals at different times. Second, there is no reactivity on the part of participants. Finally, information that may not be available anywhere else may be available in documents. Thus, document analyses can fill in gaps in observational or interview data and check the accuracy of that information. For example, suppose that a school administrator is concerned with the level of truancy in her school. She indicates that the problem is severe and that steps should be taken to correct it. However, based on records kept in the office, the truancy problem is about half that of other local schools. In this case, although truancy may be a problem, the administrator's perception of the severity of the problem may be questioned due to data in the official records.

However, document analyses have weaknesses. First, the information found in documents may be incomplete. Reports may not have been entered, or they may have been misfiled. Second, the information in the documents may be inaccurate. Just because the information is in an official document, its accuracy is not ensured. Any number of variables could make the information inaccurate, such as biased reporting by the person entering the information. Third, the

information in documents may highlight only the positive and leave out the negative, or vice versa. Finally, documents usually vary in the quality of information they contain and the specificity of that information. Again, combining other sources of data collection with document analysis improves believability of the data. Observations and interviews can verify the information obtained through documents.

Criterion 7: Disqualification of Interpretations

The final criterion has to do with the attempt made of the researcher to disqualify his/her interpretations of the data. The concern that should come to mind as one reads a qualitative investigation is whether researchers have put forth other explanations for the obtained data. Creswell (2009) notes that because researchers may never completely detach from their interpretation of events, they should describe their own potential biases, values, and personal background (e.g., gender, history, culture) as a part of the research report.

Rationalism is a central concept to science. When researchers are attempting to explain their results in a number of ways, they are practicing rationalism. For example, suppose a researcher is attempting to find out why students tend to drop out of school. The researcher visits a school with a high level of dropouts and interviews the teachers and students. The researcher also contacts other students who have dropped out of school within the past 2 years and interviews them. After analyzing the data, the researcher concludes that the reason most of the students drop out of school is a lack of understanding of the material being taught, which in turn made them feel like outcasts. The teachers indicate that the students most prone to dropout have difficulties keeping up in class. Students currently in school indicate that of the students who dropped out, most were not a part of the "in crowd." The students who dropped out indicate that school was difficult and not enjoyable. Alternative explanations the researcher considers include problems with parental support, the need for outside income for the family, and being in a large school environment. These other explanations were not supported by the data, and the researcher's explanation seems to have the greatest support from the data.

WHAT ARE THE TYPES OF TRIANGULATION METHODS?

Triangulation is defined as collecting data from multiple sources and methods in order to increase the strength of themes (Kaplan & Maxwell, 2005). When reviewing a qualitative investigation, triangulation methods should be one of the first concerns of critical research consumers. As stated by Pitman and Maxwell (1992):

> Acknowledging that qualitative research allows more scope for researchers to see what they choose and, thus, greater chance for the intentional neglect of evidence contrary to one's values or interests, Eisner argues that, *"it is especially important not only to use multiple sources of data, but also to consider disaffirming evidence and contrary interpretations or appraisals* when one presents one's own conclusions [emphasis in original]" (Eisner, 1991:111). (p. 748)

As indicated in the previous discussion, drawing from multiple data sources has the advantage of overcoming the weaknesses of using a single data source. Patton (1990) indicates that there are four types of triangulation: (1) data sources, (2) analyst, (3) theory/perspective, and (4) methods (see Figure 9.3).

Data Sources Triangulation

According to Patton (1990), triangulation of data sources means

> (1) comparing observational data with interview data, (2) comparing what people say in public with what they say in private, (3) checking for the consistency of what people say about the same thing over time, and (4) comparing the perspectives of people from other points of view—staff views, client views, funder views, and views expressed by people outside the program. (p. 467)

The main purpose of triangulation of data sources is to validate information obtained from one source by gathering information from another source. For example, to discover how satisfied secondary teachers in a large metropolitan area are, we could interview the teachers and find out that their job satisfaction is fairly low. We could also observe the teachers and see that they are not excited upon arrival at work and they leave the school building as soon as the last class has ended. The two sources of very different data seem to correspond. However, the information gathered from two or more sources may not be congruent. In other words, there are times when data from multiple sources do not support one another. Suppose that we interview not only the teachers but also administrators in regard to job satisfaction. We may find that the teachers indicate low job satisfaction but that administrators perceive the job satisfaction of teachers to be high. In this case, there is incongruence. However, a lack of correspondence is not all bad. The reason for the lack of consistent findings presents a new research question. It would be important, for example, to find out why teacher and supervisor perceptions are so different. Ultimately, critical research consumers have to judge whether conclusions based on inconsistent information from multiple data sources are compromised.

Analyst Triangulation

Analyst triangulation refers to the use of multiple analysts, such as multiple interviewers or observers (Patton, 2002). The importance of using multiple analysts is to check the accuracy of the information obtained. When a single person collects all of the data, the chance for bias is relatively strong. When multiple analysts are involved, this bias should be reduced. For example, let's say that a researcher is observing the social interactions of students in cooperative learning situations. Also suppose that the researcher is a major advocate of cooperative learning. If the researcher is the only observer, bias in the observations is a possibility. On the other hand, if there are one or more observers apart from the researcher, and the information

> **Document analysis** *involves obtaining data from any number of written or visual sources.*
>
> **Triangulation** *is defined as collecting data from multiple sources and methods.*

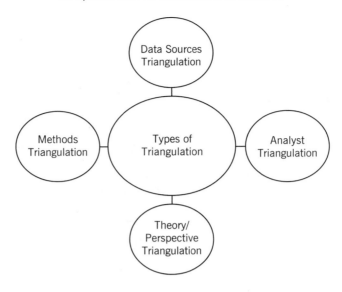

FIGURE 9.3. Four types of triangulation.

obtained from these other observers is consistent with the researcher's information, the researcher's data are more believable. Patton also recognized another form of multiple analysts. Besides using more than one observer or interviewer, two or more individuals may assess existing data and compare their conclusions. The purpose of this type of triangulation is to verify the conclusions of the researchers. However, it is unlikely that everyone will reach agreement in their conclusions. This disagreement can in fact be healthy. Since we all have different experiences, it is unlikely that we will all interpret the same thing in a similar manner. Therefore, the reasons for the differences in the interpretation can also lead to new research questions.

Theory/Perspective Triangulation

Patton (1990) suggests that triangulation can be achieved through interpreting data from different theoretical perspectives. For example, we could conduct research on teaching students how to become more independent via learning how to solve problems. Problem solving has a long research history among investigators from several theoretical positions. The data on problem solving can be gathered and interpreted

from cognitive and behavioral viewpoints, for example. A cognitive interpretation may center on how cognition changes in some manner helped the individual to process information differently. The change in the processing of information allowed the individual to solve the problems encountered. The behavioral interpretation may center on how the environment was changed to allow specific or novel responses to be emitted in response to stimuli in that environment. Patton indicates that the purpose of theory triangulation is to "understand how findings are affected by different assumptions and fundamental premises" (p. 470). Again, it is unlikely that the interpretations will agree. This disagreement is not viewed as problematic. The assumptions that led to the disagreement can become the focus of research in future investigations.

Methods Triangulation

Methods triangulation involves comparing data generated from two or more methodologies, such as qualitative and quantitative methods (Patton, 1990). The difficulty with methods triangulation is that it is not always appropriate to use any two methodologies for the same research question. However, the point with methods triangulation is that if researchers can come to the same conclusion using different methods, the conclusions are more likely to be accurate.

For example, suppose that a researcher wishes to study the effects of a compensatory reading program. The researcher may implement the reading program in one class but not in a comparable class. Pretests are given to both classes, and the pretest average reading skills are similar. A posttest is then provided to both classes after the first class concludes the reading program. The class receiving the compensatory reading program outperforms the other class. This scenario illustrates an example of a quantitative design. We could also send observers to each class to collect observational data on how students behave within the context of the classroom. We could observe, for example, how students approach the reading assignments, how they discuss the reading program with one another, and how they behave once the reading program is over for the day. We could also observe teacher behavior. Are the teachers happy and excited about the reading program? How do they treat the students? What are the teachers' nonverbal behaviors like? The information gained from the qualitative observations may indicate that there is great excitement about the program, that teachers are willing to use the program, and that students are willing to put forth effort during the program. If the researcher concluded that the reading program is more effective than the traditional program, the conclusion is more believable, with qualitative data indicating that classroom staff and students were excited about and willing to use the compensatory program. However, this agreement of the methodologies may not occur often. In fact, quantitative data might suggest that the compensatory reading program is effective, and qualitative data might suggest that a focused and structured program may restrict teachers' and students' creativity.

HOW ARE QUALITATIVE DATA ANALYZED?

Qualitative researchers have unique data analysis procedures that differ from those used by quantitative researchers. Qualitative researchers look for themes, concepts, and explanatory sets (Hart, Cramer, Harry, Klingner, & Sturges, 2010). They use coding strategies and rubrics (Quesenberry, Hemmeter, & Ostrosky, 2011). Some qualitative studies use Strauss and Corbin's (1997) process of constant comparison of data or Corbin and Strauss's (2007) coding for grounded theory. Interpretative phenomenological analysis (IPA; Smith, Osborn, & Flowers, 1999) is sometimes used as a phenomenological approach to data analysis to explore personal perceptions or experience. Consistent with the qualitative approach, these forms of data analysis produce not numerical measures of dependent variables but narrative data extracted from the research. Often the methods of analysis evolve over the course of the research. In many regards, data analysis involved with qualitative research methods is much more difficult to complete than that in quantitative research. Think of it this way. Suppose we want to identify how study guides for a social studies class affect the students in a classroom. We could use either quantitative or qualitative approaches (a combination of the two would likely be beneficial). If we select the quantitative approach, we may proceed as follows: Develop the study guides; define the student behaviors we wish to measure, such as academic performance (i.e., test scores); distribute study guides for each unit; give a unit test; determine each student's score; and get an average test score for the class. (*Note.* We are using a repeated measures design.) In a second social studies class, we do not provide study guides. At the end of the study, we see whether the class that received study guides outperforms the class that did not receive the study guides.

If we select a qualitative design, then we would most likely study one classroom. We attempt to gather data from several sources (i.e., triangulation of data) to aid in the validation of the data collection. Let's say the data we gathered are in the form of narration through journal entries. The teacher, researcher, and students are each independently writing reactions, beliefs, attitudes, expectations, interpretations, and evaluations of the study guides. Throughout the study, we continuously review the data and decide on some method of synthesizing it. Also, throughout the study, we are analyzing how the data are collected and the type of information produced. At the end of the investigation, there are mounds of journal entries. We have a coding system and begin to code the data. We look for important classes of things, persons, and events.

For instance, we may find that teachers frequently report they are anxious when instructing, since they want to cover all of the material contained in the study guide. We may find that many students report that they do not like the study guides, because they take too long to complete. We also may find that many of the teachers do not think the study guides are helping students gain information outside of what is listed on the study guide. Here, we have themes emerging, such as the length of the study guides, the type of information contained on the study guides, and the restrictiveness of the study guides. Once these themes or categories emerge, some tentative conclusions and questions can be generated, such as the study guides are too long and should be shortened. However, if we shorten them, how do we include more relevant information? Teachers should not feel constrained by the study guides when preparing their instruction, but should information contained in the instruction be represented on the study guide? The difficulty is to make sure the coding system contains all of the important information. Once the data have been coded, conclusions are made. We may wish to use numbers to help in the process of interpretation, such as the number of students who thought the journal entries were worthwhile; however, the main source of data is words.

Judgment in Qualitative Research

The analysis of qualitative data is not nearly as straightforward as that of quantitative data, and it requires a great deal more thought and effort to do well. Strauss and Corbin (1997) indicate that judgments must be made in three areas of qualitative research—reliability, validity, and credibility of the data; adequacy of the research process; and empirical grounding of the research process. Critical research consumers should consider each of the three areas to evaluate a qualitative investigation. This method of evaluation is different than the one used by quantitative researchers, in that when

looking at threats to internal and external validity, the design is paramount in the evaluation. With qualitative research, the whole process of the study is paramount, not simply the design.

In what follows, we describe how to interpret qualitative research. It is probably not useful to interpret a qualitative study using quantitative evaluation methods (Maxwell, 2010; Silverman, 2005). Qualitative and quantitative methods rest on different assumptions and have different purposes. However, since we have considered threats to internal and external validity in previous chapters, we do the same in this chapter. We also add new validity categories for analyzing the data in qualitative research.

Internal Validity

Qualitative research serves many purposes but is not specifically designed to answer cause-and-effect questions. In other words, researchers in qualitative research do not actively attempt to manipulate an independent variable. However, the question of internal validity, from a qualitative perspective, is a desirable one for many researchers (Maxwell, 2010). On the other hand, Mishler (1990) argued that to extend the concept of validity from quantitative methods to qualitative research is misguided. He indicated that validity is dependent more on researchers' judgments than on following certain procedures. As noted by Creswell (2009), "Validity does not carry the same connotations in qualitative research as it does in quantitative research, nor is it a companion of reliability or generalizability" (p. 190).

Internal validity is a quantitative concept that relies on a set of certain assumptions about how to find cause-and-effect associations. The use of specific designs and other set procedures, such as measurement, manipulation of the independent variable, and participant assignments, is critical in demonstrating internal validity for quantitative designs. On the other hand, qualitative designs rely on the understanding of the context in which participants perform and on theory that explains why something occurs. The manner in which qualitative researchers demonstrate internal validity uses logic and subjective reasoning rather than objective assessment of research methods. The problem with viewing qualitative research from a quantitative viewpoint in terms of internal validity is that qualitative research almost never meets the criteria for internal validity.

External Validity

External validity is viewed similarly by qualitative and quantitative researchers (Bogdan & Biklen, 1998). Both view external validity as an attempt to generalize results of an investigation to other individuals, in other settings, and across time. However, the role of external validity differs for different forms of research. Many times quantitative studies use sampling methods (i.e., random selection) to allow them to make external validity claims.

Qualitative research is not usually designed to allow systematic generalizations to other individuals. Qualitative researchers may use logical generalizations; they may also utilize extensions or continuations to help demonstrate generalizability of their results. Another method qualitative researchers may use to establish external validity is to develop a theory from the data that can be used in other situations or with different people. However, there are no statistical methods that can be used to achieve external validity in a qualitative investigation. Additionally, claims of external validity in qualitative research may be made by critical research consumers rather than researchers (Winter, 2000). Qualitative researchers are usually more cautious in their claims and rely on the research consumers to decide whether the results would benefit them, their students, or their setting. As with internal validity, the demonstration is more one of logical interpretation of the data than statistical manipulation of the data or special quantitative research designs aimed at these two validity types.

Analyzing Qualitative Research

Potter (1996) provides a template for analyzing these issues. Table 9.4 shows the four categories for analysis. The first category is *expectations*. Potter indicated that there are three ways in which expectations guide research—deductive, inductive, and mixed approaches. With *deduction*, researchers enter into the investigation

TABLE 9.4. Template for Analysis Issues

Issue 1: Expectations

Key question: To what extent do expectations for findings guide the selection of evidence?

Alternative answers:
1. A priori expectations: The researchers have set out a very clear goal for what data they need. With social science, theory and hypotheses are clear guides. Also, ideologies serve as a priori guides.
2. Emerging expectations: No beginning expectations, but as researchers gather data, they become more focused on searching for certain data and ignoring other data.

Issue 2: Process of analysis

Key question: To what extent does the researcher illuminate the process of using the evidence to construct arguments/findings for the written report?

Alternative answers:
1. Authors describe the steps taken in analyzing the data, that is, the step between data gathering and presenting the report.
2. Authors do not describe the steps used in analyzing their data.

Issue 3: Conceptual leverage

Key question: To what extent does the researcher extend his/her arguments/findings beyond reporting on the elements of evidence into a general conceptual level?

Alternative answers:
1. None: No attempt to move beyond describing literal events in the data. The reporting is limited to description of the actual data themselves.
2. Low level: The researcher constructs patterns (through his/her own processes of inference) to make sense of the literal data.
3. High level: Inferring a connection to an a priori construction such as a theory or ideology.

Issue 4: Generalizability

Key question: To what extent does the researcher attempt to use his/her evidence to generalize?

Alternative answers:
1. No generalizations: Researchers only present data or patterns about their observed subjects during the times and places they were observed.
2. Generalization: Researchers exhibit a large move from data to conclusion. The largeness in the degree can be due to the very small size of the sample or the very broad nature of the conclusions.

with a priori expectations. In other words, they determine before the investigation begins what they expect to find and design the collection and analysis of data around their expectations. *Induction* refers to beginning the investigation with some observations, attempting to rule out nothing from analysis. After the investigation is finished, researchers attempt to interpret the data. There are no expectations guiding the investigation. With the *mixed* approach, researchers formulate the topic, such as a research question. Most, if not all, researchers have some initial formulation before an investigation. Potter indicates that it is probably impossible for researchers to have little or no formulation, as in an inductive process. Once the investigation begins, researchers make conclusions, then test these conclusions on an ongoing basis.

The second category involves the *process* of analysis, which refers to the extent to which researchers explain or describe the methods used in the investigation to construct their arguments and/or findings. Maxwell (2010) describes this in terms of descriptive validity. The accuracy of the data collection and analysis is critical in the process.

The third category involves the *conceptual leverage* used in the analysis of the data. Potter (1996) describes three levels of conceptual leverage. The first level involves concrete description that refers to the lack of inference about the data. The data are described as observed. There is no attempt to infer to motives, beliefs, interests, or theories. The second level involves *low-level interference*, in that inferences are made in regard to those things not directly observed. This level is similar to Maxwell's (2010) interpretive validity, in which the concern is with mental rather than physical understanding. The final level involves *high-level inference*, in which a connection is made between the data and some theory or construction. There may be an attempt to determine cause-and-effect relationships through high-level inference. However, as Potter (1996) indicates, few qualitative researchers view this type of inference as desirable.

Many qualitative researchers (e.g., Cho & Trent, 2006; Maxwell, 2004) reject altogether the concept of causality based on philosophical grounds. Thus, most qualitative researchers use low-level inference. This type of inference

is similar to Maxwell's (2010) theoretical validity, which attempts to explain why something occurred rather than simply describe what occurred. High-level inference is also similar to Maxwell's evaluative validity, which attempts to make evaluative statements from an ideological framework.

The final category involves generalizability. Potter (1996) indicates that generalizability is the attempt made by researchers to extend the results of investigations to other individuals or situations. Potter suggests that many qualitative researchers do not believe that generalization is possible for a number of reasons (e.g., true objectivity is not possible and each situation is unique to itself; random sampling is not possible). Other researchers indicate that generalization is possible in the form of grounded theory and through induction. Potter states that most researchers take the middle ground, in that there are a number of definitions of generalization. Potter's generalizability is similar to the generalizability described by Maxwell (2010).

The critical point in judging qualitative research is determining the conclusions/claims made by researchers and investigating whether the data support the conclusions/claims. The subject of cause-and-effect relationships and generalizability will likely always be controversial in qualitative research. As stated by Potter (1996):

> Like with the issue of conceptual leverage, the key to appreciating generalizability is in looking for correspondence between evidence and conclusions. Whether generalization should be permissible or not within the qualitative approach is a debate that will not likely be resolved given the strongly held beliefs of the scholars on each side. So it is best to accept the range of beliefs. However, once a scholar establishes his or her position, we as readers can check to make sure that their beliefs as reflected in their design support the level of generalization in their research. (p. 133)

Computer Software for Qualitative Research

Computer software has been used by many qualitative researchers as a way to identify themes, concepts, and explanatory sets (Fielding & Lee, 1998). Some of the more popular software programs include NVivo, QDA Miner, and Ethnograph (QSR International, 2008), ATLAS.ti and Nudist (Barry, 1998), and MAX-QDA (Lu & Schulman, 2008), to name but a few. This list will undoubtedly expand and change over time. We consider one example. NVivo can perform constant comparison analysis (i.e., looking for similar themes), key words-in-context (i.e., looking for multiple words around a key word), word count (i.e., frequency of specific words), classical content analysis (counting themes or codes whether they are created a priori or a posteriori), domain analysis (i.e., symbols and semantic relationships), taxonomic analysis (i.e., how specific words are utilized by participants), and componential analysis (i.e., looking for similarities and differences in information obtained from participants) (Leech & Onwuegbuzie, 2011). Although it is beyond the scope of this book to provide detailed information on qualitative computer software, suffice it to say that many programs have been developed to analyze, organize, and present narrative data. Lu and Shulman (2008) stated,

Another important contribution of computer-assisted qualitative data analysis software results from the capability of improving rigorous analysis. Computerized qualitative data analysis, when grounded in the data itself, good theory, and appropriate research design, is often more readily accepted as legitimate research. (p. 107)

We encourage critical consumers to question this claim and would counter that while computer-assisted qualitative data analysis software assists in sorting through massive or confusing data files, the process itself does not legitimize the research. Legitimate qualitative research is founded on the extent to which methods yield data that address the research questions. The research may or may not use computer software. Others have questioned use of computer-assisted qualitative data analysis software, noting that computer-derived themes may be different from those identified by researchers (Maclean, Meyer, Estable, Kothari, & Edwards, 2010). Bassett (2004) cautions researchers to remain vigilant and not rely solely on computer software.

SUMMARY

❖ Qualitative research is defined as research concerned with understanding the context in which behavior occurs. Quantitative research, on the other hand, is concerned with the reliable and valid investigation of the impact of independent variables on dependent variables, or the relationships between or among variables.

❖ The characteristics of qualitative research are not agreed upon by all qualitative researchers. However, two characteristics are relevant: (1) Field research provides a broader perspective on theory than simply a relationship between variables; and (2) flexibility of field research allows pursuit of theory development in an effective and economical manner.

❖ There are several differences between qualitative and quantitative research: (1) source of data, (2) nature of data, (3) process of change, (4) type of reasoning, and (5) focus of research.

❖ Qualitative research procedures involve several procedures: (1) asking a research question, (2) collecting the data, (3) deciding on a sample, (4) analyzing the data, and (5) reaching conclusions or understandings.

❖ Understanding in qualitative research involves five broad categories: (1) descriptive validity, (2) interpretive validity, (3) theoretical validity, (4) generalizability validity, and (5) evaluative validity.

❖ There are seven evaluative criteria for judging the reliability and validity of qualitative research: Criterion 1 refers to the completeness of information; Criterion 2 concerns the adequacy of interpretation; Criterion 3 is the determination of inconsistencies in data; Criterion 4 refers to the adequacy of metaphors, pictures, or diagrams; Criterion 5 is the collaboration with participants; Criterion 6 involves multiple methods to gather data; and Criterion 7 concerns the disqualification of interpretations.

❖ Triangulation methods involve collecting data from a range of sources: (1) data sources, (2) analyst, (3) theory/perspective, and (4) methods.

❖ Qualitative researchers have unique data analysis procedures that differ from those used by quantitative researchers. Researchers look for themes, concepts, and explanatory sets. Qualitative research is not designed to answer internal validity questions as is quantitative research; any questions of internal validity are dependent on a researcher's judgment. External validity is viewed similarly by qualitative and quantitative researchers; however, rather than using statistical methods to make generalized claims, qualitative researchers may use logical generalization. Qualitative research may be analyzed under four categories—expectations, process of analysis, conceptual leverage, and generalizability.

DISCUSSION QUESTIONS

1. Are qualitative methods considered to be as valid as quantitative methods? Explain.

2. Is the lack of random sampling a weakness of qualitative research methods? Why or why not?

3. What are the differences between qualitative and quantitative research methods?

4. Do qualitative methods lack internal and external validity? Explain.

5. What is the problem with judging qualitative research methods from a quantitative viewpoint?

6. What evaluative criteria do Franklin and Jordan (1995) suggest when judging the reliability and validity of qualitative data? Provide a novel example for each criterion.

7. What is triangulation? In your answer, describe the different forms of triangulation.

8. How does triangulation help to increase the reliability and validity (or believability) of conclusions based on the collected data?

9. What are some of the difficulties that need to be overcome to integrate quantitative and qualitative methods?

10. How are internal and external validity viewed in qualitative methods compared to quantitative methods when analyzing data?

See Chapter 10 for an illustrative example of qualitative research.

CHAPTER 10

■ ■ ■ ■

Data Collection and Designs in Qualitative Research

OBJECTIVES

After studying this chapter, you should be able to . . .

1. Explain how defining qualitative methods is based on the method of data collection.
2. Outline the different field-oriented studies.
3. Describe what is meant by historical research and how one analyzes historical research.
4. Illustrate how mixed methods studies utilize qualitative and quantitative concepts.
5. Specify how researchers should use each qualitative research design.

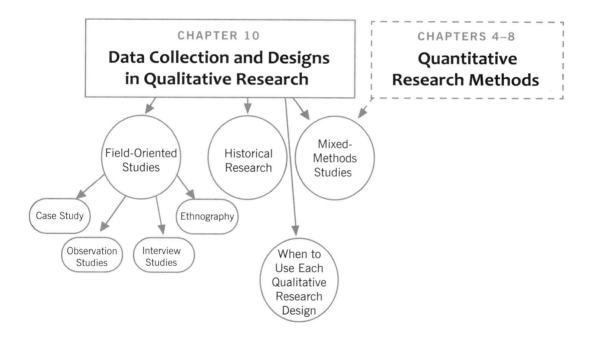

OVERVIEW

Qualitative research as a methodology has different purposes than quantitative research. In addition, validity and reliability issues are interpreted differently by many qualitative researchers than by quantitative researchers. Finally, the actual methods used differ from those used by quantitative researchers. Whereas quantitative researchers have specific designs that are rigid and defined before the collection of data, qualitative researchers' designs evolve as a result of the collection of data throughout the investigation. The methods (i.e., designs) are not as easily defined as those methods used in quantitative research. Qualitative research methods are tied to the method of data collection. For example, interview or observation studies are defined by the methods used in collecting a type of data. Quantitative research designs are independent of the data collection methods (e.g., quantitative research studies are not defined as, for example, a standardized test study).

Since qualitative research and data collection methods are so closely related, this chapter describes data collection methods in conjunction with research methods. The methods discussed in this chapter are representative of the most frequently used qualitative research methods. However, a comprehensive discussion of all qualitative research methods is beyond the scope of this chapter.

WHAT ARE FIELD-ORIENTED STUDIES?

Field-oriented studies are those conducted in applied settings wherein the researcher gathers information about a phenomenon (e.g., a person, group of people, or event), as well as all contextual factors that influence the phenomenon (Stake, 1995). Five types of field-oriented studies are reviewed in this chapter, including case studies, observation studies, interview studies, ethnographic studies, and document analysis. In practice, many qualitative research efforts combine different types of field-oriented studies. Additionally, a special form of qualitative research, historical research, is described. At the end of the chapter, an example of a qualitative investigation is presented for critique.

Case Study

Essentially, all of the designs in this chapter can be considered **case study designs**, in that each involves an intense study of the phenomenon of interest (Yin, 2009). Case study research is useful for an in-depth study of problems to understand processes or situations in context (Vennesson, 2008). A great deal of information can be learned in this way. Case study research focuses on one participant, setting, situation, or event. For example, let's say we want to study a particular elementary school due to its unusually high test scores (e.g., the average for the school is in the upper 95% nationwide). We could visit the school and assess how the students are taught. We could use any number of data collection methods, such as interview techniques aimed at teachers, parents, children, and administrators, and/or observational techniques, such as participant observations of classrooms, in which we become involved in the instruction

---

> ### Research Examples
>
> Consider these issues. Think about how you would design research to address the questions/hypotheses from these examples:
>
> - Research Example 1: How does a teacher deliver effective literacy instruction to a student who is blind and uses braille?
> - Research Example 2: In what ways do parental messages about sex influence college-age women's disclosure of sexual assault to their parents?
> - Research Example 3: What processes that intensify children's behavioral and academic difficulties contribute to their diagnosis of emotional disturbance (ED) and referral to special education?
> - Research Example 4: To what extent do Head Start policies and procedures address child guidance and challenging behaviors?
> - Research Example 5: Will a school-based psychoeducational intervention increase academic self-efficacy of urban youth enrolled in ninth grade?
>
> Research examples appear throughout the chapter.

or nonparticipant observation, in which we observe from afar.

What makes case studies different from other methods is the focus on in-depth analysis of a single case. Once we have collected and analyzed our data from the elementary school, interpretations of the data begins. One possible interpretation may be that the students have more hands-on learning opportunities or are taught in skills-intensive classrooms. The parents may come from a higher SES than the average family, or they may be more involved in their children's schooling. The administration may give teachers more autonomy with regard to curriculum decisions. The information gained from case study research can help to develop hypotheses and theories for later studies. Finally, a case narrative is written to present a holistic portrayal of the case.

Critical research consumers must have at least two general concerns when judging the adequacy of a case study. First, the information for each case must be as complete as possible. If the researcher left out critical facts or made claims that were not substantiated by data gathered in the case study, the validity of those claims must be considered carefully. Second, critical research consumers should expect the description of the case to be logical and easy to follow. If the readability of the case study is not adequate, it will be more difficult to understand and interpret the results of the investigation.

Observation Studies

An **observation study** in qualitative research, in which an observer or observers work in the field to gather information about a phenomenon, is a form of case study. It is helpful to think of observations on a continuum from complete participant (i.e., observers become involved with the participants as if they are part of the group; the participants usually do not know they are being observed) to complete observer (i.e., similar to the types of observations used in single-case research described in Chapters 11–13 [not to be confused with case study research]; when one is a complete observer, there is an attempt to remain separated from the subject matter; Bogdan & Biklen, 1998; Patton, 2002) (see Figure 10.1). In reality, qualitative research observations

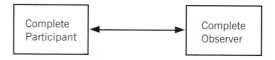

FIGURE 10.1. Continuum from complete participant to complete observer.

fall somewhere between these two extremes in the participant observation study, nonparticipant observation study, naturalistic study, or simulation.

Participant Observation Study

One purpose of observing without becoming involved with the participants is to have no effect on participants. Only those things that are directly observable are recorded when observers distance themselves from participants. However, qualitative researchers "make the assumption that behavior is purposeful and expressive of deeper beliefs and values" (Potter, 1996, p. 99). Therefore, the one method that allows consideration of these deeper beliefs and values is to become personally acquainted with participants. Researchers interact with the participants in an attempt to see whether participants say what they believe and believe what they say. In other words, they are concerned with the correspondence between what an individual says about a topic and how he/she actually views the topic. For example, think of someone you know really well. You may be able to pick up on some behaviors indicating that the person is feeling troubled about something. When you ask the person if anything is wrong, he/she says that everything is great. If you stop there, you might conclude that there is nothing wrong. However,

Field-oriented studies *are those conducted in applied settings.*

✳ **Case study designs** *involve the in-depth analysis of a single case, such as one school or one individual.*

An **observation study** *is one in which an observer or observers work in the field to gather information about a phenomenon.*

since you know the individual well, you can pick up on other signs that indicate the person is not telling you how he/she really feels. Qualitative researchers attempt to do the same thing. They try to get to know the participants well enough to pick up on these other signs. An added advantage is that once the participants get to know the researchers on an individual basis, they may begin to open up more than they would have during a nonparticipant observation.

Field Notes. Participant observations are usually recorded as *field notes.* Potter (1996) indicates that these notes usually are taken at two levels. The first level (surface) contains the facts or direct descriptions of what is seen and or overheard (this can also take the form of audio recordings). The second level involves observers writing down their thoughts about the events and interviews. The purpose of this level is to provide a context for the facts observed at the surface level and to add what the researcher thinks the facts mean. The purpose of participant observation is not only to see what is going on but also to feel what it is like to be part of the group.

Field notes are a critical part of qualitative research, because they aid researchers in collecting and remembering information from observational sessions. According to Potter (1996), notes can come in many forms, such as audiotapes, videotapes, and photographs. However, when the observer writes notes, they must be complete. One needs to include information such as who was present, what the students were doing, what the teachers were doing, what materials were used, how long each activity lasted, interruptions that occurred, arrangement of the classroom, and reactions of the students to the teachers and vice versa. In other words, field notes must include not only what is going on in a setting but also provide details about the physical setting and the reactions of the individuals present at the event. The recordings are very difficult to do well, since one is required to attend to several details at one time.

Additionally, the volume of written material can become overwhelming.

Analysis of the notes is a must in qualitative research. Observers must set up the criteria to be categorized or coded and begin to make sense of the data. They must weave together the facts from the data in a narrative story of the events observed. The difficulty of the task is represented by Potter (1996):

> When dealing with the facet of people, the qualitative researcher must develop a composite picture about how people think about things. Each person's belief may be different because people focus their attention on different things and interpret the same things differently. Also, their beliefs change over time. The researcher must make sense out of all of this seemingly conflicting information. The researcher must try to examine why there are differences in meanings. (p. 123)

Field notes are a reflection of how the observer sees the events and therefore include the observer's interpretations of the events. Potter (1996) indicates that some professionals believe field notes should be written after a period of

---

Field Notes

There must be substantial detail in field notes. Patton (1990) provides several examples of detailed field notes. He also shows how these detailed field notes can be written in a manner that loses critical information. The following example from Patton is a vague note.

> The new client was uneasy waiting for her intake interview. (p. 240)

Now, compare this note with the detailed one:

> At first the new client sat very stiffly on the chair next to the receptionist's desk. She picked up a magazine and let the pages flutter through her fingers very quickly without really looking at any of the pages. She set the magazine down, looked at her watch, pulled her skirt down, and picked up the magazine again. This time she didn't look at the magazine. She set it back down, took out a cigarette, and began smoking. She would watch the receptionist out of the corner of her eye, and then look down at the magazine, and back up at the two or three other people waiting in the room. Her eyes moved from the people to the magazine to the cigarette to the people to the magazine in rapid succession. She avoided eye contact. When her name was finally called she jumped like she was startled. (p. 24)

The point is that field notes must be detailed. They must tell a story. They must neither omit important information nor go overboard in the description of unimportant information.

time, so that the observer can reflect on what was observed. Other professionals believe field notes should include almost every detail possible and be written during the event or as soon afterward as possible. Critical research consumers should consider the level of detail provided by researchers in the investigation and consider whether there is enough information to justify researchers' conclusions. Researchers should indicate whether the notes are a description of what occurred or an interpretation or judgment of observed events. Researchers should also include their own thoughts, feelings, and experiences throughout the investigation. They should provide other evidence of the events as well, in the form of triangulation to help verify the notes taken (e.g., interviews, notes from others, documents). Direct quotes can also be used to verify some of the notes. Finally, critical research consumers should attempt to ascertain how researchers were able to synthesize the information. The synthesis provides the basis for conclusions drawn and therefore is critical in judging the adequacy of those conclusions.

Nonparticipant Observation Study

The difference between participant and nonparticipant studies has to do with the extent to which observers become involved with the participants. It is important to note that the degree to which observers are separated from the participants varies from study to study. In the purest sense, nonparticipant observations occur in a covert manner. In this way, the observer's presence is unknown to the participants. The advantage of this method of observation is clear—the reactivity associated with observations is all but eliminated. However, there are serious ethical concerns if one conducts covert observations. Another difficulty is that the ability to interact with participants and find out more about them on a personal level is limited. Only those things that are observed are recorded. Other important information that can only be obtained by interacting with participants is not considered.

Nonparticipant observations also occur when the participants are aware of the observer's presence but have little or no opportunity for interaction with the observer. There is a chance of reactivity, but the threat is reduced by effort on the part of observers not to interfere with

participants' activities. With this type of observation, there may be a time period before actual data collection when the observer is present. The purpose of this time period is to allow the participants to become used to the observer's presence. Once the observer is present for some time, data collection begins. One may check for observer bias by having a second observer also record the behaviors. An advantage of nonparticipant observations is reduced observer effects. However, a problem again stems from the type of information desired. If one wants to learn what participants feel, believe, or value, nonparticipant observations are wanting. Thus, it is important to ascertain the purpose of the investigation. If conclusions are based on beliefs of the participants, some form of interaction must take place between the observer and the participant. Nonparticipant observations likely do not allow such conclusions to be based on valid information.

Naturalistic Observation Study

A **naturalistic observation study** involves observing participants in their natural settings. There is no attempt to manipulate what goes on in the setting, and the observations are unobtrusive (Patton, 2002). Typically these are nonparticipant observations, although they can involve participants. For example, Jean Piaget (2002) interacted with the participants in his studies to a certain extent. He set up situations and observed how children responded. Piaget did not attempt to "teach" children how to respond to the situations, but he also did not sit back and observe children without manipulating the environment in some fashion. On the other hand, Fossey (2000) studied gorillas and made no attempt to interact with them in the beginning. She simply watched from afar. Later, when she began to interact with the gorillas, she changed the environment in some manner. In fact, there really is no true unobtrusive observation method unless the participants are totally unaware of the observer's presence. Whenever an observation occurs and participants are

> A **naturalistic observation study** *involves unobtrusively observing participants in their natural settings.*

aware of the observer's presence, some manipulation of the environment has taken place. However, the question of what happens when no one is present is somewhat like the question of whether the falling tree makes a sound in the forest when no one is there. Thus, critical research consumers must determine whether the obtrusiveness of the observation may have changed the situation to such an extent that "normal" behavior patterns of participants were disrupted. Obviously, in the Piaget and Fossey studies, this was not the case. If we are going to use naturalistic observation methods, we must use the most unobtrusive methods available (i.e., nonparticipant methods).

Simulations

There are times when researchers wish to obtain information on certain phenomena, but their ability to collect such information is compromised because the event does not occur frequently enough or it would be unethical to allow such an event to occur. In such cases, simulations may be used. **Simulations** involve the creation or recreation of a situation to see how participants will react under such circumstances. For example, airline pilots go through simulation training before being allowed to fly; astronauts go through simulations before embarking upon space travel; teachers may teach in front of their peers before going out "in the real world"; and children may be approached by confederates (i.e., research staff not known to the participants) during abduction prevention training. Simulations have been used in the assessment of safety skills. As stated by Gast, Wellons, and Collins (1994), "The initial teaching of safety skills may need to occur in a simulated, rather than a natural, environment" (p. 16). Therefore, researchers who are unable to observe the participants in the natural environment may be forced to set up simulations. These simulations can involve either an individual or a group of individuals. The critical concern is that the simulation resemble the natural environment as closely as possible. In order to generalize to the natural environment, the simulations must have most, if not all, of the same properties. The extent to which the simulation approaches situations encountered in the natural environment must be determined.

Determining the Observation Method to Use

The type of observation method used in qualitative research methods depends on the purpose of the investigation. If, for example, the purpose is to find out how students process information when doing math problems, participant observations may be most appropriate. If the purpose of an investigation is to determine how students interact with one another in the classroom, nonparticipant observations may be most beneficial. Critical research consumers must determine the purpose of the investigation and assess whether the observation method used was appropriate (i.e., able to generate the data necessary to answer the research question).

Determining the Method Used to Analyze Observational Data

Researchers must also determine which method to use in analyzing observational data. According to Patton (2002), researchers should determine how best to present the findings to an audience. They must determine how to get the information across, so that the audience will understand what occurred during the investigation. Providing this information is especially useful when researchers attempt to critique or replicate what was done during the investigation. Patton lists six options available to qualitative researchers who conduct analyses on observational data (see Figure 10.2). The first option is to report the chronology of what was observed over time. Essentially, the observer tells a story from beginning to end. The second option is to report key events. The reporting of key events should be in order of importance, not in order of occurrence. Reporting various settings is the third option. Here the researcher describes the various settings involved in the research, then analyzes any patterns in the data across settings. The fourth option involves reporting case studies of people involved in the investigation. Here the unit of analysis is each individual involved in the study. The fifth option is description of processes such as methods of communication observed throughout the investigation. Reporting of key issues, such as reporting how the participants were affected by something in the setting, is the sixth option. Once the researcher has decided on the best method of presenting the

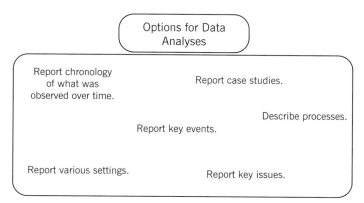

FIGURE 10.2. Options available to qualitative researchers conducting analyses on qualitative data.

data, he/she can then collect the data, paying especially close attention to variables on which he/she will report. The important point here is that once a researcher decides how he/she will present the data, the analysis of subsequent data is somewhat simplified.

Observer Effects

Observer effects refer to problems that may bias the reliability or validity of the data collected by observers (see Hawthorne effect, Chapter 2). A potential problem with observations in field settings is their effect on the behavior of the participant or participants; this is especially true with complete participation. According to Bogdan and Biklen (1998), observer effects can be minimized by working with a larger group of participants, in which the observer can blend into the crowd. When working with a small number of participants or one participant, observer effects become more likely. A method to decrease observer effects is to allow participants to become used to the observer's presence over time. For example, by being in the setting with participants for a period of time without actually gathering data, the observer allows any effects brought on by his/her presence to subside. Observer effects must always be a concern since the researcher's conclusions may be seriously compromised by these effects. Critical research consumers should attempt to find out whether and how researchers attempted to reduce observer effects throughout the investigation.

Another research strategy would be to integrate the observer effects into the investigation. For example, if observer effects are seen or suspected, the observer might document how the participant's behavior was changed by his/her presence. Data might come from the observations themselves (i.e., the participant nervously looks at the observer when the participant is teaching) or interviews with the participant. Another method of checking on observer effects is to use multiple sources of information. Data sources from individuals who are familiar with the participant's behavior or documents relating to similar information might be used (triangulation). Thus, observer effects could be a rich source of data.

Observer Bias

Observer bias is a concern whenever direct observations are conducted. Observer bias refers to inaccurately recording what is seen because of a preexisting attitude or experience. For example, let's say a researcher is a complete participant in a study on children of

---

Simulations *involve the creation or recreation of a situation to see how participants will react.*

Observer effects *refer to problems that may bias the reliability or validity of the data collected by observers.*

Observer bias *refers to recording what is seen inaccurately because of a preexisting attitude or experience.*

Mexican immigrants and is interested in the U.S.-born youth of illegal immigrants and attitudes developed by these children toward living in the United States. After developing codes and recording statements made by these youth, the researcher finds that these U.S.-born youth of illegal immigrants were denied college entry, scholarships, and many other opportunities available to other children born in the United States. In response, the researcher changed codes and developed new ones in an attempt to document prejudice and bigotry. Although the youth report several advantages to living in the United States, the researcher records only negative statements. Subjectivity is typically seen as a strength of qualitative research, because it is a basis for an observer's distinctive contribution; the data are joined with personal interpretations in collecting and analyzing the data (Marshall & Rossman, 2011). However, subjectivity in observations can also be seen as a weakness, in that the observer's recordings may not be a true reflection of what really occurred.

Qualitative observations are usually more subjective than quantitative forms of data collection; therefore, researchers should be aware of the possibility of observer bias. According to Bogdan and Biklen (1998), one way to handle observer bias is for the observer to document what he/she feels during the observations. Such data can be important when interpreting the data. Another method of preventing bias or determining whether it occurs is to obtain information from a variety of sources, such as interviews and documents.

Critical research consumers must also be aware of the possibility of bias. Researchers should provide information on the resulting bias that occurs during observations or document the methods used to prevent bias.

Recall the research question posed earlier in this chapter regarding braille literacy instruction? Read on to see how your design compares to how the actual study was designed.

Research Example 1: Case Study— Braille Literacy Instruction

A case study design was used to identify effective teaching strategies using braille procedures

(Barclay, Herlich, & Sacks, 2010). The study was part of a larger, 5-year research effort involving observation of teachers as they delivered literacy instruction to students with visual impairments (Emerson, Holbrook, & D'Andrea, 2009). Barclay et al. (2010) reported on two case studies. We review one case study here. The study focused on one teacher–student dyad (Ms. Wilson and Marco) that was purposefully selected after researchers reviewed all observational notes and found Ms. Wilson's teaching to be extraordinary. Marco entered the study as a kindergartner at age 7. He had missed considerable school during his early education due to a serious medical condition. Marco was blind due to retinal impairment. Ms. Wilson had taught students with visual impairments for 15 years. She had a strong background as a reading teacher. She worked directly with Marco on braille instruction for 75 minutes each day in a resource room. Barclay et al. used a triangulation strategy. In addition to observations and interviews, researchers administered measures of spelling and vocabulary (Brigance, 1991), passages from the Basic Reading Inventory (Johns, 2005), reading of contractions (Koenig & Farrenkopf, 1995), and words per minute of reading. These assessments, all adapted to braille, were administered once a year for the 3-year study. Ms. Wilson created tactile illustrations corresponding with various literacy activities. For example, in kindergarten, Ms. Wilson presented Marco with bags containing objects starting with different consonants (e.g., *rice, feathers, nails*). Marco removed each object, explored it, named it, and said the initial sound. In first grade, Ms. Wilson illustrated Marco's braille books with textures. By third grade, Marco was using contractions. Ms. Wilson designed an incentive system for correctly reading braille contractions from flash cards. Generally, Marco's test scores increased in successive years, although spelling and vocabulary scores decreased from third to fourth grade. Researchers noted a limitation of the research relative to relying on accuracy of the observer's interpretations.

Interview Studies

An **interview study** is one in which direct interaction between the researcher and participant involves oral questions to the interviewer and oral responses by the participant (Gall et al., 2007). According to Patton (1990), "The purpose of interviewing is to find out what is in and on someone else's mind" (p. 278). Interviewing is an alternative to observations and a compatible method of gathering information. The advantage of interviewing over observing is that because not everything can be observed, observation is either impractical (e.g., following each participant through his or her life) or impossible (e.g., finding out what someone is thinking). However, interviewing is a difficult thing to do well. Interviewers must have enough skill to access information from the interviewee in a way that allows the interviewer to understand the interviewee's world. As stated by Patton, "The quality of the information obtained during an interview is largely dependent on the interviewer" (p. 279).

Patton (1990) describes three types of interviewing: (1) the informal conversational interview, (2) the general interview guide approach, and (3) the standardized open-ended interview. Notice that the closed-, fixed-response interview is not included. According to Bogdan and Bilken (1998), qualitative interviewers should avoid closed-ended items such as "yes" or "no" questions. The problem with closed- or fixed-response interviews is that details and particulars are lost when the interviewees are not allowed to expand on their responses. Therefore, the purpose of qualitative interviewing is not met (i.e., to get inside the interviewees' world to understand more fully what those individuals are experiencing). As Patton (1990) points out:

> The purpose of qualitative interviewing in evaluation is to understand how program staff and participants view the program, to learn their terminology and judgments, and to capture the complexities of their individual perceptions and experiences. This is what distinguishes qualitative interviewing from the closed interview, questionnaire, or test typically used in quantitative evaluations. Such closed instruments force program participants to fit their knowledge, experiences, and feelings into the evaluator's categories. The fundamental principle of qualitative interviewing is to provide a framework within which respondents can express their own understandings in their own terms. (p. 290)

Informal Conversational Interview

The informal conversational interview usually involves participant observation in the field and is the most open-ended interviewing method. The interview proceeds as a conversation in which interviewers ask spontaneous questions. There is no structured format, although interviewers should have some notion of the type of information they desire. In some instances, those being interviewed may be unaware of the interview, the interviewer does not take notes during the interview but after he/she has left the situation. At times when participants are aware of the interview, interviewers usually take notes during the interview and may use a tape recorder. The disadvantage of allowing participants to know that an interview is occurring is their reactivity relative to the knowledge. On the other hand, there may be ethical concerns with not informing participants that a seemingly casual conversation is really an interview.

As the name implies, the interview format is like that of a normal conversation. Thus, interviewers must be quick on their feet, since they must generate questions spontaneously throughout the interview. A difficulty is that this type of interview may take several sessions to get the information desired, due to the inefficient nature of the interview. The indirect approach of the interview makes it much more difficult to steer the interview in the direction required to gain the needed information. On the other hand, the spontaneity of the interview allows researchers to go in any number of directions, to probe new areas that they did not think of before the interview began. New and interesting information can be generated with the informal conversational interview.

The data analysis involved with the informal conversational interview is very difficult. Since there are no general guidelines for researchers to follow, categories must be developed. The knowledge of the subject area must be in depth, and researchers must know what they

> An **interview study** is one in which direct interaction between the researcher and participant involves oral questions to the interviewer and oral responses by the participant.

are looking for, since some information must be dropped during the analysis. If important information is left out of the analysis, the validity of the conclusions must be in question.

General Interview Guide Approach

The general interview guide approach essentially involves having an outline of topics to be covered during the interview; however, the order in which topics are addressed is not set. The questions are not formulated beforehand. The purpose of outlines or guides is to aid interviewers in addressing each of the topics. The main purpose of the guides is to ensure that the same topics are covered for each participant. The main difference in the informal conversational interview is that the topics are determined beforehand. Thus, the general interview guide approach is more structured than the informal conversational interview.

This difference is also an advantage in that interviewers can be sure to cover needed topics for each participant. The questions are still generated spontaneously but within specific topics. Another difference is that whereas the informal conversational interview is more suited to individualized interviews due to the changes in coverage from session to session, the general interview guide is well suited for groups in which the same or similar information must be collected. A disadvantage of the general interview guide is that interviews are not as free flowing as the informal conversational interview. Interviewers in the informal conversational interview can cover a much wider topical area than can interviewers following the general interview guide.

Analysis of the data is slightly easier than that using the general interview guide, since topics are preselected. However, the information obtained within each topic must be coded in some manner. Researchers must integrate the information in some manner to make conclusions about the data. They may use examples of statements from participants, create categories of statements within each topic, tally the number of and type of statements made, or develop assertions that summarize the statements. Whatever method researchers decide to use to analyze the data, some information will be lost or omitted.

Standardized Open-Ended Interview

The standardized open-ended interview, perhaps the most familiar method, involves not only set topics, similar to the general interview guide, but also predeveloped questions that researchers ask throughout the interview. Each participant is exposed to the same topics and questions in the same order. The purpose of this method is to help researchers become more efficient in obtaining needed information and to reduce any interviewer effects. In other words, two interviewers who ask the same questions in the same order with the standardized open-ended interview would likely ask different questions using the general interview guide. The questions are worded in an open-ended format, with interviewers avoiding "yes" or "no" questions and fixed responses. Participants are free to provide any answer to the questions and to expand on their responses.

There are a number of strengths to the standardized open-ended interview. First, since the questions are set prior to the interview and provided in the same order, the interview instrument can be inspected by others. Second, variability in the manner in which interviewers ask questions can be minimized; thus, the interviews are standardized. Third, unlike the informal conversational interview, the interview is focused, so that a great deal of information is gained within a limited amount of time. Finally, scoring of the standardized open-ended interview is simplified, since researchers already have determined the categories for scoring in advance.

The weaknesses involve limiting information that is obtained in two ways. First, since the interview is standardized, the questions are not tailored to each participant and situation. Information is lost because interviewers cannot probe participants' reasons for particular responses or perspectives. Second, the naturalness in asking the questions is lost. In the informal conversational interview, the interview is more "free flowing"; with the standardized open-ended interview, the interview is more formal and less spontaneous. This structure may weaken or lessen explanations provided by participants. Also, since the questions are less natural and not individualized for each participant, some of the questions may lose their relevance. This irrelevance frequently occurs when interview questions are developed beforehand, but when researchers realize after the interview that the questions did not evoke anticipated responses from the participants, they say something like, "I wish I had asked her. . . . "

As with the method of observation used, the type of interview format depends on the type of research question and the type of information sought. Critical research consumers should determine the research question and assess whether researchers use an appropriate interview technique.

Types of Interview Questions

Patton (1990) indicates that researchers should make four decisions when developing an interview. First, researchers must determine the type of interview to use. Second, they must decide on the location of the interview. Many interviews are conducted in the field during participant observations. Third, they must decide on the length of the interview. Finally, researchers must at minimum decide what type of information they need to collect and at a maximum what type of questions to ask.

Patton (1990) discusses six types of questions that are asked of participants (see Figure 10.3), including (1) experience/behavior, (2) opinion/values, (3) feeling, (4) knowledge, (5) sensory, and (6) background/demographic questions. These question types can be asked in any of the interview methods and about any topic. They can also be stated in past (e.g., "What did you . . . ?"), present (e.g., "What are you . . . ?"), or future tense (e.g., "What will you . . . ?") and are considered as time-frame questions.

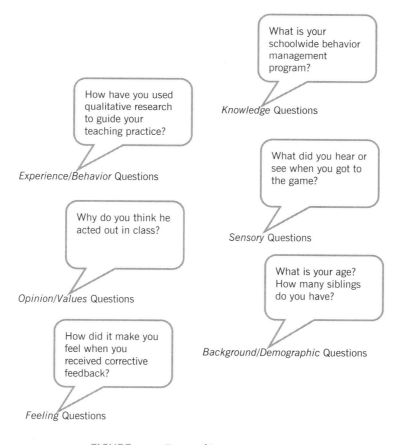

How have you used qualitative research to guide your teaching practice?

Experience/Behavior Questions

Why do you think he acted out in class?

Opinion/Values Questions

How did it make you feel when you received corrective feedback?

Feeling Questions

What is your schoolwide behavior management program?

Knowledge Questions

What did you hear or see when you got to the game?

Sensory Questions

What is your age? How many siblings do you have?

Background/Demographic Questions

FIGURE 10.3. Types of interview questions.

Experience/Behavior Questions. Experience/behavior questions refer to what one has done in the past or what one is presently doing. The purpose for experience/behavior questions is to gather information to which one would have access if one had observed the individual. The purpose for these questions is not to obtain information about phenomena that are impossible to observe (e.g., feelings, thoughts), but to obtain information that is not presently available (i.e., what has already passed). An example of an experience/behavior question is "If I had been in the teacher's lounge with you, what would I have seen you do?"

Opinion/Values Questions. Opinion/values questions seek to find out information about phenomena that are impossible to observe. We cannot directly observe the opinions or values of others; however, we can ask about a person's opinions or values. Thus, although the information may be available, it is not possible to document it directly. An example of an opinion/values question is " 'Tell me what you think is the best method of teaching reading and why?"

Feeling Questions. Feeling questions aim to find out the emotional state of others or how they respond emotionally to experiences and thoughts. As with opinion/values questions, the information may be available but not accessible directly. A feeling question may be as follows: "To what extent do the increasing illiteracy rates among our school-age population make you feel anxious about the future of our country?" Notice that the question was not "What do you think of the increasing illiteracy rates among our school-age population?" or "What do you think is the cause of the growing numbers of illiterate school-age children?" Patton (1990) makes it clear that feeling questions must not be confused with opinion/values questions. The purpose of feeling questions is to find out how people *feel* about something, not what they *think* about something.

Knowledge Questions. Knowledge questions are aimed at gathering factual information. They attempt to find out what people know, not what they think or feel about something. The information may be available from other sources,

such as asking individuals to perform a task that demonstrates knowledge, but it is more efficient to ask participants what they know about something. These questions should not be confused with feeling or opinion/values questions. An example of a knowledge question is "How many students do you have in your school who are below grade level in reading?" These questions are aimed at finding out what individuals understand to be correct.

Sensory Questions. Sensory questions involve the experiences participants have with their senses. These questions aim to find out what participants have seen, smelled, felt (in a tactile sense, not emotionally), tasted, or heard. The information here is available but not accessible directly by observers. The purpose of these questions is to find out the types of sensory experiences/behaviors to which the participants were exposed. An example of a sensory question is "When you entered into the school building, what did you hear?"

Background/Demographic Questions. Background/demographic questions are aimed at obtaining personal information about participants. Information such as the age, educational level, occupation, and living situations are important in determining how each participant fits within the sample. This information is critical for determining logical generalization (see Chapter 9). A background/demographic question might be "Where do you live?" This information is available from other sources, but the purpose of these questions is to gather the information in an efficient manner.

Recall the research question posed earlier in this chapter regarding parent messages and their influence on young women disclosing sexual assault? Read on to see how your design compares to how the actual study was designed.

Research Example 2: Interview Study— Disclosing Sexual Assault

In this study, researchers (Smith & Cook, 2008) sought to determine the influence of parental messages on college-age women in terms of whether they had disclosed being sexually assaulted to their parents. The primary research questions were whether culture and upbringing played a role in disclosure, and what motivated or discouraged women to disclose. The researchers interviewed 20 young women enrolled in an introductory psychology course who reported experiencing at least one attempted or completed act of sexual assault since age 13, in which (1) the perpetrator threatened the victim with physical harm, (2) the perpetrator used physical force, or (3) the victim was incapacitated by alcohol or drugs. Participants ranged in age from 18 to 34, were mostly single ($N = 17$) and white ($N = 10$). The individual interviews, conducted by Smith, involved open-ended experience/behavior and feeling questions focusing on the process of disclosure; that is, the interviewer asked questions relative to experiences of disclosing (or not disclosing) the incident to others, and the person to whom the participant disclosed. Participants were also asked to describe "the messages they received about sex while growing up, especially from parents, and their comfort level with discussing sexuality topics with parents and family" (Smith & Cook, 2008; p. 1333). Researchers analyzed results using a grounded theory approach. Findings indicated that participants more often disclosed sexual assault to parents who had discussed sex with them "in a frank and positive manner" (p. 1326). Three of the participants indicated they had not disclosed the incident prior to the interview. Researchers concluded that in the case of this sample of women, behaviors and attitudes of parents created a powerful climate that influenced disclosure of sexual assault. Researchers discussed findings with regard to implications for parent education to promote positive parent–child communication.

Ethnography

Everything discussed up to this point can be combined to form a special type of qualitative research method. **Ethnography** essentially combines observational methods and in-depth interview methods to investigate a phenomenon from a cultural perspective (Patton, 1990). Ethnography, an intense and in-depth study of an intact cultural group in a natural setting over a prolonged period of time, collects observational

and/or interview data (Creswell, 2009). We must point out that in this chapter ethnography refers to a particular method of gathering data. Ethnography may also refer to a philosophical paradigm to which one is committed (Marshall & Rossman, 2011). What distinguishes ethnography from the other methods described (e.g., observation and interview studies) is the combination of several data gathering methods, as well as the intensity and degree to which the data are gathered. The focus is more holistic in ethnography than in either observation or interview studies, and the involvement in the field is long term (Potter, 1996). Creswell (2009) notes that the research process is flexible and typically evolves in response to events that are encountered in the field setting.

As with much of the qualitative research previously described, ethnographic researchers enter into the field or research situation without any preconceived notion of what they will find. There are usually no specific or precise hypotheses, as there are when conducting quantitative research. The conclusions drawn from the research develop over time as the researcher becomes a part of the culture. In ethnographic research, the culture can be defined somewhat more liberally. For example, a classroom, workplace, college campus, organization, or African tribe can all be considered a culture.

When a researcher studies a culture, he/she studies all of the variables that may affect the participant(s) in a certain context. For example, if we were conducting an ethnographic study of students in a classroom, we would want to consider variables such as the teacher, other students in the school, other teachers in the school, the principal, the playground monitor, the bus driver, the cafeteria staff, and so forth.

Ethnography requires asking questions and conducting observation of all variables operating within a specific context. Let's say that a researcher is interested in studying the question "What is the school environment like in an urban high school located in a low SES area?"

> **Ethnography** *is an intense and in-depth study of an intact cultural group in a natural setting over a prolonged period of time by collecting observational and/or interview data.*

The researcher would make arrangements to visit the school to get a "feel" for the place. She would begin to talk to the students and staff. She would possibly take over some teaching duties to understand the school from a teacher's perspective. At some point, she would interact with other teachers and administrators, and take field notes. Finally, she would conduct formal and informal interviews, asking more specific questions the longer she stays in the school. The researcher begins to notice that "cliques" have developed among the students and staff. The groups seem to be organized along racial lines. Black students seem to sit alongside other black students, and white students tend to associate more with other white students. The researcher documents these and other observations. She observes how the staff interacts with the students. She notices that male students are asked different types of questions than are female students. The researcher observes the students and faculty in as many situations as possible. She interviews students and staff on an ongoing basis. The researcher audio-records many of the interviews, especially those of individuals who provide the richest information. She also videotapes the interactions in classrooms that tend to represent the school climate as a whole. The researcher continues the study for an entire school year. It is not enough to conduct the investigation for a day, a week, or a month. Data that are desirable cannot be obtained in a short time period.

Once the researcher has collected all of her field notes, interviews, and audio and video files, she is ready to interpret her data. According to Fetterman (1989), analysis of ethnographic data involves several components, including thinking (i.e., attempting to find where each piece of data fits into the big picture), triangulation (i.e., obtaining and comparing multiple sources of data), patterns (i.e., determining when thoughts and behaviors begin to be repeated), key events (i.e., determining a representative event to act as a focal point in understanding the culture), maps (i.e., developing visual representations of the culture), flowcharts (i.e., determining how activities and information flow through the system), organizational charts (i.e., laying out the hierarchy of the organization from top to bottom), matrices (i.e., establishing a picture of

behavior or thought categories), content analysis (i.e., analyzing written and electronic data), statistics (i.e., using nonparametric statistics such as nominal and ordinal scales), and crystallization (i.e., everything finally falls into place).

For example, our researcher determines that certain kinds of interactions occur in the high school. She attempts to find out how these interactions affect the overall operation of the school (thinking). She finds that most of the negative interactions between students occurs outside the school (patterns). The researcher remembers that the one event that typified the school climate was an assembly later in the year, when students were excited about the success of the football team (key event). She is able to produce a flowchart of how information about other students (rumors) moves through the school. Also, she is able to determine a hierarchy among staff and students in the school. She finds that students and staff place athletes on a higher social level.

The researcher also finds that much of the publicity about the school is about the sports teams (content analysis). She obtains information from several sources, such as faculty, students, parents, and newspapers (triangulation). She uses nominal scale data to show the school breakdown of ethnic groups. After the data analysis, the information is finally crystallized. The researcher determines that the school culture centers on sports. She finds that students are likely to segregate themselves during non-sports-related situations, but when sports are involved, the students join together. She also finds that the sports "stars" are more respected and admired by teachers and students regardless of ethnicity. However, if a student is not involved in sports, both student and teacher responses differ based on ethnicity (e.g., seating arrangements during lunch) and during instruction (e.g., types of questions asked of males and females).

The final step for the researcher is to provide a written account of what she has found that essentially tells a story. The reader should be able to visualize what the school is like. The description should be alive and rich with information. Metaphorical language should reveal degrees of understanding about the school, and the reader should obtain a holistic view of the situation.

Features

As with other qualitative research, ethnography is an inductive versus deductive approach to inquiry. Additionally, the data are open to many interpretations depending on the person making the interpretations (Potter, 2002). In this case, adequacy of conclusions may be suspect when researchers do not communicate their personal biases to readers. These personal biases are seen not necessarily as a disadvantage of ethnography but as an advantage, assuming they are revealed and analyzed by the researchers. If the researchers have communicated their personal perspectives, the reader is allowed to take these biases into consideration.

According to qualitative researchers, we all interpret our world from our own unique perspective, even quantitative researchers. The difference is that qualitative researchers are aware of their biases and integrate these into the investigation. Potter (1996) also suggests that data "are not collected in a closed set of analytical categories" (p. 51). In other words, the investigation is holistic (i.e., the investigation is not constrained by predetermined categories). Additionally, the investigation is based on a small number of cases. In the example provided earlier, the high school was seen as a single case. There was no investigation of each individual student or staff member. The school was seen as a single entity. The advantage of the intensive study of a small number of cases is that an in-depth analysis can be made. Potter also indicates that analysis of the data "is an explicit interpretation of meanings of language and human actions" (p. 51). Thus, researchers describe interpretations in a manner that is direct and clear to the reader.

However, as with all research methods, the strengths are counterbalanced by weaknesses. For example, since a small number of cases is involved, the ability to generalize findings to other cases is limited or nonexistent. From a qualitative perspective, this point may not be a weakness, since the investigation informed us about the particular case and there was no interest in generalizing. However, from another perspective, community members may ask, "What do these results mean to me?" Another problem is the subjectivity of the process. There is no way to identify whether the data

collection methods are reliable. In fact, qualitative researchers understand this not to be a particular problem, since attempting to take away subjectivity may constrain the collection of data (Maxwell, 2010). However, if there is a lack of reliability, there is also a lack of validity. Thus, it is critical for researchers to demonstrate triangulation. Critical research consumers should determine whether triangulation is present, and whether the researchers have communicated the biases they held throughout the investigation.

Recall the research question regarding students with ED posed earlier in this chapter? Read on to see how your design compares to how the actual study was designed.

Research Example 3: Ethnographic Study—Students with Emotional Disturbance

An ethnographic observational approach was used to study processes that intensified children's behavioral and academic difficulties, and contributed to their diagnosis of ED and referral to special education (Hart et al., 2010). Researchers were concerned with the "appropriateness and adequacy of the processes by which children were determined to have ED" (p. 150). The study examined data from a 3-year ethnographic study of placement processes in 12 schools in a large, diverse, urban school district. Information on 1,029 student participants was gathered, including 87 European American, 606 African American, and 336 Hispanic students. Sampling was purposeful "to investigate information-rich cases that are likely to evidence the processes being studied" (p. 150). Twelve schools were selected to represent varying SES, languages, and rates of referral to special education. Twenty-four teachers were selected to represent variations in ethnicity, years teaching, grade level, teaching skill, and referral rate. Hart et al. started with an examination of district policies and placement data, and moved to interviews and observations. Data collection strategies included recorded interviews; spontaneous conversations recorded in field notes; observations in school and home settings; and examination of school documents, files, and participant work samples. The framework for data analysis included two sets of coding systems: (1) proposed explanations of overrepresentation of African American students, and (2) description of settings, individuals, and demographics. The explanatory set comprised seven main themes that emerged from initial interviews with teachers: (1) family and community influences, (2) external pressures on schooling, (3) intrinsic child deficits, (4) teacher skills and/or biases, (5) school system or administrative policies, (6) errors or bias in psychological assessment, and (7) errors or bias in bilingual assessment. Findings indicated that all seven explanatory themes were relevant to varying degrees. However, three themes proved particularly important in creating referral of students with ED diagnoses to special education: (1) teacher skills/biases, (2) errors/bias in psychological assessment, and (3) administrative policies. A teacher's skill was important in accounting for a student's academic achievement and classroom behavior. Referral teams "generally ignored the role of school contexts in children's difficulties but focused instead on home contexts" (p. 153). Researchers recommended that the field move from a traditional focus to a more "holistic view in which the troubling behaviors of children are examined within the context of the environments in which they occur" (p. 160).

WHAT IS HISTORICAL RESEARCH?

Historical research can be regarded as quantitative or qualitative (Potter, 1996); however, given that historical research is mainly described as qualitative (Wiersma & Jurs, 2009), we describe it within qualitative research methods. Note that it is not easy to categorize historical research into any one category, mainly because historical research does not have highly developed methodology around which there is consensus (Cohen et al., 2007). Historical research is geared to describe relations, to correct inaccurate conclusions from other historical reports, or to explain what has occurred in the past.

Historical research involves a systematic process to research data from the past to help us understand what is going on now and what may occur in the future. The systematic nature of historical research makes it a scientific process.

Gall et al. (2007) described four similarities between historical research and other methodologies. First, historical research is concerned with the context under which events took place. This concern for the context of the investigation is congruent with that of qualitative and single-case researchers, for example. Second, historical researchers are concerned with all of the contextual factors surrounding a historical event or events. The emphasis, then, is on what occurred in actual situations, not artificially derived situations. Third, historical researchers appreciate the wholeness of experience. Finally, historical researchers focus on the centrality of interpretation in the research process. In other words, historical researchers focus on interpretation of their data rather than on the events themselves. Historical researchers may also use quantitative data in their research to interpret certain events. Therefore, historical research shares several characteristics with qualitative research methods, as well as quantitative and single-case research methods.

Characteristics

Historical research has several defining characteristics (Potter, 1996). First, historical research emphasizes what occurred in the past. Other methods deal with the present. Second, historical research is empirical, in that there is an attempt to obtain information from a variety of sources. Recall that empiricism is critical for the development of a science. Empiricism involves gaining information from our senses. When conducting historical research, we make observations of past events through historical sources. Finally, historical research attempts to make meaning out of the subject matter.

Purposes

Historical research can serve five purposes. First, it can answer factual questions about the past (Gall et al., 2007). For example, if we question how educators approached the instruction of students 100 years ago, we might analyze written accounts from the period, talk with individuals who had firsthand or secondhand information about the period, or analyze photos from the era.

Second, historical research may, under certain circumstances, aid us in determining what has worked in the past (or what has failed) to help us in the future (Gall et al., 2007). For example, suppose we want to determine the disciplinary methods used 25 years ago and how effective these practices were. If we find out what worked several years ago, we can use those methods today to solve some of our disciplinary problems. This is, in fact, what some people propose on a much more informal level. Many people say, "When I was growing up, the teacher would paddle us for misbehaving. We rarely had behavior problems in our classroom." However, the type of information to substantiate this claim is usually not available, since the question is one of cause and effect. It is probably not possible to determine the variables that caused something to occur or not occur in the past. Mason, McKenney, and Copeland (1997) noted, "Cause-and-effect relationships, are, of course, established precariously and with great caution in nonexperimental situations because an induction can never be proven in any formal logical system" (p. 315). (*Note.* The ability of historical research to establish cause-and-effect relationships is a philosophical argument similar to the ability of qualitative research to determine such relationships.)

In our example of disciplinary methods, suppose a researcher determines that corporal punishment seemed to decrease disciplinary problems in urban schools 25 years ago. She determined this by talking to former teachers and students, examining disciplinary records from several schools, and reviewing the concern for behavior problems in the media or in publications. The difficulty results when one considers that other variables may have been in effect at the same time, such as the type of instruction typically used in the classroom, the makeup of the students, the level of violence seen in the media, and familial support, among many others. The ability to make definitive and valid conclusions based on such historical accounts depends on contextual variables. Gall et al. (2007) state this difficulty as follows: "The validity of past research findings about education depends on the degree to which the context in which they were obtained has remained constant or has changed" (p. 533).

Third, historical research can aid us in understanding how we came to this point in time (Mason et al., 1997). For example, we may wonder how we came to teach mathematics in some manner. Historical research can aid us in answering this question. We may find that the use of manipulatives (i.e., tangible objects that can be counted) became more prevalent in the 1960s, when educators began to consider Piaget's theory of development and its educational implications. We may be surprised that time-out from positive reinforcement was first found to be an effective way to decrease behavior in laboratory research using rats (Leitenberg, 1965). We may also, for example, find that the authentic literature movement in reading instruction took hold in the 1980s, when New Zealand began to disseminate results of reading achievement using a literature-based or whole-language approach.

Fourth, historical research can aid us in seeing trends or patterns (Mason et al., 1997). For example, if a researcher investigated educational methods used during much of the 1960s, he would find that many of the techniques are being used today. There seems to be a trend in education in which one instructional technique comes into vogue, then falls out of favor, only to come back at a later time. One educational trend seen today is the back-to-basics movement that began in California and elsewhere. This movement is similar to what occurred in the 1960s and 1970s. The basics took a backseat to more progressive methods in the 1980s and early 1990s. However, a concern for teaching the basics is being seen in more communities today.

Finally, historical research can serve as a basis for later interview or observation studies (Marshall & Rossman, 2010) or the development of new hypotheses/research questions (Mason et al., 1997). For example, suppose we are interested in investigating how public schools have changed over the last 100 years. We could conduct historical research to determine the characteristics of schools of the past, then conduct an

> **Historical research** *involves a systematic process of researching data from the past that can help us understand what is going on now and what may occur in the future.*

observational study in a present-day school to see whether those characteristics determined by the historical research are still present.

Designing Historical Research

Researchers conducting historical research must complete two primary steps—develop a research question or hypothesis and collect data.

Research Question or Hypothesis

The first step in the process of historical research is the generation of a research question or hypothesis. This first step involves essentially the same process used by other researchers. Research questions or hypotheses can be generated by a desire to solve a current problem, to add to our information about the past, to satisfy a source of confusion, or to satisfy curiosity. However, a major difference between historical research and other forms of research is that much of the data may already be in existence in some form, or if not available, may be lost forever. In other forms of research, researchers go out and generate the data. Historical researchers attempt to find data that are already generated or attempt to generate data through other means, such as interviewing individuals from the era under study. For example, if a researcher wishes to investigate the extent to which multicultural practices were taught in schools in the 1950s, she would need to find information related to the question. She might search professional journals, curricular materials, books, and newspaper articles. The researcher might also interview teachers from the era to gather information on educational practices.

Data Collection Sources

The second step in the research process involves a search for relevant sources. These sources can be placed into one of two categories—primary and secondary (Marshall & Rossman, 2011). Much of the information collected through primary and secondary sources is gained through interviews and document analyses.

Primary Sources. The first category, primary sources, includes oral testimony of individuals who were present at the time, documents, records, and relics. The obvious advantage of primary sources is that the data are from sources that were present when the events took place. These sources are considered to be primary, because they were present or developed during the time period under investigation. These sources are usually considered to be the most reliable type of information. The reason these primary sources are considered more reliable than other sources is that as we go farther from the original source of information, the information tends to change. For example, a typical exercise in introduction to psychology classes is to begin a story at one side of the room. A professor may tell one student, "Research is an important endeavor because we can learn about ourselves." The first student whispers to a second student the same statement as accurately as possible. This continues until we reach the last student in the class. Finally, when the professor asks the last student what she was told, she looks puzzled and hesitant, but says, "Research is a potent river that makes us yearn about our shelves." As we go farther from the original student and what he stated, we get more and more changes in both content and meaning. People who misunderstand the original meaning may try to fill in the gaps so the message makes sense. Thus, to know what the original statement was, we should get as close to the first student, or the original source, as possible.

Secondary Sources. The second category of data includes secondary sources, which sources may include reports from individuals who relay information from people who were present during the historical period, reports from individuals who have read information from the past, and books about the period under question (e.g., history books and encyclopedias). These sources are secondary because the information did not come directly from individuals or documents from the specified historical period. The information obtained from secondary sources may not be as reliable or accurate as the data from primary sources. A critical concern is whether the researcher is able to show that other sources also reveal the same information (i.e., reliable findings; Cohen et al., 2007). If several sources, even if they are secondary, are shown to contain the same or similar information, the reliability of the information is enhanced.

Interviews. It is important to point out that interviews are important sources of data in historical research. The interviews can be from either primary or secondary sources. For example, an early educational reform advocate (Dr. Fred Keller) was interviewed just before he passed away. The information he provided during this interview included educational reform attempts and early research on alternative educational practices. These interviews were videotaped to preserve the information from a primary source.

Document Analysis. Document analysis refers to data collected as a permanent product. Document analysis involves obtaining data from any number of written or visual sources such as diaries, novels, incident reports, pictures, advertisements, speeches, official documents, files, films, audiotapes, books, newspapers, and so on. According to Potter (1996), document analysis is especially important in investigating past trends when there may not be anyone alive to provide information, or when information that exists is too limiting. Document analysis is also used when researchers want to obtain information unobtrusively, or when the information cannot be obtained in a more efficient or valid manner, such as by observation.

For example, it may be interesting to investigate attitudes in the United States during the 1960s. If we wish to do this, we might look at magazines, newspapers, art, and speeches by politicians to get a handle on the country's attitudes. In several studies, one of the authors of this text (Ron Nelson) investigated the level of disruption in schools. A primary data source was records kept by school staff on the number of students sent to the office for discipline problems. Incident reports in the school also showed the level of disruptions (i.e., the severity of the disruptive behaviors), as well as the teacher's response to the disruptions. Another example is the use of student files for programming reasons. Students with disabilities have files documenting difficulties in the classroom in terms of behavior and academic problems. One could review these documents on the students to obtain critical information to help with educational program developments.

The difficulty with document analysis is that researchers should have some idea of what they are looking for, even if only in general terms. The point here is that critical research consumers must glean from the research report what researchers were investigating, the categories used in the analysis, what was included and ignored, and the results. A major advantage of document analysis is that it allows for extensions or continuations of the research by other researchers.

Analyzing Historical Research

The analysis of historical research is unlike other forms of research, since the subject matter (i.e., past) is different from other subject matter (i.e., present). Data analysis is based on three concerns—external criticism, internal criticism, and synthesis of information (Gall et al., 2007; see Table 10.1). Before we describe the two criticisms of historical research, we should point out that internal and external criticism cannot be separated completely. Variables affecting one may, and frequently do, impact the other.

External Criticism

External criticism, which refers to the authenticity of the information obtained, has to do with historical researchers' choice of sources to read (Connors, 1992). This choice leads to concern in many debates, such as the authenticity of the Dead Sea Scrolls (Vermes, 1999). When historical evidence is found, researchers must be cautious to determine whether the evidence is indeed authentic. In order to make this determination, researchers should ask several questions (Gall et al., 2007).

First, researchers must ask, "Where was this document written?" Is it possible that the person writing this document obtained the information in a particular location? For example, suppose a researcher found a document on a method of teaching reading in the Eastern United States

> **External criticism** *refers to the authenticity of the information obtained.*

TABLE 10.1. Evaluating Historical Research

External criticism

1. Is it possible that the person writing this document would have obtained the information in the particular location?	YES	NO	?
2. Was the document written at the time the historical event occurred?	YES	NO	?
Could authentic information have been obtained at that time?	YES	NO	?
3. Who wrote the document? Did it seem authentic?	YES	NO	?
4. Could the author have written an authentic document under the prevailing conditions?	YES	NO	?
5. Is the document an original?	YES	NO	?

Overall, how authentic does the obtained information seem?

Very strong	Strong	Adequate	Weak	Nonexistent
1	2	3	4	5

Internal criticism

1. Does the author seem to be without a particular bias?	YES	NO	?
2. Were the individuals cited able to remember what occurred at a particular point in time?	YES	NO	?
3. Was the source a primary one?	YES	NO	?
4. Did the person providing the information have expertise in the area?	YES	NO	?

Overall, how accurate does the obtained information seem?

Very strong	Strong	Adequate	Weak	Nonexistent
1	2	3	4	5

Synthesis

Can generalization claims be made?	YES	NO	?

during the mid-1950s; this document might be viewed with caution if its author was from the Southern United States. The researcher would have to determine whether the author made trips to the Eastern United States, or how the individual obtained the information. It is possible that the individual was an authority on the subject even if he/she lived in another part of the country; however, the individual must have had some way of obtaining the information firsthand.

The second question refers to when the document was written. If the document in the preceding example were dated 1952, the document would be viewed with some suspicion. How could one write about a decade of instruction when the document only covers the first 2 years of the period? Similarly, if the document were dated 1990, suspicion is again aroused, since the passage of 40 years could make us question

the authenticity of the information. (Obviously, both examples make us question the accuracy of the information.)

Third, researchers should ask, "Who wrote the document?" Historical researchers are concerned with whether the documents are authentic or forgeries. *Forgeries* are documents written by someone other than the listed author. For example, suppose that a historical researcher located a document written by John Dewey. The document described the implications of approaching instruction from a more progressive manner. However, the signature on the document does not match other Dewey signatures. The historical researcher will review the document much more closely to determine its authenticity by looking at variables such as sentence structure across other documents prepared by Dewey. He/she may find that the writing style and signature do not match those of other Dewey documents; thus, the document is likely a forgery.

A fourth question is "Under what conditions was the document written?" For example, suppose that in the early 1960s a nontenured college faculty member was asked by her dean to prepare a document to describe effective instructional methods. The nontenured faculty member may present information based on what she perceived the dean and other tenured faculty to value. The document might not reflect what the author sees as effective teaching techniques, but what she thinks others view as effective. The historical researcher must try to determine whether the document is an authentic representation of the faculty member's views.

The final question asks, "Is this the original document or a copy of the original?" If the document is original, the authenticity of it is easier to determine. If the document is a copy and other versions exist, the authenticity is more difficult to determine. A concern of the historical researcher is whether the document has been altered. Given today's technology, it is difficult to determine whether a document has been altered in some manner. Thus, it is important to determine whether the document is an original.

Critical research consumers should attempt to answer these questions while considering the author's conclusions. The more researchers can present evidence that shows the authenticity of the documents, the more likely conclusions drawn from those documents will be considered to be valid.

Internal Criticism

Internal criticism refers to the accuracy of the information obtained; the documents are examined with the intent of making sure they are judged correctly (Gall et al., 2007). Determining the accuracy of the information is more difficult than determining the authenticity of the document. Furthermore, the determination of the accuracy of the information cannot occur until the authenticity of the document has been demonstrated and comparisons are made with claims in other documents.

There are several possible reasons why an authentic document may not be accurate. For example, some individuals may have particular biases that prevent them from documenting how things actually were. Suppose a school psychologist with a particular philosophical bent documented the effectiveness of a counseling method to which he was opposed on philosophical grounds. The counselor may have actually seen improvements in the students' attitudes toward school, but she documents that the students did not show any improved attitudes. In this case, the philosophical orientation of the counselor interferes with her ability to provide an accurate portrayal of what actually occurred.

Another difficulty with the accuracy of the information is the extent to which individuals can remember what occurred at a particular point in time. An example of this is the uncertainty of eyewitness testimony. Two people can view the same event but report different and sometimes conflicting information about that event. The differences may also be due to whether the individuals were participants or observers of the event. Persons who are observers may be more able to provide detailed or objective documentation of an event than can a participant.

Yet another problem has to do with whether the source was a primary or secondary one. If the person reporting the information is a secondary source, the historical researcher must be cautious about the accuracy of the information obtained. For example, suppose a person documented the advantages and disadvantages of the one-room schoolhouse. If the individual taught in such a school, the information is primary. However, if the author documented what she was told by former teachers in such schools or her own grandparents who experienced this firsthand, the information is secondary. Thus, the historical researcher must be concerned with the accuracy of the original information.

A final concern is the expertise of the person reporting. Say a person with no background in pedagogy observes several classrooms and documents what he/she sees. The concern is whether the observer has the background to understand the sometimes subtle complexities

> **Internal criticism** *refers to the accuracy of the information obtained.*

of the classroom environment. If the observer is not capable of understanding the pedagogy, the accuracy of the information is of concern.

Critical research consumers should be concerned with the internal criticism of documents reported by researchers. Simply demonstrating that documents are authentic is not sufficient. It is up to researchers also to demonstrate that the information obtained is accurate. If the information is not accurate, the researchers' conclusions will be suspect.

Synthesis of Information

Synthesis of information involves organizing the information, drawing conclusions, and, finally, making generalizations. Synthesis can be thought of as a final step in historical research (Mason et al., 1997). This step is similar in all of the research methodologies discussed throughout this text.

However, critical research consumers should be wary of generalization claims. The ability of historical research to make generalized statements is limited. The problem lies in the nature of the research. Entire populations are not likely to be investigated, nor have all of the potential variables that may account for the historical events been analyzed.

This problem is not limited only to historical research. Some researchers may mistakenly indicate that the problem with historical research is the fact that too few samples are selected for study. For example, if we study 100 one-room schools versus 10, we can make a stronger case for generalization. However, the number is not the critical variable, nor is the number of participants. What is critical are the characteristics of the schoolhouses examined. For example, location, size, ages of the students, and so on, are important factors. The conclusions are logical rather than statistical; therefore, the claims of generalization are also logical. Logical generalization suggests that we can generalize to other cases with characteristics similar to the one used in the investigation. Thus, the size of the sample is not necessarily a major obstacle in generalizing conclusions to other cases.

One difficulty with generalization claims is the validity of inferences made during the investigation and the conclusions drawn. Since it is not possible to determine a causal variable, because it cannot be manipulated or changed, it is not possible to generalize statements to other cases. These generalized statements cannot be made, because the other cases may be influenced by variables different from those in the original investigation.

Recall the research question regarding Head Start policies and procedures posed earlier in this chapter? Read on to see how your design compares to how the actual study was designed.

Research Example 4: Document Analysis— Policies and Procedures

A document analysis was used to determine to what extent Head Start policies and procedures addressed child guidance and challenging behaviors (Quesenberry et al., 2011). Researchers studied six Head Start programs to determine how they supported children's social and emotional competence and the extent to which they addressed children's challenging behavior. Quesenberry et al. noted that some children who entered Head Start programs lacked language and/or socioemotional skills, such as sharing and making friends. Socioemotional skills need to be taught, and challenging behaviors need to be addressed so that children do not develop more serious problems later (Walker, Stiller, & Golly, 1999). Three Head Start experts were asked to nominate the programs they would rate highest and lowest in relation to the quality and implementation of policies and procedures on behavior management. Selection of experts was based on unique knowledge of programs throughout the state. Six Head Start programs (three rated high, three rated low) were selected. A rubric was set up for reviewing policies and procedures. Generally, the rubric contained five items: (1) social and emotional teaching curriculum strategies; (2) screening, assessment, and ongoing monitoring of children's socioemotional development; (3) involving families in supporting their child's socioemotional development and addressing challenging behaviors; (4) supporting children with persistent challenging behavior; and (5) providing training, technical assistance, and ongoing support to staff when addressing socioemotional competence and challenging behaviors. Within each item, rating scales were developed to identify the extent to which the policies and procedures addressed the item. Researchers reviewed all policy documents of the six programs. Findings indicated that policies and procedures varied across programs. Programs rated high in one area relative to policies and procedures were rated high in all areas, and programs rated low were so rated in all areas. Some programs provided considerable attention and detail to socioemotional development and challenging behavior, while others did not. Researchers described the sample size as a limitation because results might not be representative of other Head Start programs. Rubric ratings were made by researchers who were not "blind" to initial program selection (i.e., they were aware of programs rated high and low quality by experts).

WHAT ARE MIXED-METHODS STUDIES?

Mixed-methods studies involve "a set of procedures for collecting, analyzing, and mixing both quantitative and qualitative methods in a study to understand the research problem" (Plano-Clark & Creswell, 2010, p. 299). Thus, mixed-methods research combines qualitative and quantitative methods and concepts in one study (Johnson & Onwuegbuzie, 2001). As noted by Creswell (2009), mixed-methods research involves "more than simply collecting and analyzing both kinds of data; it also involves the use of both approaches in tandem so that the overall strength of the study is greater than either qualitative or quantitative research" (p. 4). This type of research is meant to address more questions, with more depth and breadth than either approach alone. In mixed-methods studies, some research questions can be answered by only quantitative data, some others by only qualitative data, and in still other cases both methods may be required.

Mixed methods are generally accepted in educational and psychological research. Several journals accept mixed-methods research; in fact, at least one is dedicated to mixed methods (e.g.,

Journal of Mixed Methods Research). However, critical research consumers should understand the wide chasm that still exists in some circles dividing quantitative and qualitative research. As noted by Johnson and Onwuegbuzie (2001), feelings run so deep that some researchers may feel they are required to "pledge allegiance to one research school of thought or the other" (p. 14). We find this unfortunate, because it prevents research consumers from learning about a variety of research methods and thinking critically about the field. There is a vast amount of information available at the fingertips of the researcher whose only impediments are attitude and dogma.

Consider an example. Let's say we are interested in effects of a token reinforcement point system on a third-grade classroom during reading period. We decide to conduct a quasi-experimental design comparing one third-grade classroom with the point system to a matched third-grade classroom without a point system. The independent variable is the point system. The dependent measures are rates of problem behavior, words read correctly per minute during reading class, and percentage of observations during which the students are engaged in a task (vs. off-task behaviors such as talking to neighbors or looking out the classroom window). We collect data on these measures, compare them across classrooms, and draw conclusions. Now let's add a qualitative component to produce a mixed-methods design. Two graduate students play the role of participants-as-observers in an ethnographic study and join the third graders, one in the classroom with the point system and the other in the classroom without the point system. For several weeks, the participants-as-observers engage the children during reading class, recess, and lunch. The intent of the study is to find out whether introduction of the

---

Synthesis of information *involves organizing the information, drawing conclusions, and, finally, making generalizations.*

Mixed-methods studies *involve the combination of qualitative and quantitative research methods.*

point system changes student attitudes and/or confidence toward reading, satisfaction with the school experience, and degree of competition with other students. Participants-as-observers listen to students as they converse with each other and with the teacher, interact with them at recess and lunch, and ask open-ended questions. Additionally, participants-as-observers interview teachers and parents to get their perspectives. We collect and discuss field notes, code them according to themes that emerge, and draw conclusions. If we had conducted only the quasi-experimental study, we would have missed a wealth of information obtained from students and teachers. On the other hand, if we had conducted only the ethnographic study, we would have missed a wealth of information on dependent measures in the quasi-experimental study. Conducting both studies provides extensive data and perspectives from multiple sources.

As researchers plan mixed-methods research, they must first consider the research questions and how quantitative and qualitative methods will address them. Second, researchers should consider all the relevant characteristics of the design (Creswell, 2009; Johnson & Onwuegbuzie, 2001). For example, researchers must consider timing of the quantitative and qualitative phases. A key question is "Will data collection occur sequentially or concurrently?" Also, researchers should consider whether they will mix or transform data (Creswell & Plano-Clark, 2007). *Mixing data* refers to ways that researchers may examine and merge information by transforming qualitative themes into counts to create descriptive data. For example, one question is "Will there be quantitative data (e.g., a count of

the number of words identifying emotions) that can be transformed from qualitative information (interview responses)?"

Mixed-Methods Strategies

There are six strategies in mixed-methods research: concurrent triangulation, concurrent embedded, concurrent transformative, sequential explanatory, sequential exploratory, and sequential transformative strategies (see Figure 10.4). Each strategy is briefly described below. It is beyond the scope of this book to explore mixed methods in detail; the reader is referred elsewhere (e.g., Creswell, 2009; Creswell & Plano-Clark, 2007; Tashakkorie & Teddlie, 2003).

Concurrent Triangulation Strategy

In this strategy, quantitative and qualitative data are collected concurrently, then compared to determine whether there is "convergence, difference, or some combination" (Creswell, 2009, p. 213). That is, researchers examine data to determine whether there are similarities, differences, omissions, or unanswered questions. If so, additional information is collected. The concurrent triangulation strategy is the most common mixed method.

Concurrent Embedded Strategy

In this situation, data are again collected concurrently, but one method (usually qualitative) is the primary one and the other (usually quantitative) is an embedded or secondary method. The embedded strategy may address a different research question or outcome.

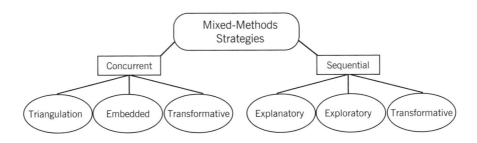

FIGURE 10.4. Concurrent and sequential mixed-methods strategies.

Concurrent Transformative Strategy

In this case, researchers are guided by a specific theoretical perspective as they collect both quantitative and qualitative data. That is, the research questions are squarely based on a particular theory or perspective. Common perspectives of some qualitative researchers are gender bias, specific positions on environmental issues, and discrimination or mistreatment toward certain groups. The theory or perspective is what drives the definition of the problem, identification of the design, source and analysis of data, interpretation, and conclusions.

Sequential Explanatory Strategy

In this strategy, quantitative data are collected in the first phase, and qualitative data are collected in a subsequent phase. Qualitative data enhance the quantitative data by providing information on similarities or differences. This strategy is particularly useful when unexpected results are found in the quantitative data. For example, the researcher can observe or interview the research participants who account for unexpected results to discover, qualitatively, reasons for the outcomes.

Sequential Exploratory Strategy

This strategy is similar to the sequential explanatory one except that phases are reversed. That is, qualitative data are collected in the first phase, and quantitative data are collected in a subsequent phase. The purpose of the research is to explore a phenomenon in the early stages. According to Morgan (1998), this design is appropriate for testing elements of an emergent theory that is the result of the qualitative phase and supplementing it with quantitative data.

Sequential Transformative Strategy

This strategy is similar to the concurrent transformative one, in that research is guided by a specific theoretical perspective. The difference is that the researcher collects quantitative and qualitative data in sequence. Either quantitative or qualitative data collection occurs first and is supplemented by the method in a second phase.

Analysis of Mixed-Methods Data

Analysis of data in mixed-methods research depends on the nature of the research questions and the strategy used. Creswell (2009) describes some of the more common analysis procedures. First, a researcher may want to mix, or transform, the data. Within a database, a researcher may create qualitative codes and themes, then examine the data for counts, percentages of totals, or other quantitative data. Second, researchers using a sequential explanatory strategy may want to observe or interview outliers who offered unusual data. Third, if using a sequential strategy, the researcher may develop an instrument. That is, if initial qualitative data suggest a theme, a second phase may call for a survey instrument that collects quantitative data. Fourth, if using a concurrent embedded strategy, a researcher may conduct a survey at one level to gather quantitative data about a sample. Concurrently, a researcher might collect qualitative data through interviews with particular survey respondents to explore a phenomenon further (i.e., to gather more information on reasons for survey responses).

Mixed-methods studies can be complex and therefore difficult to conceptualize. Creswell (2009) encourages researchers to depict a mixed-methods study using a visual diagram that shows whether data collection is concurrent or sequential, and depicts the quantitative and qualitative variables. Within both quantitative and qualitative variables, the diagram should embed the themes, categories, and/or dependent variables.

Sampling Issues in Mixed-Methods Research

One of the more knotty issues in mixed-methods research is sampling. A researcher who enters into a mixed-methods study must reconcile philosophical and pragmatic differences between quantitative and qualitative research in regard to sampling (Kemper, Stringfield, & Teddlie, 2003). Quantitative research is based on the concept of probability sampling; that is, the large sample that is drawn represents the variables of interest, so that results can be generalized to the population. See Chapter 4 for a description of probability sampling. In contrast, qualitative research is based on the concept of purposeful sampling, that is, examining one or more individuals, units, or organizations selected intentionally (see Chapter 9). In purposeful sampling, there is no intent to generalize results to the population. A researcher using a mixed-methods design must link the sampling procedure used to the research question or hypothesis in the study. If a research question or hypothesis calls for a generalization to the population regarding the effects of a variable, then one of various probability sampling procedures must be used. If a research question calls for an in-depth analysis of an individual, unit, or organization, purposeful sampling must be used. The problem occurs when a researcher makes a generalization to the population after using a purposeful sampling procedure (Kemper et al., 2003).

Recall the research question regarding academic self-efficacy posed earlier in this chapter? Read on to see how your design compares to how the actual study was designed.

Research Example 5: Mixed Methods

A concurrent triangulation mixed-methods approach was used to investigate whether a school-based psychoeducational intervention called Tools for Tomorrow (TFT) increased academic self-efficacy of ninth-grade urban youth (Perry, DeWine, Duffy, & Vance, 2007). *Academic self-efficacy* was defined as "perceived confidence in one's ability to execute actions to attain academic goals" (Perry et al., 2007, p. 104). Based on social cognitive career theory (Lent, Brown, & Hackett, 2002), self-efficacy is critical in explaining how people develop, pursue, and accomplish career and academic goals. TFT is designed to facilitate career exploration and career decision making. Its underlying premise is that if students understand that the purpose of school is to guide them to future careers, then they will be more motivated to achieve in school. In this study, 64 ninth-grade students (33 males, 31 females; 29 African American students; 26 Hispanic students; 10 students classified as ELLs) participated. All students participated in the TFT program, which included three modules (Who Am I?, Connecting School and

Career, and Identifying Resources and Barriers). TFT is designed to supplement work-based education programs. The quantitative measure was pre- and posttests using the Academic Self-Efficacy Scale (Hemond-Reuman & Moilanen, 1992), which uses a rating scale to assess self-perceived academic abilities. The qualitative measure was a semistructured interview, also administered on a pre- and postassessment basis. Results from the Academic Self-Efficacy Scale indicated no statistically significant difference between pre- and postassessments. Researchers described enhanced developmental specificity concerning academic skills and goals based on results of postinterviews.

WHEN SHOULD RESEARCHERS USE EACH QUALITATIVE RESEARCH DESIGN?

Qualitative research has many uses. It is very useful for generating both hypotheses to be tested later and grounded theories, for disproving a theory, and for describing a phenomenon in the natural world. Case studies are used when researchers wish to study an individual or "case" in depth. Researchers attempt to gain a deep understanding of a particular phenomenon under study when an in-depth examination of several individuals or cases is not practical. Researchers use an observation study when the phenomenon of interest can be investigated by assessing observable behavior. Additionally, observations allow researchers to investigate the phenomenon in context. This is to say that researchers collect data while the participants are interacting with the natural environment. When needed information cannot be obtained through observations, such as in cases where it is impossible (e.g., thinking, feelings) or improbable (e.g., observing every minute of every day), interview methods are utilized. Interviews have an advantage over observations in that they allow for the collection of data that cannot be obtained through observations; however, the weakness is that the reliability and validity of interview data are questionable. The use of ethnography allows researchers to combine several data-gathering techniques to investigate a phenomenon. In ethnography, researchers conduct in-depth interviews using participant and non-participant observational techniques to obtain a holistic picture of phenomena. The investigation occurs over an extended period of time. Researchers use ethnographies to allow for the in-depth study of a culture, be it a classroom or a workplace. Finally, document analyses are needed when researchers wish to verify data collected from other sources further, or when the data cannot be accessed any other way, such as through observations. Document analysis has the advantage of being unobtrusive, in that the data are available without researchers having to observe or interview participants.

SUMMARY

❖ Qualitative methods (designs) are not as easily defined as the methods used in quantitative research. Qualitative research methods are tied to the method of data collection, whereas quantitative research designs are independent of the data collection methods used.

❖ Field-oriented studies involve case studies, observations, interviews, and ethnographies. Case study research focuses on one participant, setting, situation, or event. An observation study is a form of a case study. It is helpful to think of observation on a continuum from complete participant to complete observer. Survey research can also be conducted in a qualitative manner through interviewing. Ethnography essentially combines observational methods and in-depth interview methods to investigate a phenomenon from a cultural perspective.

❖ Historical research can be quantitative or qualitative; however, historical research is frequently described as a form of qualitative research. Historical research has two main characteristics: (1) It emphasizes what occurred in the past, and (2) it is empirical, in that there is an attempt to obtain information from a variety of sources. Historical research also has several purposes: (1) It answers factual questions about the past; (2) it aids us in determining what has worked in the past; (3) it helps us to understand how we came to this point in time; (4) it helps us to see trends or patterns; and (5) it serves as a basis for later interview or observation studies. Designing historical research involves developing a research question or hypothesis and collecting data. Analyses of these data are based on external criticism, internal criticism, and synthesis of information.

❖ Mixed-methods studies combine qualitative and quantitative methods and concepts into one study. There are six mixed-methods strategies: (1) concurrent triangulation, (2) concurrent embedded, (3) concurrent transformative, (4) sequential explanatory, (5) sequential exploratory, and (6) sequential transformative strategies. Analyses of data and sampling issues are achieved using quantitative and qualitative approaches.

❖ Qualitative research has many uses. It is very useful for generating hypotheses to be tested later, for generating grounded theories, for disproving a theory, and for describing a phenomenon in the natural world.

DISCUSSION QUESTIONS

1. What are the different types of field-oriented studies, and what is a justification for the use of each one?

2. What are the differences between participant and nonparticipant observation studies? When would you use each type? In your answer, include the advantages and disadvantages of each type.

3. What are observer effects and observer bias in an investigation? How would you control for these?

4. What are the types of interview formats, and when would you use each type? In your answer, include the advantages and disadvantages of each type.

5. What is ethnography? What research

question might you answer with such a design?

6. When would you use historical research? In your answer, include at least one purpose of historical research and the types of sources you might access.

7. What are external and internal criticisms? Why are these criticisms important when you read historical research?

8. What is an advantage of using mixed-methods research? What research question could you answer with a mixed-methods study, and what type of data would you collect?

9. Could you have answered the question in item 8 with either a quantitative or qualitative study alone? Why or why not?

ILLUSTRATIVE EXAMPLE

Toddler Teachers' Use of *Teaching Pyramid* Practices

Diane Branson
Truckee Meadows Community College, Reno, Nevada

MaryAnn Demchak
University of Nevada, Reno

Abstract. *Effective strategies to promote social-emotional development and prevent occurrence of challenging behaviors in young children is critical. The Teaching Pyramid, a framework for supporting social-emotional development and preventing and addressing challenging behaviors, was developed for preschool children. This mixed methods study investigated toddler teachers' use of Teaching Pyramid practices and the relationship between these practices and classroom quality. Results indicated that toddler teachers used practices associated with the universal level of the Pyramid (e.g., positive relationships with children and parents). At this level, however, it was also evident that some preventive practices were missing (e.g., posted visual schedules and rules). Missing across classrooms was evidence of practices associated with the secondary level (e.g., explicitly teaching behavior expectations) and tertiary level (e.g., participating in developing behavior support plans). Implementation of Pyramid practices appeared to be associated with classrooms rated as being high quality.*

Keywords. *problem behavior, social-emotional competence, Teaching Pyramid practices*

Challenging behavior in young children has been the focus of recent research because of increasing prevalence rates and evidence that untreated problem behaviors persist into adulthood (Webster-Stratton, 1997). Moreover, disruptive behavior issues are the most common reason for referral to mental health services for young children (Kazdin & Weisz, 2003), with reported prevalence rates ranging from 7% to 25% of preschool-age children (Webster-Stratton, 2000). Children identified with aggressive behavior in preschool have a high probability of continuing with problem behavior through elementary school and into adolescence (Campbell, Spieker, Burchinal, Poe, & NICHD Early Child Care Research Network, 2006; McCartney, Burchinal, Clarke-Stewart, Bub, Owen, Belsky, & NICHD Early Child Care Research Network, 2010). In fact, the correlation between preschool-age aggression and aggression at age 10 years is higher than that for IQ (Kazdin, 1985). Shaw, Gilliom, and Giovannelli (2000) completed a longitudinal study of children identified with challenging behaviors at age 2 years and reported that 88% of the boys identified with aggressive behavior at age 2 years still showed clinical signs of aggression at age 5 years.

In addition to the long-term impact, preschool-age children with aggressive behavior face more immediate negative consequences. They are often rejected by peers (Cole & Dodge, 1998), receive less positive teacher attention (Strain, Lambert, Kerr, Stagg, & Lenkner, 1983), are less successful in kindergarten, and are at risk for later school failure (Tremblay, 2000).

Researchers document that it is important to intervene early with children with challenging behavior in order to prevent ongoing behavior problems (Campbell, 1995; Campbell et al., 2006; Shaw et al., 2000). However, the majority of behavioral intervention research focusing on young children has focused on children with disabilities who are between the ages of 3 and 6 years (Conroy, Dunlap, Clarke, & Alter, 2005). This lack of research for children under the age of 3 years is unfortunate given what we know about the importance of early experiences on brain development influencing a child's abilities to self-regulate, manage emotions, and inhibit behavioral impulses—key skills for prosocial behavior (Shonkoff & Phillips, 2000).

It is estimated that 5 million of the nation's 11 million infants and toddlers from all socioeconomic strata spend 25 or more hours each week in out-of-home care (Larner, Behrman, Young, & Reich, 2001). The National Institute of Child Health and Human Development (NICHD Early Child Care Research Network, 2001) conducted a comprehensive study of the effect of out-of-home child care on children's development and found that the amount of time spent in nonparental care was associated with poor peer interactions and behavior problems. There is also evidence that young children with challenging behavior in these out-of-home settings are 3 times as likely to be expelled for engaging in challenging behavior as school-aged children (Gilliam, 2005). Expulsion rates drop for preschoolers, however, when teachers have access to ongoing training and consultation in effective strategies for supporting children's prosocial behavior (Gilliam & Shabar, 2006). In addition to evidence that training can be effective in reducing expulsions in early childhood settings, early childhood administrators and educators identify as a high priority a need for assistance with challenging behaviors (Buscemi, Bennett, Thomas, & Deluca, 1996).

Young children are at risk for developing challenging behavior problems that if not addressed can result in long-term social and developmental consequences. This fact highlights the need to find an effective model for supporting the social-emotional development of children and methods for preventing and addressing challenging behavior in early child care settings.

Positive behavior support (PBS) is an evidence-based method that focuses on proactive, positive strategies to prevent and address challenging behavior. PBS promotes programwide use of supports through the use of environmental arrangements of antecedent stimuli, positive consequences, and the use of direct instructional strategies to teach replacement behaviors (Carr et al., 1999; Conroy et al., 2005). The *Teaching Pyramid* (Fox, Dunlap, Hemmeter, Joseph, & Strain, 2003) is an approach to providing supports at the universal level (i.e., nurturing and responsive caregiving relationships and high-quality supportive environments), secondary level (i.e., social-emotional teaching strategies), and tertiary level (i.e., individualized interventions). Hemmeter and Fox (2009) indicate that the *Teaching Pyramid* has application to children birth to 2 years even though the model was originally developed for children ages 2 to 5 years.

The purpose of this study was to examine toddler teachers' use of evidence-based practices described in the *Teaching Pyramid* (Fox et al., 2003) that are associated with supporting social-emotional development and preventing and addressing challenging behavior in young children (Hemmeter & Fox, 2009). Previous research has focused on preschool teachers' implementation of *Teaching Pyramid* practices using the *Teaching Pyramid Observation Tool* (TPOT; Hemmeter & Fox, 2006). In light of the importance of intervening early with children at risk for developing challenging behaviors (Campbell et al., 2006; Kazdin & Weisz, 2003), this study sought to understand toddler teachers' use of a range of practices associated with the *Teaching Pyramid*. An additional aim of the study was to examine the relationship between classroom quality and use of *Teaching Pyramid* practices.

Higher quality of the child care environment has been associated with positive outcomes for children (Burchinal, Roberts, Nabors, & Bryant, 1996; NICHD Early Child Care Research Network, 2003; Peisner et al., 2001) as well as fewer problem behaviors (National Scientific Council on the Developing Child, 2008; McCartney et al., & NICHD Early Child Care Research Network, 2010). The present study was designed to address gaps in knowledge about toddler teachers' use of evidence-based practices to support children's social-emotional development and prevent challenging behaviors in toddlers and the relationship between classroom quality and teachers' use of those evidence-based practices.

Two research questions guided this study: (a) To what extent are study teachers currently implementing practices associated with the *Teaching Pyramid* in their toddler classrooms? and (b) Does teachers' use of *Teaching Pyramid* practices as measured by the TPOT appear to be related to classroom quality as measured by the *Infant/Toddler Environmental Rating Scale* (ITERS; Harms, Cryer, & Clifford, 1990)?

METHOD

Design

Mixed methods research combines both quantitative and qualitative approaches in order to "provide a better understanding of research problems than either approach alone can provide" (Creswell & Plano Clark, 2007, p. 5). The four major types of mixed methods designs are Triangulation Design, Embedded Design, Explanatory Design, and Exploratory Design. These designs vary according to when data are collected, either sequentially or simultaneously, the relative weight given to each type of data, and the data analysis used (Creswell & Plano Clark, 2007). This mixed methods study used a concurrent Explanatory design in which both quantitative and qualitative data were collected and analyzed at the same time using the same collection tools (i.e., TPOT and ITERS) with an emphasis on the quantitative data. Qualitative data were used to extend and explain quantitative results. Multiple observations and in-depth interviews were used in this mixed methods study to answer the research questions.

Participants

Purposive sampling is a qualitative sampling approach where the researcher selects the most productive sample to answer the research questions (Gay, Mills, & Airasian, 2006). Given that the research questions focused on teachers' use of practices associated with preventing and managing children's challenging behaviors and classroom quality, efforts were made to (a) recruit toddler teachers who had previously expressed an interest in learning how to prevent challenging behavior in their classrooms and (b) teachers from programs that varied on variables associated with classroom quality (e.g., adult:child ratio, teacher education and training, funding source). This sampling method was used to identify four licensed toddler classrooms in a midsized city in the western United States in which the staff or director had contacted the IDEA Part C early intervention agency for help in managing children's challenging

behavior. Recruitment letters were placed in the staff rooms of two community child care centers, one child care center on a community college campus and three Early Head Start (EHS) classrooms. Two lead teachers in the EHS classrooms agreed to participate in response to the recruitment letters. The lead teachers in the toddler classroom located on the community college campus and one community child care center agreed to participate in response to a follow-up phone call. Recruitment stopped when four teachers representing maximum variation on factors associated with quality in child care settings (Phillips, McCartney, & Scarr, 1987; Vandell & Wolfe, 2000) agreed to participate. On the basis of the time commitment involved in conducting multiple observations, in-depth teacher interviews, and mixed methods data analysis for this study, recruitment stopped at four teachers who represented a range of potential participants.

Participants were lead teachers in four toddler rooms in which children aged 18 to 36 months were enrolled. It should be noted that the majority (93%) of toddlers in these rooms were aged more than 2 years. Classroom and teacher characteristics are provided in Table 1.

Data Collection

Data were collected through structured interviews with the lead teachers, participant observations in each classroom on two occasions for a total of 4 hr in each room, and completion of two instruments to measure teachers' use of *Teaching Pyramid* practices and overall classroom quality. Teachers' use of *Teaching Pyramid* practices was measured using the unpublished *Teaching Pyramid Observation Tool for Preschool Classrooms—Draft* (TPOT; Hemmeter & Fox, 2006), whereas overall classroom quality was evaluated using the *ITERS* (Harms et al., 1990). The first author conducted the observations, wrote detailed field notes during the observations, which were expanded on immediately following the observations; interviewed the lead teachers; and scored the study measures per each instrument's manual. The first author has more than 10 years' experience using the ITERS to evaluate infant–toddler classroom environments. In addition, prior to beginning the current study, the first author reviewed the ITERS training video and carefully reread through the manual to ensure accuracy in scoring. The first author achieved training in use of the TPOT by attending several workshops

TABLE 1. Classroom and Participant Characteristics

Classroom no.: description	Teacher's age	Teacher's ethnicity	Teacher's education	Teachers' years in child care	Adult:child ratio	No. of children	Ethnicity	Age range in months (*n*)
1: EHS	45	Caucasian	Some college	10	1:4	6 total; 3 boys, 3 girls	2 Caucasian 4 Latino	34–36 (6)
2: Lab	25	Latino	Some college	5	1:6	17 total; 7 boys, 10 girls	16 Caucasian 1 Latino	18 (3) 24–36 (14)
3: EHS	57	Caucasian	CDA	20	1:4	7 total; 5 boys, 2 girls	3 Caucasian 4 Latino	20 (1) 24–33 (6)
4: Private	19	Caucasian	Some college	3	1:8	24 total; 16 boys, 8 girls	22 Caucasian 2 Latino	24–36 (24)

Abbreviations: CDA, child development associates degree; EHS, Early Head Start; Lab, community college lab preschool; Private, privately owned for-profit preschool.

presented by the TPOT authors, study of the TPOT manual, and personal communication with TPOT author, Dr. Hemmeter, to clarify TPOT administration directions.

Measures

TPOT (Hemmeter & Fox, 2006)

The purpose of the TPOT, currently being field tested and used in this study with permission, is to identify which evidence-based practices associated with preventing challenging behaviors are in place in a particular classroom and to monitor fidelity of implementation of the *Teaching Pyramid* model after training (Hemmeter & Fox, 2009). The tool, completed during a 2-hr classroom observation and after a brief interview of the teacher, consists of 38 items. The first 7 items, scored as *yes* or *no* and based on observation, indicate the presence of specific classroom preventive practices. The next 15 items rated on a scale from 0 to 5 are based on observation and/or the teacher interview, with a rating of 5 indicating that the teacher demonstrated all of the behaviors for the specific indicator or item. The TPOT manual provides detailed examples of behaviors that need to be present for a specific rating to be earned for the overall item. It is important to note that within these 15 items, an item was to be scored as 0 if any of the indicators listed for a score of 1 were missing. Thus, it is possible for a classroom to receive a rating of 0 for a particular item but display "splinter" skills related to higher ratings. The final 16 items on the TPOT are rated as *yes* or *no* for the presence of "red flags" that might be indicative of areas in need of

teacher training or program policies and procedures issues. As specified by the TPOT authors, the TPOT covers the three levels of the *Teaching Pyramid* model; universal strategies (i.e., responsive interactions and classroom preventive practices), secondary strategies (i.e., social-emotional teaching strategies), and targeted strategies (i.e., individualized interventions). (See Hemmeter & Fox, 2009, for a detailed explanation of the *Teaching Pyramid* model.) Reliability and validity measures are not available for the 2006 version of the TPOT used in this study, but they have been collected on later versions (M. L. Hemmeter, personal communication, February 24, 2010).

ITERS (Harms et al., 1990)

The ITERS, used to rate the quality of child care environments, contains 35 items reflecting both the physical and social environment of infant–toddler classrooms that are rated on a 1 to 7 scale, with 7 designated as *excellent* and 1 defined as *poor*. The seven subscales on the ITERS receive a rating; the subscales are (a) furnishings and display for children, (b) personal care routines, (c) listening and talking, (d) learning activities, (e) interactions, (f) program structure, and (g) adult needs. An overall score is computed by adding up all of the individual subscale scores and dividing that number by the number of subscales. This computation yields a number, between 1 and 7, that is used as an indicator of overall classroom quality. This measure was used to rate the overall classroom quality and to then determine if there appeared to be a relationship between overall classroom and a teacher's use of classroom preventive practices. The psychometric properties of the ITERS were originally established in 1988 and showed strong interrater reliability (.84), test–retest reliability (.79), and internal consistency (.83). Criterion and content validity measures were both above 80%, indicating that the ITERS items accurately measure constructs related to the provision of quality infant–toddler care (Harms et al., 1990).

Semistructured Interview

A semistructured interview lasting between 20 and 30 min was conducted, with each teacher following the last observation in order to gather information for either ITERS or TPOT items that could not be observed (e.g., teacher's role in developing a behavior plan, opportunities for professional growth). Two of the interviews were conducted in a staff room while the teacher was released from classroom duties. The other two interviews were conducted in the EHS classrooms during free-play activities while the other teacher attended to the children. Interview questions were asked verbally and transcribed manually.

Data Analysis

Initial analysis was conducted following the guidelines and structure provided by the ITERS and TPOT. (Table 2 summarizes the research questions, data source, and data analysis.) Data were analyzed using descriptive statistics to obtain mean scores of individual components of quality of the child care environment and implementation of *Teaching Pyramid* practices. The 35 items on the ITERS were rated individually and then the overall

child care quality rating was determined by averaging the individual scores. The TPOT includes four different kinds of items that were analyzed four ways: (a) Items 1 to 7 are answered *yes* or *no* and relate to observation of preventive practices present in the classroom. A total number of preventive practices observed were calculated for this section. (b) Items 8 to 22 are based on observation and teacher interview and are scored between 0 and 5. Each item was given a score based on the indicators observed or reported for that item, and then the average TPOT rating (0-5) for each classroom was calculated by adding up the scores for each item and dividing that number by the total. The number of 0 scores was also totaled for these items. (c) Items 23 to 38 reflect "red flags" that may indicate the need for teacher training and support of program policies. The total number of red flags observed in each classroom was calculated. (d) And using the classification provided by Hemmeter and Fox (2006), the results for each room were calculated for each level of the *Teaching Pyramid:* universal, secondary, and targeted. Subsequent to this analysis, the TPOT data were then reviewed across toddler rooms to identify *Teaching Pyramid* practices implemented consistently by all teachers, practices consistently omitted, variations in implementation of practices, as well as to identify how the various levels of the *Teaching Pyramid* were addressed across rooms.

The next step in data analysis was to compare the ITERS and TPOT data to identify relationships between the two instruments in terms of patterns and themes both within rooms and across the different classrooms and to compare emerging patterns related to evidence-based practices identified in the literature. This step was achieved by coding

TABLE 2. Summary of Research Questions and Methods of Analysis

Question	Variable	Data Source	Analysis
1. To what extent are study teachers currently implementing practices associated with the *Teaching Pyramid* in their toddler classrooms?	Use of practices associated with the *Teaching Pyramid*	*Teaching Pyramid Observation Tool* (TPOT; Hemmeter & Fox, 2006)	Descriptive statistics Identification of patterns within and across classrooms
2. Is there a relationship between classroom quality as rated by the ITERS and teachers' use of the *Teaching Pyramid* practices as rated by the TPOT?	Overall program quality	*Infant/Toddler Environmental Rating Scale* (ITERS; Harms et al., 1990)	Descriptive statistics
	Use of practices associated with the *Teaching Pyramid*	*Teaching Pyramid Observation Tool* (TPOT; Hemmeter & Fox, 2006)	Qualitative analysis; coding, sorting, and categorizing data into themes

individual items on both instruments, merging codes between the instruments and developing themes based on the codes. Next, we reviewed classroom scores on both instruments for patterns related to the identified themes. For example, we looked to see if there was a relationship between scores on ITERS Items 1 to 5 (Furnishings and Displays for Children) and TPOT scores on Items 1 to 7 (presence of preventive practices). Lastly, data were reviewed to determine relationships between a room's overall quality rating, use of specific *Teaching Pyramid* practices, or the presence of red flags.

Data Validity Procedures

Research validity was achieved by collecting data from multiple sources, member checking, and an external audit (Glesne, 2006). Data were collected from participant observations using observation tools and from interviewing the teachers. Field notes and interview transcripts were shared with the teachers, with each verifying the accuracy of the notes and transcripts. The first author conducted the observations and interviews for completion of both the ITERS and TPOT and conducted the initial scoring of each instrument. Although the second author did not conduct observations for reliability purposes, efforts were taken to ensure validity of assigned scores or ratings through her review of each instrument to ensure that field notes or transcripts justified assigned ratings. If notations were not present or did not appear sufficient for a rating, the first author was asked to discuss details to ensure appropriate ratings. Item-by-item analysis resulted in an initial 96% agreement that TPOT ratings were appropriate and 100% agreement for the ITERS. At times, particular items were adjusted to ensure accuracy of scores. For example, TPOT Item 7 is a *yes–no* item asking if rules or expectations are posted and illustrated with a picture or photo. In one case, this item was rated as *no* but a subsequent item (no. 8) that pertained to schedules and rules was initially inappropriately rated; given that a schedule with visuals was not posted, it was not possible for that toddler room to be scored anything but a 0. Subsequent to such discussions, disagreements were reconciled and 100% agreement resulted for the TPOT. All items on both instruments were reviewed in this manner.

In addition, the first author independently scored each instrument to determine the overall scores and subscale scores presented in Tables 3

and 4 and Figure 1. Subsequently and independently, the second author verified all calculations, with a resulting agreement of 100%.

RESULTS

Implementation of Teaching Pyramid Practices

The results of the TPOT are reviewed for the entire instrument as well as for items within the tool; Table 3 shows the results for each toddler classroom for individual TPOT items. Toddler Room 1 was rated as having six of the seven environmental variables (Items 1–7 on the TPOT) present for classroom preventive practices at the universal level of the pyramid model. This room averaged a rating of 3.5 for Items 8 to 22 with 0 red flags present (Items 23–38). Toddler Room 2 was rated as having five of the seven environmental variables present and received an average rating of 3.1 for Items 8 to 22; two red flags were present. Toddler Room 3 was rated as having five of the seven environmental variables present, received an average rating of 3.3 (Items 8–22), and had one red flag present. Finally, Toddler Room 4 was rated as having six of the seven environmental variables present, averaged 2.1 on Items 8 to 22, and was rated as having five red flags present. Table 4 shows the results across the four toddler rooms for each level of the TPOT: universal strategies (i.e., preventive practices and

TABLE 3. Specific Item Results for *Teaching Pyramid Observation Tool* Across Toddler Classrooms

		Toddler Room 1	Toddler Room 2	Toddler Room 3	Toddler Room 4
	Environmental Arrangement Items 1–7	6	5	5	6
TPOT items	8	0	0	0	0
	9	5	4	0	2
	10	5	5	5	5
	11	5	5	5	0
	12	0	0	0	0
	13	5	5	5	2
	14	5	4	5	4
	15	2	0	4	0
	16	4	5	4	5
	17	0	0	0	0
	18	4	2	2	2
	19	2	2	5	0
	20	5	4	5	2
	21	5	5	5	4
	22	5	5	5	5
	Red Flag Items 23–38	0	2	1	5

TABLE 4. *Teaching Pyramid Observation Tool Results across Four Toddler Classrooms*

| | Universal strategies | | | | | Secondary strategies | | Targeted strategies | |
| | Classroom preventive practices | | | Responsive interactions | | Social-emotional teaching strategies | | Individualized interventions | |
Classrooms	Environmental arrangements (no. of elements present)	Mean rating of practices (maximum rating of 5)	No. of red flags present	Mean rating of practices (maximum rating of 5)	No. of red flags present	Mean rating of practices (maximum rating of 5)	No. of red flags present	Mean rating of practices (maximum rating of 5)	No. of red flags present
No. 1	6	2.5	0	5.0	0	2.5	0	3.5	0
No. 2	5	2.25	1	4.6	1	1.75	0	3.5	0
No. 3	5	1.25	1	5.0	0	2.5	0	5.0	0
No. 4	6	0.5	2	3.6	3	1.75	0	2.0	0

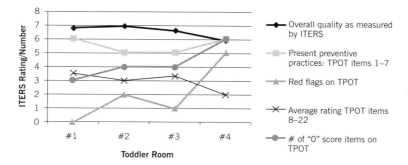

FIGURE 1. Relationship between classroom quality as measured by ITERS and various TPOT results.

Universal Strategies: Responsive Interactions

In the area of universal strategies, responsive inter-actions were consistently rated higher than were classroom preventive practices. In fact, across all levels of the TPOT and across all classrooms, responsive interactions received the highest ratings. Within the area of responsive interactions, all classrooms received a score of 5 on two items (10 and 22), indicating that all teachers demonstrated all indicators for both engaging in supportive conversations with children and building collaborative teaming relationships with other adults. Related to Item 10, teachers were observed to interact with children at eye level, greet children individually on arrival, and comfort children as needed.

Responsive interaction Item 13 (providing directions) was rated at 5 for Toddler Rooms 1, 2, and 3, whereas Toddler Room 4 received a 0 rating. Item 14 (using effective strategies to respond to challenging behavior) received a rating of 5 in Toddler Rooms 1 and 3 and a rating of 4 in Toddler Rooms 2 and 4, which indicated that all teachers did well in implementing skills in this specific area. Teachers in Toddler Rooms 1 and 4 both described and were observed responding in various ways to problem behavior. For example, Juanita (Teacher 1) described how she monitored a child prone to aggression so that she could scaffold the child's interactions with other children to avoid problems. During the observation, Alejandro, a child at risk for aggressive behavior, began to get angry when another child was standing in his way. Juanita quickly moved to Alejandro and said, "Use your

words—say 'Excuse me.'" During the interview with Jenna (Teacher 4), she described how she used interruption and redirection to avoid escalation of problem behavior. This was demonstrated during a motor activity when Jenna saw a child begin to push another child; she redirected the child to dance with the class, and when he was engaged in appropriate behavior she gave him positive attention by dancing with him.

Universal Strategies: Preventive Practices

Continuing with an examination of preventive practices, also part of the universal level, revealed Item 11 (promoting children's engagement) was rated at the highest level (5) in Toddler Rooms 1, 2, and 3; Room 4 received a rating of 0 for this item. In contrast, none of the rooms were rated as having posted rules and expectations (Item 7; all were rated *no*) or visual schedules (Item 8). Because there were no posted behavior expectations, a later item pertaining to teaching behavior expectations received a 0 rating, as it was not possible to review or remind children of the posted expectations. Similarly, each room also received a 0 rating in the area of schedules and routines for not having a classroom schedule with visuals posted. Teachers in all four classrooms were observed verbally stating expectations. Several teachers were observed saying, "Use your words," "Use gentle hands," and "Wait for your turn." When asked how children learned the rules, one teacher said, "The children just learn it through repetition." When asked if she had considered posting rules, the teacher replied, "How would you do that with toddlers who don't read?" *visuals!*

Item 9 pertained to transitions between activities. Toddler Room 2, rated 4 for this item, followed a consistent schedule, and staff provided more structure for routines and transitions than did staff in the other rooms. Two-minute transition warnings were given and then visual (lights off) and auditory (clean-up song) signals were used to help children make the transition smoothly. Toddler Room 2 used zone staffing patterns (McWilliam & Casey, 2008), where one teacher was setting up for the next activity, a second teacher was managing the current activity, and a third teacher was cleaning up from the previous activity. This arrangement facilitated child engagement and reduced waiting time. Toddler Room 4 received only a rating of 2 for Item 9 on transitions. Problems noted with this classroom's transitions included (a) too many transitions throughout the day, (b) no transition warnings given, and (c) children who followed directions and transitioned quickly being left waiting, with no positive teacher attention and nothing to do. Teachers in Toddler Room 1, the only room to receive a rating of 5 for transitions, split the class into smaller groups so that children who were ready to transition faster went with one teacher and those who were slower stayed with the other teacher. Transition warnings were not observed to be given to the whole class, but were given to individual children (e.g., one teacher told a child, "I am going to change your diaper in 2 minutes").

The universal strategies level of the *Pyramid* was the only level that reflected the presence of red flags, with Toddler Room 4 having the highest number of red flags; Toddler Room 1 had none. An analysis of the red flag items revealed that three of the four toddler rooms received red flags for teachers *not* being prepared for activities before children arrived at the activity; only in Toddler Room 1 were teachers prepared in advance.

Secondary Level: Social-Emotional Teaching Strategies

At the secondary level of the *Pyramid*, social-emotional teaching strategies, all rooms were rated 0 for Item 17 (teaching problem solving). Item 15 (teaching social skills and emotional competencies) is another item on which all received less than a full rating of 5; two rooms (2 and 4) were rated 0 whereas Room 1 was rated 2 and Room 3 received a rating of 4. Similarly, Item 18 (supporting friendship skills) was rated only 2 for Rooms 2, 3, and 4, whereas Room 1 received a rating of 4. In contrast, Item 16 (teaching children to express emotions) was rated high across all four rooms,

with Toddler Rooms 2 and 4 rated 5 and Rooms 1 and 3 rated 4, indicating that more skills were implemented across all indicators within Item 16 in comparison to other items at the secondary level of the *Pyramid*. All teachers reported using books and songs to teach children about emotions, but only one teacher (Toddler Room 2) reported using a teacher-created curriculum unit on feelings and how to be a good friend. Another teacher (Toddler Room 4) reported using puppets and role-playing to address an increase in challenging behavior related to sharing.

The four teachers reported, and it was observed, that they used naturally occurring opportunities during routines to teach social skills (e.g., taking turns, sharing toys). In one classroom, a boy tried to bite another child to get a bike from the child. The teacher came over and said, "No biting. What do you want to say? 'Anna' is using the bike right now. What can we do?" The child did not respond with a solution and so the teacher helped him engage in another activity until the bike was available. Teachers in all rooms were observed helping children generate solutions to social problems, such as that described. However, evidence of systematic teaching of problem-solving strategies and opportunities for children to reflect on the effectiveness of their problem-solving skills was lacking in all classrooms.

Tertiary Level: Individualized Interventions

The data for the final level of the *Pyramid*, the individualized interventions level, reveals that all four toddler rooms received a rating of 5 for Item 21 (focusing on involving families in supporting their child's social-emotional development and addressing problem behavior). In contrast, Item 19 (supporting children with persistent problem behavior) received variable ratings, with Room 3 rated a 5, Rooms 1 and 2 rated a 2, and Room 4 rated a 0.

Interviews revealed that the four teachers reported having worked with children with challenging behavior that required help of an "expert" in behavior management. The teachers reported that persistent aggressive behaviors (e.g., biting, hitting other children and the teacher, kicking) were the most challenging behaviors to handle. Toddler Rooms 1 and 3 had staff on-site with specialized training whom the teachers reported contacting when a child's challenging behaviors were persistent. The teachers in Toddler Rooms 2 and 4 reported requesting help from the early intervention agency with which both programs had an ongoing relationship.

Two themes emerged regarding persistent problem behavior. The first was the frustration teachers felt when children with behavior issues did not qualify for direct early intervention services under Part C of IDEA. One teacher stated, "I don't even refer children with behavior issues to early intervention services anymore, because I know that he or she won't be eligible, if the only concern is behavior." The other theme was the lack of teacher input into the behavior plans that were developed and the difficulty teachers had implementing behavior plans. Children who display persistent challenging behaviors require intensive individualized interventions composed of PBS plans. Success of PBS plans is dependent on development and implementation by a team composed of the child's family, teacher, and behavior support specialist or mental health specialist (Powell, Dunlap, & Fox, 2006).

All teachers reported providing anecdotal data regarding challenging behaviors, but that was the extent of their involvement in developing support plans. One teacher spoke about the token reward system an outside "expert" had included in a support plan for her classroom. She complained, "Giving one child a sticker for following the rules just doesn't fit with our classroom philosophy." On a positive note, another teacher reported a successful experience following suggestions two early intervention consultants had for a child at her center who had an autism spectrum disorder. She reported that a formal behavior plan was not developed, but the consultants gave her suggestions for helping the child to regulate his sensory needs and taught the teacher to use visual supports and simple sign language with this child.

All teachers reported trying "everything possible" to retain children with challenging behaviors in their programs. Although the teachers of Toddler Rooms 1, 2, and 3 reported that children with

challenging behaviors had left their programs for various reasons (e.g., mother "pulled" a child, family moved), they clearly stated, "We do not disenroll children due to challenging behavior." In contrast, the teacher for Toddler Room 4 reported that in the prior year the center in which she was employed had disenrolled one child under the age of 3 years (i.e., one toddler) because of aggressive behavior.

Relationship of Implementation of Teaching Pyramid Practices to Classroom Quality

Quality of Child Care Environment: ITERS

Table 5 presents the results for environmental quality for each toddler classroom. The two Early Head Start classrooms and the community college lab toddler classroom (i.e., Toddler Rooms 1, 2, and 3) were all rated as *excellent* in quality (6.6–6.9), whereas the privately owned community preschool (i.e., Toddler Room 4) was rated as *good* quality (5.9) according to the quality criteria defined by Harms et al. (1990).

Relationship Between Classroom Quality and TPOT Scores

Figure 1 shows the ITERS overall classroom quality scores (1–7) and TPOT results including (a) the number of preventive practices observed to be present as measured by TPOT Items 1 to 7, (b) the number of red flags observed to be present as measured by TPOT Items 23 to 38, (c) the average rating for TPOT Items 8 to 22, and (d) the number of TPOT items that were rated as 0, meaning that all the behaviors required for a score of 1 were not observed. This figure shows that Toddler Room 4, which had the lowest quality rating, also had highest number of red flags and 0 score items (meaning this room had the highest number of items for which most basic behaviors were not observed).

TABLE 5. ITERS Scores for Each Toddler Classroom

Classroom	Furnishings and display for children	Personal care routines	Listening and talking	Learning activities	Interaction	Program structure	Adult needs	Overall average item score
No. 1	7.0	7.0	7.0	6.9	7.0	7.0	5.5	6.8
No. 2	6.4	6.9	7.0	7.0	7.0	6.8	7.0	6.9
No. 3	7.0	6.9	7.0	5.4	7.0	7.0	7.0	6.6
No. 4	5.2	6.2	7.0	5.6	6.7	6.0	5.5	5.9

This room also had the lowest overall TPOT rating for Items 8 to 22, meaning that fewer *Teaching Pyramid* practices were implemented in comparison to the other rooms. In contrast to these results, Toddler Room 4 did just as well as the other three rooms in implementation of the preventive practices represented by Items 1 to 7 on the TPOT.

Specific *ITERS* items have been identified as important universal practices for preventing challenging behaviors (e.g., physical arrangement, adult–child interactions) (Hemmeter & Ostrosky, 2003) and will be discussed with anecdotal information from observations in the toddler rooms. These areas of the ITERS appear to overlap with TPOT practices.

Caregiver–Child Interactions

The ITERS defines high-quality caregiver–child interactions as frequent positive interactions initiated by the teacher throughout the day. To get an *excellent* rating, the teacher should demonstrate sensitivity to children's feelings and vary his or her interaction style based on an individual child's temperament. All four teachers were responsive to children in their care. The teachers greeted children by name and exchanged information with parents at drop-off and pick-up. One teacher, when a mother shared that her little girl was wearing "big-girl underpants," got down at eye level with the girl and said, "Look at me, I am so excited that you are wearing underwear." When children approached the teachers with requests or comments, all were observed responding to the children verbally. Teachers in all classrooms also demonstrated sensitivity to children's feelings by validating and labeling the feelings expressed. There is obvious overlap with these areas of the ITERS with the responsive interaction items of the universal level of the TPOT as well as some overlap with the secondary level of the TPOT, social-emotional teaching strategies. As was previously mentioned, the responsive interactions component of the universal strategies as measured by the TPOT received the highest ratings of all levels of the *Teaching Pyramid*. It is not surprising that similarly, the Interaction subscale of the ITERS was scored as excellent across the rooms. Although in the excellent range, Toddler Room 4 notably received the lowest rating in the Interaction area just as it received the lowest rating of the four rooms in the responsive interactions area on the TPOT. One difference noted between Toddler Room 4 and the other three toddler rooms was in teacher-initiated interactions. The teacher in Room 4 tended to provide directions and reprimands to children, rather than interactions for social purposes or to recognize positive behaviors.

Classroom Arrangement

The physical arrangement of a classroom can be used to prevent problem behavior and to encourage prosocial behaviors (Lawry, Danko, & Strain, 2000). The ITERS defines high-quality classroom arrangement as one that provides children with a variety of learning experiences in well-defined areas with separate active and quiet play areas. All four toddler rooms had well-defined play areas and clear boundaries between play areas. Toddler Rooms 2 and 4 did not have clear separations between active play and quiet areas. In addition, in Room 4 the rug for circle activities (approximately 1.8 m × 2.4 m for 12 children) was next to a cart holding manipulatives. Instead of participating in the songs and stories, several children played with building blocks, which was distracting to other children and the teacher. During this observation, nothing was used to define an individual child's physical space (e.g., carpet squares), and the rug was so small that each child was sitting directly next to another child.

DISCUSSION

This study investigated the use of *Teaching Pyramid* practices by four lead teachers in four different toddler classrooms: two EHS classrooms, one community college lab preschool classroom, and one privately owned community preschool. Overall TPOT results, reflecting the *Teaching Pyramid* model and specific practices measured by the instrument, were compared to classroom quality using the *ITERS*.

The results indicated that the toddler teachers in this study used a number of evidence-based practices across all levels of the *Teaching Pyramid*. All four teachers demonstrated the following practices associated with universal strategies: (a) having supportive conversations with children, (b) responding appropriately to problem behavior, (c) supporting families, and (d) collaborating with other staff. At the secondary level of the *Pyramid*, teaching social-emotional strategies, all teachers informally taught children to express emotions by labeling emotions for them and using books and pictures to discuss emotions. At the targeted individualized interventions level of the *Pyramid*, all teachers involved families in supporting social-emotional development and addressing problem behavior by discussing the value of social-emotional development for young children and meeting to plan informally how to address a child's challenging behavior both at home and at school.

In contrast, all four teachers either did not implement certain practices or only partially implemented indicators associated with those practices. Specifically, at the universal level of classroom preventive practices, teachers consistently did not post schedules or behavior expectations. Consistent schedules, clear rules about classroom expectations, and reliable consequences help toddlers begin to learn self-regulation skills (Powell et al., 2006). The use of pictures illustrating the behavior expectations (e.g., use walking feet, use gentle hands) could provide an understandable visual cue for teaching behavior expectation concepts. In addition, these visual supports could serve as reminders to toddlers to follow the class expectations and to teachers to reinforce children who are demonstrating class behavior expectations.

In three of the four rooms, teachers were not prepared in advance of children arriving at centers or activities. Zone defense scheduling (ZDS) for teachers is an effective way to reduce time when children are not actively engaged due to setup and clean-up preparations (Casey & McWilliam, 2005; McWilliam & Casey, 2008). Lack of preparation meant that children spent time waiting and unengaged and thus at risk for engaging in problem behaviors.

At the secondary level of social-emotional teaching strategies, these teachers did not consistently teach social skills and emotional competencies nor consistently support friendship skills. According to Joseph and Strain (2003), children who are socially competent learn the skills necessary for interacting with others positively, persisting with challenging tasks, and regulating emotional responses in the face of frustrating experiences through naturally occurring opportunities.

Children with difficult temperaments (e.g., hyperactivity, impulsivity, inattention) and children from disadvantaged backgrounds (e.g., low socioeconomic status, abuse or neglect), however, may need more explicit teaching to learn those necessary skills. Teachers in this study recognized the importance of talking about emotions and helping children negotiate social situations, but they were not aware that some children in their classrooms would need explicit instruction in social-emotional skills to become socially competent.

Young children who are competent at persisting at difficult tasks, communicating their emotions effectively, controlling their anger, and solving social problems are less likely to engage in problem behaviors (Hemmeter, Ostrosky, & Fox, 2006). Children do not necessarily learn these skills during naturally occurring activities in preschool classrooms (Eisenberg & Fabes, 1998), so it is important for teachers to intentionally teach problem solving through teaching the concept, modeling the behavior, rehearsing the behavior, and helping children reflect on their use of problem-solving strategies (Grisham-Brown, Hemmeter, & Pretti-Fontczak, 2005; Landy, 2002).

Finally, at the individualized interventions level, these teachers did not consistently support children with persistent problem behavior through their involvement in assessing problem behavior and developing support plans. Meaningful involvement in a positive behavior support plan requires ongoing coaching from a behavior support or mental health consultant during development, implementation, and evaluation of the plan (Hemmeter & Fox, 2009). Although study teachers provided anecdotal information about a child's problem behavior, they did not meaningfully participate in developing a support plan nor did they receive ongoing assistance in implementing or evaluating the behavior plan.

The TPOT (Hemmeter & Fox, 2006) was developed to assess teachers' implementation of *Teaching Pyramid* practices in classrooms. Teachers in this study used strategies to build positive relationships with children and families, but they did not use strategies to explicitly teach behavior expectations, social skills, or problem-solving skills to children. Evidence that toddler teachers demonstrated more consistent use of practices associated at the universal level of the *Teaching Pyramid* (e.g., responsive caregiving) than those associated with the secondary and tertiary levels (e.g., teaching problem-solving skills, participating in behavior plans) are consistent with results with preschool teachers reported by Hemmeter and colleagues in their research on the TPOT with 50 preschool classrooms (Hemmeter, Fox, & Synder, 2008). Even in classrooms with excellent child care quality, the teachers expected the children to learn the behavior expectations through observational learning and repetition.

There were differences noted in the use of *Teaching Pyramid* practices between the classrooms enrolled in this study. The two EHS classrooms had the highest scores for *Teaching Pyramid* practices, followed by the lab classroom at the community college. The toddler classroom in a private preschool had the lowest scores for *Teaching Pyramid* practices observed. Differences in adult:child ratio may have contributed to differences noted in classroom quality and use of *Teaching Pyramid* practices. The ratio in the privately owned preschool was 1 teacher to 8 children, with a group size of 24 children under the age of 3 years. The ratio in the EHS classroom was 1 teacher to 4 children, with a group size of 7 children. Researchers investigating the quality of child care environments related to structural measures such as adult:child ratio and group size have found that more positive caregiver–child interactions occur in smaller groups of children and in child care settings with smaller adult child ratios (Vandell & Wolfe, 2000). Another explanation may be years of experience and education level. The teacher in the private preschool was the least experienced and had the least amount of formal education.

Limitations of the Study, Implications for Practice, and Future Research Needs

The results of this study indicated that classrooms with higher overall child care quality and fewer red flags as identified by the TPOT also had fewer instances of children exhibiting challenging behaviors as reported anecdotally by teachers in response to semistructured interviews. These results could be strengthened with supporting data to verify low occurrences of problem behaviors (e.g., review of behavior incident reports). The study included only four toddler classrooms located in one state, which could affect the generalizability of the findings to classrooms in other states. In addition, given the purposive sampling used to identify toddler classrooms, the findings might not be representative of toddler classrooms in general. Given that one of the criteria for potential inclusion was that these classrooms were in centers that had previously expressed an interest in addressing problem behaviors, staff in these classrooms might not represent typical staff. It should be noted that there was no effort or intent to restrict participating classrooms to those previously determined to be of high quality. However, all the classrooms in this study were rated as *good* to *excellent* quality according to the ITERS, further potentially limiting the generalizability of the findings. Because most child care environments are not rated so favorably (Helburn, 1995), it would be important to conduct further research in classrooms that are more representative of typical child care quality. Another potential limitation is that only one author observed within each classroom and ratings were validated with the second author through reading field notes and retrospective analysis.

Teaching Pyramid practices are effective strategies for supporting prosocial behavior and preventing and addressing challenging behavior in young children (Dunlap et al., 2006; Fox, 2007; Fox, Dunlap, & Powell, 2002; Hemmeter, Fox, & Doubet, 2006; Hemmeter & Ostrosky, 2003; Horner, Sugai, Todd, & Lewis-Palmer, 2005). These practices have also been identified as easily implemented in early childhood classrooms and congruent with the early childhood emphasis on developmentally appropriate practices (Conroy, Davis, Fox, & Brown, 2002). Strategies for managing transitions and teaching rules and behavior expectations seemed too challenging for teachers in the present study to consider implementing. Teachers need training in use of visual supports to teach young children behavior expectations in toddler classrooms.

This study and others (Gilliam, 2005; Hemmeter et al., 2006; Hemmeter, Fox, Jack, & Broyles, 2007; Hemmeter et al., 2008) provide evidence that the practices described by the *Teaching Pyramid* are not always implemented in early childhood settings. Moreover, managing challenging behavior is identified as a primary training need of child care providers and early childhood educators (Dunlap et al., 2003; Hemmeter et al., 2006). There is a need for research that looks more closely at training issues related to use of *Teaching Pyramid* practices. Future research might look at (a) which *Teaching Pyramid* practices are most effective in reducing challenging behaviors in young children, particularly toddlers, (b) which *Teaching Pyramid* practices are the easiest for teachers to implement in the classroom, and (c) does training on improving child engagement improve teachers' use of *Teaching Pyramid* practices collaterally. Research is also needed to look at teacher practices that support the social development of infants and young toddlers. The Center for Social and Emotional Foundations for Early Learning Technical Assistance recently began field testing the Pyramid Infant Toddler Observation Scale (TPITOS; Hemmeter, Carta, Hunter, & Strain,

2009). This tool was developed in recognition that some *Teaching Pyramid* practices designed for older toddlers and preschoolers may not be appropriate for infants or young toddlers.

Social-emotional development is critical for positive outcomes and later school success. Young children, who fail to receive appropriate interventions for challenging behaviors, are at risk of developing persistent antisocial behavior. Research has demonstrated that both preschool and toddler teachers use some of the evidence-based *Teaching Pyramid* practices that have been shown to encourage social-emotional development and to prevent challenging behaviors in young children. It is critical to provide training and support to early childhood educators to improve the quality of child care settings and to help child care providers implement evidence-based practices that support social-emotional development and prevent and address challenging behaviors in young children.

DECLARATION OF CONFLICTING INTERESTS

The author(s) declared no conflicts of interests with respect to the authorship and/or publication of this article.

FUNDING

The author(s) received no financial support for the research and/or authorship of this article.

REFERENCES

Burchinal, M., Roberts, J., Nabors, L., & Bryant, D. (1996). Quality of center child care and infant cognitive and language development. *Child Development, 67,* 606–620.

Buscemi, L., Bennett, T., Thomas, D., & Deluca, D. (1996). Head Start: Challenges and training needs. *Journal of Early Intervention, 20,* 1–13.

Campbell, S. (1995). Behavior problems in preschool children: A review of recent research. *Journal of Child Psychology and Psychiatry, 36,* 113–149.

Campbell, S., Spieker, S., Burchinal, M., Poe, M., & NICHD Early Child Care Research Network. (2006). Trajectories of aggression from toddlerhood to age 9 predict academic and social functioning through age 12. *Journal of Child Psychology and Psychiatry, 47,* 791–800.

Carr, E., Horner, R., Turnbull, A., Marquis, J., McLaughlin, D., & McAtee, M. (1999). *Positive behavior support as an approach for dealing with problem behavior in people with developmental disabilities: A research synthesis.* Washington, DC: American Association on Mental Retardation.

Casey, A., & McWilliam, R. A. (2005). Where is everybody? Organizing adults to promote child engagement. *Young Exceptional Children, 8,* 2–10.

Cole, J., & Dodge, K. (1998). Aggression and antisocial behavior. In W. Damon & N. Eisenberg (Eds.), *Handbook of child psychology* (5th ed., Vol. 3, pp. 779–862). New York: Wiley.

Conroy, M., Davis, C., Fox, J., & Brown, W. (2002). Functional assessment of behavior and effective supports for young children with challenging behavior. *Assessment for Effective Instruction, 27,* 35–47.

Conroy, M., Dunlap, G., Clarke, S., & Alter, P. (2005). A descriptive analysis of positive behavioral intervention research with young children with challenging behavior. *Topics in Early Childhood Special Education, 25,* 157–166.

Creswell, J., & Plano Clark, V. (2007). *Designing and conducting mixed methods research.* Thousand Oaks, CA: Sage.

Dunlap, G., Conroy, M., Kern, L., Dupaul, G., VanBrakle, J., Strain, P., et al. (2003). *Research synthesis on effective intervention procedures: Executive summary.* Tampa, FL: University of Florida, Center for Evidence-Based Practice: Young Children With Challenging Behavior.

Dunlap, G., Strain, P., Fox, L., Carta, J., Conroy, M., Smith, B., et al. (2006). Prevention and intervention with young children's challenging behavior: Perspectives regarding current knowledge. *Behavioral Disorders, 32,* 29–45.

Eisenberg, N., & Fabes, R. (1998). Prosocial development. In W. Damon & N. Eisenberg (Eds.), *Handbook of child psychology: Social, emotional, and personality development* (pp. 701–778). New York: Wiley.

Fox, L. (2007). Program practices for promoting the social development of young children and addressing challenging behavior. Retrieved from *http://www.challengingbehavior.org/do/resources/documents/rph_'program_practices.pdf.*

Fox, L., Dunlap, G., Hemmeter, M., Joseph, G., & Strain, P. (2003). The *Teaching Pyramid:* A model for supporting social competence and preventing challenging behavior in young children. *Young Children, 58,* 48–52.

Fox, L., Dunlap, G., & Powell, D. (2002). Young children with challenging behavior: Issues and considerations for behavior support. *Journal of Positive Behavior Interventions, 4,* 208–217.

Gay, L., Mills, G., & Airasian, P. (2006). *Educational research: Competencies for analysis and applications* (8th ed.). Upper Saddle River, NJ: Pearson.

Gilliam, W. (2005). Prekindergartners left behind: Expulsion rates in state prekindergarten systems. Retrieved from *http://www.fed-us.org/PDFslNational-PreKExpulsionPaper03.02_newpdf.*

Gilliam, W., & Shabar, G. (2006). Preschool and child care expulsion and suspension rates and predictors in one state. *Infants and Young Children, 19,* 228–245.

Glesne, C. (2006). *Becoming a qualitative researcher: An introduction* (3rd ed.). Boston, MA: Pearson.

Grisham-Brown, J., Hemmeter, M., & Pretti-Fontczak, K. (2005). *Blended practices for teaching young children in inclusive settings.* Baltimore: Brookes.

Harms, T., Cryer, D., & Clifford, R. (1990). *Infant/toddler environmental rating scale*. New York: Teachers College Press.

Helburn, S. (1995). *Cost, quality, and child outcomes in child care centers*. Denver, CO: Department of Economics, University of Colorado at Denver.

Hemmeter, M., Carta, J., Hunter, A., & Strain, P. (2009). The Pyramid Infant Toddler Observation Scale (TPI-TOS). Retrieved August 30, 2009, from *http://www.vanderbilt.edu/csefel/states/colorado/august/itsession/session l/TPITOS _tool*.

Hemmeter, M., & Fox, L. (2006). *Teaching Pyramid observation tool for preschool classrooms* (pp. 1–10). Tampa, FL: University of South Florida, Center for Evidence-Based Practice: Young Children With Challenging Behaviors.

Hemmeter, M., & Fox, L. (2009). The *Teaching Pyramid*: A model for the implementation of classroom practices within a program-wide approach to behavior support. *NSHA Dialog, 12*, 133–147.

Hemmeter, M., Fox, L., & Doubet, S. (2006). Together we can: A program-wide approach to addressing challenging behavior. In E. Hom & H. Jones (Eds.), *Social-emotional development* (Vol. 8, pp. 1–14). Missoula, MT: DEC.

Hemmeter, M., Fox, L., Jack, S., & Broyles, L. (2007). A programwide model of positive behavior support in early childhood settings. *Journal of Early Intervention, 29*, 337–355.

Hemmeter, M., Fox, L., & Synder, P. (2008, June). *Examining the potential efficacy of a classroom-wide model for promoting social emotional development and addressing challenging behavior in preschool children*. Poster presented at the Annual Institute of Education Sciences Research Conference, Washington, DC.

Hemmeter, M., & Ostrosky, M. (2003). *Classroom preventative practices*. Tampa, FL: University of South Florida, Center for Evidence-Based Practice: Young Children With Challenging Behavior.

Hemmeter, M., Ostrosky, M., & Fox, L. (2006). Social and emotional foundations for early learning: A conceptual model for intervention. *School Psychology Review, 35*, 583–601.

Horner, R., Sugai, G., Todd, A., & Lewis-Palmer, T. (2005). Schoolwide positive behavior support. In M. Bambura & L. Kern (Eds.), *Individualized supports for students with problem behaviors: Designing positive behavior support plans* (pp. 359–390). New York: Guilford Press.

Joseph, G., & Strain, P. (2003). Comprehensive evidence-based social-emotional curricula for young children: An analysis of efficacious adoption potential. *Topics in Early Childhood Special Education, 23*, 65–76.

Kazdin, A. (1985). *Treatment of antisocial behavior in children and adolescents*. Homewood, IL: Dorsey.

Kazdin, A., & Weisz, J. (2003). *Evidence-based psychotherapies for children and adolescents*. New York: Guilford Press.

Larner, M., Behrman, R., Young, M., & Reich, K. (2001). Caring for infants and toddlers: Analysis and recommendations. *The Future of Children, 11*, 7–19.

Landy, S. (2002). *Pathways to competence: Encouraging healthy social and emotional development in young children*. Baltimore: Brookes.

Lawry, J., Danko, C., & Strain, P. (2000). Examining the role of the classroom environment in the prevention of problem behaviors. *Young Exceptional Child, 3*(2), 11–19.

McCartney, K., Burchinal, M., Clarke-Stewart, A., Bub, K., Owen, M., Belsky, J., et al. (2010). Testing a series of causal propositions relating time in child care to children's externalizing behavior. *Developmental Psychology, 46*, 1–17.

McWilliam, R. A., & Casey, A. (2008). *Engagement of every child in the preschool classroom*. Baltimore: Brookes.

National Scientific Council on the Developing Child. (2008). Mental health problems in early childhood can impair learning and behavior for life: Working paper #6 [Electronic Version], 1–16. Retrieved February 22, 2010, from *http://www.developingchild.net*.

NICHD Early Child Care Research Network. (2001, April). *Quality of child care and child care outcomes*. Paper presented at the Biennial Meeting of the Society for Research in Child Development, Minneapolis, MN.

Peisner-Feinberg, E., Burchinal, M., Clifford, R., Culkin, M., Howes, C., Kagan, S., et al. (2001). The relation of preschool child-care quality to children's cognitive and social developmental trajectories through second grade. *Child Development, 72*, 1534–1553.

Phillips, D., McCartney, K., & Scarr, S. (1987). Child-care quality and children's social development. *Developmental Psychology, 23*, 537–543.

Powell, D., Dunlap, G., & Fox, L. (2006). Prevention and intervention for the challenging behaviors of toddlers and preschoolers. *Infants and Young Children, 19*, 25–35.

Shaw, D., Gilliom, M., & Giovannelli, J. (2000). Aggressive behavior disorders. In H. Zeannah (Ed.), *Handbook of infant mental health* (pp. 397–411). New York: Guilford Press.

Shonkoff, J., & Phillips, D. (Eds.). (2000). *From neurons to neighborhoods: The science of early childhood development*. Washington, DC: National Academy Press.

Strain, P., Lambert, D., Kerr, M., Stagg, V., & Lenkner, D. (1983). Naturalistic assessment of children's compliance to teachers, requests and consequences for compliance. *Journal of Applied Behavior Analysis, 16*, 243–249.

Tremblay, R. (2000). The development of aggressive behavior during childhood: What have we learned in the past century? *International Journal of Behavioral Development, 24*, 129–141.

Vandell, D. L., & Wolfe, B. (2000). *Child care quality: Does it matter and does it need to be improved?* Report prepared for the Department for Health and Human Services, Washington, DC. Retrieved from *http://www.irp.wisc.edu/publications/sr/pdfs/sr78.pdf*.

Webster-Stratton, C. (1997). Early intervention for families of preschool children with conduct problems. In M. Guralnick (Ed.), *The effectiveness of early intervention* (pp. 429–454). Baltimore: Brookes.

Webster-Stratton, C. (2000). Oppositional-defiant and conduct disordered children. In M. Hersen & R. Ammerman (Eds.), *Advanced abnormal child psychology* (2nd ed., pp. 387–412). Mahwah, NJ: Lawrence Erlbaum.

ABOUT THE AUTHORS

Diane Branson, PhD, is a speech pathologist at Nevada Early Intervention Services and adjunct faculty at Truckee Meadows Community College, Reno, Nevada. Her current interests include early identification of autism spectrum disorders, positive behavior support, and supporting inclusion in early childhood settings.

MaryAnn Demchak, PhD, is a professor of special education at the University of Nevada, Reno.

Her current interests include positive behavior support; instructional strategies for individuals with severe, multiple disabilities; and professional development for teachers.

From Branson, D., & Demchak, M. (2011). Toddler teachers' use of teaching pyramid practices. *Topics in Early Childhood Special Education, 30,* 196–208. Copyright 2011 by the Hammill Institute on Disabilities. Reprinted by permission of SAGE.

ILLUSTRATIVE EXAMPLE QUESTIONS

1. What was the overall purpose of the investigation?
2. Who were the participants?
3. What were the characteristics of the curriculum?
4. How were the data collected?
5. How was triangulation used to increase research validity?
6. How and when did the researchers analyze the data?
7. What type of design was used? Which parts of the design were qualitative and which parts were quantitative?
8. Are the conclusions supported by the results? Do they help you come to the same conclusions?
9. Did the researchers fit their results within the framework of past research and/or theories?
10. Could there have been a problem with reactivity? What could have been tried to avoid this?

ADDITIONAL RESEARCH EXAMPLES

1. Cosier, M. E., & Causton-Theoharis, J. (2010). Economic and demographic predictors of inclusive education. *Remedial and Special Education, 31,* 1–10.

2. Hall, J. N., & Ryan, K. E. (2011). Educational accountability: A qualitatively driven mixed-methods approach. *Qualitative Inquiry, 17,* 105–115.

3. Sosu, E., McWilliam, A., & Gray, D. S. (2008). The complexities of teachers' commitment to environmental education: A mixed methods approach. *Journal of Mixed Methods Research, 2,* 169–189.

QUALITATIVE RESEARCH EXAMINATION

Circle the number corresponding to the extent to which the researcher(s) demonstrated the five analysis issues.

1 = high extent	2 = moderate extent	3 = small extent
4 = minimal extent	5 = nonexistent	NA = not applicable for this design

Expectations

a. a priori	1	2	3	4	5	NA
b. emerging	1	2	3	4	5	NA

Justification _____

_____

Process of Analysis 1   2   3   4   5   NA

Justification _____

_____

Conceptual Leverage

a. low level	1	2	3	4	5	NA
b. high level	1	2	3	4	5	NA

Justification _____

_____

Generalizability 1   2   3   4   5   NA

Justification _____

_____

Abstract: Write a one-page abstract summarizing the overall conclusions of the authors and whether or not you feel the authors' conclusions are valid based on the analysis you conducted on the investigation.

PART V

····

Single-Case
Research Methods

CHAPTER 11

Withdrawal and Associated Designs

OBJECTIVES

After studying this chapter, you should be able to . . .

1. Specify what is meant by single-case research and indicate three ways single-case research is similar to qualitative research.
2. Illustrate the graphing methods in withdrawal designs.
3. Describe each of the withdrawal and associated designs.
4. Explain when researchers should use each withdrawal and associated design.

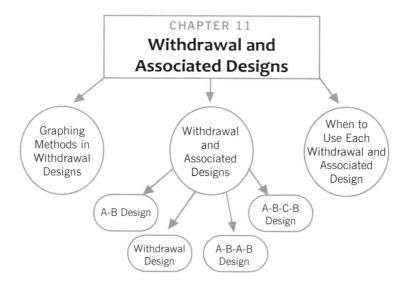

OVERVIEW

Single-case designs may be considered a combination of quantitative and qualitative research designs. (See Table 11.1 for a summary of the similarities and differences between single-case and qualitative research methods, and Table 11.2 for a summary of the similarities and differences between single-case and quantitative research methods.) Recall from Chapter 10 the five features of qualitative research: (1) The natural setting is the direct source of data, and the researcher is the key measurement instrument; (2) the research is descriptive; (3) the concern is with process rather than outcomes or products; (4) the data tend to be analyzed inductively; and (5) the meaning of the data is of essential concern (Bogdan & Biklen, 1998).

Single-case research is similar in four aspects. First, single-case researchers who operate in the applied arena usually conduct research in natural settings, and the researcher/observer is the key measurement instrument. Second, single-case researchers are as concerned with the "process" of skills acquisition as with the final outcome of an intervention. Third, single-case researchers do not develop hypotheses as do quantitative researchers. Instead, single-case researchers ask research questions and consider the process to be inductive in nature. Finally, single-case designs develop during the investigation; thus, single-case designs are flexible. This attribute is similar to qualitative designs in that the specific design is not predetermined; a research design develops throughout the investigation.

There are three major differences between single-case and qualitative methodologies. First, single-case researchers attempt to minimize subjectivity in their collection of data (see

TABLE 11.1. Similarities and Differences between Single-Case and Qualitative Research Methods

Single-case research	Qualitative research
Primary purpose is to determine cause-and-effect relationships.	Primary purpose is to describe ongoing processes.
Hypotheses are developed during the investigation; questions govern the purpose of the investigation; theories are developed inductively.	*Hypotheses are developed during the investigation; questions govern the purpose of the investigation; theories are developed inductively.*
The independent variable is controlled and manipulated.	There is no specific independent variable; the concern is to study naturally occurring phenomena without interference.
Objective collection of data is a requirement.	Objective collection of data is not a requirement; data collectors may interact with the participants.
Research design is flexible and develops throughout the investigation.	*Research design is flexible and develops throughout the investigation.*
Data are represented and summarized in numerical or graphical form.	Data are represented and summarized in narrative or verbal forms.
Reliability and validity determined through multiple sources of information (interobserver agreement).	*Reliability and validity determined through multiple sources of information (triangulation).*
Samples are purposefully selected or single cases are studied.	*Samples are purposefully selected or single cases are studied.*
Study of behavior is usually in the natural setting.	*Study of behavior is in the natural setting.*
Use of design controls for threats to internal validity.	Use of logical analyses controls or accounts for alternative explanations.
Use of similar cases to determine the generalizability of findings (logical generalization).	*Use of similar cases to determine the generalizability of findings (logical generalization) if at all.*
Rely on the researcher to control for procedural bias.	*Rely on the researcher to come to terms with procedural bias.*
Phenomena are broken down or simplified for study.	Phenomena are studied holistically, as a complex system.
Conclusions are tentative and subjected to ongoing examination (replications).	*Conclusions are tentative and subjected to ongoing examination.*

Note. Descriptions in *italics* indicate similarities or commonalities between the methodologies.

TABLE 11.2. Similarities and Differences between Single-Case and Quantitative Research Methods

Single-case research	Quantitative research
Primary purpose is to determine cause-and-effect relationships.	*Primary purpose is to determine cause-and-effect relationships.*
Hypotheses are developed during the investigation; questions govern the purpose of the investigation; theories are developed inductively.	Precise hypothesis is stated before the start of the investigation; theories govern the purpose of the investigation in a deductive manner.
The independent variable is controlled and manipulated.	*The independent variable is controlled and manipulated.*
Objective collection of data is a requirement.	*Objective collection of data is a requirement.*
Research design is flexible and develops throughout the investigation.	Research design is specified before the start of the investigation.
Data are represented and summarized in numerical or graphical form.	*Data are represented and summarized in numerical form.*
Reliability and validity are determined through multiple sources of information (interobserver agreement).	Reliability and validity are determined through statistical and logical methods.
Samples are purposefully selected or single cases are studied.	Samples are selected to represent the population.
Study of behavior is usually in the natural setting.	Study of behavior is in the natural or artificial setting.
Use of design controls for threats to internal validity.	*Use of design or statistical analyses controls for threats to internal validity.*
Use of similar cases to determine the generalizability of findings (logical generalization).	Use of inferential statistical procedures to demonstrate external validity (specifically, population validity).
Rely on the researcher to control for procedural bias.	Rely on research design and data gathering instruments to control for procedural bias.
Phenomena are broken down or simplified for study.	*Phenomena are broken down or simplified for study.*
Conclusions are tentative and subjected to ongoing examination (replications).	Conclusions are stated with a predetermined degree of certainty (i.e., a level).

Note. Descriptions in *italics* indicate similarities or commonalities between the methodologies.

Chapter 3 for interobserver agreement methods). Second, the data are quantified. Single-case researchers report their data in numerical form. However, there is a rich history of single-case researchers using descriptive analyses in the formulation of research questions and in the development of hypotheses for further study (e.g., Hammond, Iwata, Fritz, & Dempsey, 2011). Third, most single-case researchers try to avoid making inferences about internal cognitive processes and report only on observable and measurable behaviors. Thus, meaning for most single-case researchers is related to the interaction of observed environmental variables (both before and after the observed behavior) and the individual.

> **Single-case research** *is a type of research investigation that relies on the intensive examination of a single individual or a group of individuals, uses objective data collection techniques, and may be thought of as a combination of qualitative and quantitative designs.*

Single-case research is also similar to other quantitative research methods, in that the data are quantified and researchers attempt to remain objective during data collection. However, single-case designs have an advantage over the quantitative group designs discussed previously; that is, single-case designs do not require several participants (see Table 11.1). Single-case designs require at least one participant, although most studies involve two or more participants. Critical research consumers may be skeptical of studies involving a small number of participants. After all, in quantitative and some qualitative research examined thus far, large numbers of participants have been involved. In the quantitative research reviewed to this point, performance of a participant is represented by one data point. In some cases, participant performance is represented by two data points (e.g., a pretest and a posttest). Data across several participants are summed and averaged. Researchers seek to minimize variability across participants. In contrast, a participant's performance is represented by several data points in single-case research. This performance may comprise 20 or more data points across different conditions. The data are examined within and across successive conditions, much as our own behavior may be examined in a classroom or job. Researchers seek not to minimize variability but to examine why it occurs. Therefore, despite similarities between single-case and quantitative designs, significant differences exist as well.

Single-case designs are considered experimental because they can control for threats to internal validity and can be readily applied in settings in which group designs are difficult to implement. Thus, they have advantages over other methodologies. Teachers and practitioners should be clear about how to implement single-case designs in their classrooms/settings when they wish to determine the effects of instruction or management techniques. These single-case designs can be easily incorporated into ongoing activities in the form of *action research* (see Chapter 16). That is, teachers and practitioners can begin to generate their own data to guide their teaching/intervention methods rather than rely solely on the research community to supply them with answers. In a sense, single-case designs allow individuals to

---

Research Example

Consider this issue. Think about how you would design research to address the question/hypothesis from this research example:

- Research Example: To what extent will a multicomponent cognitive-behavioral intervention decrease challenging behavior and increase work completed by two 6-year-old children with traumatic brain injury?

A research example appears near the end of the chapter.

---

become scientists/practitioners. Additionally, as with other designs, critical research consumers must be able to understand what researchers do and why they do it before they can understand and apply what they read in the research literature. The designs discussed in this chapter include A-B, A-B-A, A-B-A-B, B-A-B, and A-B-C-B designs. (*Note.* The terms *withdrawal design* and *A-B-A design* are used interchangeably.)

Throughout this chapter, several types of single-case designs are presented. This chapter focuses on withdrawal and associated designs. First, graphing issues are highlighted. Since a visual analysis is crucial in withdrawal and associated designs, critical research consumers must have a high level of skill in interpreting graphs. Second, the withdrawal concept is described, along with the following associated designs: A-B, A-B-A-B, B-A-B, and A-B-C-B designs. The methods of analyzing the data follow the discussion of the different designs. Finally, research examples highlighting the different designs are presented throughout the chapter, and an illustrative investigation is included at the end of the chapter for critique. (*Note.* You should attempt to analyze the graphs presented from the research examples.)

WHAT ARE GRAPHING METHODS IN WITHDRAWAL DESIGNS?

Since this is the introductory chapter in single-case methodology, it is appropriate to discuss briefly the information contained in a graph representing performance of a participant. Single-case researchers primarily use graphs and visual analysis to demonstrate intervention (or treatment) effects. Thus, understanding how graphs are constructed is critical. Figure 11.1 shows a line graph, the most commonly used system to display data. The vertical axis (also called the y axis, or ordinate) provides a brief description of the dependent measure. The dependent measure is an indication of how we measure the dependent variable. For example, if we were teaching reading, reading comprehension might be the dependent variable. Percentage of questions answered correctly on a passage read would be the dependent measure. If we are studying this book for class, the dependent variable is probably knowledge gained in research methodology. The dependent measure might possibly be scores on tests over the material we read.

The horizontal axis (also called the x axis, or abscissa) indicates some measure of time.

For example, sessions, days, months, or trials can be measures of time passed. The term *sessions* is the most frequently used time measure in single-case research. A rule of thumb when constructing a graph is to use a ratio of vertical to horizontal axes of 1/1.6 to 1/2.2 (Tufte, 1983). In other words, if the horizontal axis is 4 inches in length, the vertical axis should be somewhere between 1.8 to 2.52 inches in length. According to Tufte, the horizontal axis should be the focus, not the vertical axis. If the vertical axis is as long or longer than the horizontal one, our attention may be focused on the wrong axis. Another reason for the ratios is that we should visually represent the data in such a manner that data items have good spacing and do not appear to be crowded.

Condition labels are located just above the graph. For example, the first condition may be "baseline" (described later) followed by the intervention. The intervention is called the independent variable. In a research methods

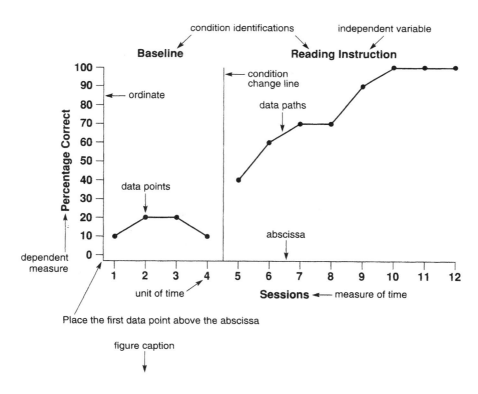

FIGURE 11.1. Line graph showing the percentage of questions answered correctly across baseline and reading instruction conditions.

class, the instruction we receive is the independent variable. Condition lines separate conditions. These lines indicate when the condition has changed. Notice in Figure 11.1 that the data points are not connected across the condition lines. The round points on the graph are the data points. These are placed on the graph by finding the time at which the data point was collected (e.g., Session 5) and the results of the measure (e.g., 50%). Data paths connect data points and help with visual analysis of the data. Trends are much easier to see if the points are connected. Finally, there is usually a figure caption under the graph. This is a summary of the figure and often lists the dependent measure and the independent variable.

Another frequently used graph is the bar graph or histogram. Figure 11.2 shows a bar graph with the same data as shown in Figure 11.1. The method of displaying the data differs across the two graphs.

WHAT ARE WITHDRAWAL AND ASSOCIATED DESIGNS?

A-B Design

When understanding single-case designs, we must learn the meaning of symbols. In single-case designs, "A" refers to baseline. A *baseline* is the repeated measurement of a behavior under natural conditions. It indicates the level at which the participant performs a behavior without the intervention. The baseline is of critical importance when considering single-case designs, since it is the best estimate of what would occur if the intervention were not applied. The baseline, then, provides a comparison to the intervention condition ("B"), the time that the independent variable is in effect. Therefore, an **A-B design** is a single-case design that combines the "A" (baseline or preintervention) condition with a "B" (intervention) condition to determine the effectiveness of an intervention.

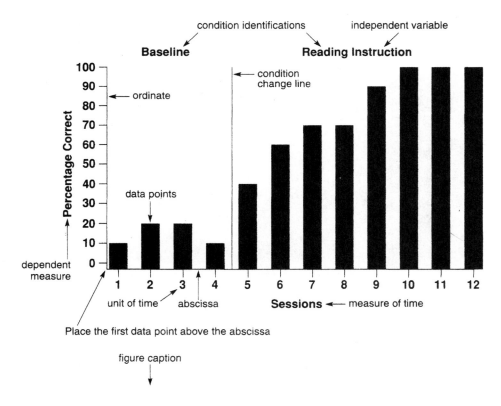

FIGURE 11.2. Bar graph showing the percentage of questions answered correctly across baseline and reading instruction conditions.

Typically, the "B" condition is used in isolation. In other words, a skill is usually taught and measured over a period of time. However, a "B" design is especially problematic, because it is not possible to indicate where the participant was before the intervention. Therefore, the comparison of assessments in "B" compared to "A" is crucial. Also, it is important to make sure that participants are not improving on their own, which would make the intervention unwarranted. Therefore, the A-B design combines the baseline or preintervention measurements with a "B" condition to determine the effectiveness of the intervention.

Figure 11.3 shows an A-B design. As can be seen, several assessments occur before the intervention, and several more occur during the intervention. Looking at the data in Figure 11.3, we can see that the intervention seems to be effective, because the frequency of fighting has decreased with the introduction of self-management. However, the major problem with A-B designs is that they fail to control for several threats to internal validity. For example, history is a critical concern, because something may have occurred during the intervention that improved the participant's performance. For this reason, the A-B design is considered to be a quasi-experimental design (Campbell & Stanley, 1963); it does not permit a complete examination of the effects of the independent variable on the dependent variable while ruling out the effects of extraneous variables. As noted by Cooper et al. (2007), an A-B comparison of a single subject's behavior does not verify levels of continued responding (i.e., stable response rate, as if an intervention had not been implemented), nor does it replicate the effects of an intervention. A more convincing demonstration of the functional relationship between variables is needed.

Withdrawal Design

The elaboration of the A-B design is the withdrawal (A-B-A) design. To verify the effects of the intervention ("B"), researchers usually withdraw the intervention to determine whether behavior returns to baseline ("A") levels. The withdrawal, or A-B-A, design is a single-case design that combines the "A" condition

(baseline/preintervention) with a "B" condition (an intervention) to determine the effectiveness of the intervention. The "B" condition is followed by a second "A" condition (baseline). The A-B-A design has been called both a withdrawal design and a reversal design (Barlow et al., 2008). However, technically, it is probably more appropriate to label the design as withdrawal rather than reversal (i.e., the reversal design may signify an active attempt on the part of the researcher to change the level of participant behavior during the "B" condition, such as reinforcing behavior that is the opposite of the desired one, rather than simply removing the intervention [Barlow et al., 2008]; see Chapter 13 for a discussion of how a reversal design can be combined with a changing criterion design to increase experimental control).

In the withdrawal design, a methodologically powerful tool in allowing for the control of threats to internal validity (Kazdin, 2003), the baseline is the first condition, followed by the intervention, followed by a return to baseline. The logic behind the withdrawal design is compelling: if a behavior changed during the "B" condition, then returned to the first baseline level during the second baseline condition, the intervention was shown to be effective. In this way, a functional relationship between the intervention and the behavior can be shown. Data in Figure 11.4 indicate a functional relationship using a withdrawal design; remember that a *functional relationship* means that when a change is produced (by the intervention) it is reliably followed by changes in the dependent variable. Of course, if the behavior had not returned to baseline levels on implementation of the second baseline, a functional relationship would not have been demonstrated.

If data were gathered as shown in Figure 11.4, the threats to internal validity would be minimized, because it is unlikely that something occurred at the precise time of the presentation of the intervention to cause an increase in the behavior, and at the precise instance of the removal of the intervention to cause a decrease

---

An **A-B design** combines the "A" condition with a "B" condition to determine the effectiveness of an intervention.

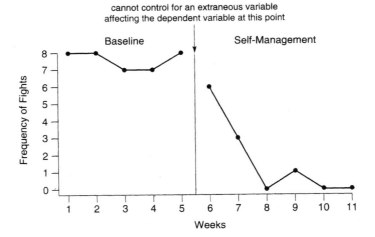

FIGURE 11.3. The frequency of fights across baseline and self-management conditions. From Martella, R. C., Nelson, J. R., Marchand-Martella, N., & O'Reilly, M. (2012). *Comprehensive behavior management: Individualized, classroom, and schoolwide approaches* (2nd ed.). Thousand Oaks, CA: Sage. Copyright 2012 by Sage Publications, Inc. Reprinted by permission of SAGE.

in the behavior. However, according to Cooper et al. (2007), the introduction and withdrawal of the intervention may coincide with natural cyclical variations of the dependent variable. This possibility is remote and can be controlled by changing the length of time a participant is

in the "B" condition and/or the second "A" condition.

The withdrawal design can be used to test the effects of interventions aimed at increasing or decreasing behaviors. As can be seen, the withdrawal design has a great deal of flexibility

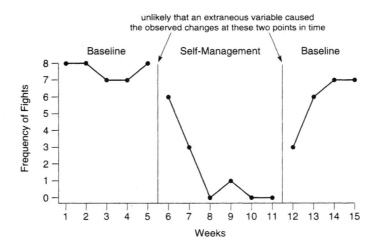

FIGURE 11.4. The frequency of fights across baseline and self-management conditions. From Martella, R. C., Nelson, J. R., Marchand-Martella, N., & O'Reilly, M. (2012). *Comprehensive behavior management: Individualized, classroom, and schoolwide approaches* (2nd ed.). Thousand Oaks, CA: Sage. Copyright 2012 by Sage Publications, Inc. Reprinted by permission of SAGE.

over a group design, in that a smaller number of participants is required, ongoing data collection is involved, and the design can be used readily in applied settings. However, the withdrawal design has a serious weakness with regard to the ethicality of leaving participants in the "A" condition. It is unlikely that researchers would be allowed to end the study without showing some final improvement. Thus, an extension of the withdrawal design is frequently applied.

A-B-A-B Design

The **A-B-A-B design** combines the "A" condition (baseline/preintervention) with a "B" condition (intervention), returns to a second baseline "A" condition, then ends with a return to the "B" intervention. The A-B-A-B design is similar to the withdrawal design in that the first three conditions (i.e., A-B-A) refer to the same activities on the part of the researcher. In fact, the A-B-A-B design may be called a withdrawal design by researchers. The difference is the final "B" condition in the A-B-A-B design. Researchers in this design end with an intervention rather than a withdrawal of treatment. The advantage of doing this is evident—the ethical problem of leaving the participant(s) without an intervention is avoided. Figure 11.5 shows data for an A-B-A-B design. Again, as in Figure 11.4, a functional relationship between the intervention and the behavior is demonstrated. In fact, the functional relationship is replicated—the second intervention (the second "B" condition) is shown to decrease fighting behavior a second time.

B-A-B Design

One potential problem with the withdrawal and A-B-A-B designs is that the initial sessions of data collection occur during a time when no intervention is present. There may be times when a participant's behavior is so severe that researchers cannot wait until enough data have been gathered to complete a baseline (Kazdin, 2003). Additionally, a **B-A-B design** may be utilized if there is an obvious lack of behavior, because the participant may have never exhibited the behavior in the past; thus, a preintervention baseline would essentially serve no

useful purpose (Kazdin, 2003). For example, if the dependent variable is to approach others and begin with a social behavior such as saying "Excuse me," and the participant had never exhibited the behavior, starting with a baseline may simply waste time. Finally, a B-A-B design may be used in applied situations where an intervention is ongoing and researchers wish to establish a functional relationship between the intervention and the dependent variable. The B-A-B design starts with the "B" condition (intervention) followed by an "A" condition (baseline), then ends with a second "B" condition.

Researchers have used the B-A-B design with much success. As with the previously discussed designs, the "B" condition refers to an intervention and the "A" condition refers to a removal of the intervention. Figure 11.6 provides data for a B-A-B design.

A-B-C-B Design

The **A-B-C-B design** is a further modification of the withdrawal design. The "A" and "B" conditions are the same as in the previous designs. The "C" condition is an addition. The "C" in this design refers to an additional intervention (i.e., one that is a variation of the first intervention in the "B" condition). In the first two conditions, the baseline and intervention data are collected. During the "C" condition, the intervention is changed to allow for the control of extra attention a participant may have received during the "B" condition. In summary, the A-B-C-B design combines the "A" condition (baseline/preintervention) with a "B" condition (intervention);

An **A-B-A-B design** *combines the "A" condition with a "B" condition, returns to a second "A" condition, then ends with a return to the "B" condition.*

A **B-A-B design** *starts with the "B" condition followed by an "A" condition, then ends with a second "B" condition.*

An **A-B-C-B design** *combines the "A" condition with a "B" condition; the first two conditions are followed by a "C" condition to allow for the control of extra attention a participant may have received during the "B" condition.*

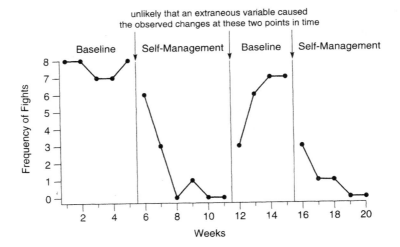

FIGURE 11.5. The frequency of fights across baseline and self-management conditions.

the first two conditions are followed by a "C" condition (a new intervention) to allow for the control of extra attention a participant may have received during the "B" condition.

For example, if a researcher were testing the effects of *contingent reinforcement* (i.e., reinforcement that is delivered only when a participant responds in a certain manner), a control for the attention may be warranted. We could safely argue that the contingent reinforcement may not be responsible for the measured effects, but that

the attention received via the contingent reinforcement is responsible. An analogous example of this problem is seen in drug studies in which there is a placebo concern. Was the drug responsible for the measured effects, or were the effects due to the reception of a pill and the expectation of results? Thus, the "C" condition serves as a type of placebo. In the example of contingent reinforcement ("B" condition), the "C" condition could be *noncontingent reinforcement* (i.e., reinforcement that is applied regardless of how

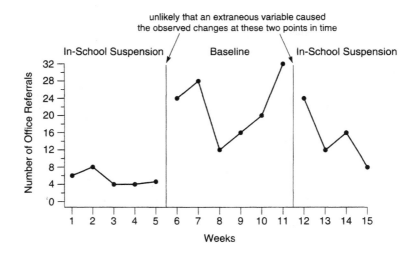

FIGURE 11.6. The number of office referrals across in-school suspension and baseline conditions.

the participant responds). Thus, if data are gathered as shown in Figure 11.7, a conclusion can be made that contingent praise is more critical for improved performance than mere increases in praise provided to the student.

Analysis of Data

Possibly the most important part of understanding withdrawal and associated designs is to understand how to analyze the data. The design, data, and presentation of the data help to control for threats to the internal validity of the investigation. Withdrawal designs present data in such a manner that a visual analysis can help critical research consumers determine whether these threats are present. To understand how to analyze the data in withdrawal and associated designs, it is critical to understand appropriate ways of displaying the data. Visual analysis is described below. (*Note.* There are statistical techniques that aid in the analysis of data; however, visual inspection is the primary method of analyzing data in withdrawal and associated designs. A description of the use of statistics is beyond the scope of this text; however, the reader is referred to Gast (2010) for information on the issue. Additionally, two critical concerns are present when analyzing the data—we must

consider the internal validity and the external validity of the investigation.

Internal Validity

When assessing the internal validity of the withdrawal and associated designs, several concerns must be taken into consideration: the condition length (including the trend of the data), changing one variable at a time, the level and rapidity of change, and whether the behavior returns to baseline levels. Table 11.3 summarizes the major threats to internal validity of the designs discussed in this chapter.

Condition Length. The *condition length* refers to how long a condition is in effect. The condition length is essentially the number of data points gathered during a condition. This number depends on a critical factor called variability. In general, researchers should see at least three stable data points or three data points moving in a countertherapeutic direction (i.e., movement in the direction opposite what is ultimately desired). Three is the minimum number of data points needed to indicate a trend. Thus, if researchers have three stable data points at the start of baseline, then three data points are all that is required. However, the more variability

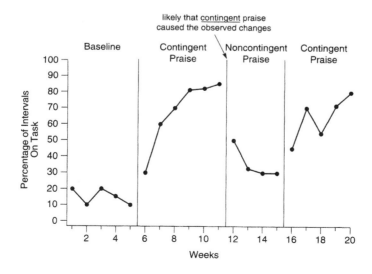

FIGURE 11.7. The percentage of intervals on-task across baseline, contingent praise, and noncontingent praise conditions.

TABLE 11.3. Threats to Internal Validity Associated with Each of the Withdrawal and Associated Designs

Threat	A-B design	A-B-A design	A-B-A-B design	B-A-B design	A-B-C-B design
1. Maturation	Possible concern	Controlled	Controlled	Controlled	Controlled
2. Selection	Not applicable	Not applicable	Not applicable	Not applicable	Not applicable
3. Selection by maturation interaction	Not applicable	Not applicable	Not applicable	Not applicable	Not applicable
4. Statistical regression	Possible concern	Controlled	Controlled	Controlled	Controlled
5. Mortality	Controlled	Controlled	Controlled	Controlled	Controlled
6. Instrumentation	Controlled	Controlled	Controlled	Controlled	Controlled
7. Testing	Controlled	Controlled	Controlled	Controlled	Controlled
8. History	Possible concern	Controlled	Controlled	Controlled	Controlled
9. Resentful demoralization of the control group	Not applicable	Not applicable	Not applicable	Not applicable	Not applicable
10. Diffusion of treatment	Not applicable	Controlled	Controlled	Controlled	Controlled
11. Compensatory rivalry by the control group	Not applicable	Not applicable	Not applicable	Not applicable	Not applicable
12. Compensatory equalization	Not applicable	Not applicable	Not applicable	Not applicable	Not applicable

Note. This table is meant only as a general guideline. Decisions with regard to threats to internal validity must be made after the specifics of an investigation are known and understood. Thus, interpretations of internal validity threats must be made on a study-by-study basis.

in the data, or if the data are moving in the ultimate desired direction, the more data points are needed. As shown in Figure 11.8(a), the data are relatively stable. There are three data points, all within a narrow range. Figure 11.8(b) shows data moving in a countertherapeutic direction, which indicates that the condition length is suitable. Figure 11.8(c) demonstrates how variable data may lengthen the condition. At the most, there are two data points moving in a countertherapeutic direction. However, the requirement is a minimum of three data points; thus, researchers must stay in the condition for a longer period of time. Figure 11.8(d) shows data moving in a therapeutic direction. If the condition were ended and the intervention started, a conclusion as to the effects of the intervention could not be made.

Of course, in the applied world, it may be difficult to achieve three stable data points or

three data points moving in a countertherapeutic trend. There may be practical problems, such as a need to get on with the intervention due to a shortage of time, or an ethical problem, such as the presence of dangerous behavior. When reading and analyzing a study, critical research consumers must always be aware of the difficulties associated with applied research. The decision as to whether the lack of stability in the data damages the integrity of the study ultimately must rest with critical research consumers. They must decide whether the researchers took the lack of stability into consideration when making claims and conclusions based on the data.

Changing One Variable at a Time. One of the most critical rules in single-case research is to change only one variable at a time when moving from one condition to the other. For example, suppose a researcher wanted to measure the

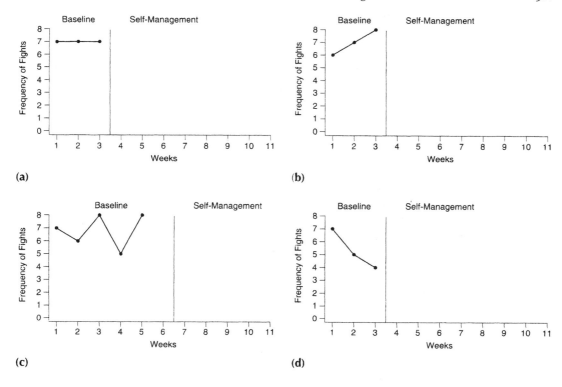

FIGURE 11.8. (a) Stable baseline; may begin instruction. (b) Data moving in a countertherapeutic direction; may begin instruction. (c) Variable data; should not begin instruction. (d) Data moving in therapeutic direction; should not begin instruction.

effects on high school students of taking notes and studying the material from science textbooks. The researcher collects several baseline data points, then introduces the students to the intervention (a note-taking strategy). After students learn to use this strategy, the researcher removes the intervention and tells students to go back to their old ways of taking notes and studying. In this case, the researcher is studying the effects of an intervention package compared to no intervention. The researcher is clearly using a withdrawal design. The researcher has also changed one variable at a time—presenting the intervention then removing the intervention. This example does not pose any problems. An assessment of the intervention package can be made, and presumably, if effective, the intervention will be reinstated.

Now suppose the researcher wanted to continue this line of research and decided to assess the combination of both procedures—note-taking strategies, or "B," and study strategies, or "C," compared to note-taking strategies ("B") in isolation. First, a baseline is conducted, followed by the intervention package (now referred to as "BC," signifying the two procedures). After the "BC" condition, a return to baseline is conducted. Next, the researcher implements the note-taking strategy ("B") in isolation. Essentially, the researcher has developed an A-BC-A-B design. The "B" condition provides us with some information. Unfortunately, the only thing the researcher can conclude in this experiment is that the "BC" condition was or was not effective (depending on the data). Note that the "BC" condition is surrounded by "A" conditions. Thus, this is the only comparison that can be made. The "B" condition is not surrounded by anything; essentially what the researcher has is an A-B design, with previous exposure to the intervention package confounding any conclusions. The second "A" condition is surrounded by the "BC" and "B" conditions, which is meaningless. Thus, the researcher put a great deal of time and effort into the study and ended up not answering the research question.

If the researcher wished to question the contributions of each component of the intervention package compared to using strategies in isolation, a variation of the withdrawal design would be required. Pay particular attention to the following design and notice how only one variable is changed—A-BC-A-BC-B-BC. Looking at the first example, the effects of the "BC" condition can be analyzed, since it is surrounded by the "A" conditions. The effects of the "B" condition can be analyzed as to its contribution to the packet, since it is surrounded by the "BC" conditions. Notice that the A-BC-B portion of the design does not provide the researcher with any meaningful information, since two variables were changed from the second "A" and "BC" conditions to the "B" condition.

Thus, when analyzing a withdrawal design or many of its variants, it is critical to determine whether only one variable was changed at a time. If this is not the case, the researcher's conclusions are most likely erroneous. Finally, be aware that the question asked by the researcher is of critical concern. If the question deals only with the intervention package, the conclusion must be based on only the intervention package, and not on the relative contributions of the package, unless an acceptable design is used.

Level and Rapidity of Change. *Level and rapidity of change* refers to the magnitude with which the data change at the time of the implementation or removal of the independent variable. Figure 11.9(a) indicates that the baseline has stability. Upon implementation of the independent variable, the participant's level of fighting does not change for a period of four sessions. This is not a convincing demonstration of experimental control. If the independent variable were effective, we would assume that the participant's behavior would change in a more timely fashion. Of course, the independent variable may have been effective but not of sufficient strength to cause an immediate change. The behavior may have been resistant to change as well. Whatever the explanation, the demonstration of experimental control is seriously weakened.

Figure 11.9(b) indicates that there was a change in the dependent variable, but the initial change was of small magnitude. Figure 11.9(c) indicates that there was a large magnitude change when the independent variable was implemented. This demonstration is much stronger than the other two. We would be more inclined to accept an argument of the effectiveness of the independent variable in this case than in the other two.

Return to Baseline Levels. When returning to baseline in Figure 11.9(d), we see that there was not a rapid change. This lack of immediate return to baseline levels detracts from the experimental control of the investigation. Essentially, we have an A-B design, since something may have occurred at the time the self-monitoring intervention was applied. The fact that the behavior did not return to baseline levels makes it probable that an extraneous variable caused the observed effects. On the other hand, Figure 11.9(e) indicates that the change was abrupt, with a return to near baseline levels. This demonstration indicates that the independent variable was likely responsible for the changes in the dependent variable.

External Validity

A major concern of single-case designs in general is external validity, because effects of an independent variable are demonstrated on such a small number of participants. Many quantitative researchers view the external validity of withdrawal designs as lacking. Thus, claims as to generalizability of the designs is said to be limited. However, single-case researchers view external validity somewhat differently than many do quantitative researchers. Single-case researchers agree that external validity is lacking with a single study; however, they take the position that one study represents isolated data and should be replicated. In other words, *any* study, whether single-case or quantitative designs are used, has a lack of external validity. This lack of validity can be viewed in degrees. Isolated data should never be thought of as valid; it is combining the data that takes on importance. Thus, withdrawal designs in isolation have the same external validity problems as quantitative designs.

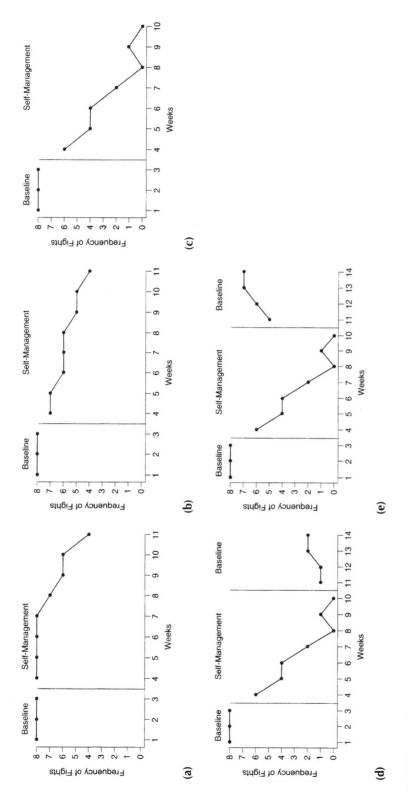

FIGURE 11.9. (a) Lack of immediate change; weak experimental control. (b) Small immediate change; better experimental control. (c) Large immediate change; better experimental control, but still weak. (c) Large immediate change; stronger experimental control. (d) Immediate change; stronger experimental control. However, there was a lack of return to near baseline levels weakening the experimental control. (e) Immediate change; stronger experimental control. Additionally, there was a return to near the baseline level adding to the experimental control.

383

Single-case researchers attempt to increase the external validity of withdrawal designs by conducting replications of the study (discussed in Chapter 1). Withdrawal designs have limited external validity; however, the lack of external validity is due to isolated data rather than the number of participants in the experiment. The experiment simply needs systematic and ongoing replication. Single-case researchers view external validity as including more than generalization across participants. Being able to generalize across settings or ecological validity is also critical. Table 11.4 summarizes the major threats to external validity of the designs discussed in this chapter.

> *Recall the research question about a multicomponent intervention posed earlier in this chapter? Read on to see how your design compares to how the actual study was designed.*

Research Example: A-B-A-B Design

Researchers (Feeney & Ylvisaker, 2008) used an A-B-A-B design to investigate the effects of a multicomponent cognitive-behavioral intervention on changing behaviors of two 6-year-old

TABLE 11.4. Threats to External Validity Associates with Each of the Withdrawal and Associated Designs

Threat	A-B design	A-B-A design	A-B-A-B design	B-A-B design	A-B-C-B design
1. Generalization across participants	Possible concern	Possible concern	Possible concern	Possible concern	Possible concern
2. Interaction of personological variables and treatment effects	Possible concern	Possible concern	Possible concern	Possible concern	Possible concern
3. Verification of independent variable	Possible concern	Possible concern	Possible concern	Possible concern	Possible concern
4. Multiple treatment interference	Controlled	Controlled	Controlled	Controlled	Controlled
5. Novelty and disruption effects	Possible concern	Possible concern	Possible concern	Possible concern	Possible concern
6. Hawthorne effect	Possible concern	Possible concern	Possible concern	Possible concern	Possible concern
7. Experimenter effects	Possible concern	Possible concern	Possible concern	Possible concern	Possible concern
8. Pretest sensitization	Not applicable	Not applicable	Not applicable	Not applicable	Not applicable
9. Posttest sensitization	Not applicable	Not applicable	Not applicable	Not applicable	Not applicable
10. Interaction of time of measurement and treatment effects	Possible concern	Possible concern	Possible concern	Possible concern	Possible concern
11. Measurement of the dependent variable	Possible concern	Possible concern	Possible concern	Possible concern	Possible concern
12. Interaction of history and treatment effects	Possible concern	Possible concern	Possible concern	Possible concern	Possible concern

Note. This table is meant only as a general guideline. Decisions with regard to threats to external validity must be made after the specifics of an investigation are known and understood. Thus, interpretations of external validity threats must be made on a study-by-study basis.

children with traumatic brain injury (TBI). Previous research has shown that TBI is often associated with challenging behavior and that the behavior worsens over time if left untreated (Anderson, Damasio, Tranel, & Damasio, 2000). Both children had experienced severe bilateral frontal lobe damage. They were in a blended kindergarten–first-grade classroom. When given high-demand academic work, Ben would become physically aggressive against his teacher or other educational staff. Challenging behavior for Joe included physical assault and refusal to complete tasks. Dependent measures were frequency and intensity of challenging behavior, and the percentage of problems completed correctly. In Baseline ("A"), the teacher provided time for independent seatwork to complete assignments as usual. The Intervention Condition ("B") was referred to in this study as the Concrete Routine Condition, which consisted of negotiation, easy tasks intermixed with hard tasks, demonstration of computation procedures, and communication skills training. After the Concrete Routine Condition ("B"), researchers returned to Baseline (the second "A" condition), followed by a second Concrete Routine Condition (the second "B" condition). Figure 11.10 presents three panels showing Ben's behavior. The top panel shows that in first Baseline Condition, Ben engaged in high levels of challenging behavior. In the Concrete Routine Condition, challenging behavior immediately dropped and remained low. In the second Baseline Condition (return to "A" condition), challenging behavior increased to baseline levels. Upon return to the Concrete Routine Condition (the second "B" condition), challenging behavior again decreased. The second panel shows that the cognitive-behavior intervention was less pronounced on intensity, because only minor decreases are apparent in the Concrete Routine Conditions. The third panel shows that in both Concrete Routine Conditions, Ben's percentage of work completed increased to 95–100%. Figure 11.11 presents three panels showing Joe's behavior. Effects were similar to those shown with Ben. Intensity of challenging behavior decreased more markedly for Joe than for Ben. Researchers described limitations of this study, including the lack of information on which components accounted for intervention effects.

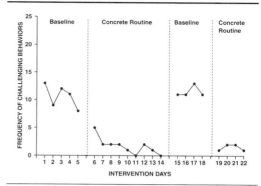

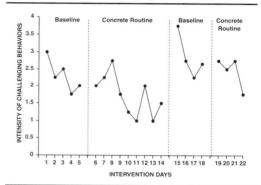

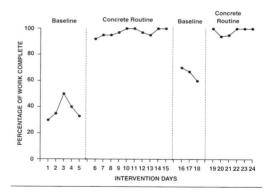

FIGURE 11.10. Frequency and intensity of challenging behavior, and percentage of work completed for Ben. From Feeney, T. J., & Ylvisaker, M. (2008). Context-sensitive cognitive-behavior supports for young children with TBI: A second replication study. *Journal of Positive Behavior Interventions, 10,* 115–128. Copyright 2008 by the Hammill Institute on Disabilities. Reprinted by permission of SAGE.

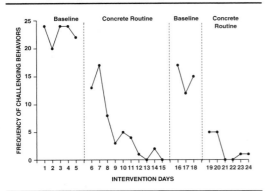

Frequency of Challenging Behavior: Joe

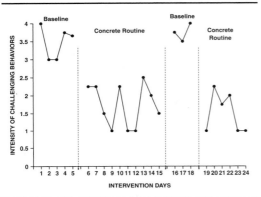

Intensity of Challenging Behavior: Joe

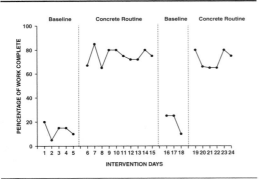

Percentage of Work Completed: Joe

FIGURE 11.11. Frequency and intensity of challenging behavior, and percentage of work completed for Joe. From Feeney, T. J., & Ylvisaker, M. (2008). Context-sensitive cognitive-behavior supports for young children with TBI: A second replication study. *Journal of Positive Behavior Interventions, 10,* 115–128. Copyright 2008 by the Hammill Institute on Disabilities. Reprinted by permission of SAGE.

WHEN SHOULD RESEARCHERS USE EACH WITHDRAWAL AND ASSOCIATED DESIGN?

Researchers must always consider what the research question is and how best to answer it. The type of research design selected is critical in the decision-making process. Researchers must consider several options before a study is initiated. For example, the first concern is whether a qualitative design is best to use, or whether a single-case design is more appropriate. If, after considering the options, researchers select a single-case design, the type of single-case design must be considered. The A-B design is usually most appropriate for practitioners not necessarily concerned with scientific rigor. However, researchers may consider the A-B design if they wish to cast doubt on theoretical assumptions, refine techniques, or provide clinical and applied examples (Barlow et al., 2008; Cooper et al., 2007).

The A-B design should not be selected if researchers want to demonstrate a functional rather than correlational relationship between the independent variable and the dependent variable. In other words, the A-B design does not control for threats to internal validity. If researchers wish to control for internal validity threats, the A-B design is not a suitable choice. However, many times researchers may not have much of an option. For example, suppose a researcher planned to use a withdrawal design and the participant was unable or unwilling to continue in the study after the "B" condition. The researcher would then have to settle for an A-B design.

If researchers wished to control for the internal validity threats, the withdrawal design is appropriate. However, according to Gast (2010), researchers rarely select the withdrawal design before beginning a study. One reason for this is that practitioners may not allow for the withdrawal of the intervention. Consider for a moment dealing with a severely disruptive student in the classroom. A researcher enters and takes baseline data, then implements a management program. You notice the student's behavior improving when the researcher informs you that the intervention will be pulled, with the expectation that the disruptive behavior will return. Your reaction would most likely be to tell the researcher that you are pleased with the results and he can go. Although researchers are usually aware that the improvement seen in the initial "B" condition will likely return if there exists a functional relationship and if a second "B" condition is added, the reality is that many practitioners are wary of a withdrawal of the intervention. Researchers may propose the A-B-A-B design to avoid ending on the "A" condition but, again, a return to baseline is required.

A second problem is that the withdrawal and associated designs (i.e., A-B-A-B and B-A-B designs) require a return to baseline levels. Thus, if we were working with a skills acquisition program, a return to baseline would not be expected (at least not initially). For example, suppose a researcher was teaching students a math problem-solving technique. During baseline, the students were less than proficient in performing the required operations. During the intervention, the students' problem-solving skills improve to near 100% levels. Then, the researcher withdraws the intervention in the hope that students' skills will return to the

less than proficient levels. However, with skills recently learned, it is unlikely that students will forget what was learned immediately after the intervention is pulled. Most likely, the students will maintain the skills for some time after the withdrawal of the intervention. If this occurs, the researcher is left with essentially an A-B design. There would be numerous threats to the internal validity of the study. Thus, if a researcher wished to study a skills acquisition intervention, the A-B-A design, or variations of the A-B-A design, would be inappropriate. Alternative designs presented in Chapter 13 overcome the problem of an inability to return to baseline levels.

As stated previously, the A-B-C-B design can be used when there is a concern about the effects of the independent variable being due to the intended intervention or to some intended side effect of the intervention, such as increased attention. However, researchers run the same risks associated with the withdrawal and associated designs.

SUMMARY

❖ Single-case research, a type of research investigation that relies on the intensive investigation of a single individual or a group of individuals, uses objective data collection techniques. Single-case research may be thought of as a combination of qualitative and quantitative designs. It is similar to qualitative research in four main ways: (1) Single-case research is usually conducted in natural settings and the researcher/observer is the key measurement instrument; (2) single-case researchers are concerned with the "process" of skills acquisition rather than the final outcome of an intervention; (3) single-case researchers ask research questions and consider the process to be inductive in nature; and (4) single-case designs develop during the investigation; thus, single-case designs are flexible.

❖ There are three major differences between single-case and qualitative methodologies: (1) Single-case researchers attempt to minimize subjectivity in their collection of data; (2) single-case data are quantified; and (3) most single-case data are quantified; and (3) most single-case

researchers try to avoid making inferences of internal cognitive processes and report only on observable and measurable behaviors.

❖ Single-case researchers primarily use graphs and visual analysis to demonstrate intervention (or treatment) effects. The line graph, the most commonly used system to display data, has four general aspects: (1) The vertical axis (also called the y axis, or ordinate) provides a brief description of the dependent measure; (2) the horizontal axis (also called the x axis, or abscissa) indicates some measure of time; the term *sessions* is the most frequently used time measure in single-case research; (3) conditional labels are located just above the graph; these conditions are separated by condition lines; and (4) a figure caption is usually located under the graph. Another frequently used graph is the bar graph, or histogram.

❖ In single-case designs, "A" refers to baseline or the behavior under natural conditions. The "A" condition provides a comparison to the intervention condition ("B").

❖ An A-B design combines the "A" (baseline or preintervention) condition with a "B" (intervention) condition to determine the effectiveness of an intervention. However, the problem is that this type of design fails to control for several threats to internal validity.

❖ The withdrawal, or A-B-A design, combines the "A" condition measurements with a "B" condition to determine the effectiveness of the intervention. The "B" condition is followed by a second "A" condition. The withdrawal design has a serious weakness with regard to the ethicality of leaving participants in the "A" condition. Thus, an extension of the withdrawal design is frequently applied.

❖ The A-B-A-B design ends with a return to intervention ("B"). There may be times when a participant's behavior is so severe that researchers cannot wait until enough data have been gathered to complete a baseline.

❖ The A-B-C-B design combines the "A" condition measurements with a "B" condition; the first two conditions are followed by a "C" condition (a new intervention) to allow for the control of extra attention a participant may have received during the "B" condition.

❖ Four concerns are present in the withdrawal and associated designs: (1) condition length (including the trend of the data), (2) changing one variable at a time, (3) level and rapidity of change, and (4) whether the behavior returns to baseline levels. Single-case researchers attempt to increase the external validity of withdrawal designs by conducting replications of the study.

❖ The A-B design is usually most appropriate for practitioners not necessarily concerned with scientific rigor. However, researchers may consider the A-B design if they wish to cast doubt on theoretical assumptions, refine techniques, or provide clinical and applied example. If researchers wish to control for the internal validity threats, then withdrawal design is appropriate. The A-B-C-B design can be used when there is concern about the effects of the independent variable being due to the intended intervention or to some intended side effect of the intervention, such as increased attention.

DISCUSSION QUESTIONS

1. How can single-case research methods be considered a combination of quantitative and qualitative methods? In your answer, explain how single-case methods are similar and dissimilar to quantitative and qualitative research methods.

2. How can an A-B design be used to provide preliminary information on the effectiveness of self-control strategies for a student with behavior problems? Provide a graph, with data showing that the self-control instruction seemed to have an effect.

3. How would the data in Question 2 look differently in a bar graph? How does the type of graph affect your interpretations, if at all?

4. What are the advantages of taking baseline data before instruction is implemented in an A-B design format?

5. Can an A-B-A design be used to determine the effectiveness of a behavior intervention? What are two potential ethical problems with such a design?

6. What design would help to avoid the problem of ending on a baseline condition when using an A-B-A design?

7. What is a problem encountered with external validity when using A-B-A designs? What is a solution to this problem?

8. Under what condition would a researcher select a B-A-B design over an A-B-A design?

9. What is a purpose of the A-B-C-B design? What conditions are compared in this design that allow for internal validity claims?

10. What is meant by each of the following when looking at withdrawal and associated designs? Explain.
    a. condition length
    b. change one variable at a time
    c. level and rapidity of change
    d. return to baseline levels

Effects of Response Cards on Disruptive Behavior and Academic Responding during Math Lessons by Fourth-Grade Urban Students

Michael Charles Lambert
Western Washington University

Gwendolyn Cartledge
William L. Heward
Ohio State University

Ya-yu Lo
University of North Carolina at Charlotte

Abstract: The authors evaluated the effects of response cards on the disruptive behavior and academic responding of students in two urban fourth-grade classrooms. Two conditions, single-student responding and write-on response cards, were alternated in an ABAB design. During single-student responding, the teacher called on one student who had raised his or her hand to answer the question. During the response-card condition, each student was provided with a white laminated board on which he or she could write a response to every question posed by the teacher. Nine students were targeted for data collection because of their history of disciplinary issues in school and frequent disruptive behavior in the classroom. Data revealed substantial reductions in disruptive behavior and increases in academic responding during the response card condition compared to single-student responding. The findings are discussed in terms of the beneficial effects of direct, high-response strategies for urban, low-achieving learners.

Consistently over the last 20 years, teachers, especially those new to the field, have reported behavior problems as one of their greatest school-related concerns and challenges (Billingsley, 2001; Billingsley & Tomchin, 1992; Darling-Hammond, 2003; Fimian & Santoro, 1983; Muscott, 1987; Pullis, 1992; Veenman, 1984). Spending classroom time managing students' behavior has a negative impact not only on teacher satisfaction and retention but also on students' academic performance. Many students who have chronic behavior problems in the classroom are significantly behind their peers academically, and the lack of instruction further accelerates the discrepancies (Coleman & Vaughn, 2000). This is especially challenging in urban schools, where even less classroom time is spent in academic instruction than in suburban schools

(Greenwood, Arreaga-Mayer, & Carta, 1994; Hart & Risley, 1995), but considerable attention is given to managing student's problem behaviors, using ineffective management strategies (Billingsley & Tomchin, 1992; Pullis, 1992).

Authorities on behavior management often point to the value of effective instruction as a means of reducing negative behavior in the classroom. Engelmann and Colvin (1983), for example, commented that students with behavior problems often are not appropriately placed in the curriculum. Acting-out, for many students, may be an effective means of escaping the academic demands of the classroom. Through careful planning and effective implementation of instructional strategies, teachers usually can eliminate as much as 90% of behavior problems that occur in their classrooms (Engelmann & Colvin, 1983). Many studies have confirmed this contention by showing that instructional techniques that promote high levels of student responding resulted in positive on-task behaviors and reduced classroom disruptions (e.g., Bullara, 1994; Carnine, 1976; Gardner, Heward, & Grossi, 1994; Heward, 1994; Lo & Cartledge, 2004b; Maheady, Michielli-Pendl, Mallette, & Harper, 2002; Sainato, Strain, & Lyon, 1987).

A particularly attractive feature of response cards is the power of peer involvement. Low-achieving students are not likely to be motivated solely by the academic content. Total class involvement, however, where students are responding enthusiastically, energetically, and rapidly, can be infectious, allowing reluctant learners to participate without feeling embarrassed in front of their peers. The use of response cards, enabling everyone in the class to participate, offers this unique benefit.

The use of response cards is one intervention with some preliminarily empirical evidence of decreasing off-task or disruptive behavior while increasing on-task behavior in the classroom. These responses occur in tandem with increased student responding and academic achievement compared to traditional whole-class lecture (e.g., Armendariz & Umbreit, 1999; Christle & Schuster, 2003; Gardner et al., 1994). Response cards are cards or signs simultaneously held up by all students in the class to display their response to a teacher-presented question or problem (Cavanaugh, Heward, & Donelson, 1996). Instead of calling on only one student to answer the question while the rest of the class sits quietly and listens, response cards enable all students in the class to participate in an active response to instruction. This allows students to be more attentive and less disruptive. However, available empirical studies showing the effects of response cards on problem classroom behavior are limited. Previous studies often relied on anecdotal observations rather than direct investigation for their conclusion as to the effects of active student responding on problem behavior in the classroom (Colvin, Greenberg, & Sherman, 1993).

Armendariz and Umbreit (1999) provided the first empirical examination of the effects of response cards on student disruptions. Response cards were used during math lessons with 22 bilingual third-grade students. The authors reported a considerable decrease in the mean percentage of intervals where students exhibited disruptive behavior during the response card condition compared to the conventional lecture/question-and-answer instruction (when only one student was called on to answer a question). All participating students had fewer occurrences of disruptive behavior during the use of response cards, with a mean reduction from 59% (the least decrease) to 100% (the greatest decrease) across the students.

Christle and Schuster (2003) evaluated the effects of response cards on student participation, academic performance, and on-task behavior of fourth-grade urban students during math instruction. Consistent with previous studies (Gardner et al., 1994; Kellum, Carr, & Dozier, 2001; Narayan, Heward, Gardner, Courson, & Omness, 1990), these authors found that the use of response cards increased active student responses as well as students' performance on weekly quizzes compared to the hand-raising (single-student responding) condition. In addition, the percentage of time on-task was higher during response cards than

during hand raising. These studies by Armendariz and Umbreit (1999) and Christle and Schuster (2003) provided promising preliminary results for using response cards to reduce disruptive behavior while improving student's time on-task.

The present study was designed to extend the findings of previous research on response cards by evaluating disruptive behavior as the primary dependent variable in addition to active student participation. The purpose of this study was to determine the effects of using response cards during math lessons in two urban fourth-grade classrooms on pupil disruptive behavior as well as the students' academic responding.

METHOD

Participants and Settings

This study was conducted in two fourth-grade general education classrooms during math lessons in a midwestern urban elementary school, preschool through fifth grade. Thirty-one students participated in this study (15 students in Classroom A and 16 students in Classroom B); however, only 9 students were targeted for data collection. The target students were nominated by the classroom teachers, who felt these students were the most disruptive, the least attentive during math lessons, and had the worst performance in math. The teachers' nominations were verified by the first author through three sessions of direct observations using the same observational procedures as in the experimental conditions, described later in this section. Of the nine target students, eight were African American and one was Caucasian. The students ranged in age from 9 years 4 months to 10 years 8 months (mean age = 9–10). All students received free or reduced-price lunch. Table 1 provides additional information on the target students.

In both classrooms, the classroom teacher provided all the instruction during the math periods with the exception of one training session where the first author taught the class the procedures for using the response cards. Students' seating was arranged in standard rows and columns, facing the chalkboard, in both classrooms. Both classroom teachers were Caucasian (male teacher in Classroom A and female teacher in Classroom B), certified in elementary education, and each had 2 years teaching experience in their current classrooms. This was the first teaching assignment for Teacher

TABLE 1. Demographic, Academic, and Prebaseline Disruption on the Target Students

Student	Gender	Age	Race	Math grade prior to study	Two-session prebaseline disruption (%)
Classroom A					
A1	F	9–7	AA	C–	75
A2	F	9–4	CA	B	80
A3	M	9–10	AA	D–	90
A4	M	9–4	AA	F	85
Classroom B					
B1	M	10–2	AA	D–	75
B2	F	10–1	AA	C–	55
B3	F	10–8	AA	F	65
B4	F	9–5	AA	D+	n/a
B5	M	10–1	AA	B	65

Note. AA = African American; CA = Caucasian.

A. Teacher B had previously taught for one-half year in a middle school. Both teachers participated in in-service training provided by the authors as one part of a larger year-long project on effective academic and behavioral interventions. However, neither of them had incorporated response cards into their lessons prior to this study.

Definitions and Measurement of Dependent Variables

Disruptive Behavior

Disruptive behavior was defined as one or more of the following: engaging in a conversation with others during teacher-directed instruction, provoking others (i.e., making faces at others, laughing at or touching others, making noises or sounds with voice, tapping objects, pounding on desk, voicing disapproval with instruction, throwing or twirling objects), attending to other stimuli (e.g., looking at or playing with other objects in desk or misusing response cards or other instructional tools), writing notes to friends or drawing pictures, spitting, sucking on fingers, or leaving assigned seat without permission (including tipping back in chair on two legs).

The first author served as the primary observer and sat at the back of the classroom when collecting data on the disruptive behavior. A partial interval recording procedure was employed to record disruptive behavior. Each target student was observed for 10 seconds, followed by 5 seconds of recording. A wristwatch was used to mark the 10-second observation periods for each interval. The observations began with Student 1, then Student 2, and Student 3 and so on until all the target students in the same classroom had been observed for 10 intervals. If the student engaged in any of the disruptive behaviors at any time during an observational interval, the interval was coded as disruptive (+). If no disruptive behavior was observed, a zero was scored for that interval. All of the observations began as soon as the question-and-answer component of the math lesson began.

Hand Raise

During the single-student responding sessions, a hand raise was scored whenever a target student's hand was lifted at least head high. However, to be scored, a student's hand raise had to occur (a) following the teacher's question, (b) prior to another student's response, and (c) before the teacher gave the answer to the question.

Academic Response

An *academic response* was defined as an observable response made by the student to the teacher's question. In this study, an academic response was scored when a student orally responded to the teacher's instructional question after raising his or her hand and being called on (during single-student responding), or when he or she wrote down the answer on the white board following the teacher's question (during response cards) during math lessons.

Correct Response

During single-student responding, a correct response was recorded if the student raised his or her hand to answer a teacher's question, the teacher called on the student, and the student gave the correct response verbally. A correct student response during response cards sessions was recorded whenever the answer written on the student's response card matched the answer provided by the teacher. Student responses were counted as correct even if any of the following spelling errors were made: reversal of letters (e.g., "divisoin"), addition of an extra letter (e.g., "divission"), omission of a single letter ("divison"), or slight distortion of a numeral due to a handwriting defect, as long as the spelling error did not produce an incorrect response (e.g., a reversal response of "01" would be scored as incorrect for a correct answer of "10" and a response of "30:0" would be scored as incorrect for its correct answer of "3:00").

The classroom teacher was the primary data collector for the students' hand raises, academic responses, and correct responses. For each condition following the baseline condition, the teacher was supplied with a data sheet located next to the overhead projector. During the single-student response condition, when a target student raised his or her hand to volunteer for a response, the teacher indicated that by placing a check mark on the data sheet for that question number. If the teacher called on one of the target students who had volunteered by raising his or her hand, the teacher recorded, next to the check mark, a plus sign for a correct response and a minus sign for an incorrect response made by the student. If no response was made, the teacher marked a zero on the data sheet. The same system was used under the response card condition except that when the teacher requested the students to display their response cards, the teacher marked a plus sign (correct), a minus sign (incorrect), or a zero (no response) for each target student. Students were informed that the teacher would be taking notes on a clipboard during the lesson, but they were unaware of the recording. Data were recorded only for the target students. Although recording responses is not a typical instructional format, it was decided that the teacher would collect this data to limit the number of observers that needed to be present in the classroom. This procedure was taught to the teachers prior to intervention

in a subject area other than math. The teachers reported no difficulty with the data collection method required during instruction.

Throughout the study, the classroom teachers were instructed to present 12 questions to the class during the 10 minutes of the question-and-answer section, thereby consistently providing approximately 1.2 opportunities per minute for students to respond. Students' responses (including hand raises, academic responses, and correct responses) per minute were calculated by dividing the total number of student responses by the length of the instructional time (i.e., 10 minutes).

Consumer Satisfaction

At the end of the study, the first author interviewed both the teachers and the target students using a teacher or a student questionnaire with eight open questions on each form. The questionnaires were developed to obtain opinions from the teachers and the students regarding their preferences on the two instructional approaches. Information concerning the effects and feasibility of response cards was also obtained from the teachers. Target students were asked the following questions about the hand raising versus the response cards:

1. Which way of answering questions did you like best?
2. Why do you like that method best?
3. Did you feel that you were better behaved in math class during one of the two ways of answering questions?
4. Which way did you think you behaved better?
5. Do you have any ideas as to why you behaved better when you were answering questions a certain way?
6. Would you like to use response cards in other classes?
7. What did you like best about using response cards?
8. What did you like least about using response cards?

The teachers were provided a questionnaire to fill out and mail into the researchers after the study concluded. The following questions were asked of the teachers:

1. Were the procedures used in this study feasible to use in your classroom?

2. Are you planning on continuing to use response cards during math class?

3. Is it likely that you will implement response cards in subjects other than math? If so, how will you use them?

4. Overall, did you think that the response cards intervention helped your students academically and behaviorally in the classroom?

5. Do you think that planning meetings as a team actually helped you prepare for the class or do you think that your time could have been better spent?

6. What was the best part of implementing this intervention in your classroom?

7. What was the worst part of implementing this intervention in your classroom?

8. What should I do differently the next time I try to have teachers implement these procedures?

Interobserver Agreement

One graduate student and one undergraduate student majoring in special education were trained as interobservers. An interobserver simultaneously, but independently, observed and recorded the disruptive behavior for 47% of the sessions and hand raising and academic responses for 29% of the sessions across all conditions. The interobserver agreement was determined as the percentage of agreement on the occurrence of the student's behavior, using an interval-by-interval or item-by-item method. Agreement was determined after each session when the observers would compare data sheets. Agreement was defined as both observers using the same code (e.g., a plus sign for target behavior present during the interval or a minus sign for an absence of the target behavior during the interval) for the same corresponding interval (e.g., Student 1, Interval 1) on the data sheet. Any other response (different codes for the same interval) was defined as a disagreement. The formula for determining the percentage of agreement among observers was the number of agreements divided by the total agreements plus disagreements multiplied by 100. The mean agreement was 98.6% (range = 98%–100%) for the disruptive behavior and 93% (range = 88%–98%) for the academic responding.

Procedural Integrity

Procedural integrity checks were conducted for 30% of the sessions within each condition to ascertain whether the teachers followed the prescribed steps for conducting the instructional sequences. Across two classrooms, the teachers averaged 95.7% (range = 91%–99%) compliance with the procedural steps during single-student responding and 97.5% (range = 96%–98%) compliance during response cards. A checklist was constructed to assess procedural integrity.

The teacher questions for each hand-raising condition were as follows:

1. Teacher presents question to the class.

2. Teacher calls on student whose hand is raised.

3. If and only if student provides correct answer, teacher provides praise statement.

4. If and only if answer was incorrect, teacher presents question again to the class and returns to Step 2.

Here are the teacher questions for each response-card condition:

1. Teacher presents question to the class.

2. Teacher provides adequate wait time for students to use response card.

3. Teacher requests students to present their cards.

4. If more than one fourth (i.e., four or five students) of the class makes an incorrect response, teacher instructs students to fix their answers to the problem and provides rationale for the answer; if fewer than one fourth of the students make an incorrect response, the teacher reveals answer to class.

5. Teacher provides praise for correct responses.

Subject Matter and Curriculum

Math was the subject matter targeted for data collection. All math lessons were designed for whole-class instruction. Lesson sequence, content, and topic duration were determined using the state's guidelines for fourth-grade proficiency. The math curriculum prescribed by the school district was the primary source of the instructional materials. A resource binder was provided to each teacher by the district containing suggested activities for each lesson as well as worksheets of math problems or extension practice. The teachers also used supplementary materials such as the math textbook *Heath Mathematics Connections* (1994) to enhance instruction and exemplars. The content areas delivered during the course of study included measurement, geometry, long division, and fractions. All of the math lessons constituted a brief lecture on a new math skill for approximately 10 minutes, followed by 10 minutes of question-and-answer practice of the skill. The math lessons concluded with 20 to 30 minutes of student independent seatwork on previous day or newly assigned homework.

Experimental Design and Procedures

An ABAB reversal design was used to demonstrate the differential effects of the two teacher presentation techniques: single-student responding and response cards.

Single-Student Responding (SSR)

Prior to this condition, the first author explained, modeled, and provided opportunities for practice to both teachers on the procedures of delivering a SSR session as well as collecting students' academic responses. The math lessons during SSR followed the typical procedures that were already used in the classrooms, including lecture on new skills, provision of skill practice using a question-and-answer format, and independent worksheets. One exception was that the teachers recorded which target students raised their hand for a particular question and which, if any, target students were called on to make a response. During the instruction, the teacher presented a question to the class either orally or visually (written on the chalkboard or on the overhead projector). Students volunteered to answer the question by raising their hand. The teacher recorded on a data sheet when the target students raised their hand to answer the question. The teacher then randomly selected a single student who raised his or her hand to answer the question for the class. If the student answered the question correctly, the teacher verified the correct response, praised the student (e.g., "Very good. The area of the square is 16 square feet"), and then moved on to the next question. If the student made an incorrect response, the teacher called on another classmate to answer the question. The correct answer was given and the math problem was explained to the whole class by

the teacher after two incorrect attempts from the students.

Response Cards (RC)

Prior to beginning the RC condition, the first author provided a 30-minute training session to both teachers on the use of response cards during math lessons through explanation, modeling, practice, and feedback. The teachers were trained to keep the instruction at a brisk pace, cue the students to write their answers on the boards, direct the students to present their responses, provide the correct answer, and either praise the students' responses or direct the students to correct their answers. In addition, the first author conducted a 1-hour training session with all of the students on the procedure for using response cards in both classrooms. The training occurred during a social studies lesson, and the response card instruction consisted of a review of a previous social studies lesson. The first author demonstrated how to use the response cards correctly through positive and negative examples; the students then practiced with praise and corrective feedback. Mastery of the procedure was determined when all the students responded on cue during the training session. No data were collected during training.

During the RC condition, each student was given a 9-inch × 12-inch shower board with one side covered with white laminate as the response card, a dry erase marker, and a piece of facial tissue or paper towel. The teacher first lectured and modeled the math skill being taught just as in the SSR condition, followed by presenting questions or problems related to the day's lesson. When the teacher asked a question, all students in the class were to respond by writing their answer on their response cards. After allocating a moment (i.e., sufficient time for answering the problem) for the students to write their answers, the teacher would say "cards up," and the students held their response cards over their head with the answer directed toward the teacher. At this point, the teacher would scan through the students' answers. If all of the students provided the correct answer, the teacher would praise the class, instruct the students to wipe off their response card with the tissue, and move onto the next question. When more than one fourth of the class failed to provide the correct answer, the teacher explained the steps involved to solve the problems and then directed the students to correct their answer. After the correction, the teacher presented the same question again for the students to practice the question correctly. If only two or three of the students responded incorrectly, the teacher gave the students the correct response, instructed the students to check their answers, then moved onto the next question without having the students present their response cards again for the same question.

RESULTS

Disruptive Behavior

The results showed moderate to high levels of responding during the SSR conditions (SSR1 and SSR2) for all of the nine target students in the two classrooms (see Figures 1 and 2). The students' disruptive behavior in the two classrooms declined to a mid and low level of responding when the response cards were employed. The behavioral

changes were dramatic, so that there existed no overlapping data points for two students (i.e., Students A2 and B2) and only one overlapping data point was observed between the SSR and RC conditions for three students (Students A1, B1, and B3). Experimental control was demonstrated in that the disruptive behavior decreased to a low level after the implementation of the RC1 condition, increased to a high level when SSR2 was reinstated, and declined again during the RC2 condition.

Table 2 presents the mean number of disruptive behaviors in the two classrooms during math lessons. The changes were consistent across students and classrooms with disruptive behavior occurring at substantially higher frequencies during the SSR conditions than during the RC conditions. On average, the mean number of disruptive behaviors decreased by 5.5 from the SSR conditions ($M = 6.8$) to the RC conditions ($M = 1.3$).

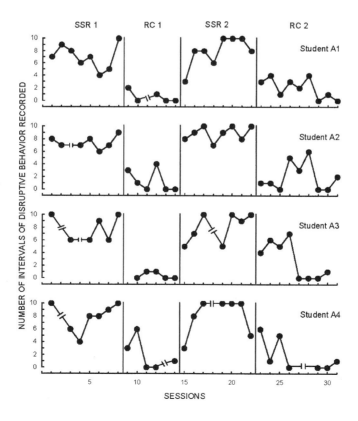

FIGURE 1. Number of disruptive behaviors during single-student responding (SSR) and response card (RC) conditions for the target students in Classroom A. Breaks in data points represent student absences.

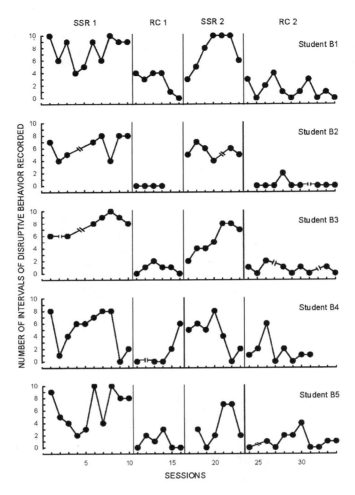

FIGURE 2. Number of disruptive behavior during single-student responding (SSR) and response card (RC) conditions for the target students in Classroom B.

Hand Raise, Academic Response, and Correct Response

Data on the hand raises, academic responses, and correct responses (see Figures 3 and 4) indicated that students were provided with more opportunities to respond to the academic materials under the RC conditions than the SSR conditions. Even with frequent hand raising (e.g., Students B4 and B5), the students received fewer opportunities to respond academically compared to when they were using response cards.

Table 3 provides the mean frequencies of hand raises, academic responses, and correct responses per minute for each student across conditions.

The mean academic responses per minute across the students were 0.12 during SSR conditions and 0.94 during the RC conditions, representing a mean increase of 0.82 academic responses per minute after the RC condition was implemented. Although the target students had higher rates of correct responding during the RC conditions as a group, the percentage of academic accuracy across conditions varied from student to student.

Consumer Satisfaction

Both classroom teachers reported that response cards increased the academic as well as social behavior of their students and that they would like

TABLE 2. Mean Number of Intervals of Disruptive Behavior by Each Student Across Experimental Conditions

Student	SSR1	RC1	SSR2	RC2
Classroom A				
A1	7.0	0.6	7.8	2.0
A2	7.4	1.3	8.9	2.0
A3	7.5	0.4	8.0	2.5
A4	7.5	2.0	8.0	1.9
Class A (M)	7.4	1.1	8.2	2.1
Classroom B				
B1	7.7	2.7	7.4	1.4
B2	6.0	0.0	5.5	0.2
B3	8.0	0.8	5.4	0.5
B4	5.6	0.4	5.1	1.5
B5	6.3	1.0	3.0	1.2
Class B (M)	6.7	1.0	5.3	1.0
Group	7.0	1.0	6.6	1.5

Note. SSR = single-student responding; RC = response cards.

to implement the easy-to-use response cards the following school year. Both teachers reported that they were especially impressed with the increased on-task behavior during the use of response cards. Although Teacher A reported that the recording of students' academic responses was somewhat difficult during instruction, he felt that it became easier for him as the sessions went on.

Of the nine target students, only seven were available to be interviewed. Five of the seven responded that they liked using response cards and they thought they learned faster and were better behaved when using response cards. Some comments from these students indicating their preference on response cards included the following: "because it was quicker than everybody yelling," "you don't have to keep raising your hand and never get called on," and "you don't talk as much and get in trouble." The remaining two students responded that they disliked the response

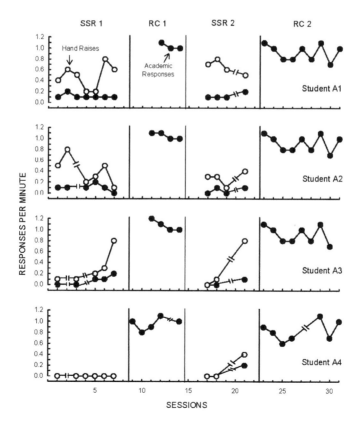

FIGURE 3. Rate of academic responses per minute during single-student responding (SSR) and response card (RC) conditions by the target students in Classroom A.

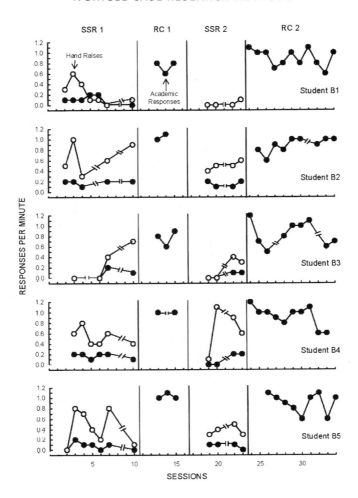

FIGURE 4. Rate of academic responses per minute during single-student responding (SSR) and response card (RC) conditions by the target students in Classroom B.

cards because "it sometimes got too noisy in there" or that he was not called on as much as he was when he raised his hand. While one of the two students only raised his hand eight times across the 16 single-student responding sessions, the other student frequently raised his hand during single-student responding.

DISCUSSION

A review of the data for each student provides a good argument for prediction, verification, and replication of the positive effects of the response cards on the students' disruptive behavior. All of the students evidenced substantial declines in disruptive behavior under the RC condition compared to SSR. Furthermore, for five of the nine target students, fewer than 10% of the data points overlapped across conditions. This means that students' disruptive behavior under the RC conditions rarely if ever reached the level of disruptions observed during SSR. When overlap did occur, it typically involved a data point in the low range of the SSR condition and a data point in the upper range of the RC condition.

In addition to an analysis of the data paths in the single-subject designs, the mean for disruptive behaviors across conditions supports a functional relationship between the dependent (disruptive

TABLE 3. Mean Number of Hand Raises and Academic Responses per Minute and Mean Percentage of Responding Accuracy by Each Student Across Experimental Conditions

Student	SSR1			RC1		SSR2			RC2	
	Hand raises	Academic responses	Accuracy (%)	Academic responses	Accuracy (%)	Hand raises	Academic responses	Accuracy (%)	Academic responses	Accuracy (%)
Classroom A										
A1	0.47	0.11	90.9	1.03	97.1	0.65	0.13	100.0	0.92	95.7
A2	0.10	0.10	100.0	1.05	95.2	0.25	0.05	100.0	0.92	96.7
A3	0.30	0.08	75.0	1.08	68.5	0.30	0.03	100.0	0.91	96.7
A4	0.00	0.00	N/A	0.96	93.8	0.13	0.07	100.0	0.83	96.4
Class A (M)	0.22	0.07	89.7	1.03	88.3	0.33	0.07	100.0	0.90	96.4
Classroom B										
B1	0.23	0.10	70.0	.073	91.8	0.03	0.03	100.0	0.90	81.1
B2	0.66	0.18	88.9	1.05	85.7	0.50	0.15	100.0	0.89	97.8
B3	0.28	0.13	100.0	0.77	100.0	0.18	0.05	60.0	0.84	72.6
B4	0.53	0.17	76.5	1.00	90.0	0.68	0.10	100.0	0.92	94.6
B5	0.43	0.07	100.0	1.03	97.1	0.38	0.08	100.0	0.98	90.8
Class B (M)	0.43	0.13	86.2	0.92	92.6	0.35	0.08	95.1	0.91	87.6
Group	0.32	0.10	87.4	0.97	90.3	0.34	0.08	97.4	0.90	92.0

Note. Accuracy was determined by dividing the number of correct responses per minute by the number of academic responses per minute then multiplying by 100. SSR = single-student responding; RC = response cards.

behavior) and independent (response cards) variables. The individual and group mean calculations consistently show higher levels of disruptive intervals during single-student responding than during response cards. One obvious explanation is that the response cards intervention required students to remain attentive throughout instruction by eliciting high levels of responding for all students in the classroom. These elements were typically absent from the teacher's traditional instructional format. Not surprisingly, as students became more engaged in instruction, there were fewer opportunities for behavior that was less conducive to learning.

The results on students' disruptive behavior in this study offer several contributions to the existing literature in this area. First, previous studies, examining response cards and problem behavior, though pioneering in their scope, lacked a strong research design. Neither Armendariz and Umbreit (1999) nor Christle and Schuster (2003) conducted a complete ABAB reversal design. Without a return to Condition B (i.e., ABA design), the evaluation of the functional relationships is limited. The current study addresses this issue. Second, a time sampling recording procedure was often used to record either the disruptive behavior (Armendariz & Umbreit, 1999) or on-task behavior (Christle & Schuster, 2003). Although appropriate,

this recording procedure often suffers from overestimation of the positive effects of the intervention (e.g., increased on-task behavior or decreased disruptive behavior). The present study used a more conservative observational method (i.e., partial interval recording) to record the disruptive behavior. The results of this study, therefore, may be even more impressive. Finally, unlike previous studies, where more experienced teachers were the implementers (e.g., Armendariz & Umbreit, 1999; Christle & Schuster, 2003; Gardner et al., 1994), two teachers in their early teaching career were trained to implement the response cards in the current study. The positive results of students' academic and social behaviors indicate that less experienced teachers can be trained successfully to implement response cards in their classrooms.

Data on students' academic responding clearly show that all the target students responded more frequently and correctly during the RC conditions than during the SSR condition. Even the most eager students (e.g., Students A1, B2, and B4), who displayed the most hand raises under the SSR condition, greatly increased their active responses with the response cards. The fact that some students failed to make any academic responses under single-student responding aligns with the data on student disruptions in that those who are not responding actively are most likely to engage in disruptive behaviors. These findings are consistent with previous studies in that the implementation of effective instructional strategies, such as response cards, that enhance high rates of active student responding, is not only beneficial but also imperative (e.g., Christle & Schuster, 2003; Gardner et al., 1994; Heward, 1994; Kellum et al., 2001; Narayan et al., 1990). Furthermore, our results support much of the research in the field on explicit teaching and the positive effects of direct instruction strategies, especially for urban learners (Bullara, 1994; Delpit, 1995). As mentioned earlier, urban students are not often competitive with their middle-class peers upon entering school. Many urban students come to school without the early learning skills needed for success. In addition, they are likely to be challenged with a curriculum that does not compensate for these deficits and to be taught by inexperienced teachers who offer students fewer opportunities to respond (Arreaga-Mayer & Greenwood, 1986; Hall, Delquadri, Greenwood, & Thurston, 1982). These factors, along with the other stressors that typically accompany poverty, converge to undermine the ideal learning environment, where students quietly attend to the teacher or wait until the teacher is available to ask questions. Strategies such as response cards engage the learners so that students are required to take an active role in their instruction. For students, having to attend to instruction means more learning as well as less distraction from other stimuli in the room and less time to disrupt others. Furthermore, the use of response cards allows teachers to receive observable responses from the students, and consequently teachers can provide constant and immediate feedback on student performance, which also enhances student learning.

Despite the positive outcomes of this study, a few limitations should be noted. First, a potentially serious methodological flaw in the current study is related to having the researchers check their wristwatches to mark the observational intervals for disruptive behavior. Requiring data collectors to attend not only to the target student but also to the time of the interval may possibly have distracted the observer enough to have missed misbehavior of the target student. It is possible that in the fraction of a second it took for the researcher to glance at his watch, the student could have engaged in disruptive behavior. Given the researchers' familiarity with the data collection procedure, it is unlikely but possible that some intervals may have been miscoded due to the data collection

procedure. However, since the observation procedures described in this study remained consistent across all phases of the study, any discrepancies due to observer distraction would remain constant. The use of an audiotape would have addressed this issue. Another related issue for future research is to reduce the duration of the partial interval observations from 10 to 5 seconds. This would result in a greater number of shorter observation intervals, and therefore provide a more precise picture of the amount of time the students are disruptive. Another possible limitation related to the data collection procedures is that the senior author served as the primary observer. A second independent observer was used for nearly a third of the academic responses and nearly half of the behavioral responses. The high mean agreements (over 90%) conducted across all conditions and variables of the study provide assurance that bias on the part of observers was unlikely.

Second, because data were only collected on the nine target students who were considered to be the most disruptive and the least attentive during math lessons, the degree to which response cards affected the academic and social behavior of the less disruptive students remains unclear. However, the anecdotal observations both from the first author and the classroom teachers indicated that all participating students were uniformly responding at higher rates and more adaptive in their behavior during response cards. Future research should extend the investigation to include students at different levels of both academic and social performance.

Third, a functional behavioral assessment/analysis (FBA) was not conducted prior to implementation of the interventions for this study. Thus, it may be assumed that the function of the disruptive behavior was connected to the students' need for stimulation that resulted from the academic engagement. Another possibility is that the response cards were powerful enough to produce changes regardless of the functions of the disruptive behaviors.

Finally, due to the varying difficulty of the content materials across sessions, the difficulty of the teacher-presented questions varied. For example, in one session the students were required to answer questions such as "What is the denominator in the fraction 3/4?" while in another session the students were asked to solve a two-digit long division problem. For the division problem, both the teacher and the first author noticed that some students who were "participating" during the RC condition were unable to produce an answer and lift their response card in the given interval provided by the teacher. A few students would still be working on the problem when the teacher requested the students to present their answers, while most of the students were finished and waiting to respond. If the student raised his or her response card without completing his answer, the response was coded as incorrect. If the student did not raise his or her response card and continued working on the problem, then no response was coded. No response was interpreted as if the student did not make any attempt to respond to the teacher's question; this would reduce the student's active student responding per minute. As a result, the academic response rate and correct responses per minute for some students during which more complicated or difficult materials were presented may have been limited on the data. Future research is encouraged not only to keep the type and difficulty of the questions more consistent across sessions, but also to evaluate how the different types of questions may contribute to student academic response rates.

CONCLUSION

All of the students targeted in the study were observed to be less disruptive, participated more in instruction, and answered more questions correctly during the response-card condition. Although further research is needed to evaluate the scope of these effects with other children, the robust change in behavior in these students suggests that response cards may have value in other classrooms not only for increasing students' academic achievement and class participation but also for reducing their negative social behavior during class instruction. Although not a definitive work, this research, along with studies by Armendariz and Umbreit (1999) and Christle and Schuster (2003), raise a compelling question about the effects that increased active student responding may have on social behavior in the classroom.

Schoolwide disciplinary data collected for this school (Lo & Cartledge, 2004a) showed that the primary reason for disciplinary referral was classroom disruption. The high levels of disruptive behavior documented in this study, combined with the school's disciplinary referral data, strongly point to the need for more effective instructional

environments that actively engage urban youth in the learning process. As these disruptive behaviors persist and continue to rule these classrooms, student learning and motivation decline correspondingly. In recent years much debate has centered on effective instructional approaches for urban learners (e.g., whole language vs. direct instruction), but the impact of these approaches on disruptive behavior rarely accompanies this discussion. This is an important consideration that deserves critical attention.

AUTHORS' NOTE

This research was supported by grants from the Ohio Department of Mental Health, Ohio Department of Education, the OSU/Urban Schools Initiative, and the Office of Special Education Programs, U.S. Department of Education (H324T010057-02).

REFERENCES

Armendariz, F., & Umbreit, J. (1999). Using active responding to reduce disruptive behavior in a general education classroom. *Journal of Positive Behavior Interventions, 1*(3), 152–158.

Arreaga-Mayer, C., & Greenwood, C. R. (1986). Environmental variables affecting the school achievement of culturally and linguistically different learners: An instructional perspective. *NABE. The Journal for the National Association for Bilingual Education, 10*(2), 113–135.

Billingsley, B. S. (2001). *Beginning special educators: Characteristics, qualifications, and experiences. SPeNSE Summary Sheet. (ERIC Document Reproduction Service No. ED467269).*

Billingsley, B. S., & Tomchin, E. M. (1992). Four beginning LD teachers: What their experiences suggest for trainers and employers. *Learning Disabilities Research and Practice, 7,* 104–112.

Bullara, D. T. (1994). *Effects of guided notes on the academic performance and off-task/disruptive behaviors of students with severe behavior handicaps during science instruction.* Unpublished doctoral dissertation, The Ohio State University.

Carnine, D. W. (1976). Effects of two teacher-presentation rates on off-task behavior, answering correctly, and participation. *Journal of Applied Behavior Analysis, 9,* 199–206.

Cavanaugh, R. A., Heward, W. L., & Donelson, F. (1996). Effects of response cards during lesson closure on the academic performance of secondary students in an earth science course. *Journal of Applied Behavior Analysis, 29,* 403–406.

Christle, C. A., & Schuster, J. W. (2003). The effects of using response cards on student participation, academic achievement, and on-task behavior during whole-class, math instruction. *Journal of Behavioral Education, 12*, 147–165.

Coleman, M., & Vaughn, S. (2000). Reading interventions for students with emotional/behavioral disorders. *Behavioral Disorders, 25*(2), 93–104.

Colvin, G. T., Greenberg, S., & Sherman, R. (1993). The forgotten variable: Improving academic skills for students with serious emotional disturbance. *Effective School Practice, 12*(1), 20–25.

Darling-Hammond, L. (2003). Keeping good teachers. *Educational Leadership, 60*(8), 6–77.

Delpit, L. (1995). *Other people's children.* New York: The New Press.

Engelmann, S., & Colvin, G. (1983). *Generalized compliance training: A direct-instruction program for managing severe behavior problems.* Austin, TX: PRO-ED.

Fimian, M. J., & Santoro, T. M. (1983). Sources and manifestations of occupational stress as reported by full-time special education teachers. *Exceptional Children, 49*, 540–543.

Gardner, R., III, Heward, W. L., & Grossi, T. A. (1994). Effects of response cards on student participation and academic achievement: A systematic replication with inner-city students during whole class science instruction. *Journal of Applied Behavior Analysis, 27*, 63–71.

Greenwood, C. R., Arreaga-Mayer, C., & Carta, J. J. (1994). Identification and translation of effective teacher-developed instructional procedures for general practice. *Remedial and Special Education, 15*(3), 140–151.

Hall, R. V., Delquadri, J., Greenwood, C. R., & Thurston, L. (1982). The importance of opportunity to respond in children's academic success. In E. B. Edgar, N. G. Haring, J. R. Jenkins, & C. G. Pious (Eds.), *Mentally handicapped children: Education and training* (pp. 107–140). Baltimore: University Park Press.

Hart, B., & Risley, T. R. (1995). *The social world of children learning to talk.* Baltimore: Brookes.

Heath mathematics connections: Grade 4. (1994). Geneva, IL: D.C. Heath.

Heward, W. L. (1994). Three "low-tech" strategies for increasing the frequency of active student response during group instruction. In R. Gardner III, D. M. Sainato, J. O. Cooper, T. E. Heron, W. L. Heward, J. Eshleman, et al. (Eds.), *Behavior analysis in education: Focus on measurably superior instruction* (pp. 283–320). Pacific Grove, CA: Brooks/Cole.

Kellum, K. K., Carr, J. E., & Dozier, C. L. (2001). Response-card instruction and student learning in a college classroom. *Teaching of Psychology (Columbia, Mo.), 28*, 101–104.

Lo, Y., & Cartledge, G. (2004a). *Office disciplinary referrals in an elementary school: Special issues for an urban population.* Manuscript submitted for publication.

Lo, Y., & Cartledge, G. (2004b). Total class peer tutoring and interdependent group oriented contingency: Improving the academic and task related behaviors of fourth-grade urban students. *Education & Treatment of Children, 27*, 235–262.

Maheady, L., Michielli-Pendl, J., Mallette, B., & Harper, G. F. (2002). A collaborative research project to improve the academic performance of a diverse sixth grade science class. *Teacher Education and Special Education, 25*, 55–70.

Muscott, H. S. (1987). Conceptualizing behavior management strategies for troubled and troubling students: A process for organizing the direction of intervention efforts in schools. *The Pointer, 31*, 15–22.

Narayan, J. S., Heward, W. L., Gardner, R., III, Courson, F. H., & Omness, C. K. (1990). Using response cards to increase student participation in an elementary classroom. *Journal of Applied Behavior Analysis, 23*, 483–490.

Pullis, M. (1992). An analysis of the occupational stress of teachers of the behaviorally disordered: Sources, effects, and strategies of coping. *Behavioral Disorders, 17*, 191–201.

Sainato, D. M., Strain, P. S., & Lyon, S. R. (1987). Increasing academic responding of handicapped preschool children during group instruction. *Journal of the Division for Early Children, 12*(1), 23–30.

Veenman, S. (1984). Perceived problems of beginning teachers. *Review of Educational Research, 54*(2), 143–178.

ABOUT THE AUTHORS

Michael Charles Lambert, PhD, is an assistant professor of special education at Western Washington University. His interests include students with disruptive behavior, the effects of academic interventions on social behavior, applied behavior analysis, and urban youth. **Gwendolyn Cartledge** is a professor in special education at The Ohio State University. Her research interests include students with behavior disorders, social skill development, and issues of urban education/special education. **William L. Heward** is professor emeritus of special education at The Ohio State University. His research interests include low-tech strategies for increasing the effectiveness of group instruction in diverse classrooms, improving the academic achievement of students with disabilities, and promoting the generalization and maintenance of newly learned skills. **Ya-yu Lo, PhD,** is an assistant professor in the Department of Special Education and Child Development, University of North Carolina at Charlotte. Her current interests include behavioral disorders, positive behavioral support, and effective instruction. Address: Gwendolyn Cartledge, Special Education Program, School of Physical Activity and Educational Services, College of Education, The Ohio State University, 371 Arps Hall, 1945 N. High St., Columbus, OH 43210; e-mail: cartledge.1@osu.edu

From Lambert, M. C., Cartledge, G., Heward, W. L., & Lo, Y. (2006). Effects of response cards on disruptive behavior and academic responding during math lessons by fourth-grade urban students. *Journal of Positive Behavior Interventions, 8*, 88–99. Copyright 2006 by the Hammill Institute on Disabilities. Reprinted by permission of SAGE.

ILLUSTRATIVE EXAMPLE QUESTIONS

1. What was the purpose of the investigation?

2. Who were the participants? Where was the setting?

3. What were the dependent and independent variables, and how was the dependent variable measured?

4. How was interobserver agreement calculated? Was it adequate?

5. What type of design was used? What occurred during each of the conditions?

6. What data were reported relative to procedural integrity? Were teachers using the procedures as prescribed?

7. Researchers interviewed students to gather data on consumer satisfaction. What additional social validity data might have been important to collect?

8. In the single-student responding (SSR) condition, the teachers recorded which target students raised their hand for a particular question and which, if any, were called on to make a response. Could this procedure have disrupted the flow of the lesson? If so, what effect would it have had on the SSR data?

9. Researchers describe as a limitation the possibility of teachers being distracted and not recording disruptive behavior. How could this have been avoided?

10. Researchers note that degree of math lesson difficulty varied across sessions. What effect would this have had on student performance and response per minute data?

ADDITIONAL RESEARCH EXAMPLES

1. Cihak, D., Fahrenkrog, C., Ayres, K. M., & Smith, C. (2010). The use of video modeling via a video iPod and a system of least prompts to improve transitional behaviors for students with autism spectrum disorders in the general education classroom. *Journal of Positive Behavior Interventions, 12*, 103–115.

2. Lane, K. L., Rogers, L. A., Parks, R. J., Weisenbach, J. L., Mau, A. C., Merwin, M. T., et al. (2007). Function-based interventions for students who are nonresponsive to primary and secondary prevention efforts: Illustrations at the elementary and middle school levels. *Journal of Emotional and Behavioral Disorders, 15*, 169–183.

3. Waller, R. D., & Higbee, T. (2010). The effects of fixed-time escape on inappropriate and appropriate classroom behavior. *Journal of Applied Behavior Analysis, 43*, 149–153.

THREATS TO INTERNAL VALIDITY

Circle the number corresponding to the likelihood of each threat to internal validity being present in the investigation and provide a justification.

1 = definitely not a threat   2 = not a likely threat   3 = somewhat likely threat
4 = likely threat   5 = definite threat   NA = not applicable for this design

Results in Differences within or between Individuals

1. Maturation   1   2   3   4   5   NA

   Justification _____

   _____

2. Selection   1   2   3   4   5   NA

   Justification _____

   _____

3. Selection by Maturation Interaction   1   2   3   4   5   NA

   Justification _____

   _____

4. Statistical Regression   1   2   3   4   5   NA

   Justification _____

   _____

5. Morality   1   2   3   4   5   NA

   Justification _____

   _____

6. Instrumentation   1   2   3   4   5   NA

   Justification _____

   _____

7. Testing   1   2   3   4   5   NA

   Justification _____

   _____

(continued)

8. History   1   2   3   4   5   NA

Justification _____

_____

9. Resentful Demoralization of the Control Group   1   2   3   4   5   NA

Justification _____

_____

Results in Similarities within or between Individuals

10. Diffusion of Treatment   1   2   3   4   5   NA

Justification _____

_____

11. Compensatory Rivalry by the Control Group   1   2   3   4   5   NA

Justification _____

_____

12. Compensatory Equalization of Treatments   1   2   3   4   5   NA

Justification _____

_____

Abstract: Write a one-page abstract summarizing the overall conclusions of the authors and whether or not you feel the authors' conclusions are valid based on the internal validity of the investigation.

THREATS TO EXTERNAL VALIDITY

Circle the number corresponding to the likelihood of each threat to external validity being present in the investigation according to the following scale:

1 = definitely not a threat   2 = not a likely threat   3 = somewhat likely threat

4 = likely threat   5 = definite threat   NA = not applicable for this design

Also, provide a justification for each rating.

Population

1. Generalization across Subjects   1 2 3 4 5 NA

   Justification _____

   _____

2. Interaction of Personological Variables and Treatment   1 2 3 4 5 NA

   Justification _____

   _____

Ecological

3. Verification of the Independent Variable   1 2 3 4 5 NA

   Justification _____

   _____

4. Multiple Treatment Interference   1 2 3 4 5 NA

   Justification _____

   _____

5. Hawthorne Effect   1 2 3 4 5 NA

   Justification _____

   _____

6. Novelty and Disruption Effects   1 2 3 4 5 NA

   Justification _____

   _____

7. Experimental Effects   1 2 3 4 5 NA

   Justification _____

   _____

(continued)

8. Pretest Sensitization   1   2   3   4   5   NA

    Justification _____

    _____

9. Posttest Sensitization   1   2   3   4   5   NA

    Justification _____

    _____

10. Interaction of Time of Measurement and Treatment Effects   1   2   3   4   5   NA

    Justification _____

    _____

11. Measurement of the Dependent Variable   1   2   3   4   5   NA

    Justification _____

    _____

12. Interaction of History and Treatment Effects   1   2   3   4   5   NA

    Justification _____

    _____

Abstract: Write a one-page abstract summarizing the overall conclusions of the authors and whether or not you feel the authors' conclusions are valid based on the external validity of the investigation.

CHAPTER 12

∎∎∎∎

Multiple-Baseline Designs

OBJECTIVES

After studying this chapter, you should be able to . . .

1. Define what is meant by a multiple-baseline design and explain three reasons why a researcher would select a multiple-baseline design over a withdrawal design.
2. Illustrate the graphing methods in multiple-baseline designs.
3. Describe each of the different multiple-baseline designs.
4. Outline when researchers should use each multiple-baseline design.

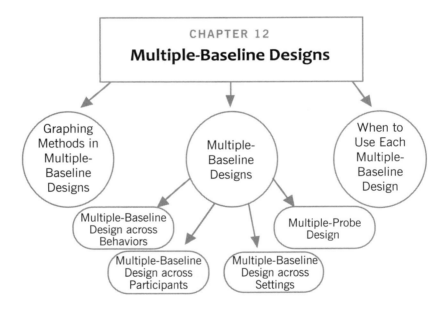

OVERVIEW

A **multiple-baseline design** is an experimental design that starts with measurement of two or more behaviors in a baseline condition, followed by application of an independent variable to one of the behaviors while baseline conditions remain in effect for other behaviors.

The independent variable is then applied in a sequential fashion to other behaviors (Cooper et al., 2007). This chapter focuses on multiple-baseline designs, which can be considered an alternative to the withdrawal design. The use of the withdrawal and associated designs has decreased in recent years. Although withdrawal designs can control for threats to internal validity, they have several disadvantages that probably account for decreased use. First, some behaviors that were changed as a function of the intervention ("B") may not immediately return to baseline levels. For example, when teaching a skill such as reading, it is unlikely that the participant's behavior will return to baseline levels when the intervention is removed. Suppose we teach a student how to decode words. At the end of the intervention ("B") condition, we return to baseline. However, because we just taught a skill, we would expect the skill to maintain for some time after we remove the independent variable. We would not expect to see an immediate return to baseline levels. We probably could not tell the student to forget what was learned. Thus, we would essentially have an A-B design.

There would be several threats to the internal validity of this investigation. Withdrawal designs are appropriate when there is a motivational problem, or when we are attempting to remove an unwanted behavior. If the lack of performance is motivational in nature, we can implement a motivational system to improve the student's performance. Upon removal of the motivational system, we would expect a return to baseline levels, because the student would no longer have the same motivation to perform the task. In this case, there would be a higher level of internal validity.

A second problem with withdrawal designs has to do with ethical concerns. Researchers may find it unethical to withdraw intervention and return to baseline conditions. As stated by Cooper et al. (2007), "One must question the appropriateness of any procedure that allows (indeed, seeks) an improved behavior to deteriorate to baseline levels of responding" (p. 186). For example, suppose we try to control the aggressive responses of a youth with behavior disorders. We implement a behavior intervention program and see a decrease in the student's aggressive behavior. Then, we decide to remove the intervention program to see whether the aggressive behavior returns to baseline levels. There is a major ethical concern here. Many staff members would not wish to return to baseline levels. We may argue that if we really want to know the scientific merits of the intervention program as the "cause" of the behavior change, we must remove the program and see

whether the behavior returns. Staff members may say, "No thanks." They may indicate that they do not really care what caused the behavior change; they only care that something happened to change the student's behavior in the desired direction. Of course, from a practical standpoint, it is critical to determine why the student's behavior changed, if for no other reason than to determine what to do in the future if the behavior returns, or if other students have similar behavior problems. However, the ethical concern must be taken into consideration when we conduct research.

A third problem deals with staff cooperation. This problem relates to the previous problem and involves ethical considerations. Staff may simply refuse to allow or be involved in the withdrawal of the intervention. Even if the behavior is not destructive or dangerous but simply annoying, staff may not be willing to allow the behavior to return. If staff members have objections to the use of a particular method used in research, then a valid measure of intervention effects is compromised and an alternative must be found.

This chapter focuses on several issues surrounding the multiple-baseline design. First, graphing issues are highlighted. Second, we discuss three types of multiple-baseline designs across behaviors, participants, and settings. A fourth design is also described. This design (i.e., multiple-probe) is a modification of the multiple-baseline design. The methods of analyzing the data follow the discussion of design types. Third, research examples highlighting the different designs are presented. (*Note.* You should attempt to analyze the graphs presented from the research examples.) Finally, an illustrative investigation is included at the end of the chapter for critique.

> A **multiple-baseline design** *starts with measurement of two or more behaviors in a baseline condition, followed by application of an independent variable to one of the behaviors while baseline conditions remain in effect for other behaviors. The independent variable is then applied in a sequential fashion to other behaviors.*

WHAT ARE GRAPHING METHODS IN MULTIPLE-BASELINE DESIGNS?

The visual display of data in multiple-baseline designs is similar to that in withdrawal and associated designs in that the descriptors (i.e., dependent measure, baseline, independent variable, time measurement, data points, data paths, condition change lines, and figure captions) are displayed in the same manner. However, instead of having one graph, the multiple-baseline display involves placing individual graphs on top of each other. Figure 12.1 demonstrates a typical multiple-baseline graph. Notice how the graphs are aligned and the placement of additional descriptors. For instance, the display in Figure 12.1 shows a multiple-baseline design across settings. If this graph displayed a multiple-baseline design across behaviors, the type of behaviors would be indicated. Likewise, if this were a multiple-baseline design across participants, the descriptors "Participant 1, Participant 2," the names of the participants, or some other form of identification would be included. Additionally, the condition change lines are drawn down to the second baseline and successive baselines to show how the conditions overlap. In Figure 12.1, the intervention took place on Session 5 in the first setting and on Session 8 in the second setting.

WHAT ARE MULTIPLE-BASELINE DESIGNS?

At a basic level, multiple-baseline designs may be thought of as a series of A-B designs

(Barlow et al., 2008). In this way, multiple-baseline designs have several advantages over withdrawal designs. For example, in a multiple-baseline design, there is not a requirement to remove or withdraw the intervention. Along these lines, there is not a need to return to baseline levels in the future. Thus, multiple-baseline designs are appropriate for investigations of skills acquisition, as well as motivational problems and the reduction of unwanted behaviors (Cooper et al., 2007). Multiple-baseline designs are in many ways more versatile than withdrawal designs, because they apply to a wide array of socially significant interventions. Additionally, multiple-baseline designs allow for the replication of interventions effects across behaviors, participants, and/or settings (discussed later). So even though the multiple-baseline design is essentially an A-B design, the effect of the independent variable is systematically replicated several times across behaviors, participants, and/or settings, making it a strong method for evaluating intervention effects.

However, multiple-baseline designs have several weaknesses. These weaknesses will be discussed throughout the chapter and include the need for two or more baselines, possible lengthy baselines for some participants, less experimental control than withdrawal designs, and more design considerations. Since the multiple-baseline designs discussed throughout this chapter have the same design considerations for gaining experimental control, a discussion will take place later on design considerations for all multiple-baselines.

Multiple-Baseline Design across Behaviors

The multiple-baseline design across behaviors requires at least two separate behaviors that are independent of one another. In other words, if a researcher applies an intervention to one behavior, there should not be a corresponding change in the other behavior (called *covariation*). Once these behaviors are targeted and a measurement system is put into place, baseline data should be collected for each behavior. Suppose a researcher is interested in investigating two behaviors (i.e., treatment of cuts and treatment of burns). The researcher begins taking baseline measurements for both of these behaviors

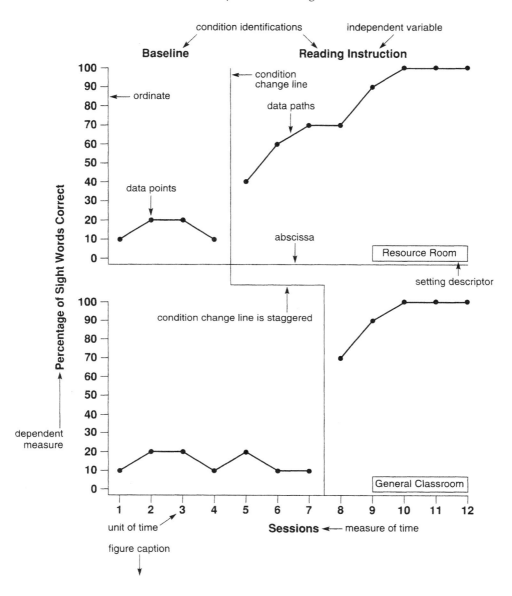

FIGURE 12.1. The percentage of sight words answered correctly across baseline and reading instruction conditions for resource room and general education settings.

simultaneously. Then, the first behavior receives the intervention and the second remains in baseline. Keeping the second behavior in baseline is critical. If the researcher implements the intervention with both behaviors at the same time, he/she would have two simultaneous A-B designs. Figure 12.2 demonstrates this problem. The researcher began taking baseline

measurements for both treatment of cuts and treatment of burns simultaneously. The participant did not perform many steps correctly. In Session 5, first-aid instruction was started to teach steps necessary to treat a cut. The participant's percentage of steps performed correctly increased. The first behavior (treatment of cuts) received the intervention and the second

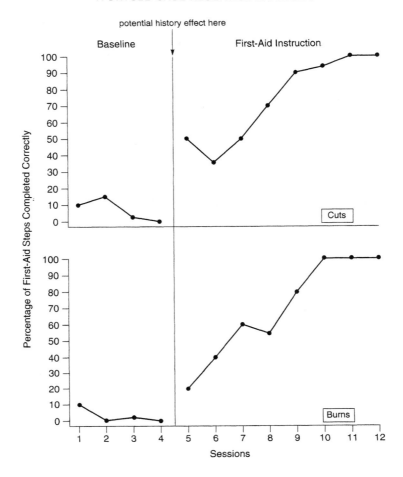

FIGURE 12.2. The percentage of first-aid steps completed correctly across baseline and first-aid instruction conditions for cuts and burns.

behavior (treatment of burns) remained in baseline. But treatment of burns increased even without treatment (i.e., covariation). In terms of internal validity, this would be an example of a history threat. It is not possible to explain away extraneous variables such as history. The resulting improvement in both behaviors may have resulted from some history effect.

The critical aspect of this design is that there are multiple behaviors with one participant or one unit of analysis in one setting. A unit of analysis is how a researcher views the participant or the makeup of the group of participants (Gall et al., 2007). In other words, even if a researcher involved several participants in a study, he/she could treat the "group" as a single

participant. For example, a researcher investigating the effects of a reading program on a single class of fourth graders (nonrandomized) could treat the class as one participant.

Multiple-Baseline Design across Participants

The multiple-baseline design across participants is similar to the multiple-baseline design across behaviors in that two or more baselines are required. However, the researcher measures behavior across two or more participants. The researcher takes frequent measures of the targeted behavior for each participant during and after baseline. Figure 12.3 shows a multiple-baseline design across participants. As can be seen, the graphs indicate the participants. Notice also how the researcher kept the second participant in baseline while the first participant received the intervention. The same procedure was used for the third participant.

There are several important aspects of this design. First, the design must include multiple participants or several groups of participants. Additionally, one behavior is measured, as opposed to several in the multiple-baseline design across behaviors. Finally, the single setting is the same as that in multiple-baseline design across behaviors.

Multiple-Baseline Design across Settings

The multiple-baseline design across settings is similar to the previous two designs except that the researcher selects two or more settings. The researcher then measures the participant's

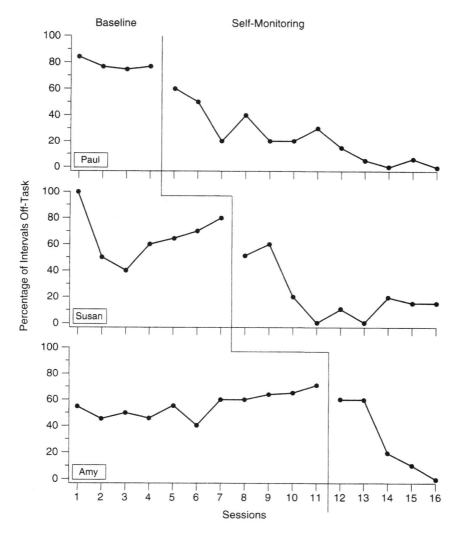

FIGURE 12.3. Percentage of intervals of off-task across baseline and self-monitoring conditions for Paul, Susan, and Amy. From Martella, R. C., Nelson, J. R., Marchand-Martella, N., & O'Reilly, M. (2012). *Comprehensive behavior management: Individualized, classroom, and schoolwide approaches* (2nd ed.). Thousand Oaks, CA: Sage. Copyright 2012 by Sage Publications, Inc. Reprinted by permission of SAGE.

behavior in each of these settings. He/she takes baseline measures in each setting, then introduces the intervention in only the first setting. The participant's behavior in the second setting is not exposed to the intervention until later. Figure 12.1 displays data for a multiple-baseline design across settings, indicating that two settings are included in the investigation.

There are several important aspects of this design. First, there should be several settings as opposed to one setting with the multiple-baseline design across behaviors or participants. Also one behavior measure is the same as that in the multiple-baseline design across participants. Recall that there are several behaviors in the multiple-baseline design across behaviors. Finally, a single participant or a single group of participants is treated as a single participant, as in the multiple-baseline design across behaviors; this is different from the multiple-baseline design across participants that requires more than one participant or group.

Multiple-Probe Design

A **multiple-probe design** is essentially a multiple-baseline design in which the measures are not collected on a frequent basis; it overcomes the problem of using repeated measurements by probing (assessing) the behavior intermittently. Multiple-probe designs can be used when effects of instruction on one skill are not likely to result in changes in performance of another skill (Cooper et al., 2007). One potential problem with multiple-baseline designs is the need for repeated measurements. At times, repeated measurements may result in reactivity during baseline (a testing problem or a change in behavior due to repetition of assessment) (Horner & Baer, 1978). There are other times that frequent assessments may not be feasible and alternative assessment methods must be used. For example, we would probably not want to administer a frequent test of vocabulary in reading (e.g., once per day) over a long period of time. First, providing such a test most likely would lead to reactivity. Second, frequent testing may be too costly and time-consuming. An alternative to frequent or repeated measurements is to "probe" the behavior every so often (e.g., once per week) during the baseline condition.

A further concern surrounding repeated measures involves the frequency with which researchers measure the behavior during the intervention condition. According to Barlow et al. (2008), if reactivity of measurement is the reason a multiple-probe design is used, then probes should also continue in the intervention condition. Barlow et al. also indicate that if the problem is the feasibility of providing frequent measures during baseline, or if researchers have reason to believe that the baseline would have been stable had frequent measures taken place, frequent measurements may be applied during the intervention condition.

Additionally, Kazdin (2003) notes that probes may be used in situations where behaviors are not the target for intervention, as in the case of assessing generalization/transfer and maintenance of intervention effects. Finally, a combination of multiple-baseline and multiple-probe designs may be used in situations where frequent measurements are applied to behaviors targeted for change and probes are conducted to assess generalization/transfer and maintenance.

Multiple-probe designs are essentially multiple-baseline designs in which the measurements are not conducted on a frequent basis. Figure 12.4 demonstrates a multiple-probe design across participants. Notice that there are fewer data points during baseline and intervention sessions. Obviously, a potential problem is a lack of data points necessary to show stability or a trend. Generally, three data points are required for such a demonstration. In the figure, only Susan and Amy had three baseline data points. However, the advantage of having fewer data points is to avoid reactivity. This is probably greater than the disadvantage of having too few data points.

Analysis of Data

As they do with withdrawal designs, critical research consumers must understand how to analyze the graphically displayed data. (*Note.* As with withdrawal and associated designs, statistics have been developed to aid in the interpretation of multiple-baseline designs; however, visual inspection is the primary method of analyzing data in multiple-baseline designs.)

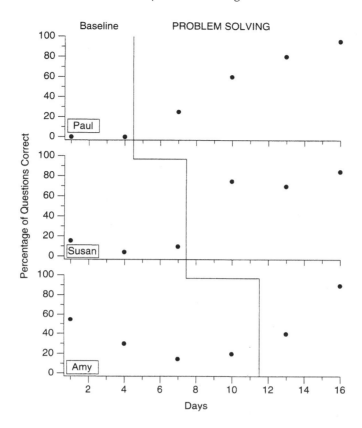

FIGURE 12.4. Percentage of questions correct across baseline and problem-solving conditions for Paul, Susan, and Amy.

Additionally, critical research consumers must consider the internal and the external validity of the investigation.

Internal Validity

When assessing the internal validity of multiple-baseline designs, the several concerns that must be taken into consideration involve the condition length; independence of behaviors; the amount of overlap of the data; the number of baselines; independence of the behaviors, participants, or settings; and the level and rapidity of change. Table 12.1 summarizes the major threats to internal validity of the designs discussed in this chapter.

Condition Length. The condition length of multiple-baseline designs is the same as that in withdrawal and associated designs. There must be at least three stable data points or a countertherapeutic trend. However, the number of data points increases as the number of baselines increases (Cooper et al., 2007). For more discussion, see the section on amount of data overlap below.

Independence of Behaviors. Possibly the most critical rule in multiple-baseline designs relates to the independence of behaviors across baselines (Cooper et al., 2007). Behaviors being measured across baselines must be independent (i.e., changes in one behavior must not coincide

> A **multiple-probe design** *is essentially a multiple-baseline design in which the measurements do not occur on a frequent basis.*

TABLE 12.1. Threats to Internal Validity Associated with Multiple-Baseline Designs

Threat	Multiple-baseline design across . . .			Multiple-probe design
	Behaviors	Participants	Settings	
1. Maturation	Controlled	Controlled	Controlled	Controlled
2. Selection	Not applicable	Not applicable	Not applicable	Not applicable
3. Selection by maturation interaction	Not applicable	Not applicable	Not applicable	Not applicable
4. Statistical regression	Possible concern	Controlled	Controlled	Controlled
5. Mortality	Controlled	Controlled	Controlled	Controlled
6. Instrumentation	Controlled	Controlled	Controlled	Controlled
7. Testing	Controlled	Controlled	Controlled	Controlled
8. History	Controlled	Controlled	Controlled	Controlled
9. Resentful demoralization of the control group	Not applicable	Not applicable	Not applicable	Not applicable
10. Diffusion of treatment	Controlled	Controlled	Controlled	Controlled
11. Compensatory rivalry by the control group	Not applicable	Not applicable	Not applicable	Not applicable
12. Compensatory equalization	Not applicable	Not applicable	Not applicable	Not applicable

Note. This table is meant only as a general guideline. Decisions with regard to threats to internal validity must be made after the specifics of an investigation are known and understood. Thus, interpretations of internal validity threats must be made on a study-by-study basis.

with changes in other behaviors). Consider a multiple-baseline design across behaviors. Suppose a researcher is investigating different methods of math instruction. The researcher defines two separate behaviors he/she is going to measure. The behaviors include adding "2" to other numbers (e.g., 2 + 1, 2 + 2, 2 + 3, etc., up to 2 + 9) and adding "3" to other numbers (e.g., 3 + 1, 3 + 2, 3 + 3, etc., up to 3 + 9). The researcher collects baseline data on each of the skills and implements the intervention by adding "2" to numbers 1 to 9. Adding "3" to numbers 1 to 9 continues in baseline. The intervention involves using blocks or manipulative objects to solve the problems. The skill of adding "2" to other numbers improves quickly and substantially. However, adding "3" to other numbers also improves. From a teaching standpoint, this may appear beneficial. However, because the skills of *adding 2* and *adding 3* are not independent, experimental control is weakened. In fact, since the skills are dependent on the same underlying math operation, the two skills improve together.

Many times, the behaviors being measured do not look the same, and one assumes that they are members of different response classes. That is, they are likely to be independent. On some occasions, behaviors may appear very different but become members of the same response class. A *response class* is a group of responses that predictably occur together (Cooper et al., 2007). Let's say a researcher wants to investigate effects of imitation training on behaviors of young children with developmental disabilities (e.g., Ledford & Wolery, 2011). After baseline, the researcher plans to implement imitation training across behaviors, such as touching one's nose, standing up from a seated position, and saying "hello." The behaviors appear different enough. But the researcher delivers an edible reinforcer after the child touches her nose following the researcher's demonstration. From that point forward, the child not only touches her nose after every demonstration but she also imitates the researcher's model in standing up from a chair and saying "hello," even when no reinforcer is provided. The researcher has become a discriminative stimulus, because he provided a reinforcer following the child's imitative response. Seemingly different behaviors are now part of the same response class. The independent variable (reinforcement for imitation) had unintended effects of increasing behaviors (standing from a chair and saying "hello") that were still in baseline. Although the child may now acquire imitative skills rapidly, the researcher can no longer demonstrate independence across behaviors.

When researchers are using a multiple-baseline design across participants, the improvements seen in the behavior of one participant may also be seen in other participants. This improvement may occur when a participant sees another participant displaying the skill and imitates the model, or when participants talk to one another. Consider teaching a particular skill such as problem solving to a class of second graders. The students are taught math strategies to use during story problems. The students display improved skills in answering math story problems that correspond to their problem-solving training. The second graders go to recess on a daily basis. On the same playground is another second-grade class that is still in baseline. The students from the first class tell the students from the second class the great things they are learning from their teacher. They tell the other students that they are learning problem-solving strategies to help with difficult math problems and are doing better as a result. The class still in baseline has been exposed to some part of the intervention. It is possible, although remote, that the class in baseline has learned enough to affect skill in problem solving and, in turn, exhibits skills in solving math story problems. Again, we have a problem with diffusion of treatment, since the participants are not independent. Researchers must attempt to ensure that their participants have as little contact with others or remain as independent as possible.

Researchers must also ensure independence of behaviors when using a multiple-baseline design across settings. There are more potential problems with this design. There may be diffusion of treatment when a participant fails to discriminate between conditions in place in one classroom and another. For example, suppose a researcher is investigating the effects of a management program for a seventh-grade student displaying aggressive outbursts. The student is taught relaxation exercises to use when he

gets angry. The researcher hopes that getting the student to concentrate on doing something else besides the aggressive act when angry will help to decrease the frequency of aggressive episodes. The researcher implements the intervention in Period 1 while keeping the behavior in baseline in Period 2. During the relaxation training, the student's aggressive behavior begins to decrease. The aggressive episodes also begin to decrease in Period 2. From a practical standpoint, what has happened is great. The student is behaving more acceptably in Period 2, without being exposed to the intervention. However, from an experimental perspective, the student's improved behavior is a problem. The behavior in Period 1 is not independent of the behavior in Period 2.

Generalization or transfer of treatment effects in this case harm the internal validity of the investigation. Again, we have diffusion of treatment. The intervention effects "leaked" into Period 2. Essentially, the researcher has an A-B design with all of its problems (see Figure 12.5). Researchers must make sure that the settings differ substantially from one another, so that independence is achieved, or they must aid the participant in discriminating when the intervention is in effect and when it is not, such as telling the student or posting this information.

Amount of Data Overlap. The amount of data overlap is important in multiple-baseline designs. As with a baseline in a withdrawal design, there should be a minimum of three stable data points or three data points moving in a countertherapeutic direction to show a trend. This is also true with the baseline in a multiple-baseline design. However, one additional feature with multiple baselines adds to the complexity of condition length. The successive baselines (e.g., each one after the initial baseline) during the intervention of the previous behavior should have at least three data points, in other words, a minimum of three overlapping data points for the first baseline, and a minimum of three for the second baseline plus three additional data points of overlap during the intervention of the first behavior. In all, there should be a minimum of six data points for the second baseline.

Figure 12.6(a) shows a multiple-baseline design across participants in which there is

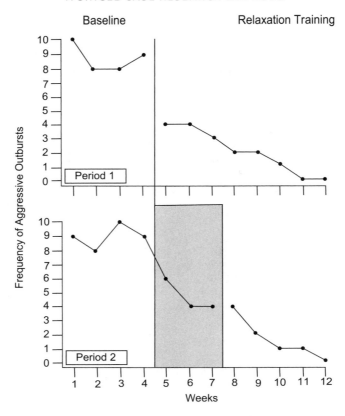

FIGURE 12.5. The frequency of aggressive outbursts across baseline and relaxation training conditions for Periods 1 and 2.

only one data point of overlap. Self-monitoring starts in Session 5 for Paul. Look straight down to Susan's data. She remains in baseline for Session 5 but then receives the self-monitoring intervention in Session 6 (see gray area showing overlap between baselines). There is only one point of overlap when comparing the self-monitoring condition for Paul and the baseline condition for Susan. Only one session of overlap between baselines can hinder the experimental demonstration of the effects of the independent variable. Draw the condition line straight down from the previous participant. The control comes from demonstrating that the previous participant's behavior would not have changed if the intervention were not implemented. This demonstration comes from the other participant's behavior remaining stable. The least amount of data needed to detect a trend is three data points. Thus, the way researchers can demonstrate

stability or a countertherapeutic trend is to generate three data points. An argument that can be made about the data in Figure 12.6(a) is that one data point is not enough to demonstrate that the first behavior would have gone unchanged if the intervention were not provided.

Figure 12.6(b) shows the overlap of three data points (see the gray area of Susan's behavior). This overlap is clearly a better demonstration of experimental control, since a therapeutic trend is not detected in the following behavior. Thus, when interpreting the data of a multiple-baseline design, critical research consumers must look at the amount of data overlap, as well as the trend in the data for the behavior(s) that follows.

Number of Baselines. In order to have a multiple-baseline design, researchers must have at least two baselines. However, the question to ask is whether two baselines are sufficient to

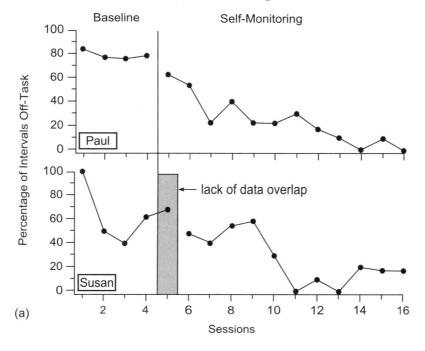

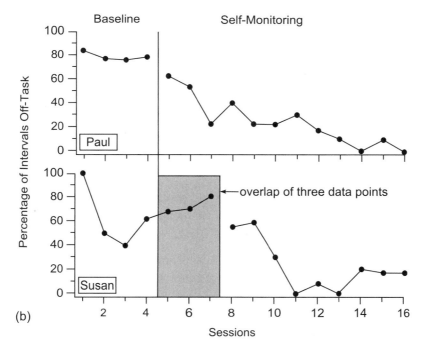

FIGURE 12.6. (a) Percentage of intervals off-task across baseline and self-monitoring conditions for Paul and Susan. (b) Percentage of intervals off-task across baseline and self-monitoring conditions for Paul and Susan.

demonstrate experimental control. In order to answer this question, we must first look at how experimental control comes from the multiple-baseline design. As stated in the previous section, we must project the data down from the previous behavior(s); see Figure 12.6(b). Notice that we must infer whether the behavior would have remained at baseline levels if the intervention had not taken place. On the other hand, in the withdrawal design, the participant serves as his/her own control. We can claim that the behavior would have stayed the same or changed little since the behavior returns to near baseline levels. The amount of inference is considerably less with the withdrawal design than with the multiple-baseline design. For this reason, the withdrawal design is considered to have a higher level of internal validity than the multiple-baseline design (Barlow et al., 2008). Multiple-baseline designs are weaker, because the participant does not serve as his/her own control; different behaviors, participants, or settings that follow the initial baseline serve as the control.

Recall that a multiple-baseline design is simply a series of A-B designs. The experimental control of an A-B design is not considered to be especially strong (see Chapter 11). However, when a multiple-baseline design is implemented, the A-B designs are combined so that the baselines begin at the same time but the interventions occur at different times. Thus, the number of baselines is critical for the demonstration of experimental control. The chances that history or some other extraneous variable caused the change in the independent variable is fairly high with the A-B design; see Figure 12.7(a). The chances that an extraneous variable caused the results with a multiple-baseline design across two behaviors, participants, or settings is lessened, because it is less likely that the same extraneous event caused the observed changes for behaviors/participants/settings at different points in time; see Figure 12.7(b). The chances that an extraneous event caused the changes in a multiple-baseline design across three behaviors, participants, or settings are even less; see Figure 12.7(c). Finally, the chances that an extraneous variable caused the changes in a multiple-baseline design across four behaviors, participants, or settings, are much lower; see Figure 12.7(d).

In summary, the larger the number of baselines, the higher the level of experimental control, simply because the probability that an extraneous variable caused the observed changes in each of the behaviors becomes less likely the more behaviors, participants, or settings we have. Barlow et al. (2008) recommend that there be a minimum of three to four baselines, and Kazdin (2003) recommends more than three baselines to clarify the effects of the independent variable.

Thus, it would seem that four or more baselines should be the goal of researchers. However, there is a major problem with a higher number of baselines; that is, the more baselines, the longer the later behaviors remain in baseline or are kept from receiving the intervention. For example, if we use the three data point overlap rule, the first behavior is in baseline for at least three sessions, the second is in baseline for six sessions, the third occurs for nine sessions, and the fourth for 12 sessions. Thus, there is a minimum of 12 sessions for the fourth baseline. If there is any variability or if a behavior is moving in a therapeutic direction, the researcher may need to add even more sessions to examine for stable data. Thus, there are times when less than three data points of overlap are used, or when fewer than four baselines are included. Critical research consumers should remember the following general guidelines: The fewer baselines, the weaker the experimental control; the fewer the number of data points with overlap, the weaker the experimental control.

A further advantage of more baselines is that if we have, say, five baselines and the intervention does not work as intended for one of these, or if the behavior begins to improve before the intervention, there are still four more baselines to demonstrate experimental control (see the data in Figure 12.8 for Amy). Of course, the experimental control demonstration is weakened in such a situation. The more "failures" in the multiple-baseline design (e.g., two or more behaviors failing to improve or improving too soon), the weaker the control. Consider the researcher who has only two baselines and the second behavior does not respond to intervention or improve before the intervention. The experimental control is weak, since the researcher is left with an A-B design. On the one

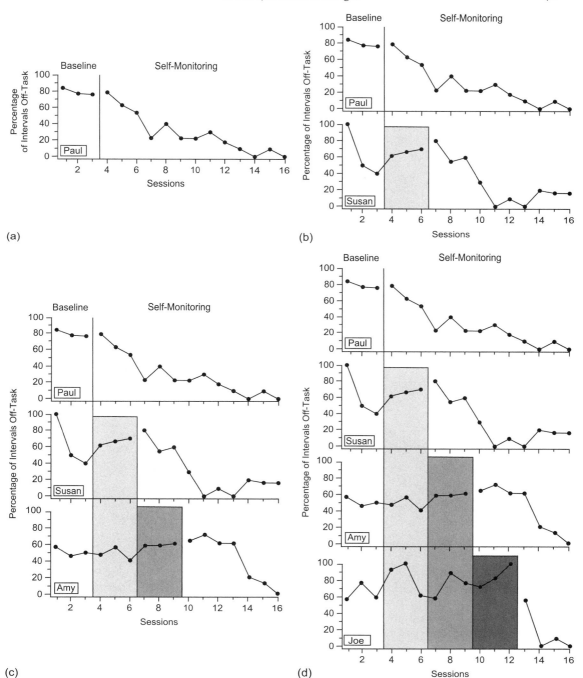

FIGURE 12.7. (a) Percentage of intervals off-task across baseline and self-monitoring conditions. (b) Percentage of intervals off-task across baseline and self-monitoring conditions for Paul and Susan. (c) Percentage of intervals off-task across baseline and self-monitoring conditions for Paul, Susan, and Amy. (d) Percentage of intervals off-task across baseline and self-monitoring conditions for Paul, Susan, and Joe.

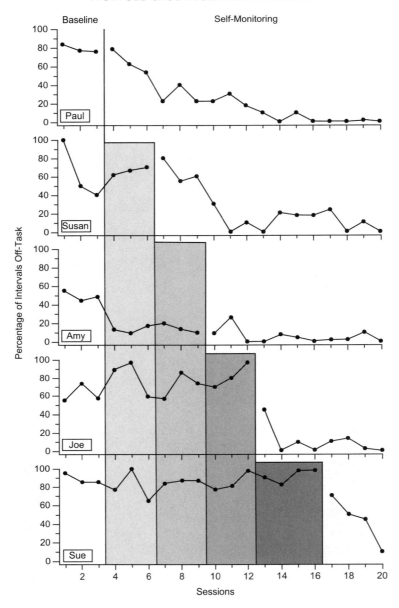

FIGURE 12.8. Percentage of intervals off-task across baseline and self-monitoring conditions for Paul, Susan, Amy, Joe, and Sue.

hand, there are advantages to many baselines; on the other hand, the amount of time needed to conduct several baselines may be prohibitive. However, if researchers use only two baselines, the levels and rapidity of change and the stability of the data must be especially clear (Kazdin, 2003).

Level and Rapidity of Change. The concept of level and rapidity of change is the same as that in the withdrawal design. However, the level and rapidity of change are critical for all of the behaviors in a multiple-baseline design. For example, Figure 12.9 shows a multiple-baseline design across participants.

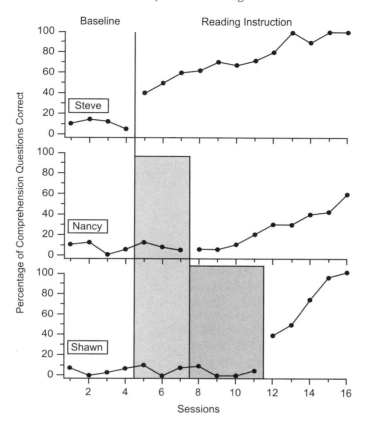

FIGURE 12.9. Percentage of reading comprehension questions correct across baseline and reading instruction conditions for Steve, Nancy, and Shawn.

The first participant showed rapid and significant improvements in reading. The second participant had difficulty obtaining the skill, and acquisition was slower and not as pronounced at first. The third student had a similar response to that of the first participant. The behavior change was rapid and substantial. Notice that if the researcher only had two baselines, the experimental control would have been much weaker. Essentially, with two baselines and the data presented in Figure 12.9, the researcher would have had an A-B design. Thus, the change should be substantial and rapid for each of the behaviors if strong experimental control is to be achieved.

Withdrawal. One method to increase the internal validity of multiple-baseline designs is to withdraw the intervention from each of the behaviors/participants/settings. In other words, we would return to the baseline condition after seeing an effect during the intervention condition. Essentially, the multiple baseline remains by staggering the implementation of conditions, but each baseline also includes a withdrawal condition. Of course, all of the disadvantages associated with withdrawal designs are present when a return-to-baseline condition is implemented. Return-to-baseline levels of behavior may not occur for skills acquisitions; it may be unethical in some instances to remove the intervention; or it may not be ethically defensible to end on a baseline condition (of course, this problem is easily rectified with an additional "B" condition). A primary reason researchers would opt for a multiple-baseline design over a withdrawal design is the difficulties associated with the withdrawal design.

External Validity

The external validity of multiple-baseline designs can best be assessed by reviewing what is meant by external validity. *External validity* is essentially the generalization of the treatment effects to other people (population validity) or different situations (ecological validity). There is no standard that suggests how many participants the researchers must have, or how many settings or measures, to claim external validity. Researchers frequently determine the number of participants required to increase power; however, this is an internal validity concern, not specifically an external one.

Recall the primary problem with the withdrawal design—there is typically one participant in one setting with one behavior of concern. Of course, as indicated previously, single-case studies are not limited to one participant. However, the withdrawal design generally has a lack of external validity. The primary advantage that multiple-baseline designs have over the withdrawal design is that they represent the real world more closely. We can have several participants at one time as in a multiple-baseline design across participants; several settings available, as in a multiple-baseline design across settings; and several behaviors under investigation at one time, as in a multiple-baseline design across behaviors; or we can have behaviors not under explicit investigation (i.e., not a primary dependent variable) assessed for carryover or generalization effects, as in a multiple-probe design (Kazdin, 2003). Thus, the external validity of multiple-baseline designs (including the multiple-probe design) is stronger than that of the withdrawal design. However, the primary purpose of multiple-baseline designs is to control for threats to internal validity, not external validity. We should view multiple-baseline designs as alternatives to withdrawal designs in determining the effects of the independent variable on the dependent variable, not as a method of demonstrating the generalizability of treatment effects. Single-case researchers attempt to determine the generalization of treatment effects through replications (see Chapter 1). Table 12.2 summarizes the major threats to external validity of the designs discussed in this chapter.

Recall the research question about youth learning grocery skills posed in an earlier chapter? Read on to see how your design compares to how the actual study was designed.

Research Example: Multiple-Baseline Design

A multiple-baseline design across participants to teach grocery store purchasing skills to students with intellectual disabilities used a computer-based instructional program (Hansen & Morgan, 2008). Three participants with intellectual disabilities were chosen from a high school classroom. A pretest determined that these students usually responded incorrectly on steps involved in purchasing items from a community grocery (i.e., selecting the shortest checkout line; placing items on conveyor; providing the correct number of dollar bills, plus one, to the cashier; responding to the cashier's question about bagging preference; and taking coin change, receipt, and groceries). The study took place in a high school computer laboratory and community supermarkets. Dependent measures included percentages of correct scores on computer-based instruction assessments and correct scores in community grocery store probes (i.e., assessment in grocery stores but without on-site training). The independent variable was the effect of a computer-based instructional program on grocery shopping skills. The computer-based video program showed correct and incorrect ways to shop and to purchase groceries (Ayres, Langone, Boon, & Norman, 2006). The program comprised 36 videos showing different cashiers asking for various amounts of money up to $9.93. As shown in Figure 12.10, baseline measures comprised grocery store probes (black squares) exclusively. Correct responses across the five purchasing steps ranged from 60% ("Mr. Red") to 0% ("Mr. Green"). Training in computer-based instruction (white triangles) started with Mr. Red and was implemented successively across the remaining participants. Performance on computer-based instruction assessments started and maintained at 100% for two participants (Mr. Red and Mr. Green) and increased over time for Mr. Blue. Grocery store probes showed similar performance, with percentage correct occurring higher than baseline for all three participants and reaching

TABLE 12.2. Threats to External Validity Associated with Multiple-Baseline Designs

Threat	Multiple-baseline design across . . .			
	Behaviors	Participants	Settings	Multiple-probe design
1. Generalization across participants	Possible concern	Possible concern[a]	Possible concern	Possible concern
2. Interaction of participant-specific variables and treatment effects	Possible concern	Possible concern[a]	Possible concern	Possible concern
3. Verification of independent variable possible concern	Possible concern	Possible concern	Possible concern	Possible concern
4. Multiple treatment interference	Controlled	Controlled	Controlled	Controlled
5. Novelty and disruption effects	Possible concern	Possible concern	Possible concern	Possible concern
6. Hawthorne effect	Possible concern	Possible concern	Possible concern	Possible concern
7. Experimenter effects	Possible concern	Possible concern	Possible concern	Possible concern
8. Pretest sensitization	Not applicable	Not applicable	Not applicable	Not applicable
9. Posttest sensitization	Not applicable	Not applicable	Not applicable	Not applicable
10. Interaction of time of measurement and treatment effects	Possible concern	Possible concern	Possible concern	Possible concern
11. Measurement of the dependent variable	Possible concern[b]	Possible concern	Possible concern	Possible concern
12. Interaction of history and treatment effects	Possible concern	Possible concern	Possible concern	Possible concern

Note. This table is meant only as a general guideline. Decisions with regard to threats to external validity must be made after the specifics of an investigation are known and understood. Thus, interpretations of external validity threats must be made on a study-by-study basis.

[a]Could be stronger than other single-case designs depending on the number of participants; however, most likely, the participants are not representative of the general population.

[b]Could be stronger since there are multiple behaviors being measured.

100% soon after computer-based instruction was implemented. In probes of different stores with various configurations of checkout stands (and without training), all three participants performed well. Upon return to the original grocery store in a 30-day follow-up, participants continued to perform at 100%.

WHEN SHOULD RESEARCHERS USE EACH MULTIPLE-BASELINE DESIGN?

We can choose from several options when conducting single-case research. To determine the type of design to use, we must consider the research question(s). For example, suppose we were interested in investigating the effects of a behavior intervention program on an individual with autism spectrum disorder. The procedure that we wish to use allows the individual to engage in self-stimulatory behavior (e.g., rocking back and forth) if he first sits still for 30 seconds. In this way, we make rocking contingent on sitting still. In this case, we are only concerned with one particular individual and one behavior. Suppose we were also concerned with the intervention effects across several settings, such as school and home. Also, suppose that teachers and parents are concerned with the return to baseline that would likely result

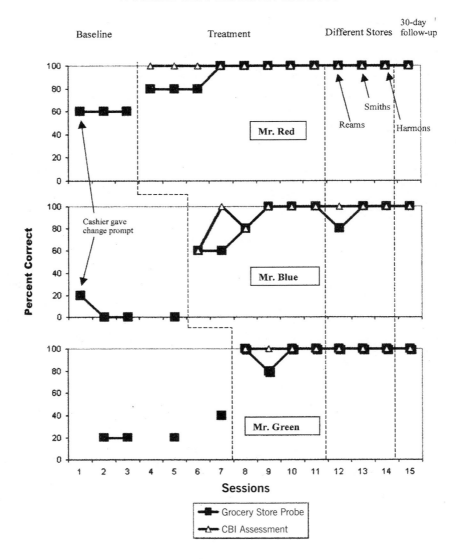

FIGURE 12.10. Grocery store and CBI performance mastery assessments in baseline, treatment, different grocery stores, and 30-day follow-up. From Hansen, D. L., & Morgan, R. L. (2008). Teaching grocery store purchasing skills to students with intellectual disabilities using a computer-based instruction program. *Education and Training in Developmental Disabilities, 43,* 431–442. Copyright 2008 by the Council for Exceptional Children, Division on Autism and Developmental Disabilities. Reprinted by permission.

in a withdrawal design. The most appropriate design would clearly be the multiple-baseline design across settings.

Now suppose we are interested in teaching self-instructional skills to students in a mathematics class. We hypothesize that the self-instructions would help students solve problems, because they would acquire a

metacognitive technique that would aid in the prompting of appropriate math calculations. The focus at this point is in only the mathematics skill and in only one setting. We have three classrooms at the same level of mathematics instruction. Thus, the most appropriate single-case design would be the multiple-baseline design across participants. We would conduct baseline measures in all three classrooms and implement the self-instructional training in a staggered fashion.

Consider a situation in which we are concerned with the effect of teacher's behavior on the performance of students in a class. We are concerned with one set of students, one teacher, and only one setting. However, teachers display several behaviors that can affect the behavior of students. For example, type of instructions provided, error corrections used, and frequency and type of praise can all influence student behavior. Thus, we define three instructional behaviors of interest: appropriate instructions, effective error correction methods, and meaningful praise. In this example the most appropriate single-case design is the multiple-baseline design across behaviors (in this case, teacher behaviors).

Finally, assume that a researcher is interested in measuring the effects of learning letter–sound combinations on the comprehension skills of young children (age 5–6 years). Several children from different classrooms are involved in the investigation. The researcher is interested in only one primary dependent variable (i.e., letter–sound combinations) in only one setting (i.e., a public elementary school). However, the generalization of learning letter–sound combinations is of concern. Thus, the researcher decides to use a multiple-probe design (actually, the design would be a combination of a multiple-baseline design across participants and a multiple-probe design), with the probes conducted on comprehension skills. The researcher does not wish to intervene on comprehension directly but to see whether learning letter–sound combinations aids in the understanding of reading material. Thus, as conceived by the researcher, comprehension may be affected by, or be a generalized skill of, letter–sound combinations. The

researcher does not wish to conduct frequent and consistent measurements of passages comprehension because he is concerned with practice effects. Therefore, the multiple-probe design is most appropriate.

As shown in the previous scenarios, the questions posed by the researchers are critical in determining the most appropriate single-case design to use. Additionally, ethical or practical concerns; the availability of other behaviors, participants, or settings; the possibility of carryover effects; or the likelihood of practice effects due to frequent measures will help to determine the best design. For example, if there are ethical or practical concerns, a multiple-baseline design should be considered, not a withdrawal design. If only one participant is available, a multiple-baseline design across participants is not appropriate. With several participants available but in only one setting, a multiple-baseline design across settings would not be possible. If there is only one behavior of concern, a multiple-baseline across behaviors would not be of interest. If carryover effects or diffusion of treatment due to participants' communication with one another, generalization of behavior change across settings, or non-independence of behaviors are likely, multiple-baseline designs are probably not appropriate. Finally, if there is a likelihood of practice effects, a multiple-probe design is appropriate. Ultimately, the decision as to which design to use lies with the researcher; however, the decision must not be made lightly. The decision could increase or decrease internal validity.

The decisions described here pertain to only multiple-baseline and multiple-probe designs. Researchers with research questions that suggest use of single-case designs should also consider withdrawal designs (Chapter 11) and additional designs described in this chapter.

SUMMARY

❖ A multiple-baseline design is an experimental design that starts with measurement of two or more behaviors in a baseline condition, followed by application of an independent variable to one of the behaviors while baseline conditions remain in effect for other behaviors. The independent variable is then applied

in a sequential fashion to other behaviors. Multiple-baseline designs may be preferable to withdrawal designs because of four main disadvantages with withdrawal designs: (1) Some behaviors were changed as a function of the intervention; (2) behaviors may not immediately return to baseline levels; (3) researchers may find it unethical to withdraw intervention and return to baseline conditions; and (4) staff cooperation may be a problem due to the previous ethical considerations.

❖ The visual display of data in multiple-baseline designs is similar to withdrawal and associated designs in that descriptors (i.e., dependent measure, baseline, independent variable, time measurement, data points, data paths, condition change lines, and figure captions) are displayed in the same manner. However, instead of having one graph, the multiple-baseline display involves placing individual graphs on top of each other.

❖ Multiple-baseline designs can be thought of as a series of A-B designs and have several advantages over withdrawal designs: (1) There is not a requirement to remove or withdraw the intervention and, thus, no need to return to baseline levels in the future; (2) multiple-baseline designs are in many ways more versatile than withdrawal designs because they apply to a wide array of socially significant interventions; and (3) multiple-baseline designs allow for the replication of intervention effects across behaviors, participants, and/or settings.

❖ Multiple-baseline designs have several weaknesses: (1) the need for two or more baselines, (2) possible lengthy baselines for some participants, (3) less experimental control than withdrawal designs, and (4) more design considerations.

❖ The multiple-baseline design across behaviors requires at least two separate behaviors that are independent of one another. The researcher conducts measures on two or more behaviors of one participant in one setting.

❖ The multiple-baseline design across participants is similar to the multiple-baseline design across behaviors in that two or more baselines are required. However, the researcher measures a single behavior across two or more participants in one setting.

❖ The multiple-baseline design across settings is similar to the previous two designs except that the researcher measures a single behavior or a single participant across two or more settings.

❖ A multiple-probe design is essentially a multiple-baseline design in which the measures are not collected on a frequent basis; it overcomes the problem of using repeated measurements by probing (assessing) the behavior intermittently. A multiple-probe design also allows for the assessment of the generalization/transfer and maintenance of learned skills.

❖ When assessing the internal validity of multiple-baseline designs, several concerns must be taken into consideration: (1) condition length; (2) independence of behaviors; (3) the amount of overlap of the data; (4) the number of baselines; (5) independence of the behaviors, participants, or settings; and (6) and the level and rapidity of change.

❖ The external validity of multiple-baseline designs (including the multiple-probe design) is stronger than that of the withdrawal design. However, the primary purpose of multiple-baseline designs is to control for threats to internal, not external, validity. Single-case researchers attempt to determine the generalization of treatment effects through replications.

❖ The selection of a multiple-baseline design depends on the research question and the availability of behaviors, participants, and settings. If the effect of an intervention on two or more behaviors is of interest, a multiple-baseline design across behaviors may be appropriate as long as the behaviors are independent of each other. If the effect of an intervention across two or more participants is of interest, a multiple-baseline design across participants may be appropriate as long as two or more participants are available and independent of each other. If the effect of an intervention on a behavior across two or more settings is of interest, a multiple-baseline design across settings may be appropriate if two or more settings are available and the behavior is independent across the settings. If non-independence of behaviors, carryover effects or diffusion of treatment due to participants' communication with one another, or generalization of behavior change across settings are likely, multiple-baseline designs are probably not appropriate. If there is a likelihood of practice effects, a multiple-probe design would be appropriate.

DISCUSSION QUESTIONS

1. How could you use the three types of multiple-baseline designs (i.e., across behaviors, participants, and settings) to examine the effectiveness of using study guides? Explain.

2. For each of the multiple-baseline designs in Question 1, draw a graph with fictitious data showing that study guides are effective.

3. Why would you use a multiple-baseline design rather than a withdrawal design? In your answer, describe advantages and disadvantages of multiple-baseline and withdrawal designs.

4. How is experimental control achieved with a multiple-baseline design?

5. How can you establish external validity with multiple-baseline designs?

6. All things being equal, are multiple-baseline designs as strong experimentally (i.e., controlling for threats to internal validity) as withdrawal designs? Why or why not?

7. What alternative is available to being exposed to the same measurement several times during baseline? Explain how this alternative allows exposure to the same measurement.

8. How could you increase the interval validity of multiple-baseline designs to make the level of control the same as withdrawal designs? What are some problems with doing this?

9. What are the concerns surrounding the following issues?
   a. condition length
   b. independence of behaviors
   c. the amount of overlap of the data
   d. the number of baselines
   e. independence of the behaviors, participants, or settings
   f. the level and rapidity of change

10. For the six issues listed in Question 9, which issue(s) are a specific concern for multiple-baseline designs?

ILLUSTRATIVE EXAMPLE

Improving the Writing Performance of Struggling Writers in Second Grade

Torri Ortiz Lienemann
University of Nebraska–Lincoln

Steve Graham
Vanderbilt University

Beth Leader-Janssen and Robert Reid
University of Nebraska–Lincoln

An important goal in preventing writing disabilities is to provide effective early instruction to at-risk students to maximize their writing development. This study examined whether or not explicitly teaching six at-risk second-grade writers, including children with disabilities, how to plan and draft stories would improve their story writing as well as their recall of narrative reading material. The self-regulated strategy development model was used to teach these strategies; the impact of this instruction was evaluated via a multiple-baseline design. Instruction had a positive impact on students' writing, as their stories were longer, more complete, and, with the exception of one student, qualitatively better. Instructional effects also transferred to the recall of narrative reading material for four of the six students. These findings were generally maintained over time.

Writing is a difficult and demanding task. It is a conscious and self-directed activity, involving the intelligent use of a variety of mental operations and skills to satisfy the writer's goals and meet the needs of the reader (Graham, in press b). As a result, a writer must deal with many demands at once. As Hayes and Flower (1980) noted, skilled writers caught in the act look very much like busy switchboard operators as they try to juggle a number of demands on their attention simultaneously (e.g., making plans, drawing ideas from memory, developing concepts, or creating an image of the reader). In fact, skilled writing does "not simply unfold automatically and effortlessly in the manner of a well learned motor skill . . . writing anything but the most routine and brief pieces is the mental equivalent of digging ditches" (Kellogg, 1993, p. 17). It involves a high degree of self-regulation, cognitive effort, and attentional control (Graham & Harris, 2003).

Writing is a difficult and demanding task that many children find difficult to master. This observation is supported by data from the National Assessment of Educational Progress (Persky, Daane, & Jin, 2003). Three out of every four 4th-, 8th-, and 12th-grade students achieve only partial mastery of the writing skills and knowledge they need at their respective grade levels. Only 1 in 100 students attains "advanced" writing skills. Difficulties mastering the writing process are even more prevalent for students with special needs or disabilities (e.g., Graham, Harris, & Larsen, 2001; Harris & Graham, 1999; Resta & Eliot, 1994). These students' papers contain fewer ideas, are more poorly organized, and are of lower quality compared with compositions produced by their typically achieving peers (Graham & Harris, 2002).

Children's difficulties with learning to write led the National Commission on Writing (NCW; 2003) to recommend that writing become a central focus of school reform efforts, as students' educational and occupational success will be impeded if they do not learn to write well. The NCW's efforts have convinced both the general public and policymakers of the importance of writing (see also NCW, 2004, 2005), as well as the need to take action now. The success of reform efforts in writing, however, depends in large part on the application of instructional practices that are effective in enhancing writing development. The identification of effective instructional practices for young beginning writers, particularly students at risk for writing difficulties and students with special needs, is especially critical. Addressing these children's writing problems early in the educational process is advantageous for two reasons (Graham, Harris,

& Mason, 2005). First, waiting until later grades to address literacy problems that originated in the primary grades has not been very successful (Slavin, Karweit, & Madden, 1989). Second, early intervention should help to maximize the writing development of young at-risk writers, minimizing the number of students who develop long-term difficulties with writing.

One approach to early writing intervention with at-risk students and children with special needs is to provide additional or specialized instruction in basic text transcription skills, such as handwriting and spelling. These efforts have resulted in improvements in the writing output, writing quality, and sentence construction skills of these children (Berninger et al., 1997; Berninger et al., 1998; Graham, Harris, & Fink, 2000; Graham, Harris, & Fink-Chorzempa, 2002; Jones & Christensen, 1999). A second approach is captured by the work of Englert and her colleagues (1995). They examined the effectiveness of a curricular approach that tied writing and reading instruction together, made writing and reading strategies visible, involved teacher–student discussion about these strategies, provided procedural facilitators (such as a semantic map) around which this dialogue occurred, and encouraged students to share their knowledge with others. This program had a positive impact on both the reading and writing performance of primary-grade students with mild disabilities. Berninger and her colleagues (Berninger, Abbott, Whitaker, Sylvester, & Nolen, 1995) illustrate a third approach to early intervention. They taught handwriting and spelling to third-grade struggling writers individually and also modeled the composing processes of planning, writing, reviewing, and revising. This had a positive impact on these young students' writing skills.

Another approach to early writing intervention with young struggling writers is illustrated in the work of Graham and Harris (see Graham & Harris, 2005a). Although their primary instructional focus was on teaching children strategies for carrying out specific composing processes (e.g., planning), they also taught them how to apply the target strategies, better understand the writing task, and regulate their behavior during writing. Their instruction was further designed to enhance specific aspects of motivation, such as self-efficacy and effort. This approach is consistent with theories on how competence and expertise develop in subject-matter domains (see Alexander, 1992; Pintrich & Schunk, 1996). These conceptualizations emphasize that learning depends, in large part, on changes that occur in strategic knowledge, domain-specific knowledge, and motivation.

This early writing intervention research by Graham and Harris (2005a) draws on their instructional work with older struggling writers (Grades 4–8). Starting in the 1980s (Harris & Graham, 1985), they began investigating the effectiveness of an instructional approach they initially called *self-instructional strategy training*. They later changed the name to *self-regulated strategy development* (SRSD; Harris & Graham, 1996, 1999) to capture the emphasis their instruction placed on students' development of self-regulatory skills. SRSD involves explicitly teaching students strategies for accomplishing specific writing tasks, such as composing a persuasive essay. Students are also taught any skills or knowledge (e.g., the attributes and elements of a convincing argument) needed to apply the strategies effectively. Students further learn to use a variety of self-regulation procedures (self-instructions, goal setting, self-monitoring, and self-reinforcement) to enhance motivation and regulate their use of the target strategies, the writing task, and their behavior during writing. The emphasis of this instruction is on students' independent, effective, and flexible use of the target strategies. Consequently, procedures for promoting maintenance and generalization are embedded throughout the instructional regime.

The effectiveness of SRSD was established in several recent meta-analyses. In a comprehensive review of writing intervention literature with students in Grades 4 through 12, Graham and Perrin (in press) reported that SRSD had a strong and positive impact on the quality of students' writing. The average weighted effect size was 1.14 (based on eight large-group studies; five of these were conducted with struggling writers). In fact, SRSD yielded the highest average weighted effect size of any of the writing interventions that were studied. These findings were replicated in another meta-analysis with students at all grade levels (Graham, in press a).

Because SRSD had been successful with older children, including students with disabilities, Graham and Harris (2005a) believed that it might be equally successful with younger students who were at risk for writing difficulties. In an initial study, they taught pairs of third-grade struggling writers (about one third of the students had special needs) strategies for planning and drafting a story and a persuasive essay (Graham et al., 2005).

They made some modifications in their instructional materials and procedures to make them more appropriate for younger students. They further sought to find out if the addition of a peer-support component to promote maintenance and generalization of strategy use would enhance performance. When compared with a control condition involving process writing instruction, SRSD with and without the peer-support component increased students' knowledge of writing and improved their performance on the two instructed genres (stories and persuasive writing) as well as on one uninstructed genre (informative writing). The addition of the peer support component to the SRSD approach resulted in an increase in students' knowledge of writing and facilitated transfer to two uninstructed genres (informative and personal narrative).

Saddler, Moran, Graham, and Harris (2004) examined the effectiveness of SRSD instruction with even younger children as they taught three pairs of second-grade struggling writers strategies for planning and drafting a story. They evaluated the effects of this treatment using a multiple-baseline design. As a result of SRSD instruction, students' stories became longer, more complete, and qualitatively better. The positive effects of instruction were generally maintained over time and also generalized to a similar but uninstructed genre (personal narrative writing).

A study on a larger scale was then conducted to examine the effects of SRSD instruction, as well as the additive benefits of the peer support component, when teaching strategies for planning and drafting stories and persuasive essays to pairs of second-grade struggling writers, about one fifth of whom had special needs (Harris, Graham, & Mason, in press). The findings from this study generally replicated those from the earlier study by Graham et al. (2005) that involved slightly older children. When compared with process writing, SRSD instruction with and without peer support increased students' knowledge of writing and improved their writing on the two instructed genres (stories and persuasive essays) as well as on two uninstructed ones (informative writing and personal narrative). The inclusion of the peer support component further enhanced children's writing, as it helped them write better papers for all tested genres (story, persuasive, informative, and personal narrative).

This study replicates and extends the early writing intervention research of Graham and

Harris. Like the Saddler et al. (2004) investigation, six struggling writers in second grade were taught strategies for writing and drafting stories. We extend the work of Saddler et al., however, by examining the effectiveness of this instruction with a more diverse set of struggling writers. In the prior investigation, the primary problem for most of the participating students was difficulty with writing (two students had mild speech and language difficulties, with one of them experiencing difficulty with reading). In our study, writing was a problem for all of the students, each child had difficulty with reading (according to their teachers and confirmed by a norm-referenced reading measure for five of the six students), and all but two of the children experienced other challenges, such as learning disabilities, language difficulties, orthopedic impairments, and attention-deficit/hyperactivity disorder (ADHD)/reactive attachment disorder/bipolar disorder. Although the Graham et al. (2005) and Harris et al. (in press) large-group investigations included students with special needs, it was not possible to tease out the effects of SRSD on these particular children, as the unit of analysis was the average score for each student pair (pairs may or may not have included students with special needs). As De La Paz and Graham (1997) noted, research is needed that examines the effectiveness of SRSD with a broader range of students.

We also extended previous work in terms of the context in which our study took place. All of the previous early intervention investigations by Graham and Harris (Graham et al., 2005; Harris et al., in press; Saddler et al., 2004) took place in urban schools that were overwhelmingly populated by African American children from economically disadvantaged families. This study occurred in a rural setting in a school with mostly European American children who were not economically disadvantaged. As Horner et al. (2005) noted, the external validity of research is enhanced through replication of the effects across different participants and conditions.

The current study also differed from the previous investigations in terms of the type of writing instruction that occurred in the participating schools. In Graham et al. (2005), Harris et al. (in press), and Saddler et al. (2004), the schools used a process approach to writing instruction that emphasized the importance of writing processes, such as planning, drafting, and revising. Thus,

students already had considerable exposure to the importance of planning and drafting (the processes emphasized in the previous studies). In the current study, the participating school employed a different approach to teaching writing to young children, which involved teaching basic writing skills, such as handwriting and spelling, with little emphasis on the process of writing. Establishing that SRSD was effective in a more restrictive writing environment would provide additional evidence of its external validity (Horner et al., 2005).

A final and especially important extension made by the current study involved examining whether or not the effects of SRSD instruction on writing resulted in improvements in reading. Part of the planning strategy that students were taught to use involved generating ideas for each of the basic parts of a story (Stein & Glenn, 1979) before writing. Although a number of SRSD studies have used this story grammar strategy (e.g., Danoff, Harris, & Graham, 1993; Graham et al., 2005; Graham & Harris, 1989; Harris et al., in press; Saddler et al., 2004; Sawyer, Graham, & Harris, 1992), no one has examined the possible carryover effects to reading. We anticipated that learning about the parts of a story and how to generate ideas for each of these parts would make students more attentive to these markers when reading narrative material, which would increase their recall of this material. SRSD instruction in writing is likely to be more attractive to teachers if it enhances reading as well as writing.

We further anticipated that SRSD instruction would enhance the length, structure, and quality of the story writing of the participating children. Children with writing disabilities and those at risk for them typically produce incomplete stories of poor quality that contain few ideas (Graham & Harris, 2003). Furthermore, they often minimize the role of planning when they write (Graham, 1990; McCutchen, 1988), converting the writing task into simply telling what they know. Text is generated as ideas come to mind, with each preceding idea serving as the stimulus for the next idea. Consequently, little attention is directed to whole-text organization or the constraints imposed by the genre. The instruction that students received in this study was responsive to these shortcomings, as they were taught how to plan in advance of writing and they learned about the attributes and elements of a good story as well as how to generate ideas for each of these elements.

METHOD

Design

The design used in this study was multiple base-line across participants with multiple probes during baseline and independent performance (Kazdin, 1982). To avoid prolonged baselines, the six participating students were divided into two cohorts, with three students in each cohort. For each cohort, SRSD instruction was systematically and sequentially introduced to one participant at a time. Prior to the introduction of SRSD instruction, each student's writing performance was measured over time to establish a baseline of typical writing performance. A functional relationship between the independent variable and partici-pants' progress was established if the target behav-ior improved only after the completion of SRSD instruction and if the noninstructed participants' performance stayed at or near preintervention lev-els across baseline.

Setting

The study was conducted during the fall semes-ter in a rural elementary school in a midwestern state. The demographics of the school district were as follows: 96% European American, 1% African American, 2% Hispanic, and 1% Asian. A total of 8% of the students received free or reduced-price lunch. Writing instruction for students in second grade consisted of teaching basic skills, such as handwriting and spelling.

Participants

Three second-grade teachers were asked to identify students whom they considered at risk for writing failure and who also struggled with reading. A total of 10 students were identified. These students then completed the *Story Construction* subtest from the *Test of Written Language–3* (TOWL-3; Hammill & Larsen, 1996) to verify that they were at risk for a writing disability. *At risk* was defined as fall-ing at the 25th percentile or below in comparison with the normative test sample. This test assesses a child's ability to write a complete and interest-ing story. Reliability of the test for second-grade children is .89. Four girls and two boys from two second-grade classrooms qualified for the study. Table 1 provides the descriptive information for these students, including their standard scores on the TOWL-3 (a standard score of 8 is equivalent to a score at the 25th percentile) and grade-equivalent scores for the *Gates-MacGinitie Reading Test* (Mac-Ginitie & MacGinitie, 1992). The reading test con-firms that all but one child (Tim) were functioning below grade level in reading.

The first cohort consisted of Tim, Sarah, and Kristina. Tim had not been referred for special education services. Sarah was diagnosed with ADHD, reactive attachment disorder, and bipolar disorder. Medical records also indicated the pos-sibility of fetal alcohol syndrome. On the *Univer-sal Nonverbal Intelligence Test* (UNIT; Bracken & McCallum, 1998), she had a Full Scale IQ of 82. She was receiving special education services for read-ing and language arts. Kristina was identified as

TABLE 1. Student Information

Item	Tim	Sarah	Kristina	Katie	Trevor	Skylar
Age	7 years 11 months	7 years 5 months	8 years 0 months	7 years 3 months	7 years 4 months	7 years 11 months
Race	European American	African American	European American	Hispanic American	European American	European American
Test of Written Language–3 percentile rank	8	7	7	8	8	7
Gates–MacGinitie grade equivalent	Total: 3.2 Comp.: 2.7	Total: 1.6 Comp.: 1.5	Total: 1.5 Comp.: 1.3	Total: 1.4 Comp.: 1.1	Total: 1.8 Comp.: 2.0	Total: 1.6 Comp.: 1.7
IQ	NA	82	100	NA	NA	"Normal"

Note. The mean standard score for the *Test of Written Language–3* (Hammill & Larsen, 1996) is 10 and the standard deviation is 3. Comp. = comprehension; NA = Not Available.

having a learning disability in the area of reading. Her *Wechsler Individual Achievement Test* scores (Psychological Corporation, 2002) were as follows: reading comprehension = 76; word reading = 82; written expression = 87; spelling = 93. This test has a mean of 100 and a standard deviation of 15. Her IQ was 100 as measured by UNIT.

The second cohort consisted of Katie, Trevor, and Skylar. Katie was born in Mexico; German, however, was the language predominately spoken in her home. Katie's teacher had concerns about her language development and had referred her for a language evaluation, but she had not been tested at the time of the study. Trevor has not been referred for special education services. Skylar was identified as having orthopedic impairments due to a stroke she had when she was 3 months old, which resulted in right hemiparesis. She had minimal use of her arm but was very functional with her leg. Her pediatric neurologist had warned that these problems could lead to developmental delay, learning disabilities, or seizures.

Procedure

Students were taught in two cohorts. The 6 participants were randomly assigned to one of the two instructors. Instruction was individually administered by either the first or third author. Both authors have M.Ed. degrees in special education and extensive classroom experience. Prior to implementing the intervention, the instructors received training in the SRSD model and practiced implementing the instructional procedures until they mastered them.

Baseline Probes

During baseline, each child wrote three or more stories to establish pretreatment performance.

Treatment

Instruction was initiated for the first student in each cohort after the children established a stable baseline for number of elements in their stories. Instruction continued until the first child in the cohort demonstrated independent mastery of the strategy, resulting in a story with all of the basic story elements. Instruction did not begin for the next child in the cohort until the first student's independent or posttreatment performance reached a criterion level of 5 story parts (out of a possible 7). These same procedures were used with the third student in each cohort.

Independent Performance

Each student wrote three to four stories immediately following SRSD instruction. These writing probes were completed under the same conditions as during baseline.

Maintenance

Maintenance probes were conducted 2 and 4 weeks after the end of the independent performance phase. These writing probes were completed under the same conditions as baseline and independent performance.

Generalization Reading Probes

To assess generalization related to reading comprehension, students were asked to read and retell narrative stories during baseline, instruction, independent performance, and maintenance phases. All stories were at the students' instructional reading level. The school reading specialist conducted all story retells.

Testing Materials

Story-Writing Prompts

We used the black-and-white line-drawn pictures employed by Saddler et al. (2004) as prompts for writing stories during the baseline, independent performance, and maintenance phases of this study. Each of these pictures had previously been evaluated by a second-grade student and one former second-grade teacher. All of the pictures were judged to be interesting and easy to write about by both the student and the teacher. The story-writing prompts were presented in randomized order. They were also administered in the same order to all participants. When presented with a story-writing prompt, students were asked to look at the picture and write a story. They were told to plan their story, include all the elements of a good story, and write as much as they could.

Generalization Reading Probes

To assess the extent to which SRSD instruction generalized to reading comprehension, a story-retell probe was administered during baseline, instruction, independent performance, and maintenance. Stories from the *Qualitative Reading Inventory* (Leslie & Caldwell, 2001) were modified so that they contained all 7 of the story elements students were taught to use when writing. All stories were at the students' instructional reading level. Participants read the stories and then were asked to retell what had happened. The retell task was administered by the school reading specialist, who was unaware of the study hypotheses and conditions. All retells were transcribed and scored by the first and third authors.

Dependent Measures

Each story was scored for number of story elements, number of words, and overall quality. The generalization reading probes were scored for the number of story elements included.

Number of Story Elements

Number of story elements was scored by tabulating students' inclusion of the following 7 common elements in their papers: main characters, locale, time, what the main characters want to do, what they did, how they felt, and how it all ended (see Stein & Glenn, 1979). Students were taught to generate ideas for these elements or parts during instruction. Consequently, we used this measure to make decisions about when to start and end instruction for students (see "Procedure"). Interrater agreement (agreements divided by agreements plus disagreements) for two independent raters was .93.

Number of Words

Each story was entered into a word processing program. Spelling and punctuation were corrected. The number of words written was computed by using the word processing program's word count function. Because this measure was machine scored, no reliability was computed.

Quality Ratings

Raters evaluated quality of stories using a 7-point holistic scale (with a score of 1 representing the lowest quality and a score of 7 the highest quality). They were asked to read each paper attentively, but not laboriously, to obtain a general impression of overall writing quality. To guide the raters in the scoring process, we used anchor points for second grade developed by Saddler et al. (2004). These anchor points provided a representative paper for scores of 2, 4, and 6 for both stories and personal narratives.

Two raters independently scored each paper for overall quality. The raters were graduate students (one at the master's level and one at the doctoral level), and both were unaware of study hypotheses. Before papers were scored, they were typed and entered into a word processor. All spelling and punctuation errors were corrected prior to scoring. Interobserver agreement for the stories was .83.

Story Retells

Each story retell was scored for the number of story elements that were included. Interobserver agreement (agreements divided by agreements plus disagreements) between two independent scorers was 100%.

General Instructional Procedures

SRSD was used to teach a story planning and writing strategy. With this approach (Harris & Graham, 1996), students are explicitly and systematically taught a task-specific strategy for accomplishing an academic task or problem (e.g., story writing). Self-regulation is advanced by teaching students how to use goal setting, self-monitoring, self-instructions, and self-reinforcement to manage their use of the strategy, the task, and their behaviors. Knowledge is enhanced by teaching any information (or skills) students need to use the strategy. Motivation is boosted through a variety of procedures, including emphasizing the role of effort in learning, making the positive effects of instruction concrete and visible (through self-monitoring and graphing), and promoting an "I can do" attitude.

The emphasis during SRSD instruction is on students' independent use of the strategy and accompanying self-regulation procedures. This includes learning when, where, and how to apply these procedures. Instruction is scaffolded so that responsibility for applying and recruiting the strategy and self-regulation procedures gradually shifts from the instructor to students. The level and type of feedback and instructional support are individualized so that they are responsive to children's needs. Students are treated as active collaborators in the learning process. Furthermore, instruction is criterion based rather than time based, as students move through each instructional stage at their own pace and do not proceed to later stages of instruction until they have met criteria for doing so.

Detailed lesson plans were used during each stage of instruction (these are available at *http://kc.vanderbilt.edu/casl/srsd.html*). Each participant received 30- to 45-min individualized instructional sessions until mastery was achieved. Mastery was defined as independently writing a story with all 7 elements. Tim and Skylar achieved mastery in six sessions. Katie, Sarah, and Trevor required seven sessions to reach mastery. Due to illness and school vacations, Kristina required eight sessions before achieving mastery.

Instructional Procedures for Teaching the Planning and Story-Writing Strategy

The planning and story-writing strategies applied in this study were used in previous studies with second-grade students (Harris et al., in press; Saddler et al., 2004). These included POW, a mnemonic device designed to help students organize the planning and writing process by reminding them to *"Pick My Ideas"* (i.e., decide what to write about), *"Organize My Notes"* (i.e., develop an advanced writing plan), and *"Write and Say More"* (i.e., expand the plan while writing). A second mnemonic, WWW, What = 2, How = 2, reminded students to generate notes for each of the 7 basic parts of a story during the second step of POW (i.e., "Organize My Notes"). Each letter of the mnemonic stood for a question for which students were to generate notes before writing their stories: Who are the main characters? When does the story take place? Where does the story take place? *What* do the main characters want to do? *What* happens when the main characters try to do it? *How* does the story end? *How* do the main characters feel?

In the first stage of instruction, "Develop Background Knowledge," each student acquired the knowledge and skills needed to apply the planning and writing strategies. First, POW and its steps were introduced, and the instructor and student discussed what it stood for and why each step was important. Before moving to the next activity, the student explained the three steps and the importance of each step. The student was then asked, "What is a good story?" In discussing what makes a good story, the instructor emphasized that a good story has many characteristics, and

students should remember that a good story (a) makes sense, (b) is fun to write and read, (c) uses interesting vocabulary or "million-dollar" words, and (d) includes all 7 story elements. To help students remember these 7 parts, the mnemonic device WWW, What = 2, How = 2 was introduced as a "trick" for remembering them. The student then listened along as the instructor read a story, and the child identified each of the 7 elements. As the student identified and described each element, the instructor wrote it in the appropriate section of a chart with the story element reminder. This continued with additional stories until the student could identify all parts accurately. Finally, the term "transfer" was introduced to explain how a strategy could be moved or used in other places or situations. The child was asked to identify where he or she could use these types of strategies and to set a goal to use what had been learned before the next session. A few minutes were spent during each succeeding lesson rehearsing POW and the story part mnemonic, as well as what they stood for, until they were memorized.

In the second stage of instruction, "Discuss It," students further discussed the rationale for using the strategy. Self-monitoring procedures were also introduced. The child analyzed a previously written story from baseline to determine how many basic story elements were included in it (this represents self-monitoring). The student then graphed the number of elements in the story by coloring in the corresponding number of segments on a rocket ship with seven segments. Next, the teacher and child discussed which parts were and were not included. The instructor established that the goal in writing a story is to include all 7 parts and emphasized that even if a story part was included, it could be improved (e.g., fleshed out). Most important, the instructor and student discussed how using POW and the WWW mnemonic could improve story writing. At the end of the session, the instructor asked the student to identify how he or she had used some aspect of this material since the previous session. They discussed the responses and wrote them on a chart. The student then set a new goal to use what he or she had learned outside of the instructional setting. This process of identifying instances of transfer, discussion, and goal setting continued in all subsequent sessions.

In the third stage of instruction, "Model It," the instructor showed the student how to apply the strategies and introduced the concept of self-instructions. The instructor first discussed with the student the goal of writing a story: It should make sense, use "million-dollar" words, be fun to write, and include all 7 elements. The instructor then modeled, while "talking out loud," how to plan and write a story using POW and the story parts reminder (i.e., the WWW mnemonic). The child helped the instructor by generating ideas for the parts of the story as well as additional ideas while writing it. They recorded their notes for the story on a graphic organizer that included a prompt for each part of the WWW mnemonic. While modeling, the instructor used a variety of self statements to assist with problem definition (e.g., What do I have to do here?), planning (e.g., What comes next?), self-evaluation (e.g., Does that make sense?), self-reinforcement (e.g., I really like that part!), and coping (e.g., I'm almost finished!). Once the story was completed, the importance of what we say to ourselves was discussed and the types of self statements used by the instructor were identified. The student then identified at least three self statements that he or she would use while writing and recorded them on a small chart. The instructor and student also verified that all 7 elements were included in the story, highlighting each element and graphing the results.

The next stage, "Support It," began with a collaborative writing experience. First, the instructor and student set a goal to include all 7 elements in the story. Second, they planned the story together using POW, the story element reminder, the graphic organizer, and the student's self statements. However, this time the student directed the process and the instructor only provided support as needed. Third, using the collaboratively generated notes, the student wrote a story. Fourth, after the story was completed, the student identified each story element by highlighting it. Then the student determined if they had met their goal and graphed the results. Fifth, the instructor and student discussed how the strategies helped the child write a better story.

In subsequent sessions, the student was gradually weaned from relying on the planning graphic organizer. The instructor explained that the graphic organizer was helpful but would not always be readily accessible when the child wanted to write a story. The student was taught to write the story part reminder (Who, When, Where, What, What, How, How) at the top of the page to assist him or her in planning and writing a complete story. The student continued to set a goal to include all 7 parts and graphed his or her success in doing so.

For all of the papers written during this stage, the instructor provided support and encouragement as needed, but the level of assistance was faded.

The final stage, "Independent Performance," was reached when the student could successfully write a story with all 7 story elements independently without assistance from the instructor.

Fidelity of Treatment

To ensure consistency in implementation of the SRSD treatment, we employed the following procedures. First, the instructors were trained in how to apply instructional procedures until they could implement them without error. Second, each instructor had a checklist with step-by-step instructions for each lesson. Third, 25% of all lessons were observed by two individuals. The observers also had the same step-by-step checklist as the instructors to determine implementation fidelity. Fidelity was 100%.

RESULTS

Figures 1 and 2 show the number of story elements included in each story composed by students as well as the number of story elements included in each story retell in all conditions (i.e., baseline, independent performance, and maintenance). For Katie and Tim, the last data point in baseline and independent performance for writing and reading story elements are the same. Table 2 provides the means and standard deviations for the average length and quality of students' compositions in baseline, independent performance, and maintenance.

Baseline

Prior to instruction, students' compositions were short, incomplete, and of poor quality (see Figures 1 and 2; Table 2). They contained an average of only 2.1 story elements and 28 words, and they scored an average of 1.8 on a 7-point quality scale. None of the students showed any evidence of planning, as they immediately began writing as soon as the directions for the story prompt were finished. This was generally consistent with the writing behavior in the Saddler et al. (2004) study, except that our students produced even less text (28 vs. 41 words).

Students' scores on the story retell measure during baseline were similar to their writing

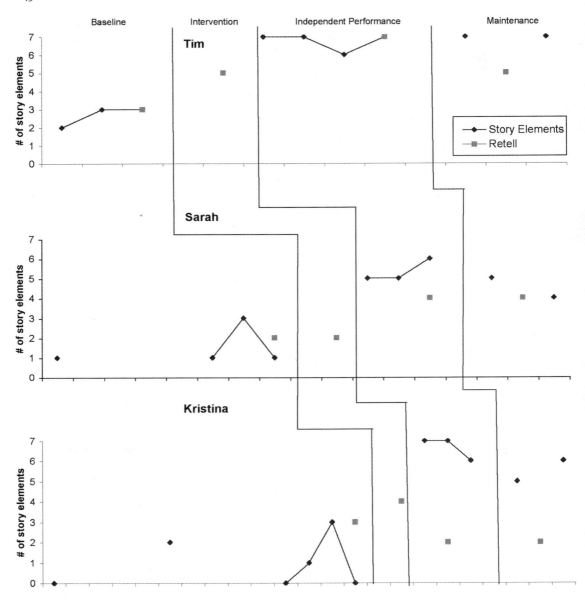

FIGURE 1. Number of story elements for writing and reading retells for Cohort 1.

performance (see Figures 1 and 2). As a group, their recall of basic story elements was incomplete, as their retellings averaged only 2.5 parts.

Instruction

No story-writing probes were collected during instruction. However, each student completed a story-retelling probe toward the end of instruction. Four students (Katie, Trevor, Tim, and Kristina) recalled more story parts during instruction than they did during baseline (see Figures 1 and 2). Two of these students (Trevor and Tim) recalled two more parts when retelling a story during instruction than they did during baseline, whereas the other two students (Katie and Kristina) recalled just one additional element. One student (Sarah) showed no increase in the number of elements recalled between baseline and instruction. The final student (Skylar) recalled one less element during instruction than she did during baseline. It is interesting to note that she had the highest retell score during baseline, recalling 5 of the 7 elements.

Independent Performance

Following instruction, all students' stories improved markedly on the independent performance writing probes (see Figures 1 and 2; Table 2). Four students (Trevor, Skylar, Tim, and Kristina) included all 7 story elements in all or all but one of their independent performance stories.

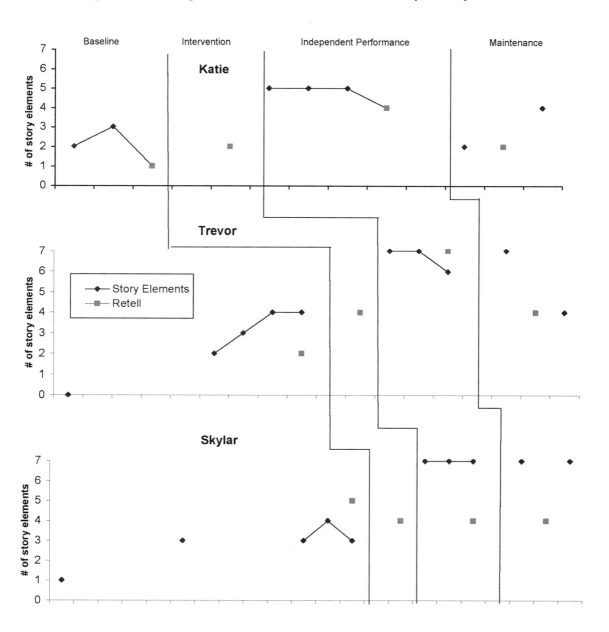

FIGURE 2. Number of story elements for writing and reading retells for Cohort 2.

TABLE 2. Average Length and Quality of Stories

Student (number of compositions)	Story			
	Length	SD	Quality	SD
Katie				
Baseline (3)	10.3	2.08	1.2	0.29
Independent performance (4)	61.8	14.66	3.1	0.95
Maintenance (2)	23	8.49	1.5	0.71
Trevor				
Baseline (5)	43.4	18.37	2.3	0.57
Independent performance (3)	43.3	7.51	2.7	0.29
Maintenance (2)	33.5	7.78	2.75	0.71
Skylar				
Baseline (5)	27.6	12.05	2.2	0.45
Independent performance (3)	56	18.73	3.7	0.76
Maintenance (2)	42	5.66	3.5	1.41
Tim				
Baseline (3)	13.7	2.52	1.3	0.29
Independent performance (4)	51	6.06	3.6	0.25
Maintenance (2)	64	9.90	4.8	0.35
Sarah				
Baseline (4)	48.3	30.31	2.7	0.50
Independent performance (3)	82	1.00	3.7	0.76
Maintenance (2)	72	26.87	3	0.35
Kristina				
Baseline (6)	16.2	4.88	1.3	0.61
Independent performance (3)	41	6.93	2.8	0.58
Maintenance (2)	50	7.07	3.75	0.35

Tim included all 7 elements in three out of four independent performance stories. His stories became almost 4 times longer, and his quality scores improved nearly threefold. Kristina's stories included all 7 elements in two out of three stories. Her stories were also 2.5 times longer, and the average quality of her stories more than doubled. Skylar included all 7 story elements in each of her independent performance stories, nearly doubled the average length of her stories, and made a 168% improvement in her mean quality scores. Trevor's stories included all 7 story elements in two out of three independent performance writing probes. In contrast to the other students, however, his story length stayed about the same and the quality of his stories improved only slightly.

Although Sarah and Katie did not include all 7 story elements in their independent performance stories, they still made improvements (see Figures 1 and 2). Sarah went from a mean of 2 elements in baseline to a mean of 5.3 elements during independent performance; the length of her stories nearly doubled, and story quality improved by 1 point on a 7-point scale (see Table 2). Katie's stories went from a mean of 2 elements in baseline to a mean of 4.8 elements during independent performance. Her stories became more than 6 times longer, and quality scores improved nearly threefold.

Three of the students (Katie, Trevor, and Skylar) provided overt evidence of using the story-planning strategy they had been taught. Katie consistently wrote the story part reminder at the top of each of her independent performance stories. Trevor wrote the story part reminder on his first and second independent performance stories. Skylar wrote the story part reminder at the top of her first independent performance story. The relationship between writing the reminder on the paper and performance was unclear, however, as the student who did this most consistently (Katie) did not include all story parts, and all 7 story elements were included by some students when this was not done (see, e.g., Tim; Figure 2). It must also be noted that all three of the students who overtly wrote the story part reminder on one or more stories had the same instructor.

Students' story retells at the independent performance phase generally showed improvements over baseline and instruction (see Figures 1 and 2). The performance of three students (Katie, Trevor, and Tim), who recalled more story elements during instruction than they did during baseline, continued to improve, as they included even more parts when they retold their independent performance story. In addition, Sarah, who showed no improvement from baseline to instruction, recalled twice as many parts when retelling her independent performance story. In contrast, Skylar still recalled one less element than she did during baseline, and Kristina's performance, which had shown a small gain from baseline to instruction, declined below baseline levels.

Maintenance

Four of the six students (Skylar, Tim, Sarah, and Kristina) maintained improvements in the number of story elements across the 2- and 4-week maintenance probes (see Figures 1 and 2). Katie returned to baseline levels on her first maintenance probe but increased above baseline levels on the second one. Trevor included all 7 elements at the first maintenance probe but decreased markedly to baseline levels on the second probe. All but one student maintained improvements in the length of stories (see Table 2). The exception was Trevor, whose average story length dropped below baseline levels. Nevertheless, the quality of all students' stories was above baseline levels at maintenance. For three students (Trevor, Skylar, and Sarah), there was little change in story quality from independent performance to maintenance. For two other students (Tim and Kristina), story quality improved at maintenance, but it declined for Katie, staying only marginally better than baseline. There was little overt evidence that the students used the story-planning strategy at maintenance, as only Katie and Trevor wrote the story part reminder at the top of any maintenance story (this occurred on the first maintenance story).

DISCUSSION

This study demonstrated that explicitly teaching young struggling writers, including those with special needs, strategies for planning and writing text, the knowledge needed to apply these strategies, and procedures for fostering self-regulation and motivation was an effective instructional approach with these children. We found that providing such instruction for story writing had a strong impact, as all of the participating students wrote more complete stories immediately following instruction and, with the exception of one child, produced papers that were much longer. Even more important, the quality of these students' writing improved. For five of the six students, quality scores for story writing increased by 137% to 277%. The smallest average change in quality scores was 113%, and this occurred for the student who evidenced no increase in story length as a result of instruction. These findings add to a small but growing body of literature (Graham et al., 2005; Harris et al., in press; Saddler et al., 2004) showing that an early intervention designed to enhance strategic behavior, knowledge, and motivation can have a positive impact on young students who are at risk for writing disabilities.

These findings do more than replicate the earlier studies by Graham, Harris, and colleagues (Graham et al., 2005; Harris et al., in press; Saddler et al., 2004), as they extend them in three important ways. First, our study provides evidence that this instructional approach can have a positive impact on the writing of a group of young struggling writers who evidenced a broader range of difficulties than the children involved in the previous investigations. Second, we showed that such instruction is effective in a rural setting where most of the children are not economically disadvantaged. The three previous studies were all conducted in urban schools where the majority of the students were African American children from economically disadvantaged families. Third, this instruction was also effective in an instructional environment in which the teaching of basic writing skills was emphasized but little emphasis was placed on the process of writing. The previous studies all occurred within the context of a writing environment where the writing process was stressed. These three extensions enhance the external validity of this approach by replicating its positive effects across different participants and conditions.

An especially important extension in the current study was that SRSD instruction in writing resulted in improvement on a reading task for four of the six students. Learning about the parts of a story and how to generate writing ideas for these elements appeared to facilitate these students' recall of these parts when they retold stories they had read. Although there was some decline for three of these four students on the retell measure administered at maintenance, all of them still recalled more elements than they did on the baseline probe. To date, more than 25 large-group and single-subject design SRSD writing studies have been conducted (see Graham, in press a; Graham & Harris, 2003; Graham & Perrin, in press), and none of these investigations have examined possible carryover effects to reading. Shanahan (in press) has argued that it should be possible to teach writing in a manner that promotes reading development. Clearly, additional research is needed to examine the extent of carryover that occurs when knowledge that can be used in both reading and writing is taught in one subject or the other (Fitzgerald & Shanahan, 2000). In addition, research is needed to explore how such carryover can be maximized.

One concern about the effects of early intervention in general, and strategy instruction in particular, is whether the gains obtained immediately following instruction are maintained over time (Graham & Harris, 1989; Slavin et al., 1989). With regard to SRSD instruction, a recent meta-analysis (Graham & Harris, 2003) reported that gains at maintenance are not as large as those obtained immediately following instruction, but they remain well above preinstructional levels. The findings from the current study were generally consistent with this observation. On the variable that was most directly related to the instructional intervention (i.e., number of story grammar elements in stories), one student's average score rose slightly on the maintenance probes, another student's average score stayed the same, and four students showed a decline in comparison with the writing probes taken immediately after instruction ended. Nevertheless, the average number of elements in all students' maintenance stories exceeded baseline stories (average increases above baseline ranged from 150% to 458%). With the exception of one student, similar findings were obtained for story length. In terms of story quality, the average maintenance scores for all six students exceeded their mean baseline performance, but this was a marginal advantage in the case of three

children. It must be noted that maintenance probes were only taken at 2 and 4 weeks. As a result, this study does not provide a strong test of maintenance effects. This is also a problem for research on the SRSD approach in general, as maintenance probes have never exceeded 15 weeks. Thus, future research should examine whether or not SRSD effects are maintained over a longer period of time.

Despite the generally positive effects for maintenance, it must be noted that two of the students produced maintenance stories with the same or fewer elements than their best stories during baseline. Although there was some indication that concurrent school activities may have influenced the maintenance performance of at least one of these students, it is possible that our mastery criteria were too lenient. Before instruction ended, students had to demonstrate only once that they could independently use the strategy to write a story containing all 7 parts. These two children may have needed additional practice to fully master these strategies. It is also not clear if the decline in writing performance that occurred for most students at maintenance was simply a reflection of normal variability in performance, as little is known about how well children maintain what they are taught over time. In any event, teachers should not view strategy instruction as once-and-done. Strategies such as the ones taught in this study should be periodically revisited and even upgraded over time (Graham & Harris, 2005a).

It is also important to note that there was little overt evidence that students actually used the strategies they were taught. By the end of instruction, students were taught to write the mnemonic for the story grammar questions at the top of their papers, as a reminder to plan for and include these parts in their stories. Nevertheless, students did this on only 28% of their independent performance and maintenance stories combined. Students' failure to write the reminder does not mean that they did not apply what they had learned, as they averaged 6.2 and 5.4 story parts on the independent performance and maintenance probes, respectively (vs. 2.1 elements during baseline). A more likely explanation, given these findings, is that the mnemonic was no longer necessary, as instructed students knew that they should include these elements in their stories.

In addition to limitations involving the relatively small sample size and maintenance probes that spanned only 4 weeks, our instructional regime only concentrated on planning and drafting. Other important writing processes, such as revising, editing, and publishing, were not included, nor did children have the opportunity to share what they had done with their peers. Even so, the effects of instruction were pronounced, and we anticipate that they would be improved by including these other components (see Graham & Harris, 2005b, for other examples of validated writing strategies).

Another limitation of the current study is that not all of the students had identified disabilities at the time the study was conducted. Thus, there is a need to conduct additional research with young children with disabilities. Even though SRSD instruction has been an effective intervention with students of varying ability levels (Graham & Harris, 2003), additional research is needed to determine if this is the case with primary-grade children. All current work with these children has involved struggling writers (Graham et al., 2005; Harris et al., in press; Saddler et al., 2004). Furthermore, the current study involved one-on-one instruction conducted outside of the general education classroom. Additional research is needed to examine the effects of such instruction when it is delivered directly by teachers in primary-grade classrooms. It is interesting to note that the findings from this study and earlier investigations with struggling writers in the primary grades (Graham et al., 2005; Harris et al., in press; Saddler et al., 2004) suggest that SRSD provides a potentially useful Tier 2 response-to-intervention treatment in the area of writing. In this and previous studies, students who were experiencing difficulty learning to write showed strong gains in writing performance when individual or small-group SRSD instruction was provided by a specially trained instructor. It must be noted, however, that no attempt was made in this or previous studies to determine if students were already receiving quality writing instruction prior to the implementation of SRSD. Research is needed to examine more directly the effectiveness of SRSD as a Tier 2 intervention and to identify other writing interventions that are effective prevention and early intervention techniques with young struggling writers.

In summary, the results from this study and previous research (Berninger et al., 1995; Berninger et al., 1997; Berninger et al., 1998; Englert et al., 1995; Graham et al., 2000; Graham et al., 2002; Graham et al., 2005; Harris et al., in press; Saddler et al., 2004) provide support for the importance of providing early intervention to students who are at risk for writing disabilities. Even relatively brief interventions, such as the one studied here, can have a marked effect on these children's writing performance. Additional research is needed, however, to develop and study other options for early intervention for students who struggle with writing.

REFERENCES

Alexander, P. (1992). Domain knowledge: Evolving issues and emerging concerns. *Educational Psychologist, 27*, 33–51.

Berninger, V., Abbott, R., Whitaker, D., Sylvester, L., & Nolen, S. (1995). Integrating low- and high-level skills in instructional protocols for writing disabilities. *Learning Disability Quarterly, 18*, 293–309.

Berninger, V., Vaughn, K., Abbott, R., Abbott, S., Rogan, L., Brooks, A., et al. (1997). Treatment of handwriting problems in beginning writers: Transfer from handwriting to composition. *Journal of Educational Psychology, 89*, 652–666.

Berninger, V., Vaughn, K., Abbott, R., Brooks, A., Abbott, S., Rogan, L., et al. (1998). Early intervention for spelling problems: Teaching functional spelling units of varying size with a multiple-connections framework. *Journal of Educational Psychology, 90*, 587–605.

Bracken, B. A., & McCallum, R. S. (1998). *Universal nonverbal intelligence test*. Itasca, IL: Riverside.

Danoff, B., Harris, K. R., & Graham, S. (1993). Incorporating strategy instruction within the writing process in the regular classroom: Effects on normally achieving and learning disabled students' writing. *Journal of Reading Behavior, 25*, 295–322.

De La Paz, S., & Graham, S. (1997). Strategy instruction in planning: Effects on the writing performance and behavior of students with learning difficulties. *Exceptional Children, 63*, 167–182.

Englert, C., Garmon, A., Mariage, T., Rozendal, M., Tarrant, K., & Urba, J. (1995). The early literacy project: Connecting across the literacy curriculum. *Learning Disability Quarterly, 18*, 253–275.

Fitzgerald, J., & Shanahan, T. (2000). Reading and writing relations and their development. *Educational Psychologist, 35*, 39–50.

Graham, S. (1990). The role of production factors in learning disabled students' compositions. *Journal of Educational Psychology, 82*, 781–791.

Graham, S. (in press a). Strategy instruction and the teaching of writing. In C. MacArthur, S. Graham, & J. Fitzgerald (Eds.), *Handbook of writing research*. New York: Guilford Press.

Graham, S. (in press b). Writing. In P. Alexander & P. Winne (Eds.), *Handbook of educational psychology*. Mahwah, NJ: Erlbaum.

Graham, S., & Harris, K. R. (1989). A components analysis of cognitive strategy training: Effects on learning disabled students' compositions and self-efficacy. *Journal of Educational Psychology, 81*, 353–361.

Graham, S., & Harris, K. R. (2002). Prevention and

intervention for struggling writers. In M. Shinn, G. Stoner, & H. Walker (Eds.), *Interventions for academic and behavior problems: Vol. 2. Preventive and remedial techniques* (pp. 589–610). Washington, DC: National Association of School Psychologists.

Graham, S., & Harris, K. R. (2003). Students with learning disabilities and the process of writing: A meta-analysis of SRSD studies. In H. L. Swanson, K. R. Harris, & S. Graham (Eds.), *Handbook of learning disabilities* (pp. 323–344). New York: Guilford Press.

Graham, S., & Harris, K. R. (2005a). Improving the writing performance of young struggling writers: Theoretical and programmatic research from the Center to Accelerate Student Learning. *The Journal of Special Education, 39*, 19–33.

Graham, S., & Harris, K. R. (2005b). *Writing better: Effective strategies for teaching students with learning disabilities.* Baltimore: Brookes.

Graham, S., Harris, K. R., & Fink, B. (2000). Is handwriting causally related to learning to write? Treatment of handwriting problems in beginning writers. *Journal of Educational Psychology, 92*, 620–633.

Graham, S., Harris, K. R., & Fink-Chorzempa, B. (2002). Contributions of spelling instruction to the spelling, writing, and reading of poor spellers. *Journal of Educational Psychology, 94*, 291–304.

Graham, S., Harris, K. R., & Larsen, L. (2001). Prevention and intervention of writing difficulties with students with learning disabilities. *Learning Disabilities Research and Practice, 16*, 74–84.

Graham, S., Harris, K. R., & Mason, L. H. (2005). Improving the writing performance, knowledge, and self-efficacy of struggling young writers: The effects of self-regulated strategy development. *Contemporary Educational Psychology, 30*, 207–241.

Graham, S., & Perrin, D. (in press). Improving the writing ability of adolescent students: A cumulative meta-analysis. In A. Henriquez (Ed.), *Annual report on adolescent literacy.* New York: Carnegie Foundation.

Hammill, D., & Larsen, S. (1996). *Test of written language (TOWL-3).* Circle Pines, MN: AGS.

Harris, K. R., & Graham, S. (1985). Improving learning disabled students' composition skills: Self-control strategy training. *Learning Disability Quarterly, 8*, 27–36.

Harris, K. R., & Graham, S. (1996). *Making the writing process work: Strategies for composition and self-regulation.* Cambridge, MA: Brookline Books.

Harris, K. R., & Graham, S. (1999). Programmatic intervention research: Illustrations from the evolution of self-regulated strategy development. *Learning Disability Quarterly, 22*, 251–262.

Harris, K. H., Graham, S., & Mason, L. H. (in press). Improving the writing performance, knowledge, and motivation of struggling writers in second grade: The effects of self-regulated strategy development. *American Educational Research Journal.*

Hayes, J., & Flower, L. (1980). Identifying the organization of writing processes. In L. Gregg & E. Steinberg (Eds.), *Cognitive processes in writing* (pp. 3–30). Hillsdale, NJ: Erlbaum.

Horner, R., Carr, E., Halle, J., McGee, G., Odom, S., &

Wolery, M. (2005). The use of single-subject research to identify evidence-based practices in special education. *Exceptional Children, 71*, 165–180.

Jones, D., & Christensen, C. (1999). The relationship between automaticity in handwriting and students' ability to generate written text. *Journal of Educational Psychology, 91*, 44–49.

Kazdin, A. E. (1982). *Single case research designs: Methods for clinical and applied settings.* New York: Oxford University Press.

Kellogg, R. (1993). *The psychology of writing.* New York: Oxford University Press.

Leslie, L., & Caldwell, J. (2002). *Qualitative reading inventory–3* (3rd ed.). New York: Allyn & Bacon.

MacGinitie, W. H., & MacGinitie, R. K. (1992). *Gates-MacGinitie reading tests* (3rd ed.). Itasca, IL: Riverside.

McCutchen, D. (1988). "Functional automaticity" in children's writing: A problem of metacognitive control. *Written Communication, 5*, 306–324.

National Commission on Writing. (2003). *The neglected "R."* New York: College Entrance Examination Board.

National Commission on Writing. (2004). *Writing: A ticket to work . . . or a ticket out: A survey of business leaders.* Available at *www.collegeboard.com.*

National Commission on Writing. (2005). *Writing: A powerful message from state government.* Available at *www. collegeboard.com.*

Persky, H., Daane, M., & Jin, Y. (2003). *The nation's report card: Writing.* Washington, DC: U.S. Department of Education.

Pintrich, P., & Schunk, D. (1996). *Motivation in education.* Englewood Cliffs, NJ: Prentice-Hall.

Psychological Corporation (The). (2002). *Wechsler individual achievement test* (2nd ed.). San Antonio, TX: Author.

Resta, S., & Eliot, J. (1994). Written expression in boys with attention deficit disorder. *Perceptual and Motor Skills, 79*, 1131–1138.

Saddler, B., Moran, S., Graham, S., & Harris, K. R. (2004). Preventing writing difficulties: The effects of planning strategy instruction on the writing performance of struggling writers. *Exceptionality, 12*(1), 3–7.

Sawyer, R., Graham, S., & Harris, K. R. (1992). Direct teaching, strategy instruction, and strategy instruction with explicit self-regulation: Effects on learning disabled students' composition skills and self-efficacy. *Journal of Educational Psychology, 84*, 340–352.

Shanahan, T. (in press). Relations among oral language, reading, and writing development. In C. MacArthur, S. Graham, & J. Fitzgerald (Eds.), *Handbook of writing research.* New York: Guilford Press.

Slavin, R., Karweit, N., & Madden, N. (1989). *Effective programs for students at-risk.* Boston: Allyn & Bacon.

Stein, N., & Glenn, C. (1979). An analysis of story comprehension in elementary school children. In R. Freedle (Ed.), *Advances in discourse processes: Vol. 2. New directions in discourse processing.* Norwood, NJ: Ablex.

ILLUSTRATIVE EXAMPLE QUESTIONS

1. What was the purpose of the study?

2. Who were the participants (students and peer tutors)? What were the settings?

3. How were the data collected, what were the dependent variables, and how were the dependent variables measured?

4. Describe how the independent variable was presented.

5. What were the conditions and what type of design was used?

6. Why did researchers divide the six participants into cohorts of three students? How was fidelity of intervention assessed? Why is it necessary to have two observers determine agreement on fidelity of intervention?

7. Using the performance figures of the six participants (but without referring to the results), how would you describe the performance of participants in terms of number of story elements? In terms of retelling?

8. Using the table showing performance of the six participants (but without referring to the results), how would you describe the performance of participants in terms of average length of stories? In terms of story quality?

9. Authors note that maintenance data (see the figures) were above baseline levels for all participants. However, performance was variable across participants and across maintenance probes. How would you account for the variability?

10. What recommendations would you make for strengthening this research investigation to demonstrate more convincingly a functional relationship between variables and to control for extraneous factors?

ADDITIONAL RESEARCH EXAMPLES

1. Chariana, S. M., LeBlanc, L. A., Sabanathan, N., Ktaech, I. A., Carr, J. E., & Gunby, K. (2010). Teaching effective hand raising to children with autism during group instruction. *Journal of Applied Behavior Analysis, 43*, 493–497.

2. DiGennaro-Reed, F. D., Codding, R., Catania, C. N., & Maguire, H. (2010). Effects of video modeling on treatment integrity of behavioral interventions. *Journal of Applied Behavior Analysis, 43*, 291–295.

3. Levingston, H. B., Neef, N. A., & Cohon, T. M. (2009). The effects of teaching precurrent behaviors on children's solution of multiplication and division word problems. *Journal of Applied Behavior Analysis, 42*, 361–367.

THREATS TO INTERNAL VALIDITY

Circle the number corresponding to the likelihood of each threat to internal validity being present in the investigation and provide a justification.

1 = definitely not a threat   2 = not a likely threat   3 = somewhat likely threat

4 = likely threat   5 = definite threat   NA = not applicable for this design

Results in Differences within or between Individuals

1. Maturation   1 2 3 4 5 NA

   Justification _____

   _____

2. Selection   1 2 3 4 5 NA

   Justification _____

   _____

3. Selection by Maturation Interaction   1 2 3 4 5 NA

   Justification _____

   _____

4. Statistical Regression   1 2 3 4 5 NA

   Justification _____

   _____

5. Morality   1 2 3 4 5 NA

   Justification _____

   _____

6. Instrumentation   1 2 3 4 5 NA

   Justification _____

   _____

7. Testing   1 2 3 4 5 NA

   Justification _____

   _____

(continued)

8. History   1   2   3   4   5   NA

Justification _____

_____

9. Resentful Demoralization of the Control Group   1   2   3   4   5   NA

Justification _____

_____

Results in Similarities within or between Individuals

10. Diffusion of Treatment   1   2   3   4   5   NA

Justification _____

_____

11. Compensatory Rivalry by the Control Group   1   2   3   4   5   NA

Justification _____

_____

12. Compensatory Equalization of Treatments   1   2   3   4   5   NA

Justification _____

_____

Abstract: Write a one-page abstract summarizing the overall conclusions of the authors and whether or not you feel the authors' conclusions are valid based on the internal validity of the investigation.

THREATS TO EXTERNAL VALIDITY

Circle the number corresponding to the likelihood of each threat to external validity being present in the investigation according to the following scale:

1 = definitely not a threat   2 = not a likely threat   3 = somewhat likely threat

4 = likely threat   5 = definite threat   NA = not applicable for this design

Also, provide a justification for each rating.

Population

1. Generalization across Subjects   1   2   3   4   5   NA

   Justification _____

   _____

2. Interaction of Personological Variables and Treatment   1   2   3   4   5   NA

   Justification _____

   _____

Ecological

3. Verification of the Independent Variable   1   2   3   4   5   NA

   Justification _____

   _____

4. Multiple Treatment Interference   1   2   3   4   5   NA

   Justification _____

   _____

5. Hawthorne Effect   1   2   3   4   5   NA

   Justification _____

   _____

6. Novelty and Disruption Effects   1   2   3   4   5   NA

   Justification _____

   _____

7. Experimental Effects   1   2   3   4   5   NA

   Justification _____

   _____

(continued)

8. Pretest Sensitization   1   2   3   4   5   NA

Justification _____

_____

9. Posttest Sensitization   1   2   3   4   5   NA

Justification _____

_____

10. Interaction of Time of Measurement and Treatment Effects   1   2   3   4   5   NA

Justification _____

_____

11. Measurement of the Dependent Variable   1   2   3   4   5   NA

Justification _____

_____

12. Interaction of History and Treatment Effects   1   2   3   4   5   NA

Justification _____

_____

Abstract: Write a one-page abstract summarizing the overall conclusions of the authors and whether or not you feel the authors' conclusions are valid based on the external validity of the investigation.

CHAPTER 13
■ ■ ■ ■

Additional Single-Case Designs

OBJECTIVES

After studying this chapter, you should be able to . . .

1. List the three considerations on which additional single-case designs are selected.
2. Illustrate a changing-criterion design.
3. Depict a multitreatment design.
4. Explain what is meant by an alternating treatments design.
5. Specify the features of combination designs.
6. Describe when researchers should use each of the additional single-case designs.

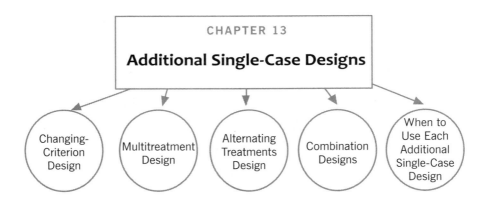

OVERVIEW

Although the mainstays of single-case research are the withdrawal and multiple-baseline designs, other designs are used as well. Selection of these designs is based on the behavior to be changed, the type of research question asked (e.g., what is the most effective method of teaching reading?), or the constraints present (e.g., ethical issues surrounding the use of withdrawal designs, lack of multiple behaviors, participants, or settings).

This chapter focuses on additional single-case designs. Changing-criterion, multitreatment, alternating treatments, and combination

designs are described in detail. Concerns with the analysis of data are described within each design. Research examples demonstrating each design are highlighted throughout the chapter. (*Note*. You should attempt to analyze the graphs presented in the research examples.) Finally, an illustrative investigation is included at the end of the chapter for critique.

WHAT IS A CHANGING-CRITERION DESIGN?

The **changing-criterion** design is an experimental design in which an initial baseline is

Research Examples

Consider these issues. Think about how you would design research to address the questions/hypotheses from these research examples:

- Research Example 1: To what extent will an intervention increase responsiveness across successive requirements for participation for a first grader who is unresponsive during classroom group activities?
- Research Example 2: To what extent will a function-based intervention improve behavior with four elementary students in special education or at risk for referral to special education?
- Research Example 3: To what extent will working in a self-selected, high-preference job result in higher levels of on-task behavior in community-based work settings in comparison to low preference jobs for youth with intellectual disability?
- Research Example 4: To what extent will a self-monitoring program decrease a 12-year-old student's disruptive, negative remarks?

Research examples appear throughout the chapter.

followed by a series of intervention phases with successive and gradually changing criteria (Cooper et al., 2007). The changing-criterion design has not been a popular design in single-case research (Barlow et al., 2008; Gast, 2010). Researchers have used alternative designs to demonstrate experimental control. However, the changing-criterion design is an important design that researchers can use under the appropriate circumstances (Nevin, 2006). In Figure 13.1, a fictional changing-criterion design, a baseline condition is followed by the intervention condition. Essentially, without the "phase" lines (i.e., changes within the intervention condition), the design looks the same as an A-B design. The difference between a changing-criterion design and an A-B design is the use of a criterion within each phase. As shown in Figure 13.1, the horizontal lines between phase lines depict the behavioral criteria. Think of a changing-criterion design as an attempt to reduce or increase some dependent variable in a stepwise manner. In fact, this is what the design

is intended to do—to increase or decrease a dependent variable gradually. Thus, the changing-criterion design is useful for dealing with addictive behaviors such as caffeine consumption or smoking. In many smoking cessation programs, we attempt to fade out the use of nicotine. The changing-criterion design is specially suited for such an attempt. Additionally, the changing-criterion design may be useful in monitoring other dependent variables (Cooper et al., 2007) such as classroom management problems or academic difficulties.

The method of implementing a changing-criterion design is a combination of planning and good guessing. This means that researchers should plan as they would in other investigations. The independent and dependent variables must be well defined, the method of data collection must be determined, and the participant(s) must be prepared to become involved in the investigation. Researchers need to rely on good guessing, in that they must determine the level of criterion changes throughout the investigation and hope that the steps are not too large or too small. To implement a changing-criterion design, researchers must do the following. First, they must collect baseline data. Second, the first criterion level should be set around the average of the baseline (Cooper et al., 2007). Third, once the participant meets some predetermined level such as three data points at or below (in cases where the behavior is to decrease) or above (in cases where the behavior is to increase) the criterion, the criterion should be changed to a new level.

The difficulty with this final step is determining how large the change should be. For example, if the change is too large, the participant may not be able to meet the new level. Consider attempting to decrease the number of cigarettes one smokes per day. Suppose an individual smokes an average of 40 cigarettes per day. The first criterion is then set at 40 cigarettes. Once the participant smokes 40 or less cigarettes per day for 5 consecutive days, we decide to change

> A **changing-criterion** design is achieved by following the initial baseline with a series of intervention phases with successive and gradually changing criteria.

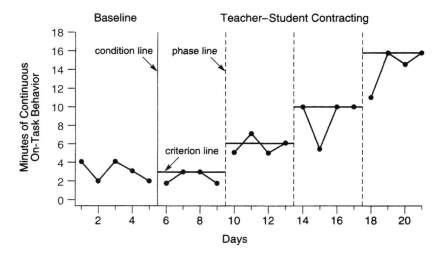

FIGURE 13.1. Minutes of continuous on-task behavior across baseline and teacher–student contracting conditions.

the criterion to 10 cigarettes per day. If you said to yourself "big mistake," you are probably right. The step may be too much. The researcher is doomed to fail by requiring the behavior to be decreased too rapidly. Figure 13.2 demonstrates what happens when a criterion is changed too fast. As can be seen, the participant cannot meet the required criterion. On the other hand, if

the researcher decided to go from 40 to 39 cigarettes after 5 consecutive days, the move may be too small. It will take too long to get down to zero cigarettes per day. Thus, researchers must determine how quickly to reduce or increase the dependent variable. This determination is a difficult one to make, since experimental control depends on it.

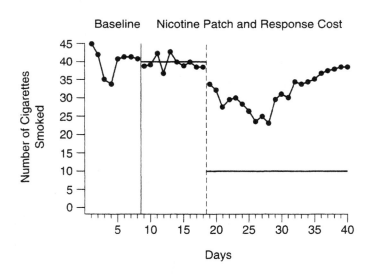

FIGURE 13.2. Number of cigarettes smoked across baseline and nicotine patch and response cost conditions.

Analysis of Data

In this section, we consider internal validity, condition length, criterion level, stability and immediacy of change, number of criterion levels, and other control procedures. We also consider external validity.

Internal Validity

When assessing the internal validity of the changing-criterion design, several concerns must be taken into consideration. These concerns involve the condition length (including the trend of the data), whether the behavior stays near the criterion level, the stability and immediacy of data change, the number of criterion levels, and other control procedures. Table 13.1 summarizes the major threats to internal validity of the changing-criterion design.

Condition Length. The consideration of condition length for a changing-criterion design is similar to that in withdrawal and multiple-baseline designs. During the baseline condition, at least three data points should demonstrate stability or show the behavior moving in a countertherapeutic direction. If there are less than three data points or the data are moving in a therapeutic direction, experimental control is weakened considerably.

After the intervention is implemented, the critical concern is whether the data are clustered around the criterion line. Researchers generally set a criterion that must be met before the participant moves to the next phase (i.e., before the criterion line is changed). The critical demonstration in each phase is controlling the behavior at the criterion line for at least three consecutive sessions. Thus, the three-data-point rule holds here as well. Researchers may require more than three data points at each phase before changing the criterion. For example, Martella, Leonard, Marchand-Martella, and Agran (1993) required four data points at or below the criterion line for problem behavior. As shown in Figure 13.3, three data points in baseline show stable performance; however, in the second teacher–student

TABLE 13.1. Threats to Internal Validity Associated with Additional Single-Case Designs

Threat	Changing-criterion design	Multitreatment design	Alternating treatments design	Combination designs
1. Maturation	Controlled	Controlled	Controlled	Controlled
2. Selection	Not applicable	Not applicable	Not applicable	Not applicable
3. Selection by maturation interaction	Not applicable	Not applicable	Not applicable	Not applicable
4. Statistical regression	Controlled	Controlled	Controlled	Controlled
5. Mortality	Controlled	Controlled	Controlled	Controlled
6. Instrumentation	Controlled	Controlled	Controlled	Controlled
7. Testing	Controlled	Controlled	Controlled	Controlled
8. History	Controlled	Controlled	Controlled	Controlled
9. Resentful demoralization of the control group	Not applicable	Not applicable	Not applicable	Not applicable
10. Diffusion of treatment	Controlled	Possible concern	Possible concern	Controlled
11. Compensatory rivalry by the control group	Not applicable	Not applicable	Not applicable	Not applicable
12. Compensatory equalization	Not applicable	Not applicable	Not applicable	Not applicable

Note. This table is meant only as a general guideline. Decisions with regard to threats to internal validity must be made after the specifics of an investigation are known and understood. Thus, interpretations of internal validity threats must be made on a study-by-study basis.

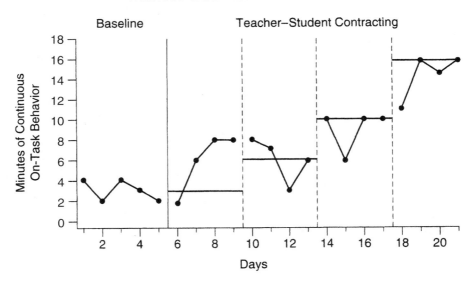

FIGURE 13.3. Minutes of continuous on-task behavior across baseline and teacher–student contracting conditions. From Martella, R. C., Nelson, J. R., Marchand-Martella, N., & O'Reilly, M. (2012). *Comprehensive behavior management: Individualized, classroom, and schoolwide approaches* (2nd ed.). Thousand Oaks, CA: Sage. Copyright 2012 by Sage Publications, Inc. Reprinted by permission of SAGE.

contracting phase of the intervention (Sessions 10 through 13), three consecutive data points are not clustered at or above the criterion line. This demonstration makes claiming internal validity more difficult. If there were three consecutive data points clustered around the criterion line, the experimental demonstration would have been greater.

Criterion Level. Initially, the criterion level should be set at a level that is attainable. This level may be set at the mean level of baseline or just below or above this level (depending on whether one decreases or increases a behavior). Once the participant has met the criterion at this initial level, there should be a change in the next criterion. The difficulty here is that the level change should neither be so small as to "overreinforce" the participant at a previous level nor so large that the participant is unable to meet this level. In these cases, the participant's behavior in meeting the level and/or his/ her effort in doing so may extinguish or cease. Thus, researchers must be especially cautious when changing levels of criteria throughout the investigation. Although a given intervention

may be effective, a mistake in the level of criterion change could lead to a conclusion that the intervention is inadequate.

Stability and Immediacy of Change. A critical concern with changing-criterion designs is the stability and immediacy of change. Experimental control comes from demonstrating that the participant's behavior is held at a certain level. If the behavior is held at each criterion level as in Figure 13.1, we can conclude that the researcher had experimental control over the behavior. However, suppose that the data look like those in Figure 13.4. The problem here is that the researcher essentially has an A-B design with all of its associated weaknesses.

One way to think of a changing-criterion design is to conceptualize it as a series of A-B designs. Essentially, the logic of the changing-criterion design is a series of A-B replications. Even though A-B designs are considered weak in internal validity, a series of A-B designs increases confidence that the independent variable is responsible for the measured changes in the dependent variable. As shown in Figure 13.5, each phase acts as both an "A" and a "B"

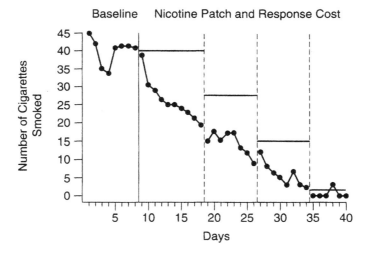

FIGURE 13.4. Number of cigarettes smoked across baseline and nicotine patch and response cost conditions.

condition; that is, each phase is an "A" condition for the following phase and a "B" condition for the previous phase. If there is an inability to keep the dependent variable at the criterion level in one or more of the criterion phases, the internal validity is weakened. The extent of the threat to internal validity is dependent on how far the data venture from the criterion line, as well as the number of phases in which there is an inability to control the behavior.

Another concern has to do with the immediacy of change. When a criterion is changed, there should be an immediate change in the level of the dependent variable. The longer it takes for

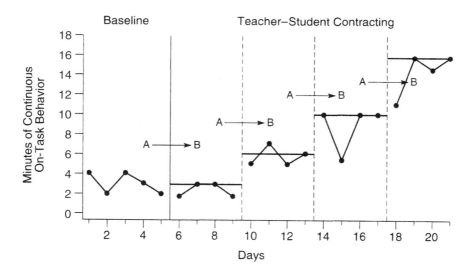

FIGURE 13.5. Minutes of continuous on-task behavior across baseline and teacher–student contracting conditions.

the data to cluster around the criterion level, the more likely it is that there is a potential threat to the internal validity of the investigation. Again, the purpose of the changing-criterion design is to demonstrate that there is control over the dependent variable. Whenever there is an inability to control the dependent variable, the demonstrated experimental control is compromised. Thus, critical research consumers analyzing a changing-criterion design must look at how quickly the dependent variable changes in response to a change in the criterion level.

Number of Criterion Levels (Replications). According to Cooper et al. (2007), the more times the target behavior changes to meet new criteria, the more convincing the experimental control. The purpose of this is to replicate the behavior changes frequently enough to show that changes did not occur by chance. The rule is similar to the rule stated by Kazdin (2003) for multiple-baseline designs; that is, four or more A-B replications are required to replicate the effects of the independent variable on the dependent variable to make a determination of the internal validity of the investigation. Thus, if there are fewer than four criterion change phases in an experiment, the internal validity of the investigation is weakened, much as it is with a multiple-baseline design.

Other Control Procedures. Overall, the changing-criterion design is not considered one of the stronger designs, since it is simply a series of A-B designs. The inference of experimental control is greater with the changing-criterion design than with other single-case designs. Researchers must infer that the control is coming from the independent variable; however, some of the control certainly comes from the criterion level. Additionally, the control may come from a history factor, for example, in combination with the criterion level. The independent variable may have very little to do with the observed changes if the intervention is separated from the changing-criterion levels. In other words, there is no direct investigation of the independent variable's effects on the dependent variable.

Threats to internal validity are difficult to rule out with this design. However, there are steps researchers can take to improve the internal

validity of the changing-criterion design. The first technique is to vary the level of changes in the criterion level. For example, researchers could decrease or increase (depending on the dependent variable to be changed) the criterion level by 25% in the first phase, 10% in the second, and 50% in the third phase. Varying the level of changes aids in the demonstration of control over the dependent variable. Along these lines, researchers could also vary the length of each criterion phase. Rather than requiring four consecutive data points at or near the criterion line, five or six consecutive data points may be required.

A more rigorous demonstration that directly measures the effects of the independent variable over the dependent variable is to reverse the criterion. Recall that the influence of history is difficult to rule out with a changing-criterion design. Suppose the researcher has two phases of decreasing criteria (phases two and three), as shown in Figure 13.6. Then, the researcher reverses the dependent variable by increasing the criterion in the fourth phase. Then, the fifth phase shows a decrease in the criterion. Notice that this combines two designs—a changing-criterion design and a reversal (not a withdrawal) design. The strength of the reversal design is combined with the changing-criterion design to produce a powerful demonstration of experimental control.

External Validity

Clearly, the external validity of the changing-criterion design is fairly weak. There is typically one participant in one setting with one measure of the dependent variable. There is also a difficulty with the method of changing the dependent variable. It is probably not too common to decrease or increase behaviors in such a stepwise manner. This is not to say that doing so is not effective, only that it does not occur frequently in many applied settings such as a classroom. As explained before, single-case researchers look to replications to demonstrate external validity in a systematic manner. Many researchers do not see how a single investigation can demonstrate external validity. Table 13.2 summarizes the major threats to external validity of the changing-criterion design.

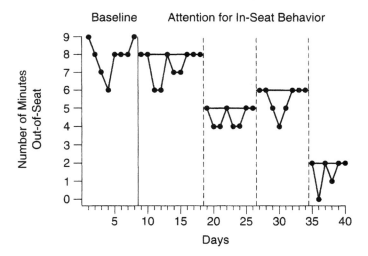

FIGURE 13.6. Number of minutes out-of-seat across baseline and attention for in-seat behavior conditions.

TABLE 13.2. Threats to External Validity Associated with Additional Single-Case Designs

Threat	Changing-criterion design	Multitreatment design	Alternating treatments design	Combination designs
1. Generalization across participants	Possible concern	Possible concern	Possible concern	Possible concern
2. Interaction of participant-specific variables and treatment effects	Possible concern	Possible concern	Possible concern	Possible concern
3. Verification of independent variable possible concern	Possible concern	Possible concern	Possible concern	Possible concern
4. Multiple treatment interference	Controlled	Possible concern	Possible concern	Controlled
5. Novelty and disruption effects	Possible concern	Possible concern	Possible concern	Possible concern
6. Hawthorne effect	Possible concern	Possible concern	Possible concern	Possible concern
7. Experimenter effects	Possible concern	Possible concern	Possible concern	Possible concern
8. Pretest sensitization	Not applicable	Not applicable	Not applicable	Not applicable
9. Posttest sensitization	Not applicable	Not applicable	Not applicable	Not applicable
10. Interaction of time of measurement and treatment effects	Possible concern	Possible concern	Possible concern	Possible concern
11. Measurement of the dependent variable	Possible concern	Possible concern	Possible concern	Possible concern
12. Interaction of history and treatment effects	Possible concern	Possible concern	Possible concern	Possible concern

Note. This table is meant only as a general guideline. Decisions with regard to threats to external validity must be made after the specifics of an investigation are known and understood. Thus, interpretations of external validity threats must be made on a study-by-study basis.

Recall the research question posed earlier in this chapter about the unresponsive first grader? Read on to see how your design compares to how the actual study was designed.

Research Example 1:
Changing-Criterion Design

A changing-criterion design was used to increase participation of a first-grade student in a general education classroom (Lane, Rogers, et al., 2007). "Claire" was a 7-year-old, typically developing European American girl in a first-grade class with 21 students. She was identified as non-responsive and at risk for referral to special education. When the teacher asked a question, Claire looked away and did not respond. Nonresponsiveness occurred mostly during academic tasks. A functional behavior assessment identified antecedents and consequences surrounding the nonresponsive behavior in an effort to identify its purpose or function. Interviews with the

teacher, the mother, and Claire, as well as direct observations, suggested that Claire was afraid of getting the wrong answers (i.e., the function of the behavior was to escape attention). An intervention was developed to increase the probability of responding. Each morning, Claire and her teacher set a goal for the number of times Claire would participate in whole-class activity. If she met her goal, she was allowed a break from participation (i.e., sitting out the remainder of the session). Baseline data were collected and indicated that Claire participated an average of only twice per 30-minute session. The initial criterion for participation was set at three occurrences per session. If Claire's participation equaled or exceeded the criterion for three consecutive sessions, successive increments were arranged up to six occurrences per 30-minute session. As shown in Figure 13.7, Claire's participation exceeded criteria on most days, even as criteria changed from three to six occurrences. In a

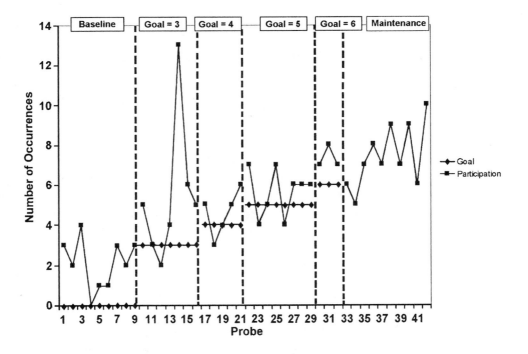

FIGURE 13.7. Claire's intervention outcomes. From Lane, Rogers, et al. (2007). Function-based interventions for students who are nonresponsive to primary and secondary prevention efforts: Illustrations at the elementary and middle school levels. *Journal of Emotional and Behavioral Disorders, 15*, 169–183. Copyright 2007 by the Hammill Institute on Disabilities. Reprinted by permission of SAGE.

final maintenance condition, the intervention was discontinued and regular practices were used. During maintenance, Claire's participation remained at a high rate. The study illustrates that function-based interventions can be implemented in general education settings. As noted by Lane, Rogers, et al., "the nature of the changing criterion design . . . allows a student to gradually gain fluency in a particular behavior while being positively reinforced" (p. 177).

WHAT IS A MULTITREATMENT DESIGN?

The **multitreatment design** is planned in such a way as to allow comparison of two or more interventions or the additive components of an intervention. The multitreatment design is an associate of the withdrawal design discussed in Chapter 11. This design is an alternative to group designs that allow the same type of comparisons to be made. Several possible variations of the withdrawal design demonstrate the effects of several interventions or components of an intervention. For example, if two interventions are compared, an A-B-A-C-A design might be used. In this case, it is possible to determine which intervention is more successful at changing the dependent variable in comparison to the baseline condition. What is critical to understand here is that this design is consistent with the "change one variable at a time" rule. As shown in Figure 13.8, the token economy system was more effective than the warning condition in reducing talk outs in comparison to baseline. The difficulty with this design is that interpreting the relative effectiveness of "B" and "C" is a problem. Conditions "B" and "C" are never directly compared. A related problem is the possibility of sequencing effects. In other words, was the "C" condition more or less effective than the "B" condition because the "B" condition preceded it?

Another variation of the withdrawal design compares interaction effects of intervention components. For example, the A-B-A-B-BC-B-BC design compares the "B" intervention with the addition of the "C" intervention. The advantage of this design is obvious; that is, additive effects of interventions are important to test, since in effect rarely is one variable in isolation in applied settings. The comparisons come from "BC" being surrounded by "B," and "B" being surrounded by "BC."

A researcher who wishes to compare the addition of different components in an intervention uses a similar design. For example, suppose she wants to use a self-management program containing two separate variables ("B" and "C") with a student who has difficulty staying in his seat. Most self-management programs contain several components, such as self-reinforcement, self-monitoring, and self-evaluation. Now suppose the self-management program contains two instructional components (i.e., self-monitoring and self-instruction). The researcher implements the self-management program and finds that the dependent variable decreases immediately after implementation of the independent variable. The question of the contributions of the components to the package is raised. Thus, the researcher implements the self-management package without the self-instruction (C). She also implements the package without self-monitoring (B). Thus, an A-BC-A-B-A-C-A design can be used. To compare the relative effectiveness of each the researcher could do the following: A-BC-A-BC-B-BC-C-BC-B-C-B. Several combinations are compared in this example—the comparisons of "BC" with baseline, "B" with "BC," "C" with "BC," and "C" with "B." A sample investigation, shown in Figure 13.9, indicates that the combination of the two components is effective at increasing in-seat behavior. The relative effectiveness of the self-instruction is also apparent. The self-monitoring alone is almost as effective as the combination intervention; the self-instruction condition alone is clearly less effective than the self-monitoring. Thus, the self-instruction component adds little to the effectiveness of the self-management program.

Analysis of Data

In this section, we consider internal validity, condition length, changing of one variable at a time, level and rapidity of change, returning to

> A **multitreatment design** *allows for the comparison of two or more interventions or the additive components of an intervention.*

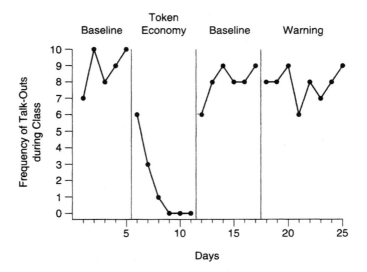

FIGURE 13.8. The frequency of talk outs during class across baseline, token-economy, and warning conditions.

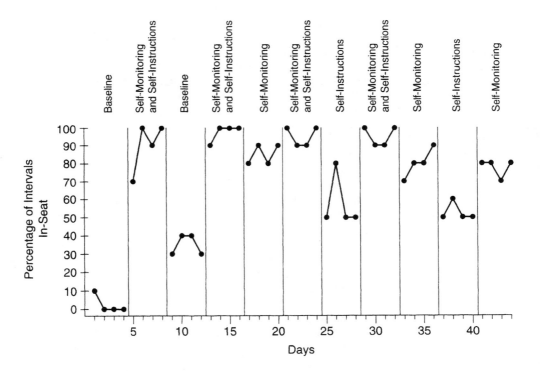

FIGURE 13.9. Percentage of intervals in-seat across baseline, self-monitoring and self-instruction, self-monitoring alone, and self-instruction alone conditions.

baseline level, and time of implementation. We also consider external validity.

Internal Validity

The threats to internal validity of the multi-treatment design are similar to threats in other designs discussed thus far. The threats especially critical to control are history and maturation. The following all have an impact on the control of threats to internal validity: condition length, changing one variable at a time, level and rapidity of change, return to baseline levels, and time of implementation. Table 13.1 summarizes the major threats to internal validity of the multitreatment design.

Condition Length. The condition length criterion is the same as that in other designs discussed thus far. There must be a minimum of three consecutive stable data points or three consecutive data points moving in a counter-therapeutic direction.

Changing One Variable at a Time. As indicated in Chapter 11, there must be a change in one variable at a time to demonstrate the effectiveness of each intervention compared to the baseline condition, or to determine the relative effectiveness of multiple interventions. Additionally, a design such as an A-BC-B-A-B-BC design does not demonstrate experimental control. The reason for this lack of control is that no comparisons are being made. Notice that the two "BC" conditions are not surrounded by an "A" or a "B" condition. Likewise, the "B" conditions are not surrounded by an "A" or a "BC" condition.

In order to demonstrate the effectiveness of the interventions as compared to the baseline, an A-BC-A-B-A design is appropriate. To compare the relative effectiveness of the interventions together versus one intervention in isolation, an A-BC-A-BC-B-BC-B design can be used. In the last example, the critical comparisons are as follows: A-BC-A, BC-A-BC, BC-B-BC, and B-BC-B. Unfortunately, when researchers make a mistake with the "change one variable at a time" rule, some experimental control is lost, and conclusions made should be viewed the same as the conclusion drawn when using an A-B design.

Level and Rapidity of Change. The level and rapidity of change is the same as explained in previous chapters. The change in level of the dependent variable should be fairly substantial and occur as soon as possible once the condition change occurs. If there is a lack of change, or a very small one, the demonstration of experimental control is weakened. Likewise, the demonstration of experimental control is compromised if there is a delay in the change of the dependent variable.

Return to Baseline Levels. An inability to return to baseline levels is also referred to as a *problem with reversibility*. As with the withdrawal design, if the dependent variable does not return to baseline levels in a design such as the A-BC-A-B-A design, the experimental control is compromised. There must be a return to baseline or near baseline levels to make firm conclusions about effects of the independent variable on the dependent variable.

When a design allows for direct comparisons between or among multiple interventions, the rule is changed somewhat. For example, in an A-B-A-B-BC-B-BC design, there should be a return to baseline levels in the two baseline conditions; however, what is required for the adjacent "B" and "BC" conditions is a difference in the levels of performance. If no changes occur in the dependent variable when conditions are changed, the conclusion as to the differential effectiveness of the "B" and "BC" conditions becomes more difficult.

Suppose there was little or no change between the conditions, as shown in Figure 13.10. In this case, self-instruction with self-reinforcement intervention showed no advantages over the self-instructional intervention alone. However, what can we conclude? The addition of self-reinforcement adds little to nothing to the overall effects of the self-instructional intervention. However, we cannot conclude that the self-instructional component ("B") is more effective than the self-reinforcement component ("C"). In order to make this comparison, we would have to add something like the following to the design: C-B-C. Now a direct comparison is being made. In the earlier design, the "B" and "C" components are not directly compared. Although the self-reinforcement component

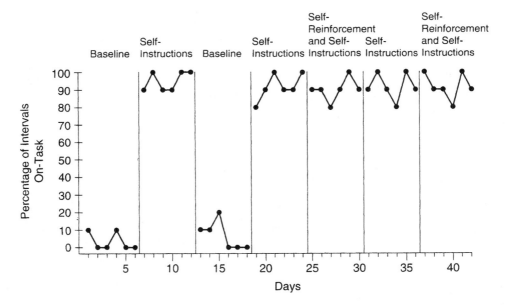

FIGURE 13.10. Percentage of intervals on-task across baseline, self-instruction and self-reinforcement, and self-instruction alone conditions.

adds nothing to the overall impact of the intervention, the self-instruction component may actually suppress the effects of the self-reinforcement component. In other words, when combined with self-instruction, self-reinforcement loses its effectiveness, but when viewed alone, it is more effective than self-instruction alone. Again, researchers must be careful what conclusions they make, and critical research consumers must also be careful in interpreting the results of investigations, especially the conclusions based on those investigations.

Time of Implementation. A final concern is the amount of time it takes to implement a multitreatment design (Gast, 2010). Consider an A-B-A-C-A design. There are five conditions. Thus, a minimum of 15 data points must be gathered (three consecutive stable data points or data points moving in a countertherapeutic direction per condition). Now consider the A-B-A-BC-B-BC-B design. There are seven conditions, for a minimum of 21 data points. What if three interventions are compared? Suppose we compare the relative effectiveness of extrinsic reinforcement (B), intrinsic reinforcement

(C), and a combination of the two (BC) on the motivation of school children. We would use a design such as: A-B-A-B-C-B-C-BC-C-BC-B-BC-B. We can compare the following: A-B-A, B-A-B, B-C-B, C-B-C, C-BC-C, BC-C-BC, BC-B-BC, and B-BC-B. There are 13 conditions, with a minimum of 39 data points. Not only is the multitreatment design cumbersome, but it also takes a great deal of time to implement. The problem is that taking such a long time to implement a design increases the potential for history and maturation to have an effect.

External Validity

The external validity of the multitreatment design is weak. It is no different than other single-case designs. A major threat to external validity is multiple-treatment interference (Gast, 2010). Since a participant is exposed to a number of interventions, there is concern that if others, outside of the investigation, are not exposed to the interventions in the same order, the generalizability of the results may be suspect. For example, if the "B" condition comes before the "BC" condition in the investigation, does it also need to occur before a combination intervention outside of the investigation? Suppose we again implement a self-management procedure. The "B" condition is self-instruction and the "C" condition is self-reinforcement. The question that should be addressed is whether the self-instruction intervention must come before the combination of both interventions to make the combination more effective. What if a teacher attempts to use the combination without implementing the self-instruction intervention alone first? Would her results be different than those reported by the researchers? Table 13.2 summarizes the major threats of the multitreatment design to external validity.

All of the other threats to external validity are present in this design. As with other single-case designs, replications are required to increase our confidence in the generalizability of the results.

Recall the research question posed earlier in this chapter about four elementary school students at risk for referral to special education? Read on to see how your design compares to how the actual study was designed.

Research Example 2: Multitreatment Design

A multitreatment design was used to examine the efficacy of a function-based intervention with four elementary school students in special education or at risk for referral to special education (Payne, Scott, & Conroy, 2007). One participant, "Julie," an 11-year-old girl in third grade, had repeated first and third grades. She had been diagnosed with specific learning disabilities. Data indicated high rates of off-task behavior and noncompliance. Researchers performed a functional assessment (FA) to identify the function of the problem behavior and hypothesized that Julie was off task to access attention from a specific peer (i.e., a classroom friend). However, to confirm the hypothesized function, researchers performed an experimental analysis that comprised systematic presentation and withdrawal of the functional consequence (i.e., the attention of a specific peer). To do so, researchers measured off-task behavior when Julie (1) had access to the specific peer, (2) limited access to the specific peer, and (3) access to

nonspecific peers. Differences in off-task behavior across these successive conditions would verify the function of the problem behavior. During 10-minute sessions, activities, teacher interaction, and setting were held constant. As shown in the top panel of Figure 13.11, higher rates of off-task behavior were exhibited when Julie had access to the specific peer. Given these functional analysis results, an intervention was developed to provide Julie access to the specific peer contingent on only low levels of off-task behavior. Julie earned a break with her friend that was contingent on attending to academic tasks and following teacher instructions. A second intervention was also developed. In a functionally unrelated intervention, Julie received prompts to return to task (i.e., teacher attention) when she was off task. Researchers compared interventions using an A-B-C-B-C design. As shown in the bottom panel of Figure 13.11, in a baseline condition ("A") involving no specific intervention, Julie was off task between 20 and 25% of intervals observed. In the first presentation of the non-function-based intervention ("B"), off-task increased to 26 to 30% of intervals. The non-function-based intervention was followed by the function-based intervention ("C") and resulted in an immediate decrease in off-task behavior ranging from 8 to 16% of intervals. The "B" condition was reintroduced and off-task behavior increased to about 50% of intervals. Finally, a "C" condition was reintroduced and off-task behavior decreased to less than 5% of intervals. Results were similar for three additional participants and demonstrated the value of function-based interventions.

WHAT IS AN ALTERNATING TREATMENTS DESIGN?

An **alternating treatments design** (ATD), or multielement design, is an experimental design in which two or more conditions are presented

---

*An **alternating treatments design** involves presenting two or more conditions in rapidly alternating succession (e.g., on alternating days) to determine differences between the conditions.*

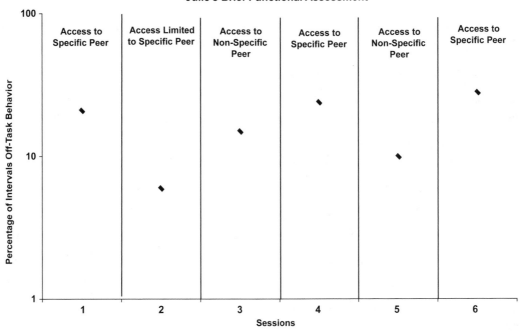

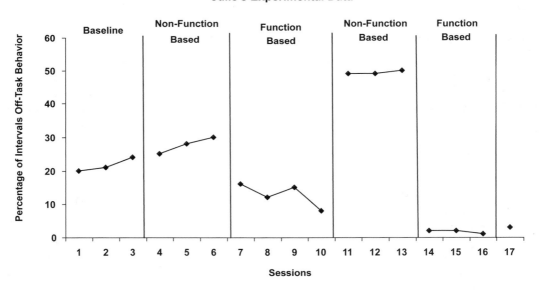

FIGURE 13.11. Brief FA and experimental analysis results: Julie. From Payne, L. D., Scott, T. M., and Conroy, M. (2007). A school-based examination of the efficacy of function-based intervention. *Behavioral Disorders*, 32, 158–174. Copyright 2007 by the Council for Children with Behavioral Disorders, Council for Exceptional Children. Reprinted by permission.

in rapidly alternating succession (e.g., on alternating days) to determine differences between the conditions (Cooper et al., 2007). One of the conditions may be a no-treatment condition, or there may be multiple treatment conditions. Although the multitreatment design is adequate for comparing components of intervention packages or interventions, the disadvantages are difficult to overcome. An alternative to the use of multitreatment designs is the ATD, also called the multielement design (Cooper et al., 2007).

The main purpose of the ATD is to make comparisons between or among two or more conditions or interventions such as baseline and intervention(s) or multiple interventions. A secondary function is to determine experimental control. Whereas other single-case designs discussed thus far (with the possible exception of the multitreatment design) are planned to control only for the threats to internal validity, the ATD attempts to demonstrate the superiority of one intervention over the other. Thus, for most purposes, the ATD is used both to compare two or more conditions or interventions and to control for the threats to internal validity.

The ATD is the single-case alternative to the factorial design used in group research. The experimental control achieved through this design can be quite extensive, since one way to increase statistical power is by eliminating intersubject variability or unsystematic variance. Essentially, the ATD splits the participant into equal parts and provides the different interventions to each part. Thus, if a participant is exposed to a historical situation, such as difficulty at home, the history will affect all of the interventions equally (Barlow et al., 2008). Any differences between or among the conditions or interventions are the differential effects of the interventions.

The ATD achieves this ability to overcome threats to internal validity and to make equal comparisons between or among conditions or interventions by alternating the presentation of each condition or intervention. For example, suppose we wish to compare two methods of classroom management such as in-class time-out and reprimands. We alternate the interventions to see the relative effects of each on the classroom behavior of the students. The manner in which we alternate the interventions can

vary. For example, we could split the day in half and run one intervention in the morning and the other in the afternoon. We could also run one intervention on Monday, Wednesday, and Friday during the first week, on Tuesday and Thursday during the second week, and then repeat the sequence. We could then run the other intervention on the other days. To control for threats such as maturation (e.g., students may be tired in the afternoon, which leads to more difficulties), we must randomly determine when each intervention is in effect.

Suppose we elect to alternate days rather than time of day. We randomly determine when each intervention is in effect. Researchers may set a rule on the number of consecutive times the same intervention can occur. Due to the chance factor, it would be possible to have an entire week with the same intervention. Thus, a rule may be made, such as a maximum of 2 consecutive days with the same intervention. Once it is determined when each intervention will be implemented, data can be collected on the effects of each intervention. In Figure 13.12, an example of the ATD, no more than 2 consecutive days of the same intervention are allowed. The interventions are alternated on a daily basis. Conclusions can be drawn based on the data in Figure 13.12. It seems as though time-out are more effective than reprimands. We can determine this by looking at the spread in the data. The wider the spread, the greater the differential effects of the interventions. Notice that there is no baseline condition shown. The investigation sought to determine which intervention was more effective; therefore, the baseline condition was not needed.

As stated previously, a formal baseline condition is not required with an ATD. In fact, we could alternate an intervention with a baseline as opposed to two interventions. The comparison would then be between intervention and no intervention. However, many times a formal baseline condition is initiated. Figure 13.13 shows an ATD with such a baseline condition and also shows a comparison between two interventions.

On completion of the comparison between or among conditions or interventions, a visual analysis is conducted. The amount of spread between or among the conditions or

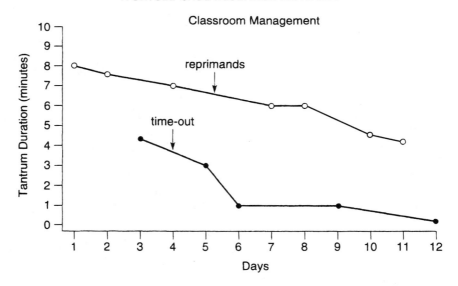

FIGURE 13.12. The daily duration of tantrums across time-out and reprimand conditions. From Martella, R. C., Nelson, J. R., Marchand-Martella, N., & O'Reilly, M. (2012). *Comprehensive behavior management: Individualized, classroom, and schoolwide approaches* (2nd ed.). Thousand Oaks, CA: Sage. Copyright 2012 by Sage Publications, Inc. Reprinted by permission of SAGE.

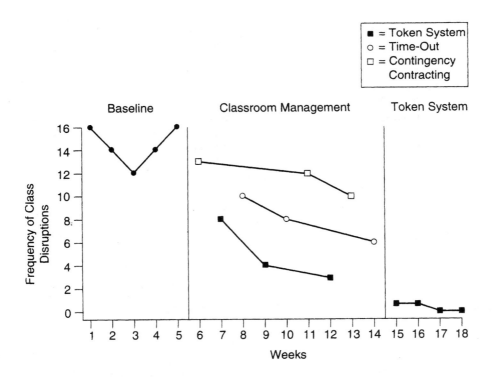

FIGURE 13.13. The frequency of class disruptions across baseline, token system, time-out, and contingency contracting conditions.

interventions indicates the level of differential effectiveness. For example, in Figure 13.13, a token system was clearly found to be superior to the time-out condition, which was more effective than contingency contracting in reducing classroom disruptions. If there were a lack of spread between or among the data, the conclusion would be that there were few or no differences between or among the conditions or interventions.

Once a determination has been made with regard to the relative effectiveness of the conditions or interventions, a final condition may be added to the design (Cooper et al., 2007). Figure 13.13 demonstrates this added condition. Many times, researchers implement the condition or intervention singularly. The most effective condition or intervention would be implemented at all times, such as every day, rather than alternating days. This final condition demonstrates that the condition or intervention can sustain the dependent variable change across other times or situations.

Skills Acquisition Program

Recall that a major problem with the withdrawal design is that the dependent variable must be reversible. That is, the dependent variable must return to baseline levels when the intervention is removed. Acquiring skills is an example of a nonreversible dependent variable. Researchers who teach problem-solving skills cannot tell the participant to forget everything he/she has learned. The multiple-baseline design corrects for this problem by not requiring the dependent variable to revert to baseline levels. A problem with the multiple-baseline design is that direct comparisons between or among several independent variables cannot be made. The multitreatment design and the ATD allow for such a comparison. The multitreatment design requires the dependent variable to be reversible; however, the ATD does not require this (Cooper et al., 2007). Unfortunately, the ATD allows for only one dependent variable. This fact raises a problem with skills acquisition programs. How can a researcher teach problem solving using two separate teaching techniques and still determine the relative contributions of each teaching method? This determination is not possible.

Thus, Sindelar, Rosenberg, and Wilson (1985) proposed the adapted alternating treatments design (AATD) for instructional research, and Gast and Wolery (1988) proposed the parallel treatments design (PTD) as an alternative. (It is not our purpose to explain the similarities and differences of these two designs; they are similar in most respects but do have some specific differences. For our purposes, an overall general discussion of the key points made by Sindelar and colleagues [1985] and Gast and Wolery [1988] suffices.)

Essentially, the AATD and PTD are modifications of the ATD. These designs help to solve the problem of investigating the relative effectiveness of different instructional methods on skill acquisition dependent variables. The AATD and PTD require that two or more "sets" of dependent variables or behaviors be developed. These dependent variables or behaviors should be similar in difficulty and effort to perform. For example, suppose a researcher is teaching reading skills. She would take two aspects of reading that are equal in difficulty and randomly assign these aspects to the different instructional methods. The difficulty here is that the sets of dependent variables must be independent. If one method of instruction is effective in teaching some aspect of reading, there should be no carryover to the other behaviors or aspects involved in reading. Researchers may attempt to find two parallel dependent variables or behaviors, or take a set of behaviors and randomly assign these to the instructional methods. When two sets of dependent variables are used in this manner, the difficulty seen with the ATD with regard to identifying the more effective instructional method for skills acquisition is overcome.

Likins, Salzberg, Stowitschek, Lignugaris/Kraft, and Curl (1989) used a PTD to investigate relative effectiveness of coincidental teaching with versus without quality-control checking when teaching students with mild or moderate intellectual disability to make a salad. The salad-making task was broken into 16 steps, ordered in terms of their level of difficulty (assessed in an earlier study). These 16 steps were then assigned alternately to the first or second instructional method. With this design, the researchers were able to determine that coincidental teaching with quality-control checking was more effective than teaching without quality-control checking. Notice that a standard ATD would not be appropriate for this study. If all 16 steps to making a salad were taught one of two ways on alternating days, there would most likely be carryover effects. Thus, a modification of the ATD is appropriate in cases such as this.

Analysis of Data

In this section, we consider internal validity, condition length, carryover effects, and external validity issues in regards to ATD designs.

Internal Validity

When assessing the internal validity of ATD and its variations, several concerns must be taken into consideration. These concerns involve condition length and carryover effects (i.e., diffusion or treatment). Table 13.1 summarizes the major threats to internal validity of the ATD.

Condition Length. As with all of the other designs discussed here and in Chapters 11 and 12, the length of the baseline condition should be at least three consecutive stable data points or three consecutive data points moving in a countertherapeutic direction. This concern is valid when there is a formal baseline condition. For the intervention condition, there should be at least two data points per condition or intervention (Barlow et al., 2008); however, the larger the number of data points collected, the better. Obviously, this is a major advantage of the ATD; it takes only a minimum of four sessions to compare two conditions or interventions. If a study has fewer than two data points per condition or intervention, the experimental control is seriously weakened. A trend must be demonstrated in single-case research, and fewer than two data points per condition or intervention cannot establish a trend when using the ATD.

Carryover Effects. One major threat comes from carryover problems. **Carryover effects** occur when the effect of an intervention used in one experimental condition influences behavior in an adjacent condition (Gast, 2010). If an intervention has an effect on the other intervention,

irrespective of how the interventions were sequenced, the differences between the interventions may be either minimal or nonexistent, or greater than would otherwise occur, not because the interventions are equal in effectiveness or one intervention is clearly less effective than the other, but because the effectiveness of one intervention improves or harms the performance of the other. The conclusion that one intervention is not superior to another or that one intervention may be superior to the other, may be incorrect due to this threat. This was the justification for proposing the AATD and the PTD. Carryover effects are expected to be present under some conditions, such as when teaching a skill.

There are two types of carryover effects—positive and negative (Gast, 2010). *Positive carryover effects* occur when the effects of one intervention are enhanced when alternated with the other intervention. *Negative carryover effects* occur when one intervention is less effective when alternated with the other intervention. Both carryover effects compromise the ability to make adequate conclusions with regard to the effects of each independent variable on the dependent variable. To prevent carryover effects, researchers should do the following:

1. Counterbalance the order of interventions (i.e., ensure an equal number of instances of the first intervention before and after the second intervention).

2. Separate interventions with a time interval. This interval aids the participant in discriminating when one intervention as opposed to the other is in effect. The participant must be able to tell when one intervention is in effect, since an inability to do so results in a lack of differential responding to the different interventions.

3. Be careful that the speed of alterations is not too rapid. For example, if interventions are rotated every hour, the participant may again have difficulty in discriminating when each intervention is in effect.

If critical research consumers suspect carryover effects, the conclusions made by the researcher may be compromised. These threats may lead to erroneous conclusions about the internal validity of the investigation.

External Validity

The ATD has the same difficulties as other single-case designs with regard to external validity. An added threat to external validity is multiple-treatment interference. However, participants in applied research rarely go without experiencing some multiple-treatment interference. If an intervention is used in an applied setting, it may have to compete with other factors such as history, maturation, and so on. Thus, when looking at several conditions or interventions, one can determine the effects of the intervention when the participant is also exposed to other conditions or interventions.

Specifically, a threat associated with multiple-treatment interference is *sequential confounding*, which occurs when one intervention may be more or less effective since it always follows the other intervention. Thus, the reason for randomly alternating the interventions is to prevent such a result. This is a threat to the external validity of the investigation, since the conclusion about the generalizability of an intervention's effectiveness may be incorrect if it is tied to how that intervention was ordered.

When considering the external validity of the ATD, we must realize that it can be improved with replications of the investigation's results. The researcher should report enough information in sufficient detail to allow for replications and logical generalization. Table 13.2 summarizes the major threats to external validity of the ATD.

Recall the research question about job preferences posed earlier in this chapter? Read on to see how your design compares to how the actual study was designed.

Research Example 3: Alternating Treatments Design

An ATD was used to investigate whether working on a self-selected, high-preference job was associated with higher levels of on-task behavior in community-based work settings in comparison to self-selected, low-preference jobs

(Morgan & Horrocks, 2011). Three young adults with moderate intellectual disabilities participated. Before the research began, participants identified high- and low-preference jobs using a video Web-based assessment program. Participants were then taken to community settings and taught by researchers to perform high- and low-preference job tasks. All work was performed in community locations representing individual participant selections. High- and low-preference job sessions, lasting 25 minutes, were performed each day. The order of sessions was randomized. A third daily session provided participants the opportunity to choose which job they wanted to perform. Two data collectors were unaware of participants' high- and low-preference job choices. They recorded observations and calculated the percentage of on-task behavior. The performance of one participant ("Diego"), an 18-year-old Hispanic male with Down syndrome, is shown in Figure 13.14. Diego's high-preference job was stocking shelves at a supermarket (white triangle). In all choice sessions, he selected the supermarket (shaded triangle; i.e., the same job as the previously selected high-preference job). His low-preference job was stripping and cutting wires at an assistive technology lab. Diego's levels of on-task behavior at the high-preference job ranged from 72 to 96% (mean = 87.4%). Choice sessions were always performed at the supermarket, with levels of on-task behavior similar to high-preference levels. His on-task behavior at the low-preference job ranged from 29 to 90% (mean = 63.9%). Figure 13.14 shows that no overlapping data are found when comparing high-preference to low-preference choice sessions. Data from four of 10 high-preference sessions overlap with data from low-preference sessions. Generally, Diego's on-task behavior was higher in the high-preference job. Researchers discuss limitations of this study, including absence of measures of productivity on the job and the need for more extensive pretraining before starting jobs.

Carryover effects *occur when the effect of an intervention used in one experimental condition influences behavior in an adjacent condition.*

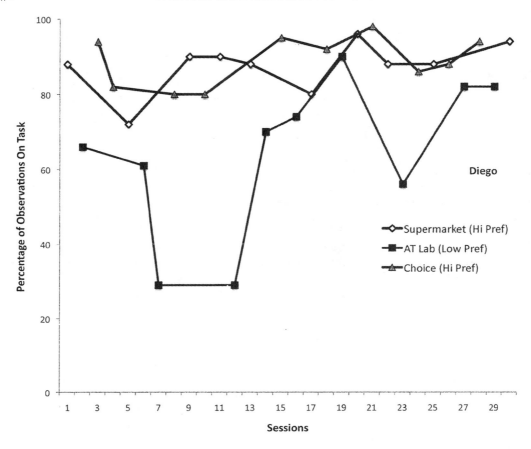

FIGURE 13.14. Percentage of observations on task for Diego in high-preference (supermarket), low-preference (AT lab), and choice conditions. Correspondence between video-based preference assessment and subsequent community job performance. *Education and Training in Autism and Developmental Disabilities*, 46, 52–61. Copyright 2011 by the Division on Autism and Developmental Disabilities, Council for Exceptional Children. Reprinted by permission.

WHAT ARE COMBINATION DESIGNS?

Combination designs, because of complex research questions about effects of variables and the need to minimize threats to internal validity, require researchers to combine single-case designs, such as embedding A-B-A-B conditions within a multiple-baseline design across participants. One advantage of single-case designs is the ability to combine two or more designs readily. As we mentioned in Chapter 12, multiple-probe designs can be combined with multiple-baseline designs to assess the generalizability of the dependent variable. Other combination designs that have appeared in the literature include changing-design criterion within a multiple-baseline design alternating treatments design within a multiple-baseline design, withdrawal design within a multiple-baseline design and within a changing-criterion design, and a multiple-baseline design across participants within a multiple-baseline design across behaviors (see Gast, 2010, for more examples).

The advantage of combination designs is that they can improve the internal validity of the investigation. For example, suppose we are working with a single participant who has difficulty reading and doing math. We can implement a study strategy that we hope will help her reading and math skills. We implement the intervention in a staggered fashion (i.e., a multiple-baseline design across behaviors). However, there is a weakness with a multiple-baseline design across two behaviors. Thus, we can combine the design with another, such as a withdrawal design, in such a way that the intervention is removed (i.e., the participant is no longer supplied with the materials necessary for study strategy behavior). If the behavior (e.g., reading) maintains after the intervention is removed, we still have a multiple-baseline design across two behaviors. On the other hand, if the behavior (e.g., reading) decreases to baseline levels, we have a stronger demonstration of experimental control.

Another example involves the difficulty of having only two participants in one setting. We can use a multiple-baseline design across two participants; however, we still have a weakness. Suppose we want to test the effects of compliance instruction in the classroom for the two participants. We cannot only use the multiple-baseline design across participants but also test the intervention in other settings, as shown in Figure 13.15. Notice how the combination of the designs increases the internal validity of the investigation. The addition of one more setting improves the research design substantially.

Combination designs can also add information to designs that may not have been set up to probe for such additional information. Recall the primary purpose of the ATD is to compare two or more conditions or interventions. Suppose we want to compare one instructional method of teaching problem solving to another. The first method involves a standard problem-solving format, such that a participant is taught to recognize the problem, define the problem, generate solutions, compare each solution to the predicted consequences, apply the solution, and assess the results. The second method involves a new method that adds self-instruction, such that each participant is required to talk him-/herself through the problem to reach a solution. We decide to use an ATD in which two sets of different but comparable (in terms of difficulty level) problem situations are developed. In addition to measuring the relative effects of the interventions, we are interested in seeing whether the same results hold true for others. Thus, we combine the ATD with a multiple-baseline

design across participants. Figure 13.16 demonstrates the case in which the self-instruction problem-solving format is superior to the standard format for all four participants. This finding is important, since the superiority of the self-instruction format is replicated across four individuals. This replication increases our confidence in the superiority of adding self-instructions to a standard problem-solving format.

Combination designs can also be used to increase the internal validity of single-case designs that are initially considered to be weaker from the start, such as the changing-criterion design. As previously described, a withdrawal design can be added to a changing-criterion design, and a changing-criterion design can be placed within a multiple-baseline design.

Analysis of Data

In this section, we consider internal validity and external validity issues related to combination designs.

Internal Validity

As mentioned, the combination of single-case designs may improve the internal validity of the investigation and/or gather additional information. When conducted appropriately, the combination of two or more designs can increase the internal validity of the investigation. The control issues (e.g., level of change, return to baseline, carryover or sequential confounding effects) discussed here and in Chapters 11 and 12 are all in effect here.

External Validity

Threats to external validity are always a problem with single-case designs when considering isolated investigations. However, combinations of designs can improve the external validity in some ways. For example, the combination of single-case designs within multiple-baseline designs can increase the external validity across behaviors, participants, and settings. The

> **Combination designs** *are those that involve the combination of at least two single-case designs.*

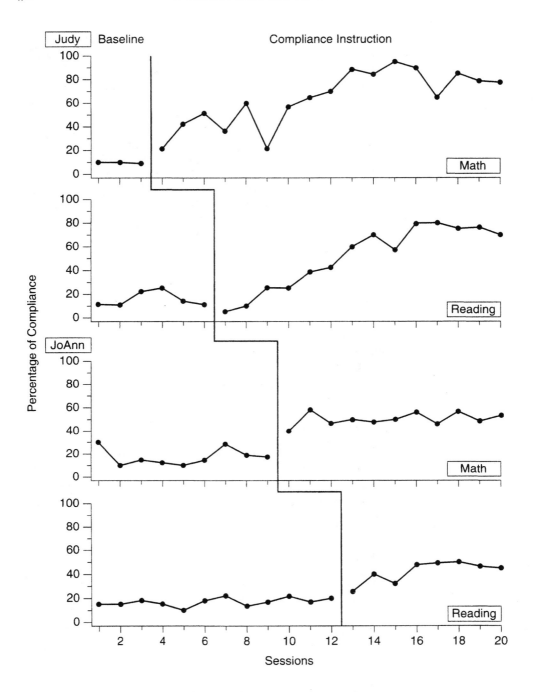

FIGURE 13.15. Percentage of compliance across baseline and compliance instruction conditions for Judy and JoAnn for math and reading classes.

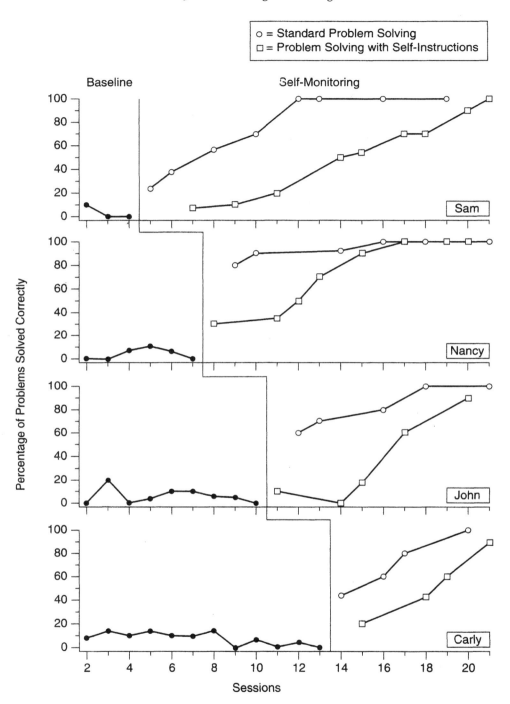

FIGURE 13.16. Percentage of problems solved correctly across baseline, standard problem solving, and problem solving with self-instruction conditions for Sam, Nancy, John, and Carly.

combination of other single-case designs with an ATD can increase the external validity across multiple treatments (more like real life, in which many extraneous variables are constantly present). The combination of multiple-probe designs with other single-case designs can increase external validity across response measures. Thus, the combination of several single-case designs can have important advantages over isolated single-case designs in terms of external validity.

Recall the research question about a self-monitoring program posed earlier in this chapter? Read on to see how your design compares to how the actual study was designed.

Research Example 4: Combination Designs

Martella et al. (1993) used a combination of a changing-criterion design within a multiple-baseline design across settings to investigate the effects of a self-monitoring program on a student's negative verbalizations. The student, a 12-year-old male with mild intellectual disabilities, received special educational services in a self-contained classroom. His verbal behaviors (derogatory to self and/or others) were so disruptive in the classroom that educational staff considered placing him in a classroom for youth with behavior disorders.

The independent variable comprised self-monitoring, self-charting, and reinforcement for reaching daily goals (i.e., behavior criteria). The dependent variable was negative statements. Positive statements were also measured to determine the collateral effects of the intervention. The dependent measures were the rates of negative and positive statements in two different periods. During the baseline condition, pretraining on how to self-monitor took place to ensure that changes were due not to the student learning how to self-monitor but due to contingencies set in place for his self-monitoring.

As shown in Figure 13.17, the student's negative statements (black squares) decreased when the intervention program was implemented. The negative statements were reduced in a stepwise fashion. The teacher in the classroom did not believe the student's negative verbalizations would be reduced over the long run unless they

were reduced gradually. The student's negative statements decreased to a final level of 0.0 and maintained at that level over 8 weeks of follow-up. The positive statements (white circles) increased to a level of approximately 0.5 statements per minute in Period 2 and 1.0 statement per minute in Period 1.

WHEN SHOULD RESEARCHERS USE EACH OF THE ADDITIONAL SINGLE-CASE DESIGNS?

As with the designs in Chapters 11 and 12, the designs discussed in this chapter serve special purposes in research. Depending on the research question, one design may be more appropriate than the others. For example, for a researcher attempting to reduce an addictive behavior, one that is resistant to quick changes, the changing-criterion design is appropriate. Similarly, if a researcher is teaching a skill that is best acquired in stages, the changing-criterion design is appropriate. However, the experimental control exerted by a changing-criterion design is more difficult to demonstrate. The dependent variable must cluster around the criterion level during each change in the criterion phase. If not, the experimental control is seriously weakened. Thus, researchers must be careful to use the changing-criterion design at appropriate times, and to set and change the criterion at appropriate times and at appropriate levels.

For researchers who want to compare components of an intervention package or multiple interventions, the multitreatment design or ATD is acceptable. If they decided to use the multitreatment design, the problem of irreversibility must be taken into account. If it is not possible to reverse the dependent variable, or if it would be unethical to do so, the multitreatment design should not be used. Additionally, carryover or sequential confounding effects are also problems that may preclude the use of the multitreatment design. Finally, since it is cumbersome and can take a great deal of time to complete, it is unwise to use the multitreatment design when simplicity or timely decision making is desired. In this case, researchers would select the ATD. However, if researchers are

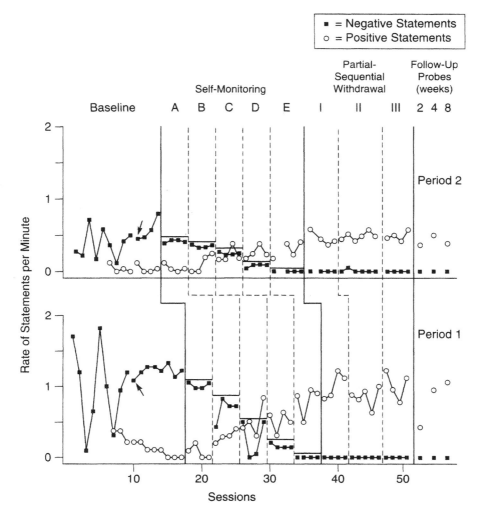

FIGURE 13.17. The rate of negative and positive statements per minute for an adolescent student with mild mental retardation across Periods 2 and 1. The arrows indicate when pretraining began. From Martella, R. C., Leonard, L. J., Marchand-Martella, N. E., & Agran, M. (1993). Self-monitoring negative statements. *Journal of Behavioral Education, 3*, 77–86. Copyright 1993 by Human Sciences Press. Reprinted by permission.

worried about carryover and sequential confounding effects, the ATD may not be appropriate. In this case, the only option may be a group factorial design.

If researchers are interested in investigating the effects of an intervention on some dependent variable but the proposed design has obvious weaknesses, such as only two settings, they can combine the multiple-baseline design across settings with another design. If researchers are interested in generalization issues, a multiple-probe design can be combined with other designs. The use of combined single-case designs is not always the result of overcoming the weaknesses of another stand-alone design, but the combinations can provide additional experimental control and produce additional information. The decision to use a combined design comes about as a result of the research question and the most appropriate method to answer that research question, as is true with the other designs.

SUMMARY

❖ Selection of additional single-case designs is based on several considerations: (1) the behavior to be changed, (2) the type of research question asked, or (3) the constraints present (e.g., ethical issues surrounding the use of withdrawal designs; lack of multiple behaviors, participants, or settings).

❖ The changing-criterion design is an experimental design in which an initial baseline is followed by a series of intervention phases with successive and gradually changing criteria. Without the "phase" lines (i.e., changes within the intervention condition), the design looks the same as an A-B design. The difference between a changing-criterion design and an A-B design is the use of a criterion within each phase. To implement a changing-criterion design, researchers must do the following: (1) Collect baseline data; (2) set the first criterion level around the average of the baseline; and (3) change the criterion to a new level once the participant meets some predetermined level, such as three data points at or below (in cases where the behavior is to decrease) or above (in cases where the behavior is to increase) the criterion. When assessing the internal validity of the changing-criterion design, several concerns must be taken into consideration: (1) the condition length (including the trend of the data), (2) whether the behavior stays near the criterion level, (3) the stability and immediacy of change, (4) the number of criterion levels, and (5) other control procedures. The external validity of the changing-criterion design is fairly weak; thus, single-case researchers look to replications to demonstrate external validity in a systematic manner.

❖ The multitreatment design allows for the comparison of two or more interventions or the additive components of an intervention. The multitreatment design is an associate of the withdrawal design. Several of the possible variations of the withdrawal design demonstrate the effects of several interventions or components of an intervention. The following all have an impact on the control of threats to internal validity: (1) condition length, (2) changing one variable at a time, (3) level and rapidity

of change, (4) return to baseline levels, and (5) time of implementation. The external validity of the multitreatment design is weak, so replications must be conducted to increase confidence in the generalizability of the results.

❖ An ATD, or multielement design, is an experimental design in which two or more conditions are presented in rapidly alternating succession (e.g., on alternating days) to determine differences between the conditions. One of the conditions may be a no-treatment condition, or there may be multiple treatment conditions.

❖ The ATD is an alternative to the multitreatment design.

❖ The main purpose of the ATD is to make comparisons between or among two or more conditions or interventions, such as baseline and intervention(s) or multiple interventions. A secondary function is to determine experimental control.

❖ The ATD is also the single-case alternative to the factorial design used in group research. On completion of the comparison between or among conditions or interventions, a visual analysis is conducted. The amount of spread between or among the conditions or interventions indicates the level of differential effectiveness. Once a determination has been made with regard to the relative effectiveness of the conditions or interventions, a final condition may be added to the design.

❖ The AATD and PTD are modifications of the ATD. These designs help to solve the problem of investigating the relative effectiveness of different instructional methods on skill acquisition dependent variables. The AATD and PTD require that two or more "sets" of dependent variables or behaviors be developed. These dependent variables or behaviors should be similar in difficulty and effort to perform. Concerns of the AATD and PTD are (1) condition length and (2) carryover effects. The ATD has the same difficulties as other single-case designs with regard to external validity. An added threat to external validity is multiple-treatment interference. When considering the external validity of the ATD, we must realize that it can be improved with replications.

❖ One advantage of single-case designs is the ability to combine two or more designs readily. Combination designs, because of complex research questions about effects of variables and the need to minimize threats to internal validity, require researchers to combine single-case designs. Combination designs can also be used to increase the internal validity of single-case designs that are initially considered to be weaker from the start, such as the changing-criterion design. These designs can also add information to designs that may not have been set up to probe for such additional information. The control issues (e.g., level of change, return to baseline, carryover or sequential confounding effects) discussed here and in Chapters 11 and 12

are all in effect. The threats to external validity are always a problem with single-case designs when researchers consider isolated investigations. However, combinations of designs can improve the external validity in some ways.

❖ Depending on the research question, one design may be more appropriate than the others. For example, if the research question is to determine the comparative effects of three interventions across several students, a combined ATD and multiple-baseline design across participants might be appropriate. If the research question is to determine the effects of an intervention for several students across several settings, a combined multiple-baseline design across participants within a multiple-baseline design across settings might be appropriate.

DISCUSSION QUESTIONS

1. What type of design can be used for a student who frequently interrupts instruction by blurting out answers to questions and making comments? (In your answer, assume you want to reduce the interruptions gradually.) Explain how you would implement the design.

2. For each of the designs in Question 1, what would a graph look like with fictitious data showing that a self-control procedure was effective when implemented? Show the graph and data.

3. Would a multiple-baseline design be appropriate if one wanted to compare the effectiveness of two separate interventions? Why or why not? If not, what would have been an appropriate design for the researcher to use?

4. How can the experimental control of a changing-criterion design be improved? Describe two ways.

5. What design would you use to show the most efficient instructional method for teaching spelling? Explain.

6. You are aware of the weaknesses of the multitreatment design. What is an alternative design to the multitreatment design? Explain why this design is a better alternative.

7. How would you use a combination design to increase the experimental control of a multiple-baseline design across only two subjects? Explain how this would be done.

8. How can a multiple-probe design and a multiple-baseline design across behaviors be combined to assess generalization? Explain.

9. What are the internal validity concerns with the following?
   a. changing-criterion design
   b. multitreatment design
   c. alternating treatments design

10. How can two single-case designs be combined to form a new design in order to answer the following research question: What is the most effective instructional procedure to use when teaching basic math facts to students in the general education classroom and to those located in a resource room? Explain.

ILLUSTRATIVE EXAMPLE

A Comparison of Picture and Video Prompts to Teach Daily Living Skills to Individuals with Autism

Toni Van Laarhoven and Erika Kraus
Northern Illinois University, DeKalb, IL

Keri Karpman, Rosemary Nizzi, and Joe Valentino
North DuPage Special Education Cooperative, Bloomingdale, IL

Abstract. *This study was conducted to compare the effectiveness of video prompting and picture prompting when used as antecedents for teaching daily living skills to two adolescents with autism. Participants were taught two different skills, and the effects of the instructional conditions were compared and evaluated using an adapted alternating-treatments design. The results can be interpreted to conclude that video prompting was slightly more effective in terms of independent correct responding, fewer external prompts for task completion, and fewer prompts to use instructional materials. In addition, when efficiency scores were calculated by considering the ratio of each participant's growth (from pretest to posttest) to the measured "cost" of minutes required to create instructional materials, video prompting was considerably more efficient than picture prompting.*

Keywords. *autism, picture prompting, video prompting, daily living skills, efficiency*

Individuals with autism spectrum disorders (ASD) frequently use visual supports to make sense of the environments in which they function (Rogers, 2005). Visual supports may include text, line drawings, photographs, or video-based materials that are used to assist individuals become more independent. The use of visual supports to teach individuals with ASD typically results in positive outcomes for a broad range of learners and is considered to be an evidence-based practice (Myles, Grossman, Aspy, Henry, & Coffin, 2007; Odom et al., 2003). Learners can use visual supports to help them communicate, establish predictability in carrying out daily routines, acquire new skills, and become more independent in and across a variety of environments.

Some of the most widely used visual supports include photographs or line drawings (Lancioni & O'Reilly, 2001, 2002). Photographs or illustrated pictures are relatively easy to create and often are used to teach or prompt individuals with ASD or other developmental disabilities to complete complex or multistep skill sequences. For example, photographed and/or illustrated task analyses have been used effectively to teach food preparation skills (Bergstrom, Pattavina, Martella, & Marchand-Martella, 1995; Book, Paul, Gwalla-Ogisi, & Test, 1990; Johnson, & Cuvo, 1981; Martin, Rusch, James, Decker, & Tritol, 1982; Singh, Oswald, Ellis, & Singh, 1995), vocational skills (Martin, Mithaug, & Frazier, 1992; Wacker & Berg, 1983), daily living skills (Pierce & Schreibman, 1994), and community skills (Alberto, Cihak, & Gama, 2005; Cihak, Alberto, Taber-Doughty, & Gama, 2006). When used in this way, skill sequences are typically task analyzed and pictures are used to represent each step. For example, Pierce and Schreibman (1994) used multistep pictures based on task analyses to teach daily living skills such as making lunch, getting dressed, and setting the table to three young children with autism. Each step in the task analyses was represented with picture prompts and was used while the participants completed the tasks. The authors reported that each child acquired the targeted skill and was able to complete the tasks independently by following the picture prompts, even when the order of pictures was changed. In another study, Copeland and Hughes (2000) taught two high school students vocational skills in a hotel using a two-part picture prompt strategy. Participants were expected to touch a picture to initiate tasks and to turn pages to indicate task completion. Both participants increased their number of independent task initiations, but only one of the participants improved his ability to complete tasks.

Although picture prompting strategies have been shown to be effective for teaching or prompting complex behaviors, many researchers also have investigated the efficiency and effectiveness of using video-based instructional materials to prompt responses. Much of the research that has been conducted on video-based instruction involves *video modeling*. Video modeling refers to an instructional approach whereby learners view an entire video skill sequence prior to engaging in a task. This also has been referred to as "video priming" (Schreibman, Whalen, & Stahmer, 2000) or "video rehearsal" (Van Laarhoven & Van Laarhoven-Myers, 2006). *Video prompting*, on the other hand, is an instructional approach that involves showing each *step* in a skill sequence on video, followed immediately by task engagement with that particular step (Sigafoos et al., 2005). This requires that learners have access to a television, computer, or handheld device in the environment where the skill is being practiced so that they can watch a clip, go perform the step, and then return to the television or computer to complete the remainder of the steps. Several researchers have successfully used a combination of video modeling and video prompting to teach skill sequences to individuals with developmental disabilities (Graves, Collins, Schuster, & Kleinert, 2005; Norman, Collins, & Schuster, 2001).

In a comparative study, Van Laarhoven and Van Laarhoven-Myers (2006) used three different video-based instructional methods (video modeling alone, video modeling plus in vivo picture prompting, and video modeling plus video prompting) to teach three daily living skills to three high school-aged participants with moderate intellectual disabilities. All three methods were effective for increasing independent correct responding, but the video modeling plus video prompting and video modeling plus picture prompting conditions resulted in quicker acquisition and in higher independent correct responding, suggesting that the addition of in vivo antecedent prompting techniques resulted in more efficient and effective skill acquisition. Cannella-Malone et al. (2006) had somewhat similar findings when they compared video modeling with video prompting to teach six adults with developmental disabilities how to set a table and put away groceries. They found that video prompting was much more effective than video modeling for five of the six participants, which also suggests that in vivo prompting may be necessary for promoting rapid skill acquisition. Although it has been demonstrated that video prompting can be a very powerful instructional method, some researchers have suggested that it can be even more effective when used in conjunction with video feedback (referencing) error correction procedures (Goodson, Sigafoos, O'Reilly,

Cannella, & Lancioni, 2007; Martin et al., 1992; Van Laarhoven, Johnson, Van Laarhoven-Myers, Grider, & Grider, 2009). Video referencing or feedback, when used as an error correction procedure, involves having participants refer back to video clips in the event of an error or no response during task engagement.

A few researchers have conducted studies to compare picture versus video prompts. For example, Alberto et al. (2005) and Cihak et al. (2006) compared the effectiveness of static picture prompts and video models or video prompts, respectively, but the instructional prompting strategies were used by individual students in a simulated setting approximately 90 min before the participants engaged in community-based skill sequences. Alberto et al. concluded that both techniques were effective and were not functionally different when independent correct responses and the number of sessions to criterion were considered. Cihak et al. provided instruction to groups of students in simulated settings in the classroom. They also found no functional differences between the two conditions. Although there were no functional differences between the conditions when independent correct responding and number of sessions to criterion were considered, both groups of researchers indicated that students with attention difficulties seemed to perform better with static picture prompts.

The purpose of this study was to compare the effectiveness of in vivo picture prompting and video prompting strategies on the independent functioning of two adolescents with autism who were learning daily living skills. Unlike the comparative studies conducted by Alberto et al. (2005) and Cihak et al. (2006), the picture and video prompts were used as antecedent prompts during in vivo task engagement rather than as simulation techniques that were temporally distant. In addition, the prompting systems were manipulated by the participants and data were collected on the number of prompts needed to use the technologies to determine if the participants could use them independently. Cost-benefit or "efficiency" analyses of the amount of time required to develop each set of instructional materials were measured to assess the practical utility of each intervention. The conditions that were compared included (a) picture prompts presented in a booklet and (b) video prompts presented on a laptop computer. The prompting strategies were used in conjunction with error correction or feedback procedures that included picture feedback (Martin et al., 1992) and video feedback procedures (Goodson et al., 2007; Van Laarhoven, Johnson, et al., 2009; Van Laarhoven, Van Laarhoven-Myers, & Zurita, 2007) by having the participants refer back to the visual systems if they made errors.

METHOD

Participants

Participants were recruited from a special education cooperative located in the suburbs of Chicago. An e-mail was sent to special education teachers employed in the cooperative to inform them of the research study. A questionnaire was sent to the teachers who volunteered to (a) identify specific skills for instruction, (b) determine availability of the participant, and (c) obtain personal information for the students who were eligible to participate. A description of the study was sent home to those parents to obtain informed consent and assent. Participants were selected from the pool of respondents on the basis of the level of intellectual functioning (i.e., mild or moderate), skills requiring instruction (indicated on a survey from parents and teachers), and scores on pretests that were given to the initial pool of participants to determine daily living skills to be targeted for instruction. All intelligence testing had been conducted by school psychologists hired by the special education cooperative.

Two male students with autism and mild to moderate intellectual disabilities participated in the study. Both participants were enrolled in a public middle school where they received educational programming in both self-contained and integrated classrooms. The program in which they were enrolled provided academic, functional, and community-based educational programming. Both participants had similar skills requiring instruction, including daily living skills as well as vocational skills, which were identified as instructional priorities by their teacher and parents.

At the time the study was conducted, Marvin was 13 years old. He was a very pleasant young man who liked to move quickly. He was verbal and spoke in short sentences to communicate his wants and needs. He also engaged in some echolalic speech and often recited scenes from movies or lyrics from songs when he was not engaged in tasks. On the basis of the Stanford–Binet Intelligence Scale, Marvin's full-scale IQ score was 39, which placed him in the low moderate range of intellectual disability. Scores on the Woodcock–Johnson test of achievement indicated that he was at the readiness or early first grade level in reading and had some letter recognition and sight word vocabulary. Marvin had previous exposure to using the Picture Exchange Communication System and also used picture schedules and other visual supports within the structure of his day. He had some experience using picture-based task analyses but primarily used visual supports to prompt changes in schedules or to promote communication. He used the computer in the classroom independently to navigate educational software used primarily for drill and practice; however, he had no previous experience with video-based instruction.

Gary was 14 years old at the time of the study and was in the same classroom as Marvin. He also was a very pleasant young man who spoke in short sentences using a slow rate of speech with unique intonation and stress patterns. His previous full-scale IQ score on the Wechsler Intelligence Scale for Children was 52, while a more recent test, the Kaufman Brief Intelligence Scale, resulted in a composite score of 65, placing him in the mild to moderate range of intellectual functioning. Scores on the Woodcock–Johnson test of achievement placed him at the first to second grade level in reading. His teacher indicated that Gary knew approximately 65 sight words and performed better with reading tasks when pictures were paired with text. Gary used picture schedules and other visual supports throughout the day and enjoyed using the computer in the classroom, but he had no prior exposure to video-based instruction.

Skills Selected for Instruction

Each participant was taught two different skills in each of the instructional conditions (i.e., one skill taught with picture prompts and one taught with video prompts). The targeted skills fell within the vocational or daily living domains (folding laundry and meal preparation). The skill sequences were selected on the basis of parent and teacher priorities, the students' preferences, and participants' pretest scores. First, teachers and parents were provided with a list of potential tasks to be taught and asked to indicate which tasks were high priorities. Tasks that did not share any common features with each other were selected to ensure that the responses across the skill sequences were mutually exclusive and independent of one another to prevent any carryover effects from one condition to the next. Marvin and Gary were taught the same two skills: making microwave pasta and folding laundry using a flip-and-fold. The two tasks were similar in difficulty and length or number of steps (i.e., 22 steps for pasta and 23 steps for folding clothes).

Setting

Instructional sessions were conducted in the faculty lounge at the middle school. The room had a sink with a long countertop that held the microwave, cabinets above and below the counter, and a refrigerator along the adjacent wall. The room had several round tables scattered around the center of the room and one long table that was pushed against a wall near the sink and microwave. The sessions took place at the long table that was located near the sink.

Generalization sessions, which were only conducted during pre-, post-, and maintenance sessions, were conducted in another area of the school that was located behind the stage or in a faculty office that was not being used. In addition to being conducted in different settings, the materials that were used in the instructional and generalization conditions differed across stimulus dimensions. For example, different pasta dishes (i.e., microwave spaghetti vs. microwave lasagna), utensils that varied in size and color, and different microwaves, laundry baskets, clothing items, and flip-and-folds were used in instructional versus generalization sessions. No video- or picture-based prompting systems were developed for generalization sessions.

Design

A within-subject adapted alternating-treatments design (Wolery, Bailey, & Sugai, 1988) was used in this study. In an adapted alternating-treatments design, the treatments are applied to different but equally difficult, independent behaviors or skills, whereas in the alternating-treatments design, the treatments are applied to the same behavior or skill. In the adapted alternating-treatments design, two or more treatment conditions are introduced in a rapidly alternating fashion with a randomized order of presentation. Each participant was taught

a different skill within each condition, and the skills were counterbalanced across conditions and subjects to control for task difficulty. Marvin was taught to fold clothes using picture prompts and to make microwave pasta using video prompts. Gary was taught to cook microwave pasta using picture prompts and to fold clothes using video prompts.

Data Analysis

Experimental control was determined primarily through visual inspection of the data and through comparisons of means for each condition. With the adapted alternating-treatments design, experimental control is demonstrated by a consistent level and/or trend difference between the interventions (Wolery et al., 1988). At a quick glance, one can determine if one intervention is better than the other if there is little or no overlap between the data paths. In addition, although baseline measures are not necessary with the alternating-treatments design, the pretest and posttest scores for each condition were compared using both instructional and generalization materials.

Independent Variables

All video-based and picture-based materials were created by the first author, who had experience with all of the technologies, in the setting where instructional sessions took place (i.e., the faculty lounge). A man who was a teaching assistant in the classroom acted as the model in both of the tasks, and the photos and videos displayed him engaging in the skill sequence using both zoom and wide-angle shots (i.e., combination of "other" model and subjective or first-person viewpoint for zoom shots). To create the materials, the model engaged in each skill sequence twice; the first time through, video segments of each step were shot, and the second time through, photographs were taken of each step, and the number of seconds required to gather the shots under both conditions was recorded. Both video segments and photographs were shot with a combination of wide-angle (full view of the model) and a few zoom shots (showing the arm of the model setting the microwave). Zoom shots for both the picture- and video-based materials were used to ensure that participants attended to the critical aspects of the steps (e.g., setting the microwave for 4 min). In addition, some text was added to both prompting conditions to encourage sight reading, but the text was treated as nontargeted information and not measured.

Condition 1: Picture Prompts

After the photographs were taken, they were captured using the built-in scanner and camera wizard loaded on the laptop. They were cropped if necessary and saved in a folder on the desktop. Sometimes more than one picture was needed to depict a step. For example, to demonstrate the step for "Fold," it was necessary to show three pictures: (a) fold in side A, (b) fold in side B, and (c) fold up C using the flip-and-fold. Or, for "Gather Materials," it was necessary to show pictures of each needed item. After saving the pictures to the desktop, they were imported into Microsoft Power-Point, with one step in the task analysis per slide. A short description of each step was placed on the top of each slide (e.g., "Set Microwave"), and the picture(s) was placed below. When more than one picture was presented on the slide, a text box with a sequenced number was placed on each picture to indicate the correct order of substeps. The Power-Point presentation was then printed, with one slide per page. After the materials were printed, they were laminated, sequenced, hole-punched in the top left corner, and held together with a notebook ring to create a booklet. A stopwatch was used to calculate how long it took to create the materials (including photography, capturing, cropping, creating the PowerPoint presentation, printing, laminating, etc.). During the intervention, the participants looked at the picture(s) on one page, engaged in the step, went back to the booklet, turned the page, engaged in the next step, and so forth until the skill sequence was completed.

Condition 2: Video Prompts

After videos were filmed, they were captured, and each segment was edited using Pinnacle Studio 10.1. Skill sequences (e.g., making microwave pasta) were broken into short video segments (for each step). Photos of the most salient feature of the steps (e.g., a still shot of "4:00" on the microwave) were "grabbed" out of the video and placed at the beginning of each video segment. Voiceover narrations were then added to each segment to describe the actions being depicted in each segment and to cover the background noise that was present in the setting during filming (e.g., the bell ringing, announcements over the intercom). Each step of

the task was edited and saved as a separate file and placed in a PowerPoint presentation. Each slide in the PowerPoint presentation had a short description of the step on the top of the screen and the grabbed photo visible in the middle of the screen. The slide show was set so that the participants had to move the cursor to the photo and use a mouse click to view the video prior to completing the step. After completing the step, the participants clicked on a hyperlinked "Next" button at the bottom right of the screen to advance to the next slide. Again, a stopwatch was used to determine how long it took to create the materials, including videotaping, capturing, editing, narrating, creating Power-Point presentations, and burning presentations to CDs. During intervention, participants viewed the video segment of each step on a laptop computer prior to engaging in each step until the task was completed.

Procedures

Pretests

During the pretesting phase, several tasks were selected as potential skills to be targeted for instruction. Task analyses were written and evaluated by four veteran teachers (each had been teaching for at least 5 years), who rated the task analyses according to complexity and difficulty (easy, moderately difficult, or difficult) and then ranked the steps within each difficulty level to verify that the skills were equivalent in terms of complexity. During the 1st week of the study, initial pretests using instructional materials were given to potential participants (i.e., those with consent who had given assent) in the setting where instruction was to take place. Potential participants were tested without the use of video or picture prompts to determine their current levels of independent functioning with various tasks.

For pretest sessions, participants were brought to the instructional area and were told what task they were going to perform. They were asked to do their best and told that if they did not know what to do at any point, they could ask the researchers to complete the step for them. Each participant was given an instructional cue, such as "fold clothes," "cook the spaghetti," "wash the dishes," and so forth; the verbal cue was used throughout the session. If participants made errors during the testing phases or did not respond within 10 s, the experimenter asked them to turn away or close their eyes, and the step with the error was completed for them. The researcher then gave the next instructional cue to get the participant to continue with the task. This protocol was repeated until the task was completed, and no feedback related to task performance was given; however, praise statements were delivered for staying on task and working hard.

All potential participants were pretested again the following week using generalization materials and settings for the same tasks. The assessment protocol was delivered in the same format as the original pretests. Potential participants who scored 50% or less on both pretests were included in the study. To control for participant skill level prior to instruction, the scores for instructional pretests and generalization pretests were averaged and ranked. Each participant's task with the highest score was randomly assigned to one of the different conditions. Intervention began 2 weeks after the pretesting phase to allow time for training the participants to use the technologies and to create the instructional materials.

Training Participants to Use Technology and Photos

Prior to engaging in instructional sessions, each participant was taught to use each of the prompting systems via a model-lead-test format until he could use the prompting systems independently to complete a task that was unrelated to the instructional tasks (i.e., cleaning a desk). They were taught to use a picture booklet and taught to operate the laptop to navigate through the PowerPoint presentation until they could independently use the materials to prompt responses for three consecutive sessions. The first author taught both participants to operate the prompting systems during initial training sessions and also taught a teaching assistant (another certified teacher) to conduct the training sessions on days when she could not be present. Although it may take more time, we believe that training participants to use the technologies independently is important, because it can result in true independence during task engagement and result in less reliance on caregivers or staff.

Instructional Sessions

During instruction, the picture prompting booklet or laptop was placed on the long table next to the counter in the faculty lounge. When the participants entered the faculty lounge, they were told which task they were going to do for the day and shown the prompting system. They were then given the instructional cue of either "fold clothes" or "cook pasta." Participants used the prompting devices by looking at the picture in the booklet or playing the video segment on the laptop prior to performing each step in the skill sequence. They then returned to the booklet or computer to prompt the next step until the entire sequence was completed. Researchers intervened only if participants made an error or needed a prompt to use the technology. Praise statements were delivered to reinforce correct responding during task engagement, and high fives or knuckle bumps were given following the completion of the tasks. In addition, participants were allowed to eat the pasta dishes or give them to peers or faculty of their choosing.

Posttests

One week after participants met criteria in the intervention (i.e., three consecutive sessions with 85% correct responding or higher with both tasks), they were given a posttest using materials used during instruction. Posttests were given in the same manner as the pretests to determine if the participants could independently complete the tasks without the use of video or picture prompts. Two days later, they were given posttests in different environments using different materials to determine if they could generalize their skills to different settings and materials. The generalization posttests were conducted again 6 weeks later to determine if skills were maintained.

Data Collection Procedures

During pre- and posttesting, instruction, and generalization testing, task analytic data were collected with correct and incorrect performance being reported on each step of the skill sequence. A "+" was recorded for independent correct responses, a "–" was recorded for incorrect attempts, "N–" was recorded for no attempt, and "S–" was recorded for a sequence error. Data were collected on prompt levels during instruction; a check mark was recorded for each prompt given at each step (with a maximum of two per step). To obtain data on prompt levels, a two-level prompting hierarchy was used. In the event of an error or no attempt within 8 s of seeing the step, participants were instructed to refer back to the visual prompt (booklet or computer) and review the step. If this did not result in a correct response, a gestural or physical prompt was provided (depending on what was necessary for the particular step) to ensure correct responding. Data also were collected on prompts necessary for the participants to use the technologies to determine if they could use the technologies independently during task engagement. In the event that the student did not refer to the prompting system prior to performing the step, he was reminded to "look at" the picture or video clip, and the prompt to use the technology was recorded by circling the step on the data sheet.

Dependent Measures

Percentage of Independent Correct Responses

Participants were assessed on how independently they performed the skills selected for instruction prior to engaging in the instructional sequences (pretest), during instruction, and following instruction (posttest). The score was determined by dividing the number of steps with independent responding by the total number of steps in the skill sequence and multiplying by 100%.

Percentage of Error Correction Prompts

Participants were assessed on the number of external prompts needed to complete the skill sequence during the instructional phase of the study. The score was determined by dividing the number of prompts given by the total number of prompts possible (i.e., two per step) and multiplying by 100%.

Percentage of Prompts to Use Technology

Participants were assessed on the number of prompts they needed to use the booklet or computer. The score was determined by dividing the number of prompts given by the total number of steps in the skill sequence and multiplying by 100%.

Number of Sessions to Reach Criterion

The acquisition criterion for each skill sequence was a score of 85% independent correct responses for three consecutive sessions. The number of instructional sessions required for the participant to reach criterion was counted to determine if either of the instructional conditions resulted

in faster acquisition. Participants engaged in skill sequences until criteria were met on both tasks.

Percentage of Independent Correct Responses on Measures of Generalization

Prior to and following instruction (at 1 and 6 weeks), participants performed the skills in novel environments, using different stimulus materials, without the aid of prompting systems to determine if their skills generalized to untrained environments and novel materials following instruction.

Efficiency Measures

It is important in comparative studies to assess the amount of time and effort expended in preparing materials, teacher and student preferences for intervention strategies, and student outcomes. Van Laarhoven, Zurita, Johnson, Grider, & Grider (2009) did this when they compared the effectiveness of self-, other-, and subjective-video (i.e., first-person) modeling packages on teaching daily living skills to three students with disabilities. The authors reported that all models were effective in terms of student outcomes, but the amount of time required to develop the self-modeling materials was almost double the time required to develop the other- and subjective-modeling materials. As a result, the other- and subjective-model videotape packages were more efficient in addition to being somewhat more effective. The authors recommended that future comparative researchers evaluate the cost-effectiveness of interventions in terms of time needed to create materials and student outcomes.

In this study, an efficiency score was computed by considering the ratio of each participant's growth (from pretest to posttest) to the measured "cost" of minutes required to create instructional materials (i.e., [posttest – pretest]/minutes of preparation) to get a score representing the percentage increase per minute of preparation. To determine the number of minutes of preparation, a stopwatch was used to calculate the number of minutes required to prepare the picture books and video-based instructional sequences.

Reliability

The first or second author and/or the instructional assistant simultaneously collected data for 28% of all sessions (including pre- and posttests and instructional sessions). The percentage agreement index (i.e., the number of agreements divided by number of agreements plus disagreements times 100%) was used to calculate interobserver agreement. Agreement for independent correct responses averaged 99% (range = 99%–100%). Agreement for error correction prompts and prompts to use technologies resulted in a mean score of 96% (range = 88%–100%). In addition, the second observer collected procedural reliability data (Billingsley, White, & Munson, 1980). These measures included the following: (a) checking to ensure that the correct condition was being applied to the intended task for each participant, (b) checking to determine if the order of tasks were presented as stated in the research protocol, (c) checking to make sure that the correct materials were used, and (d) checking that the prompting system was delivered as intended. Procedural reliability was calculated by dividing number of correct measures by the total number of assessed variables and multiplying by 100%. Procedural reliability agreement was 100%.

RESULTS

Both of the instructional procedures were effective in increasing independent responding and/or decreasing external prompts and prompts to use technology during instruction for both participants, but some differentiated effects were observed between the conditions. Video prompting appeared to be somewhat more effective than picture prompting across most dependent measures, especially when efficiency measures were analyzed.

Percentage of Independent Correct Responses

When the percentage of independent correct responses was measured across conditions and tasks, the data were interpreted to conclude that both conditions and prompting systems were effective in increasing independent responding for both participants. During the instructional phase, both students engaged in more independent correct responding with the video prompting condition, with Marvin having the clearest results (see Figure 1). Gary engaged in more independent correct responding when the video prompting condition was used ($M = 91\%$) than with the picture prompting condition ($M = 83\%$), but there was

some overlap in his data paths, suggesting that there was no functional relation between conditions. Marvin also had higher independent correct responding when the video prompting materials were used ($M = 90\%$) than in the picture prompting condition ($M = 76\%$), and there was a clear separation in data paths, suggesting the presence of a functional relation. When the change in the level of data was analyzed from the pretest scores to the first instructional session, both participants demonstrated much steeper increases in independent responding with the video prompting condition, suggesting that it may be a more powerful intervention, particularly during initial sessions.

During posttest phases, participants no longer used the prompting materials during task engagement. This was done to determine if the participants improved their independent correct responding without antecedent prompting supports. They were tested using instructional materials in the initial posttest 1 or 2 days after reaching criterion on both tasks ("Inst. Post" in Figure 1). They were given a generalization posttest ("Gen. Post" in Figure 1) 1 week later and again at 6 weeks ("6-wk Maint." in Figure 1). Both of the participants demonstrated that they could independently perform the skill sequences without technology supports after reaching criterion as measured by the postinstruction tests. Using 85% as the criterion, they were able to generalize their skills to untrained settings with novel materials as measured by the postgeneralization tests that were conducted 1 week after the instructional phase ended, with both doing better with the skill taught via video. Six weeks after instruction ended, Marvin demonstrated generalization and maintenance of his skills with both prompting techniques, but Gary only maintained the skill that was taught with video prompting (i.e., his score was above 85% correct).

Percentage of Error Correction Prompts

As seen in Figure 2, participants received fewer error correction prompts in the conditions in which they had the most independent correct responding, which was the video prompting condition. Gary had a mean of 6% of external prompts for the video prompting condition and a mean of 14% for the picture prompting condition. Marvin had similar findings, with a mean of 9% external prompts for the video prompting condition and a mean 17% for the picture prompting condition.

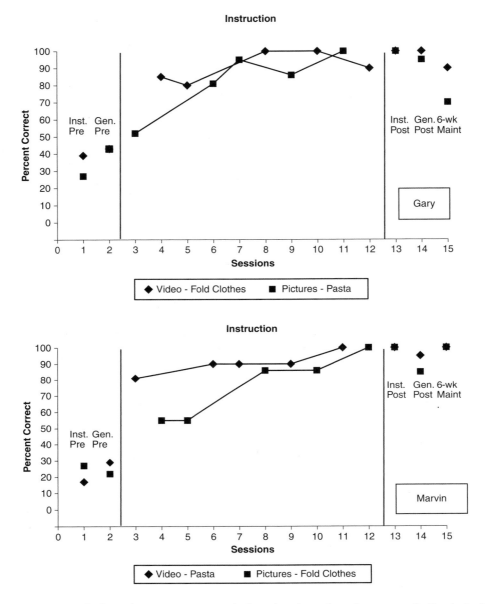

FIGURE 1. Percentage of independent correct responses in the task analyses. Note: Gen. = generalization; Inst. = instructional materials; Maint. = maintenance.

Percentage of Prompts to Use Technology

Figure 3 presents the percentage of prompts needed for the participants to use the technology across sessions and tasks. Because the prompting systems were not used during baseline or post-testing phases, only the instructional data are presented. Although there was some variability in the percentage of prompts to use the different technologies, there was a steady decrease in prompts across prompting systems for both participants, with the exception of Gary's last two sessions. Both participants required fewer prompts to use the technologies when the video prompting condition was in place. For Gary, the mean percentage of prompts to use technology across conditions was as follows: $M = 7\%$ for video prompts and $M = 13\%$ for picture prompts. Marvin also required fewer prompts to use the technologies with the videos ($M = 2\%$) compared with the pictures ($M = 7\%$).

Number of Sessions to Criterion

Gary reached criterion on both tasks within five sessions, while Marvin reached criterion within four sessions when the video prompting condition was in place and five sessions when the picture

prompting condition was in place. In terms of efficiency related to number of sessions to criterion, there was very little difference between the two prompting systems.

Efficiency Measures Related to Time to Create Materials

When the growth from pre- to posttest was considered across instructional, generalization, and maintenance measures, the video prompting condition was more efficient for each participant

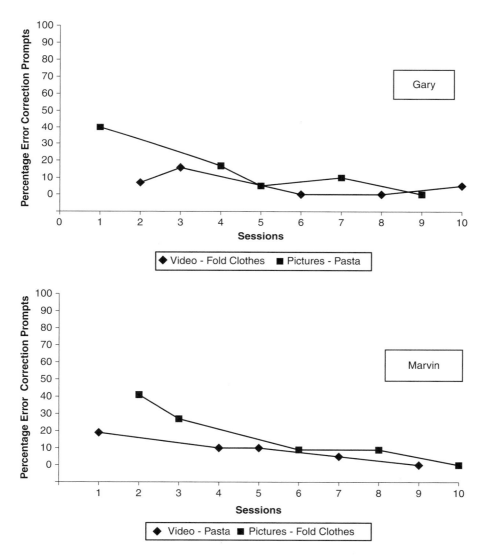

FIGURE 2. Percentage of error correction prompts used during instruction.

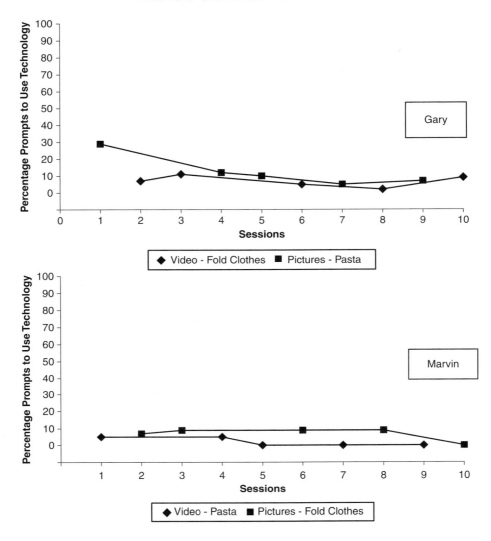

FIGURE 3. Percentage of prompts to use technology during instruction.

across all measures (see Figure 4). Gary had efficiency scores of 2.03 for the video prompting condition and 1.38 for the picture prompting condition when the instructional materials were used. When the generalization materials were used, Gary had efficiency scores of 1.9 for video prompting and 0.98 for picture prompting for the 1-week tests and 1.7 for video prompting and 0.81 for picture prompting at the 6-week tests. Marvin had similar results. When efficiency scores were calculated for instructional materials, he had efficiency scores of 2.44 for the video prompting condition and 1.38 for the picture prompting condition. When the generalization materials were used, Marvin had

efficiency scores of 1.94 for video prompting and 1.19 for picture prompting at the 1-week tests and efficiency scores of 2.15 for video prompting and 1.57 for picture prompting at the 6-week tests. When the means were combined across measures, conditions, and participants, the video prompting condition was more efficient. In essence, each minute of time spent creating the materials "bought" an average increase of 2.03 percentage points for the video prompting condition and an average increase of 1.22 percentage points for the picture prompting condition, indicating that the video prompting condition was the most efficient in terms of amount of growth from pre- to

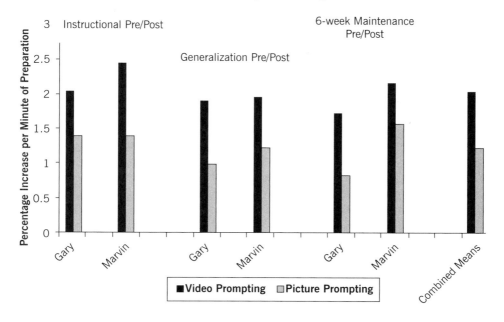

FIGURE 4. Efficiency measures for independent variables.

postmeasures relative to the time needed to create the instructional materials.

Social Validity

Informal interviews were conducted with the participants and some of the school staff members following the intervention. During their interviews, Marvin and Gary were asked (a) if they liked using the pictures and videos during instruction, (b) if they thought the pictures and videos were helpful in assisting them to perform tasks, (c) if they preferred using pictures or videos, and (d) to indicate what prompting system they would like to use in the future. Both Marvin and Gary indicated that they liked using both of the prompting systems and that they found them to be helpful for learning the different tasks. When asked which system they preferred and which system they would like using in the future, both indicated that they preferred using the videos and would like to use them again in the future.

At the conclusion of the study, the results were shared with the teacher and one of the teaching assistants, who were asked which prompting system they would be most likely to use in the future. Although both agreed that the video prompts were somewhat more effective, they indicated that they would be more likely to use picture prompting

systems because they were more familiar with using them. They also indicated that they would probably use pictures because they were more portable than the laptop. However, they were impressed with the effectiveness of video-based instruction and indicated that they would like more information or instruction on how to develop video-based instructional prompts.

DISCUSSION

The purpose of this research was to compare the effectiveness and efficiency of picture versus video prompting in teaching daily living skills to two adolescents with ASD. The effectiveness of the interventions were measured by comparing the percentage of independent correct responses during the instructional phase and growth from pre- to postmeasures using instructional as well as generalization materials and settings. The efficiency of the interventions was measured by comparing the number of sessions to criterion and the "cost" of minutes required to create the instructional materials relative to growth. In addition, to determine if the prompting procedures promoted independence while reducing reliance on practitioners, the percentage of external prompts, and prompts to use the technology were measured. In summary, both of the prompting systems were effective at increasing independent correct responding for both participants, but the video prompting system appeared to be somewhat more effective and efficient than the picture prompting system across all dependent measures, with clearer results being present for Marvin. The video prompting condition was associated with the highest percentage of independent correct responding, fewer external prompts, and fewer prompts to use technology for both participants. When the efficiency related to the time required to create materials (relative to growth) was measured, the video prompting strategy was more efficient in terms of the percentage increase obtained relative to the number of minutes required for material preparation.

Although the results are promising, there were several limitations to this study. First, the generalizability of the findings is limited, because there were only two participants. The results would have been strengthened if another replication could have been conducted through the addition of two additional participants and counterbalancing across tasks. Additionally, the results may have been stronger if an extended baseline phase had been conducted to establish low levels of student responding prior to instruction. Although a baseline phase would have been preferable, a relatively low level of correct responding was demonstrated for both participants as they had two pretests, or baseline probes, with one pretest involving materials presented during instruction and the other pretest using materials used during generalization sessions. Although it would have been preferable to have an extended baseline, it was still possible to demonstrate a change in the level of the data when the pretest scores were compared with the 1st day of instruction for both conditions. When independent correct responding was considered, there was a much steeper change in the level of data when the video prompting condition was in place for both participants, indicating that video prompting may have been more powerful than picture prompting during initial instructional sessions. However, a possible limitation in this comparison is related to the voiceover narration that was added to the video prompts. It cannot be stated that the video alone was responsible for the rapid increase in independent correct responding, because students may have been responding to the auditory prompts.

Overall, the most substantial finding of this research was in relation to the cost-effectiveness of each prompting strategy when the ratio of growth per minute of preparation was considered.

Considering the efficiency of instructional methods is very important, especially in relation to the rate of skill acquisition and teachers' or caregivers' willingness to prepare the instructional materials. The time required to create instructional materials is a very real concern because teachers have many other responsibilities that demand a great deal of their time. Although many teachers and/or direct care providers often operate under the assumption that working with video requires too much time, it can actually be comparable with or require less time than creating picture-based visual supports. Creating picture sequences often requires extensive printing, cutting, and laminating, which not only adds time needed to create the materials but also can add monetary cost over time. Taking the actual pictures can take longer than videotaping, because the "model" or person who is performing the skill sequence has to stop and pose for each step, whereas with video, the steps can be performed more fluidly, and there is less starting and stopping, which reduces the amount of time needed to videotape. In many cases, more pictures need to be taken to communicate the response requirements of various steps that easily could be represented by one short video clip. For example, at least three pictures were needed to demonstrate folding laundry and setting the time on the microwave for the pasta task. Each of these steps was easily demonstrated with one video clip, which made it easier to model the fluidity of the response requirements. We believe that is why the participants may have needed more external prompting when the picture prompting strategies were in place. Perhaps the pictures did not provide enough information for the participants, and it was necessary to provide additional supports to teach the response requirements, whereas with the video prompts, more complete models were provided to allow the participants to perform the steps more independently.

Although video prompts with this study resulted in increased student independence and less reliance on direct care providers, in many cases, the teacher or direct care providers will be the ones to determine which instructional materials will be used. For example, when the teacher in Alberto et al.'s (2005) study was asked which prompting system he preferred, he indicated that he preferred creating the video-based materials because they took less time to develop. The teachers in Cihak et al.'s (2006) study, however, indicated that they preferred the picture prompting strategies because they believed that pictures took less time to develop. Maybe the preferences indicated by the teachers were related more to their comfort level with using the technologies rather than the actual time required to create the instructional materials. Picture prompting strategies have been used for more than two decades, whereas video-based strategies are relatively new, and there are not as many people adept at using this technology. It is possible that with more training or professional development opportunities, teachers, parents, and direct care providers will be more likely to integrate video-based instruction into skills training.

Although the time required to create the materials is important in terms of teacher or caregivers' willingness to create various prompting systems, the most important consideration is the student and his or her ability to gain independence using methods that are effective. Video prompting was somewhat more effective than picture prompting for both of the participants in this study, and these findings are closely aligned to those found by Mechling and Gustafson (2008). However, another variable that must be considered is the students' preference for the various technologies. When the students in this study were asked which type of prompting system they preferred, both indicated that they preferred the video prompts. Marvin, in particular, seemed to enjoy viewing the videos and would often mimic the voiceover narrations while he was completing the task, essentially using self-prompting while engaged in the skill sequences. Perhaps students who have preferences for watching videos or who frequently recite lines to movies perform better or are more interested in video-based models. Gary, on the other hand, had a preference for quieter settings and often wore earplugs to reduce the noise in his environment. Because of this, it was somewhat surprising that he preferred the video-based prompting system, because it introduced more "noise" into the environment than the picture prompting system. Maybe there are certain student characteristics, student preferences, or task requirements that influence the effectiveness of the various interventions. For example, Alberto et al. (2005) and Cihak et al. (2006) suggested that students with attentional difficulties may perform better when static picture prompts are used. This makes sense because students with attentional difficulties may miss some of the relevant stimuli that are presented in video-based materials if their attention is diverted.

Although the video-based prompting systems appeared to be somewhat more effective for these participants, the bottom line is that all students

are different. Different individuals will have different preferences across the types of instructional materials being used, how the instructional materials are presented (e.g., video prompts vs. video models), as well as the types of tasks that are being taught. In addition, the feasibility of using various prompting systems in vocational and/or community-based environments must be considered. In this study, a laptop computer was used to present video prompts; however, as the practitioners involved in this study expressed, more portable systems may need to be used to make the presentation of videos possible in vocational or community-based settings. There currently is very limited research available regarding the use of handhelds or portable systems for delivering video-based instructional materials (Taber-Doughty, Patton, & Brennan, 2008; Van Laarhoven et al., 2007; Van Laarhoven et al., 2009), and much more research needs to be done in this area. Future researchers should investigate methods for training personnel and caregivers to use video technology so that it is used more widely in applied settings, and cost-benefit analyses should be conducted to determine if handheld devices can reduce costs associated with hiring additional personnel, particularly in employment settings. Hopefully, with additional research and increased professional development opportunities for teachers, parents, and preservice educators, video-based instruction can become a more common educational tool for promoting independence among individuals with autism and other developmental disabilities.

DECLARATION OF CONFLICTING INTERESTS

The author(s) declared no potential conflicts of interests with respect to the authorship and/or publication of this article.

FINANCIAL DISCLOSURE/FUNDING

This research was partially funded by Northern Illinois University's Undergraduate Special Opportunities in Artistry and Research (USOAR) award.

REFERENCES

Alberto, P., Cihak, D., & Gama, R. (2005). Use of static picture prompts versus video modeling during simulation instruction. *Research in Developmental Disabilities, 26,* 327–339.

Bergstrom, T., Pattavina, S., Martella, R. C., &

Marchand-Martella, N. E. (1995). Microwave fun: User-friendly recipe cards. *Teaching Exceptional Children, 28*, 61–63.

Billingsley, F. F., White, O. R., & Munson, R. (1980). Procedural reliability: A rationale and an example. *Behavioral Assessment, 2*, 229–241.

Book, D., Paul, T. L., Gwalla-Ogisi, N., & Test, D. T. (1990). No more bologna sandwiches. *Teaching Exceptional Children, 22*, 62–64.

Cannella-Malone, H., Sigafoos, J., O'Reilly, M., de la Cruz, B., Edrisinha, C., & Lancioni, G. E. (2006). Comparing video prompting to video modeling for teaching daily living skills to six adults with developmental disabilities. *Education and Training in Developmental Disabilities, 41*, 344–356.

Cihak, D., Alberto, P., Taber-Doughty, T., & Gama, R. (2006). A comparison of static picture prompting and video prompting simulation strategies using group instructional procedures. *Focus on Autism and Other Developmental Disabilities, 21*, 89–99.

Copeland, S. R., & Hughes, C. (2000). Acquisition of a picture prompt strategy to increase independent performance. *Education and Training in Mental Retardation and Developmental Disabilities, 35*, 294–305.

Goodson, J., Sigafoos, J., O'Reilly, M., Cannella, H., & Lancioni, G. E. (2007). Evaluation of a video-based error correction procedure for teaching a domestic skill to individuals with developmental disabilities. *Research in Developmental Disabilities, 28*, 458–467.

Graves, T. B., Collins, B. C., Schuster, J. W., & Kleinert, H. (2005). Using video prompting to teach cooking skills to secondary students with moderate disabilities. *Education and Training in Developmental Disabilities, 40*, 34–46.

Johnson, B. F., & Cuvo, A. J. (1981). Teaching mentally retarded adults to cook. *Behavior Modification, 5*, 187–202.

Lancioni, G. E., & O'Reilly, M. F. (2001). Self-management of instruction cues for occupation: Review of studies with people with severe and profound disabilities. *Research in Developmental Disabilities, 22*, 41–65.

Lancioni, G. E., & O'Reilly, M. F. (2002). Teaching food preparation skills to people with intellectual disabilities: A literature overview. *Journal of Applied Research in Intellectual Disabilities, 15*, 236–253.

Martin, J. E., Mithaug, D. E., & Frazier, E. S. (1992). Effects of picture referencing on PVC chair, loveseat, and settee assemblies by students with mental retardation. *Research in Developmental Disabilities, 13*, 267–286.

Martin, J. E., Rusch, F. R., James, B. L., Decker, P. J., & Tritol, A. (1982). The use of picture cues to establish self-control in the preparation of complex meals by mentally retarded adults. *Applied Research in Mental Retardation, 3*, 105–119.

Mechling, L. C., & Gustafson, M. R. (2008). Comparison of static picture and video prompting on the performance of cooking-related tasks by students with autism. *Journal of Special Education Technology, 21*, 31–45.

Myles, B., Grossman, B., Aspy, R., Henry, S., & Coffin, A. (2007). Planning a comprehensive program for students with autism spectrum disorders using evidence-based practices. *Education and Training in Developmental Disabilities, 42*, 398–409.

Norman, J. M., Collins, B. C., & Schuster, J. W. (2001). Using an instructional package including video technology to teach self-help skills to elementary students with mental disabilities. *Journal of Special Education Technology, 16*, 5–18.

Odom, S., Brown, W., Frey, T., Karasu, N., Smith-Canter, L., & Strain, P. (2003). Evidence-based practices for young children with autism: Contributions for single-subject design research. *Focus on Autism and Other Developmental Disabilities, 18*, 166–175.

Pierce, K., & Schreibman, L. (1994). Teaching daily living skills to children with autism in unsupervised settings through pictorial self-management. *Journal of Applied Behavior Analysis, 27*, 471–481.

Rogers, L. (2005). *Supporting students with autism spectrum disorders: Visual strategies for visual learners.* Retrieved June 24, 2008, from *www.atpe.org/Resources/Professional Development/_private/Autism/austism.asp.*

Schreibman, L., Whalen, C., & Stahmer, A. C. (2000). The use of video priming to reduce disruptive behavior in children with autism. *Journal of Positive Behavior Interventions, 2*, 3–11.

Sigafoos, J., O'Reilly, M., Cannella, H., Upadhyaya, M., Edrisinha, C., Lancioni, G. E., et al. (2005). Computer-presented video prompting for teaching microwave oven use to three adults with developmental disabilities. *Journal of Behavioral Education, 14*, 189–201.

Singh, N. N., Oswald, D. P., Ellis, C. R., & Singh, S. D. (1995). Community-based instruction for independent meal preparation by adults with profound mental retardation. *Journal of Behavioral Education, 5*, 77–92.

Taber-Doughty, T., Patton, S. E., & Brennan, S. (2008). Simultaneous and delayed video modeling: An examination of system effectiveness and student preferences. *Journal of Special Education Technology, 23*, 1–18.

Van Laarhoven, T., Johnson, J., Van Laarhoven-Myers, T., Grider, K., & Grider, K. (2009). The effectiveness of using a video iPod as a prompting device in employment settings. *Journal of Behavioral Education, 18*, 119–141.

Van Laarhoven, T., & Van Laarhoven-Myers, T. (2006). Comparison of three video-based instructional procedures for teaching daily living skills to persons with developmental disabilities. *Education and Training in Developmental Disabilities, 41*, 365–381.

Van Laarhoven, T., Van Laarhoven-Myers, T., & Zurita, L.M. (2007). The effectiveness of using a pocket PC as a video modeling and feedback device for individuals with developmental disabilities in vocational settings. *Assistive Technology Outcomes and Benefits, 4*, 28–45.

Van Laarhoven, T., Zurita, L. M., Johnson, J. W., Grider, K. M., & Grider, K. L. (2009). A comparison of self, other, and subjective video models for teaching daily living skills to individuals with developmental disabilities. *Education and Training in Developmental Disabilities, 44*, 509–522.

Wacker, D. P., & Berg, W. K. (1983). Effects of picture prompts on the acquisition of complex vocational tasks by mentally retarded adolescents. *Journal of Applied Behavior Analysis, 16,* 417–433.

Wolery, M., Bailey, D. B., & Sugai, G. M. (1988). *Effective teaching: Principles and procedures of applied behavior analysis with exceptional students.* Needham, MA: Allyn & Bacon.

ABOUT THE AUTHORS

Toni Van Laarhoven is an associate professor in the Department of Teaching and Learning at Northern Illinois University. She teaches courses in the areas of developmental disabilities, assistive technology, and applied behavior analysis. Her research interests include video-based instruction, assistive technology, functional assessment, and technology integration in teacher education.

Erika Kraus conducted this research while a student at Northern Illinois University. Currently, she works at Streamwood Behavioral Healthcare System in Streamwood, Illinois, on the Pervasive Developmental Disorder/Autism Inpatient Unit as an inpatient education coordinator and teacher.

Keri Karpman has been in the field of special education for the past 17 years. She is currently the multineeds coordinator for North DuPage Special Education Cooperative in Bloomingdale, Illinois. She has been an adjunct professor for Northern Illinois University for the past 5 years, teaching methods courses for the Department of Teaching and Learning.

Rosemary Nizzi is a multineeds and transition coordinator for North DuPage Special Education Cooperative in Bloomingdale, Illinois.

Joe Valentino has experience teaching students with multiple disabilities at the elementary, middle, and high school levels. At the time this study was conducted, he was a middle school teacher with North DuPage Special Education Cooperative. Much of his work involves teaching academics and life skills, supporting inclusion and mainstream activities, and fostering peer relationships.

ILLUSTRATIVE EXAMPLE QUESTIONS

1. What was the purpose of the investigation?
2. Who were the participants in the study? What was the setting?
3. What was the dependent variable, and how was it measured?
4. What were the independent variables?
5. What type of design was used?
6. What were the levels of interobserver agreement and procedural reliability?
7. How do posttest results compare to pretest results?
8. Is one procedure clearly more effective than the other procedure? Why or why not?
9. Describe the efficiency measure? Which procedure was more efficient?
10. What was the social validity procedure? What measures did it yield?

ADDITIONAL RESEARCH EXAMPLES

1. Ganz, J. B., & Flores, M. M. (2009). The effectiveness of direct instruction for teaching language to children with autism spectrum disorders: Identifying materials. *Journal of Autism and Developmental Disorders, 39,* 75–83.

2. Mann, T. B., Bushell, D., & Morris, E. K. (2010). Use of sounding out to improve spelling in young children. *Journal of Applied Behavior Analysis, 43,* 89–93.

3. Rehfeldt, R. A., Walker, B., Garcia, Y., Lovett, S., & Filipiak, S. (2010). A point contingency for homework submission in the graduate school classroom. *Journal of Applied Behavior Analysis, 43,* 499–502.

THREATS TO INTERNAL VALIDITY

Circle the number corresponding to the likelihood of each threat to internal validity being present in the investigation and provide a justification.

1 = definitely not a threat   2 = not a likely threat   3 = somewhat likely threat

4 = likely threat   5 = definite threat   NA = not applicable for this design

Results in Differences within or between Individuals

1. Maturation   1   2   3   4   5   NA

   Justification _____

   _____

2. Selection   1   2   3   4   5   NA

   Justification _____

   _____

3. Selection by Maturation Interaction   1   2   3   4   5   NA

   Justification _____

   _____

4. Statistical Regression   1   2   3   4   5   NA

   Justification _____

   _____

5. Morality   1   2   3   4   5   NA

   Justification _____

   _____

6. Instrumentation   1   2   3   4   5   NA

   Justification _____

   _____

7. Testing   1   2   3   4   5   NA

   Justification _____

   _____

(continued)

8. History   1   2   3   4   5   NA

Justification _____

_____

9. Resentful Demoralization of the Control Group   1   2   3   4   5   NA

Justification _____

_____

Results in Similarities within or between Individuals

10. Diffusion of Treatment   1   2   3   4   5   NA

Justification _____

_____

11. Compensatory Rivalry by the Control Group   1   2   3   4   5   NA

Justification _____

_____

12. Compensatory Equalization of Treatments   1   2   3   4   5   NA

Justification _____

_____

Abstract: Write a one-page abstract summarizing the overall conclusions of the authors and whether or not you feel the authors' conclusions are valid based on the internal validity of the investigation.

THREATS TO EXTERNAL VALIDITY

Circle the number corresponding to the likelihood of each threat to external validity being present in the investigation according to the following scale:

1 = definitely not a threat   2 = not a likely threat   3 = somewhat likely threat
4 = likely threat   5 = definite threat   NA = not applicable for this design

Also, provide a justification for each rating.

Population

1. Generalization across Subjects   1   2   3   4   5   NA

   Justification _____

   _____

2. Interaction of Personological Variables and Treatment   1   2   3   4   5   NA

   Justification _____

   _____

Ecological

3. Verification of the Independent Variable   1   2   3   4   5   NA

   Justification _____

   _____

4. Multiple Treatment Interference   1   2   3   4   5   NA

   Justification _____

   _____

5. Hawthorne Effect   1   2   3   4   5   NA

   Justification _____

   _____

6. Novelty and Disruption Effects   1   2   3   4   5   NA

   Justification _____

   _____

7. Experimental Effects   1   2   3   4   5   NA

   Justification _____

   _____

(continued)

8. Pretest Sensitization   1   2   3   4   5   NA

Justification _____

_____

9. Posttest Sensitization   1   2   3   4   5   NA

Justification _____

_____

10. Interaction of Time of Measurement and Treatment Effects   1   2   3   4   5   NA

Justification _____

_____

11. Measurement of the Dependent Variable   1   2   3   4   5   NA

Justification _____

_____

12. Interaction of History and Treatment Effects   1   2   3   4   5   NA

Justification _____

_____

Abstract: Write a one-page abstract summarizing the overall conclusions of the authors and whether or not you feel the authors' conclusions are valid based on the external validity of the investigation.

PART VI

····

Evaluation Research

CHAPTER 14

∎∎∎∎

Program Evaluation

OBJECTIVES

After studying this chapter, you should be able to . . .

1. Trace the history of program evaluation.
2. Illustrate the goal and objectives of program evaluations.
3. Describe the types of program evaluations.
4. Explain how a program evaluation is conducted.
5. Outline when program evaluations should be conducted.

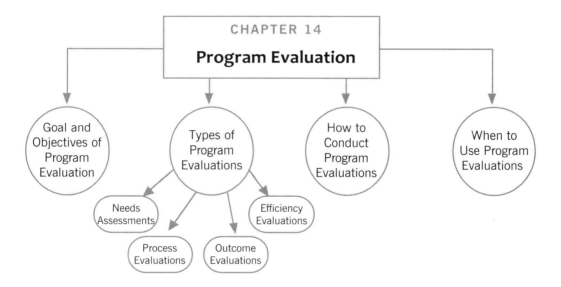

OVERVIEW

Evaluation is a part of everyday life. Athletes continually evaluate their performance to decide where they need to make improvements. Teachers assess whether their students acquire various academic skills. Similarly, social service and education programs use evaluations not only to improve services but also to document effectiveness of the provided services. Although social service and education programs have been in existence for many years, the relatively young field of program evaluation is continually evolving. **Program evaluation** (sometimes

> **Program evaluation** *is a systematic process of collecting and analyzing data on the quality or effectiveness of programs, products, or practices for purpose of making decisions.*

501

called *evaluation research*) refers to a systematic process of collecting and analyzing data on the quality or effectiveness of programs, products, or practices for purpose of making decisions (Gay, Mills, & Airasian, 2009).

The field of program evaluation has evolved based on the particular needs of society. In the late 1960s and early 1970s, program evaluations emphasized experimental methods, standardized data collection, large samples, and provision of scientific data (Maddaus & Stufflebeam, 2002). It was believed that experimental methods would provide not only unequivocal evidence of the effectiveness of programs but also a sound rationale for social service programs. This type of information was critical at the time, because policymakers believed social service programs could eliminate most problems facing society. However, soon experimental methods were considered unresponsive to the unique characteristics of local programs; thus, evaluators began to focus on those unique characteristics and processes within local settings and issues perceived to be important to stakeholders (i.e., program participants, staff, site administrators, governing board, and community members). Such evaluations were designed on the premise that social service programs are often complex and vary significantly from one community to another. These responsive program evaluations stress the importance of using qualitative methods to understand how a program is run and its effects on program participants.

Today, public pressure demands that programs demonstrate their effectiveness in producing desired outcomes and to do so efficiently (i.e., use the minimum resources necessary to obtain maximum outcomes). Both quantitative and qualitative procedures may be used to produce the measures necessary to evaluate a particular project. No single approach evaluates all projects, so the researcher must examine the characteristics of a project and select the most appropriate and sensitive evaluation measures.

There are a number of models or approaches used by program evaluators. Table 14.1 presents some of the more common evaluation models used by program evaluators. In looking over the table, it is important to note that these program evaluation models are not mutually exclusive.

TABLE 14.1. Program Evaluation Models

- *Participant-oriented.* Focus is on program processes and the perspectives of stakeholders
- *Objectives-oriented.* Focus is on the extent to which a program meets its established objectives
- *Management-oriented.* Focus is on providing program managers information to aid decision making
- *Expertise-oriented.* Focus is on the judgment of an expert
- *Adversary-oriented.* Focus is on incorporating negative and positive views in the evaluation
- *Logic-oriented.* Focus is on providing stakeholders with a visual map describing a sequence of related events (resources/inputs and activities) leading to intended results (outputs, outcomes, and impacts)

That is, the methods employed under each of the models are similar. We do not discuss any particular program evaluation model or approach in the remainder of this section because we have drawn, at least in part, from all of the models. For more specific information, see other sources (Kellogg Foundation, 2004; Posavac & Carey, 2003; Royce, Thyer, & Padgett, 2010).

We begin this section with a discussion of the varying goals and objectives of program evaluations. This discussion is followed by a description of the types of program evaluations used by evaluators and others. The remainder of this section includes a description of the general process used to conduct a program evaluation, to evaluate program evaluation data, and to decide when program evaluations are to be conducted.

Research Example

Consider this issue. Think about how you would design research to address the question/hypothesis from this research example:

- Research example: How would you design research to evaluate the benefits of an educational program for stepfamilies?

A research example appears near the end of the chapter.

WHAT ARE THE GOALS AND OBJECTIVES OF PROGRAM EVALUATION?

An important aspect of program evaluations is the consideration of its goal and objectives (see Figure 14.1).

Goal

The overall goal of program evaluation is to make good decisions about social and human service programs using rigorous procedures and providing feedback (Royce et al., 2010). Program evaluation provides feedback to professionals who decide which social services are to be offered, what new programs are to be designed, or what changes in existing approaches are needed (Posavac & Carey, 2003). Feedback, as with any activity, is critical to the success of social service and education programs and practices. As noted before, the practice of evaluating one's own efforts is commonplace.

Objectives

Within the overall goal of providing feedback, there are five general objectives of program evaluation: (1) meet existing needs, (2) provide services, (3) determine effectiveness of services, (4) determine relative effectiveness of programs, and (5) maintain and improve programs.

Meet Existing Needs

The first objective is to ensure that social service and education programs meet existing needs. Social service and education programs must be designed to target the most critical of these existing needs. It is not uncommon to develop programs with little thought as to whether they truly meet an existing need, much less a critical one. Thus, it is important that program evaluations be used to establish social service and education programs that meet a specified existing need.

Provide Services

The second objective of program evaluations is to verify that planned programs do provide services. Once social service and education programs are developed, it is crucial to see whether they were implemented as prescribed. Consequently, program evaluations should monitor whether social service and education programs have been implemented as specified. Although it may seem unnecessary for program evaluations to be concerned with the monitoring of programs, programs must be implemented if results are to be obtained and assessed.

Determine Effectiveness of Programs

The third objective of program evaluation is to determine whether a social service and

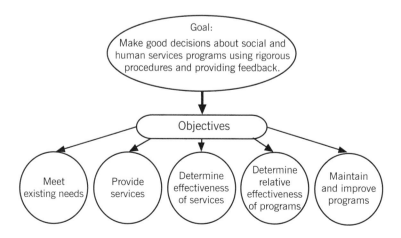

FIGURE 14.1. The goal and objectives of program evaluation.

education program is effective. Although many program managers believe that providing services is equivalent to rendering quality services, program evaluations must be conducted to determine whether a program leads to improved outcomes for program participants. Additionally, program evaluations aimed at assessing the effectiveness of social service and education programs should determine whether such programs have any unplanned side effects. For example, social service programs aimed at moving people off welfare may place greater demands on other social service agencies, such as churches and food banks.

Determine Relative Effectiveness of Programs

The fourth objective of program evaluation is to determine which particular program produces the best outcomes. Social service and education programs designed to meet a specified need often can be constructed in a number of ways. For example, a tutoring program for students at risk for school failure might be provided one-on-one or in a small-group format. Program evaluations enable social service and education providers to choose among potential programs.

Maintain and Improve Programs

The fifth objective of program evaluation is to provide information to maintain and improve social service and education programs. The focus here is not necessarily on determining whether a social service or education program works (see the third objective). Rather, the goal is to provide information that leads to improvements in the services offered. Such program evaluations are especially important when the social service and education program is mandated (e.g., bilingual and special education).

WHAT ARE THE TYPES OF PROGRAM EVALUATION?

Program evaluation efforts help organizations focus on important needs, develop effective programs, and assess and monitor the quality of programs (Royce et al., 2010). The four major

types of program evaluation include (1) needs assessment, (2) process evaluation, (3) outcome evaluation, and (4) efficiency evaluation. Program evaluations may utilize a combination of method types. For example, program evaluators exploring the effectiveness of an afterschool academic and social program for students at risk for school failure might assess the quality of the program and any existing needs within the program. Figure 14.2 depicts the relationship among the four major types of program evaluations conducted throughout the life of a program.

Before describing the four types of program evaluations, it is important to note that program evaluations are often categorized as either formative or summative, depending on the goal of the evaluation (Gall et al., 2007). **Formative evaluation** refers to measures taken during the development of a project to improve effectiveness and use resources efficiently. The goal of formative evaluations is to measure the implementation of a new social service or education program, or to changes in an existing one. **Summative evaluation** refers to measures taken to determine the worth of a fully developed program. The goal of summative evaluations is to describe the implementation of a program and

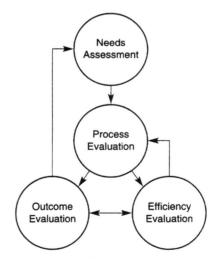

FIGURE 14.2. Relationship among the major types of program evaluations conducted throughout the life of a program.

its effects on program participants. Although we have chosen not to categorize program evaluations as formative or summative, you might want to consider these categories as you read the descriptions of the different types of program evaluations.

Needs Assessment

Stevens and Gillam (1998) state that the purpose of a **needs assessment** is to gather information required to bring about a beneficial change, usually within the context of finite resources. Social service and education programs are developed to serve a need. The goal of needs assessments is to identify the level of existing need within an organization or program. In other words, the goal is to look for potential but unavailable services for an identified population of individuals. An important part of conducting needs assessments entails defining what is meant by "needs." *Needs* can be defined as discrepancies between an actual state and a (1) normative, (2) minimum, or (3) desired or expected state. For example, needs assessments of programs for students at risk for school failure are often based on discrepancies from a norm. Gall et al. (2007) defined a *need* as "a discrepancy between an existing set of conditions and a desired set of conditions" (p. 575). Needs differ depending on the organization or program. A need refers to something (X) that people must have to be in a satisfactory state. Without X, they would be in an unsatisfactory state; with X, they achieve but do not exceed a satisfactory state. This definition of need provides a useful framework for structuring needs assessments.

It is important to distinguish between the incidence and the prevalence of an existing need or problem. *Incidence* refers to the number of people experiencing a problem during a specified time period, whereas *prevalence* refers to the number of people who have a problem at a given time. Making a distinction between the incidence and the prevalence of a problem is important, because a program designed to address a widespread temporary problem will differ from one designed to address a less widespread, long-lasting problem. For example, attempts to help children who experience a traumatic life event (e.g., death of a parent) differ from those that help children who experience ongoing life events (e.g., low SES).

Once the needs are defined for a given population, program evaluators should identify what resources are currently available to these individuals as part of their effort to assess existing needs. Program evaluators conducting needs assessments typically study a wide range of needs-relevant information, which might include objective data about the social and economic conditions of the population (e.g., school dropout rates, crime, levels of physical illness) and the opinions of both members of the population and experts, obtained through surveys and focus groups.

Finally, needs assessments should lead to program planning. Needs assessments are meaningless if they are not used to develop or restructure a program or organization. Consistent with the definition of needs, program evaluators use information gained from a needs assessment to develop a program to help members of the population obtain a satisfactory state. Program evaluators typically begin the program development or restructuring process by defining *outcome goals* (e.g., desired or normative state). Next, they develop a series of intermediate and long-term goals that need to be achieved to reach the outcome goals. Program evaluators use a variety of strategies to develop programs that meet the needs of members of the population. What does not change dramatically is the process of working in a backward direction throughout the planning process; that is, program evaluators identify the existing need *prior* to developing a program to meet it.

Formative evaluation *refers to measures taken during the development of a project to improve effectiveness and use resources efficiently.*

Summative evaluation *refers to measures taken to determine the worth of a fully developed program.*

Needs assessment *involves identifying the level of existing needs within an organization or program; the goal is to look for potential but unavailable services for an identified population of individuals.*

Process Evaluation

After a social service or education program has been developed or restructured, program evaluators should assess the extent to which the program has been implemented, serves the identified population, and operates as expected. **Process evaluations** are as important to program evaluation as assessment of treatment fidelity in research studies. The outcomes of a program evaluation, like those in a research study, are meaningful only to the extent that one understands a program's activities, how it works, and the population it serves. There is little reason to assess outcomes associated with a program if the program has not been implemented as planned.

When conducting a process evaluation, evaluators must discriminate between the program as described and the program as administered. This discrimination is critical, because the actual services provided by a social service or education program may differ substantially from its description. For example, as part of an effort to evaluate parent education programs provided by a variety of social service agencies, we visited the programs when the parent education programs were officially scheduled, only to find that the program was not being offered due to a lack of participation. If we had based our evaluation on the program descriptions, we would have concluded that parent education programs were being offered as planned.

Information collected for a process evaluation is often available from a program's information system. Of course, the information may be recorded in a way that is hard to use. For example, information on program participants is often not summarized, and records of services received may not be recorded. Thus, it may be necessary for program evaluators to work with program managers to develop an information tracking system that is easy to use and provides critical information with which to conduct a process evaluation.

Although information collected through a process evaluation varies depending on the particular social service or education program, two general types of information are generally considered. The first centers on the program participants. Social service and education programs are generally designed to meet the existing needs of a specific population. As a result, the population to be served should have been well defined during the conception of the program. Information describing the program participants who are actually served should be assessed to determine the degree to which it matches the original description of the population.

The second type of information focuses on the program itself. As noted before, programs are designed to achieve a desired or expected outcome. Thus, program evaluators must establish whether the program is being carried out as conceived. Program evaluators typically have the greatest difficulty assessing the degree to which a program is being implemented, because program managers often do not collect information on implementation.

A common strategy used by evaluators is called "to follow the course of services"; that is, tracking forms are developed to document the types and intensity of services provided to program participants. For example, a therapist working in a program that provides mental health services to students with behavioral problems might document her total caseload, including active and inactive cases, the average number of sessions provided to participants, a description of the focus of sessions, and ratings of the functional status of students when they exit the program. Information collected with the tracking forms are then compared to descriptions of how the services were originally conceived.

Outcome Evaluation

Outcome evaluation refers to using person- and organization-referenced outcomes to determine the extent to which a program meets goals and objectives, and whether a program made a difference (Schalock, 2001). Outcome evaluation, the most common type of evaluation, is often referred to as *summative evaluation*, because the primary goal is to develop summary statements and judgments about the program and its value. Furthermore, outcome evaluations can take on several levels of complexity. At the first level, an outcome evaluation might be designed only to determine whether program participants have improved. At the second level, an outcome evaluation may be designed to determine whether program participants have improved relative to a similar group not receiving services. At the third level, an outcome evaluation might be designed to determine whether there is a cause-and-effect relationship between program services and the outcomes of program participants. Finally, an outcome evaluation might be designed to determine whether program effects generalize across agencies, time, and other conditions.

Efficiency Evaluation

An **efficiency evaluation** examines whether the programs are operated in a cost-effective way; that is, it evaluates whether activities consume the least possible volume of resources in order to achieve the maximum production (Lorenzo & Garcia Sanchez, 2007). Although programs might help program participants, they often must show that they do so in a cost-effective way. Efficiency evaluations deal with questions of cost related to resources used. Even programs that produce significant improvements in the lives of program participants may be judged negatively if the costs necessary to achieve the improvements exceed what communities are willing to pay. Such programs might also be judged negatively if alternative approaches that are less costly can be implemented. In today's climate of dwindling resources, examining the cost-effectiveness of programs is becoming more important.

According to Gall et al. (2007), evaluators use the term *cost analysis* to refer to either (1) comparison of costs of a program to benefits (called *cost–benefit ratio*), or (2) the relationship between costs of different interventions in relation to their measured effectiveness in achieving a desired outcome (called *cost-effectiveness*).

Efficiency evaluations commonly place costs into categories to identify what is needed to run or support a program (Levin & McEwan, 2000). For example, one way of looking at costs is to categorize them into fixed and variable. *Fixed costs* (e.g., rent, lights, telephones, and secretarial support) are costs that are necessary to open the doors to the first program participant. Such costs are fixed because they do not change, regardless of whether one individual or

a maximum number of individuals accesses the program. On the other hand, some costs vary depending on the level of program activity or number of program participants. These costs are considered *variable costs* and include costs such as staff salaries and supplies.

Once the costs associated with running a program have been established, several levels of analysis can be conducted. On one level, evaluators might compare program outcomes to costs. The question is, "Are the program outcomes worth the costs?" This level of analysis requires the evaluator to consider what the outcome would be if the program had not been implemented. For example, say we develop a program to increase the vocational success of students with behavioral disorders in transitioning from school to employment. Prior to implementation of the program, approximately 30% of the students were employed 1 year after graduation and their median income was $8,500. Following the implementation of the program with 50 students, at a total cost of $200,000, we find that 40% of the students were employed 1 year after graduation, and their median income was $8,500. The question in an efficiency evaluation is, "Are the program outcomes worth the costs?" In this case, we are spending $200,000 to improve the vocational outcomes by 10% (a difference of five students), with no increase in median income. The results of this efficiency analysis might lead one to judge the program negatively even though it has increased the vocational outcomes achieved by students with behavioral disorders. Cost-efficiency experts often create units of measurement to gauge cost–benefit ratios, usually dollars spent per unit (e.g., one student) to reach a desired benefit. For example, in this

---

Process evaluation *refers to examining the extent to which the program has been implemented, serves the identified population, and operates as expected.*

Outcome evaluation *is the use of current and desired person- and organization-referenced outcomes to determine the extent to which a program meets goals and objectives, and whether a program has made a difference.*

An **efficiency evaluation** *examines whether a program is conducted in a cost-effective way.*

case, we may say the program required $200,000 ÷ 5 students = $40,000 per student to achieve employment.

HOW IS A PROGRAM EVALUATION CONDUCTED?

The process of conducting a program evaluation, like a research study, can be quite complex. Program evaluations are often emotionally sensitive processes in which many obstacles may (will) be encountered. It is important to keep in mind that many of the key stakeholders may not fully understand or may be threatened by the evaluation process. Thus, program evaluators must work closely with the key stakeholders throughout the evaluation process.

Program evaluations typically include four phases (see Figure 14.3): (1) establishing the boundaries of the evaluation; (2) selecting the evaluation methods; (3) collecting and analyzing data; and (4) reporting the findings (Fitz-Gibbon, 2003).

Establishing Boundaries

Establishing boundaries of the evaluation involves determining the purpose of the evaluation (e.g., outcome evaluation) and focusing the evaluation. The program evaluator begins by meeting with key stakeholders to determine what type of evaluation needs to be conducted. This step is crucial, because it is not uncommon for the key stakeholders to be unclear about the type of evaluation needed. Once the type of evaluation has been established, the program evaluator must focus the evaluation. Focusing an evaluation involves a number of wide-ranging tasks, such as learning about the program through program descriptions and talking with staff and program participants. Focusing an evaluation also involves determining what tasks need to be accomplished, establishing specific objectives for the evaluation, and identifying

any potential barriers to conducting the program evaluation (e.g., lack of a control group in an outcome evaluation).

Selecting Evaluation Methods

The next step, selecting the evaluation methods, is much like laying out a research study. Depending on the type of program evaluation, the program evaluator must select the data collection procedures, develop a sampling strategy, and establish how the data will be analyzed. As in a research study, selection of the evaluation methods is dependent on not only the objectives of the program evaluation but also constraints associated with the program itself (e.g., monies available to conduct the program evaluation, access to a control group, and organizational arrangements). The program evaluator must be adept at weighing all of the issues and selecting appropriate evaluation methods.

The research methods discussed throughout this volume may be useful evaluation methods. Outcome evaluations that focus only on determining whether program participants have improved may rely on preexperimental (e.g., one-shot case study) and qualitative designs. In contrast, outcome evaluations that center on determining whether program participants have improved relative to a group of individuals that did not receive services may rely on quasi-(e.g., nonequivalent control-group design) and true-experimental (e.g., pretest and posttest control group design) designs. The particular research design used in an outcome evaluation, as in a research study, is dependent on the question being addressed.

Although experimental designs have traditionally been used in outcome evaluations, qualitative methods should not be overlooked. In qualitative program evaluations, the evaluator strives to describe and understand the program or particular aspects of it. The evaluator tries to understand the meaning of the program and its outcomes from participants' perspectives. The

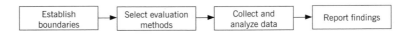

FIGURE 14.3. Program evaluation phases.

emphasis is on detailed descriptions and on in-depth understanding that emerges from direct contact and experience with the program and its participants. Qualitative outcome evaluations rely on observations, interviews, case studies, and other fieldwork techniques.

Collecting and Analyzing Data

After the evaluation methods have been selected, the program evaluator collects and analyzes the data. The key to efficient data collection and analyses is to establish a time frame that is both clear and reasonable for collecting and analyzing the data. The time frame for data collection must be clear, so that program staff and participants can structure the data collection into their busy days. The time frame for data collection must be reasonable, because program staff and participants involved in the evaluation tend to be very busy. Again, the program evaluator must be adept at weighing all of the issues and choosing an appropriate time frame for data collection and analysis.

Reporting the Findings

The program evaluator must report the findings. Although one might assume that reporting the findings of a program evaluation is straightforward, this often is not the case. The program evaluator begins by considering the different audiences that will view the findings, and deciding what presentation mode is most appropriate (e.g., oral or written; formal or informal). Program evaluators often have to prepare several reports because the findings must be reported to several different audiences.

Analysis of Data

The analysis of data in program evaluations is the same as the evaluation of data in the other research methods discussed throughout the text. The first step is to determine the type of research method used in the evaluation. Was the method quantitative or qualitative? If the evaluation was quantitative, was the design experimental, quasi-experimental, preexperimental, causal–comparative, or correlational? If the method was qualitative, was an ethnographic,

observation, questionnaire, or case study design used? Did the evaluation use document analyses? Were surveys used? Once these questions have been answered, critical research consumers should determine the most appropriate method of considering the internal validity (if appropriate) and external validity (if appropriate). The review forms presented throughout this volume can aid in the analysis of a program evaluation.

Recall the research question about stepfamily education posed earlier in this chapter? Read on to see how your design compares to how the actual study was designed.

Research Example: Evaluation—Stepfamily Education

Skogard, Torres, and Higginbotham (2010) evaluated a relationship education (RE) program for stepfamilies to determine specific benefits. The program was based on the theory that social support is critical to the success of stepfamilies (Michaels, 2000). This evaluation was part of a larger project exploring the experiences of participants in Smart Steps, an RE program addressing the relationship skills needed for successful stepfamilies (Adler-Baeder, 2007). Group sessions for stepfamilies lasted 6 weeks. Parents met in one room to take a class for 90 minutes. Children and youth ages 6–17 met in another room. Families met together for a 15- to 30-minute activity at the end. Program evaluation sought to discover the benefits that step-parents received from taking classes with other stepfamilies. From a pool of 230 adults, interviews were conducted with 40 stepparent participants (30 from English-speaking classes and 10 from Spanish-speaking classes). The 40 interview respondents represented a convenience sample. Ages of interviewees ranged from 22 to 47 ($M = 36$). The interviewees included 17 males and 23 females. Examples of questions included "What was your experience of taking this course with other stepfamilies?" and "What was the best part of the stepfamily course for you?" Interviews were recorded. Researchers identified coding categories for the general evaluation question. Then, researchers developed coding categories reflecting the themes described by participants. When they identified differences in coding categories, researchers went back to the data and established consensus. Findings indicated four themes. First, the benefit most frequently reported by stepparents was learning from others. Second, stepparents reported benefiting from *normalization* (i.e., recognition that other stepfamilies had similar experiences). Two other benefits included social support and teaching others.

WHEN SHOULD PROGRAM EVALUATIONS BE CONDUCTED?

Program evaluations continue to be used and most likely will become more important in the current context of dwindling resources. Such activities are undertaken to help plan and refine programs, to assess their effectiveness, and to make changes in ongoing services. Unlike other research methods that may develop from a researcher's interest in a phenomenon, program evaluations usually result from a specific need of a program. For example, federal granting agencies require an evaluation section that describes how the project will be evaluated. Universities and programs within universities have evaluations of their programs. You will most likely be involved in one of these evaluations during your studies at your university/college or once you graduate. Therefore, program evaluations result from a need to determine the effectiveness of a program. They serve a specific purpose and help to meet current and future needs of those receiving services from programs.

SUMMARY

❖ In the late 1960s and early 1970s, program evaluations emphasized experimental methods, standardized data collection, large samples, and provision of scientific data. When experimental methods were considered unresponsive to the unique characteristics of local programs, evaluators began to focus on unique characteristics and processes perceived to be important to stakeholders within local settings and issues. These responsive program evaluations stress the importance of using qualitative methods for understanding how a program is run and its effects on program participants. Today, public pressure demands that programs demonstrate effectiveness in producing desired outcomes, and to do so efficiently. Thus, both quantitative and qualitative procedures may be used to produce the measures necessary to evaluate a particular project.

❖ The overall goal of program evaluation is to make good decisions about social and human service programs using rigorous procedures and providing feedback. Within the overall goal of providing feedback, there are five general objectives of program evaluation: (1) meet existing needs, (2) provide services, (3) determine effectiveness of services, (4) determine relative effectiveness of programs, and (5) maintain and improve programs.

❖ There are four major types of program evaluations: (1) needs assessments (gathering information required to bring about a beneficial change), (2) process evaluations (examining the extent to which the program has been implemented, serves the identified population, and operates as expected), (3) outcome evaluations (using person- and organization-referenced outcomes to determine the extent to which a program meets goals and objectives, and whether a program made a difference), and (4) efficiency evaluations (examining whether the programs are operated in a cost-effective way). Program evaluations may utilize a combination of method types.

❖ Program evaluations typically include four phases: (1) establishing the boundaries of the evaluation (determining the purpose of the evaluation); (2) selecting the evaluation methods (selection of data collection procedures, development of a sampling strategy, and establishing how the data will be analyzed); (3) collecting and analyzing data; and (4) reporting the findings.

❖ Program evaluations are undertaken to help plan and refine programs, to assess their effectiveness, and to make changes in ongoing services.

DISCUSSION QUESTIONS

1. What is meant by the term *program evaluations*? Why are they important?

2. How have the methods of program evaluation changed over the years and why?

3. What are the common evaluation models used by program evaluators? Summarize the focus of each.

4. What are the overall goal and objectives of program evaluations? In your answer, explain what is meant by each of the objectives.

5. What is the difference between formative and summative evaluations?

6. What are the types of program evaluations? When would you use each?

7. Why must program evaluators work closely with the key stakeholders throughout the evaluation process? How does establishing boundaries aid in this process?

8. What are the four phases of program evaluations? Describe each.

9. What questions should we ask when analyzing the data in program evaluations?

10. When should program evaluations be conducted?

Note. **Read this before starting the illustrative example article**. Positive behavior support (PBS) is based on the systematic organization of school environments and routines that enables educators to increase the capacity to adopt, use, and sustain effective behavioral practices and processes for all students (Horner, Sugai, & Lewis-Palmer, 2005). PBS proposes positive approaches to intervention, such as teaching appropriate behaviors as opposed to relying on punishment alone. PBS utilizes a three-tiered system of behavioral support (Horner et al., 2005) referred to as universal, secondary, and tertiary prevention. Tier 1, or universal prevention (described in this article), is designed to address the entire school population. Applied to the entire school, the focus is on reaching the approximately 80–90% of students who do not have serious behavior problems or mental health needs. The focus of universal strategies is to maximize achievement, prevent problem behavior, and increase positive peer interactions and teacher–student interactions. Tier 2, or secondary prevention, focused on the 5–10% of students considered at risk for developing behavioral disorders or mental illness. These students carry significant risk factors and may be unresponsive to universal prevention strategies alone. In Tier 2, the goal is to decrease opportunities in which high-risk behaviors may develop, and to establish effective and efficient prosocial skills that would increase their responsiveness to universal interventions. Tier 3, or tertiary prevention, targets the remaining 1–5% of students who display severe and/or chronic problem behavior. In Tier 3, the goal is to reduce the frequency, intensity, and complexity of students' maladaptive behavior patterns and provide them with suitable, efficient, and effective replacement behaviors.

A Model for Statewide Evaluation
of a Universal Positive Behavior Support Initiative

Karen Elfner Childs, Don Kincaid, and Heather Peshak George
University of South Florida, Louis de la Parte Florida Mental Health Institute, Tampa, FL

Abstract. *Several statewide evaluations of Tier 1/Universal Level Positive Behavior Support (PBS) implementation efforts have been conducted, adhering to the evaluation template developed by Horner, Sugai, and Lewis-Palmer in 2005. Building on these examples, Florida's Positive Behavior Support Project developed a comprehensive evaluation system that sought to answer critical questions about building a scalable and sustainable PBS system at the state level that also provides data for decision making at the school and district levels. This article describes Florida's evaluation system as a model driven by 12 questions, including topics of implementation fidelity as both a dependent and independent variable, and expanding traditional questions of statewide evaluations to include consumer satisfaction, team processes, barriers and facilitators to implementation, and attrition. The data indicated that implementing Tier 1/ Universal Level PBS with fidelity was associated with improved student outcomes. Additional findings are described as are considerations for future directions.*

Keywords. *positive behavior support, program evaluation, implementation, scale up, systems change*

Program evaluation is defined as "applied research" that systematically examines human service programs for pragmatic reasons (Royse, Thyer, Padgett, & Logan, 2001). These reasons include determining whether the program is accomplishing its goals, should be funded in the future, is meeting the needs of its consumers, or is experiencing barriers to implementation. Early in the maturity of Tier 1/Universal Level of School-Wide Positive Behavior Support (PBS), several researchers and education agency personnel began to identify a need for evaluation of implementation and outcomes of Tier 1/Universal Level PBS (Chapman & Hofweber, 2000; Lohrmann-O'Rourke et al., 2000; Nakusato, 2000; Nersesian, Todd, Lehmann, & Watson, 2000; Sadler, 2000). However, most of these implementation efforts were in their infancy, so evaluation efforts did not include data from large numbers of schools or for multiple years.

Over the past decade, a consensus about the core features of Tier 1/Universal Level PBS has solidified and includes the following: (a) a committed team leading all PBS efforts, (b) positively stated school-wide behavior expectations and rules, (c) a method for identifying current problems through ongoing self-assessment, (d) lesson plans to teach the expectations and rules, (e) procedures for encouraging expected behaviors, (f) procedures for discouraging violations of school-wide expectations and rules, and (g) a plan for monitoring implementation and effectiveness (George, Kincaid, & Pollard-Sage, 2009). Although a plan for monitoring implementation and effectiveness at the school level is evident in most, if not all, PBS efforts, district- and state-level evaluation efforts have not grown to a level to address the more than 9,000 documented schools that are implementing Tier 1/Universal Level PBS across the country (*Office of Special Education Programs*, 2008).

Following initial efforts at district and state-wide evaluation, Horner, Sugai, and Lewis-Palmer (2005) provided an evaluation template and formal structure to evaluate the degree to which Tier 1/ Universal Level PBS are occurring as planned, resulting in change in schools and producing improvement in student outcomes. The authors identified the critical questions and some useful instruments and assessments to assist in answering those questions. These instruments and assessments include the Team Implementation Checklist (TIC), Effective Behavior Support Self-Assessment Survey (EBS), Systems-wide Evaluation Tool (SET), School-Wide Benchmarks of Quality (BoQ), School Safety Survey, and the School-Wide Information System (SWIS™; May et al., 2002), as well as other tools that are being developed to assist schools, districts, and states with evaluation processes. By adhering to that template and using these tools, several state-wide evaluations of implementation efforts have addressed the critical areas of consumer outcomes (students, teachers, schools, etc.) and implementation fidelity.

Mass-Galloway, Panyan, Smith, and Wessendorf (2008) conducted a statewide evaluation of universal school-wide positive behavioral supports (SWPBS) utilizing SET, TIC, and office discipline referral (ODR) data to assess fidelity of implementation and student outcomes. The authors found that most schools in Iowa were implementing universal SWPBS with fidelity (score over 80% on the SET and TIC). Furthermore, 75% of schools in three cohorts also showed a 42% decrease in ODRs over a 2-year period.

Irwin and Algozzine (2005) conducted an extensive evaluation of the statewide PBS system in North Carolina. In addition to measuring the spread of the PBS efforts across the state (53% of local education agencies), they also assessed the impact of PBS efforts on student outcomes and implementation fidelity of the PBS activities. However, further analysis was only available for a dozen schools with multiple years of data, and the implementation results for those schools were mixed. During 2004–2005, it was reported that 46 schools began baseline measures of implementation. Sixteen of those schools utilized the SET to evaluate implementation fidelity, with 9 of the schools scoring at least 80% on total implementation and 80% on behavioral expectations taught. It is anticipated that North Carolina's evaluation system has likely grown since the published statewide evaluation, as the number of schools implementing Tier 1/Universal Level PBS has increased to several hundred schools across the state.

Muscott, Mann, and LeBrun (2007) evaluated the effect of large-scale Tier 1/Universal Level PBS implementation on school discipline and academic outcomes. Twenty-eight schools were evaluated for implementation using the Universal Team Checklist, the EBS Survey, and the SET. After 1 year, 21 of 24 teams (88%) were scoring at or above the 80/80 criteria on the SET. Schools averaged a 28% reduction in ODR, a 31% reduction in in-school suspensions (ISS), and a 19% reduction in out-of-school suspensions (OSS). Decreases in ISS and ODR accounted for significant time savings for instruction, whereas implementation was also associated with math gains for the majority of schools.

Perhaps no state has a documented evaluation process as extensive as Maryland's (Barrett, Bradshaw, & Lewis-Palmer, 2008). More than 400 schools have been trained on Tier 1/Universal Level PBS, and a corresponding multiple-tiered evaluation plan has been applied to all of the schools. Fidelity of implementation was assessed with the TIC, the Coaches Checklist, the SET, and the Implementation Phases Inventory. In the past 2 years, Maryland's PBIS Project has also started to utilize the BoQ to measure team implementation of Tier 1/Universal Level PBS (S. B. Barrett, personal communication, August 4, 2007). Outcome measures gathered in Maryland include ODR, suspension rates, and a staff survey (Lewis-Palmer & Barrett, 2007). Training and support needs were assessed with periodic needs assessments. Preliminary results from 467 schools trained in Tier 1/Universal Level PBS suggest that Maryland has developed an effective and efficient structure to measure and promote statewide implementation.

These early evaluation efforts reflect the first attempts of states to develop comprehensive protocols and processes for evaluation of their Tier 1/Universal Level PBS efforts. These evaluation efforts allow states and funded initiatives to answer critical questions about whether the allocation of funds is sufficient to produce and sustain large-scale systems change and whether and where to target programmatic changes (e.g., training, technical assistance, products, etc.) to produce better outcomes for schools. Building on these examples, Florida's Positive Behavior Support Project has developed a comprehensive evaluation system that seeks to answer critical questions about building a scalable and sustainable PBS system at the state level that simultaneously provides data for decision making at the school and district levels.

This article presents a model for conducting a comprehensive statewide evaluation of PBS training and technical assistance efforts at the Tier 1/Universal Level PBS. Figure 1 provides an illustration of the service delivery and evaluation model utilized by Florida's PBS Project. The described evaluation process is ongoing, and some of the critical questions will not be answered with sufficient data for several more years. We encourage the reader to critically examine the model and process for evaluation and consider the types of evaluation questions that are asked, the data required to answer those questions, and the process for gathering those data. We describe here where sufficient data exist in the current evaluation process to derive conclusions about the effectiveness of Tier 1/Universal Level PBS. We also alert the reader to additional data necessary to warrant further conclusions.

This article addresses the statewide evaluation of the PBS process in more than 300 schools. Many of the data sources utilized to answer program

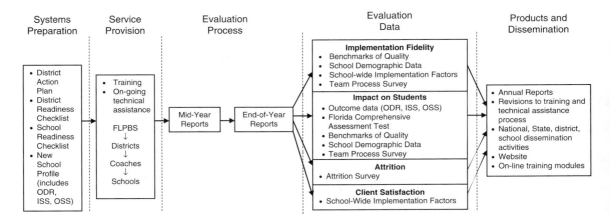

FIGURE 1. Florida's Positive Behavior Support (FLPBS) Project's Service Delivery and Evaluation Model.

evaluation questions at a state level are also critical for evaluation and data-based decision making at the district and school levels. Florida's PBS evaluation process follows many of the inquiries in the Horner et al. (2005) template and expands its statewide evaluations by addressing additional questions about consumer satisfaction, team processes, barriers and facilitators to implementation, and attrition. Furthermore, the Florida evaluation process examines the critical issue of implementation fidelity as both a dependent variable (e.g., How well are trained schools implementing the Tier 1/Universal Level PBS process?) and an independent variable (e.g., Is the level of implementation at a school related to differences in the outcomes achieved for the school?). Table 1 contains a list of the evaluation questions asked, along with the measures used to answer the questions.

PARTICIPANTS AND SETTINGS

Florida's PBS Project is funded by the Florida Department of Education to increase the capacity of Florida's school districts to provide PBS at the Tier 1/Universal, Tier 2/Supplemental or Targeted Group, and Tier 3/Intensive or Individual levels. Project staff initially train school and district teams at Tier 1/Universal Level PBS throughout the school year at varying times, dependent on the district schedules.

Florida public schools are eligible for voluntary participation in training at the Tier 1/Universal Level PBS as guided by a required district action plan developed by their local district leadership teams. Florida's PBS Project facilitates this action-planning meeting (see George & Kincaid, 2008) prior to any school participating in training in order to secure district commitment in supporting the schools interested in Tier 1/Universal Level PBS. Once commitment is secured, local schools complete the *School Readiness Checklist* (see *http://flpbs.fmhi.usf.edu*) within a specified time frame, which assesses the school's commitment to training and implementation and determines eligibility for training participation in its district. From school year 2002–2003 to school year 2003–2004 only 25% of schools continued implementation (George & Kincaid, 2008). As a result of these enhanced readiness requirements for schools, by the end of the 2006–2007 school year more than 85% of trained schools remained active.

A critical prerequisite to attendance in Tier 1/Universal Level PBS training is the active participation of the school's administration (e.g., the principal, assistant principal, or dean who is responsible for discipline on campus) throughout the entire training. The Tier 1/Universal Level PBS training typically occurs for 3 consecutive days and may occur at any time during the calendar year as determined by the district. Because participating schools receive training after district and school readiness items have been completed, yearly cohorts are not created within the state (i.e., schools or districts enter training at different times). For example, although schools may be considered in Year 1 of implementation, their onset of

TABLE 1. Summary of Evaluation Questions and Sources of Data

Evaluation Question	Data Source
Implementation fidelity	
Are schools trained in Universal school-wide positive behavioral support (SWPBS) implementing with fidelity?[a] Across years? Across school types?	Benchmarks of Quality (BoQ), school demographic data
What factors are related to implementing with fidelity?	School-Wide Implementation Factors (SWIF) survey, BoQ
Do teams that work well together implement with greater fidelity?	Team Process Evaluation, BoQ
Impact on student behavior	
Do schools implementing SWPBS decrease office discipline referrals (ODRs), days of in-school suspensions (ISS), and days of out-of-school suspensions (OSS)?[a]	ODRs, ISS, OSS
Do schools implementing SWPBS realize an increase in academic achievement?[a]	Florida Comprehensive Assessment Test (FCAT) scores
Is there a difference in outcomes across school types?	ODRs, ISS, OSS, FCAT scores, school demographic data
Do schools implementing with high fidelity have greater outcomes than do implementers with low fidelity?	BoQ, ODRs, ISS, OSS
Do teams that work well together have greater outcomes than those that do not work as well together?	Team Process Evaluation, ODRs, ISS, OSS
Attrition	
Why do schools discontinue implementation of SWPBS?	Attrition Survey
Consumer satisfaction	
Are our consumers satisfied with the training, technical assistance, products, and support received?	SWIF survey

[a]Questions also found in the *School-Wide Positive Behavior Support Evaluation Template* (Horner, Sugai, & Lewis-Palmer, 2005).

implementation varies depending on when they received the training (e.g., spring, summer, winter, etc.). School teams participate in lectures and team activities and view videotapes of actual schools to assist in visualizing implementation on their campuses, and the teams complete a comprehensive action plan to guide implementation activities throughout the school year. Tier 1/Universal Level PBS training components include establishing a team, understanding basic behavioral principles, building faculty buy in, establishing a data-based decision-making system (e.g., including behavioral definitions, behavior tracking forms, coherent discipline referral process, and effective consequences), identifying expectations, establishing rules for specific settings, developing reward systems, and implementing and evaluating the Tier 1/Universal Level PBS system. As of August 2008, more than 500 Florida schools in 42 (out of 67) districts had been trained in Tier 1/Universal Level PBS. This represents approximately 20% of the public schools in Florida. It is important to note

that the number of schools completing the assorted midyear and end-of-year evaluation measures varies by year and by measure.

PROCESS AND OUTCOME MEASURES

Evaluation instruments measure all intervention efforts including training impact and satisfaction, technical assistance efforts, team processes, implementation activities, and student outcomes. Reports generated from these evaluation measures are used by Florida's PBS Project and the state funding source to assess the effectiveness of Florida's PBS Project activities. All data are entered online two times annually (midyear in December and end of year in June), and evaluation summaries are automatically generated and immediately available for viewing and downloading by school and district. All instruments and protocols for use are available at the Florida PBS Project's Web site (*http://flpbs.fmhi.usf.edu*).

New School Profile

The New School Profile is a two-page form designed to collect basic demographic information about the school prior to receiving initial training. These data assist Florida's PBS Project staff in providing support and demonstrating effectiveness across the state. Basic contact information, demographics (e.g., ethnicity, attendance, percentage of students on individualized education programs, staff stability, etc.), baseline behavior, and academic data are requested and self-reported on the form by participating schools. These baseline data are used to investigate how implementation may differ across participating schools with various characteristics.

School Profile

After a school receives Tier 1/Universal Level PBS training, the PBS Project asks the school to provide demographic data on an annual basis using the School Profile. This profile is identical to the New School Profile except that it does not include behavior or academic data. For existing schools, these data are automatically collected at the end of the year through the Outcome Data Summary. The PBS coach (i.e., the team facilitator with additional training in PBS) completes this form midyear with assistance from school personnel (i.e., the school administrator and/or data clerk).

Team Process Evaluation

This 20-item survey evaluates the PBS team's functioning and effectiveness. Items are divided into the following four domains that correspond with best practice in team building and functioning: (a) trust building, (b) communication/distributive leadership, (c) problem solving, and (d) conflict management. Participants score each item on a Likert-type scale from 1 (*we never do*) to 3 (*we sometimes do*) to 5 (*we always do*). A sample item is "We arrive at meetings on time and stay for the duration of the meeting." Each member of the PBS team (including the coach) completes a Team Process Evaluation. The coach then calculates the average response for each item (to the nearest 10th, i.e., 4.2) and records this as the final score for each item, which is then entered online. Data are collected mid-year, and the results are used to identify areas of needed support for teams and to assist coaches in effective PBS implementation.

Benchmarks of Quality

This evaluation instrument assesses the fidelity of Tier 1/Universal Level PBS implementation by listing 53 benchmarks of quality that address 10 critical elements (Kincaid, Childs, & George, 2005). Validation study results indicate that the BoQ is a reliable, valid, efficient, and useful instrument for measuring the fidelity of implementation of the primary or universal level of PBS application in individual schools (Cohen, Kincaid, & Childs, 2007). The BoQ is completed annually each spring and requires the coach to complete the Benchmarks Scoring Form (100-point scale) after the PBS team members have completed and returned the Team Member Rating. The Benchmarks Scoring Guide describes the administration process of the instrument and provides a rubric for scoring each item. The results are used to evaluate the extent to which teams are implementing Tier 1/Universal Level PBS, to identify potential model schools (i.e., demonstrations or exemplars), and to provide a mechanism for school teams to identify areas of strength and weakness for establishing future action plans. The project considers high implementers (those with strong fidelity) to be schools scoring a 70 or higher on the BoQ, whereas schools scoring below 70 are considered low implementers. This distinction is based on an average score of 69 for the instrument during validation (Cohen et al., 2007); however, for clarity, a cutoff of 70 is used by the project. It is important to note that a BoQ score may not be reflective of a full year of implementation. For example, a school initially trained in January and another trained the same year in September will each complete the BoQ for Year 1 implementation when evaluated the following spring. Therefore, first-year implementation scores could be indicative of 16 months or 8 months of implementation, respectively. All information derived from the BoQ is summarized and reported back to the school-based PBS team. A comparison of BoQ scores for all of Florida's reporting schools since 2004 is reported to Florida's Department of Education each year (Kincaid, George, & Childs, 2007).

Outcome Data Summary

The Outcome Data Summary provides basic outcome data related to attendance, behavior referrals, and academic achievement. More specifically, teams complete these end-of-year data on ODR, ISS,

OSS, and certain academic data (e.g., *Florida Comprehensive Assessment Test*, or FCAT, the statewide assessment test). The FCAT is part of Florida's overall plan to increase student achievement by implementing higher standards and is administered to students in Grades 3 to 11 (Florida Department of Education, 2008). It contains two basic components: criterion-referenced tests, which measure selected benchmarks in mathematics, reading, science, and writing, and norm-referenced tests in reading and mathematics, which measure individual student performance against national norms. Yearly improvements on the FCAT are critical variables in determining whether the state judges a school to have made adequate yearly progress and therefore is of particular importance to Florida schools. FCAT student results are reported by achievement levels from the lowest level (Level 1) to the highest level (Level 5). Level 3 indicates that a student's performance is on grade level. Furthermore, student progress can be tracked over time and across grade levels, indicated as student learning gains.

The coach completes this self-report form with assistance and input from the school-based PBS team and data-entry personnel. The combined results are used to identify whether the implementation of Tier 1/Universal Level PBS has had an impact on the outcome data variables such as academics. Completion of this form for ongoing data analysis is essential because only 25% of Tier 1/Universal Level PBS-trained schools utilize SWIS™ (the Web-based gold-standard data system for Tiers 1 and 2), and the project has no other way to access this data.

School-Wide Implementation Factors

The School-Wide Implementation Factors (SWIF) is a Web-based survey that gathers information from PBS team members, coaches, and district coordinators on the facilitators and barriers to Tier 1/Universal Level PBS implementation. The items on the SWIF survey were derived from the nominal group process technique conducted with implementers from Florida's PBS schools as described by Kincaid, Childs, Blasé, et al. (2007) and Kincaid, George, et al. (2007). The SWIF also assesses consumer satisfaction with training, technical assistance, or product development activities provided by Florida's PBS Project. Data are entered at the end of the year, and the results are used to direct the future training and technical assistance activities of Florida's PBS Project. To date, 211 individuals representing 91 schools in their first, second, and third year of implementation have completed the SWIF survey.

Attrition Survey

This is a Web-based exit survey that gathers information from participants from school PBS teams to identify factors contributing to the discontinuation of participation in PBS. Respondents to the Attrition Survey rated items on a 4-point Likert-type scale from contributed significantly to did not contribute at all. Domains examined include knowledge, motivation, support, and the participant selection processes. The Attrition Survey is completed by team members whose schools are no longer implementing Tier 1 PBS. Data will be utilized to assist in preventing future discontinuation of participants. To date, 32 individuals representing 18 schools have responded to the Attrition Survey.

PROCEDURES

Baseline data were collected with the New School Profile at least 2 weeks prior to the onset of the initial Tier 1/Universal Level PBS training. Midyear data were requested in the fall and collected by mid-December each year. These data included the School Profile, School Team Update, and the Team Process Evaluation. Results were provided in early January, which assisted in midyear action planning, the delivery of appropriate technical assistance, and training for ongoing skill building. End-of-year data were requested in late spring and collected by mid-June each year. These data included the BoQ and the Outcome Data Summary that assist in determining model school status (i.e., exemplar schools), overall outcomes, and future action planning. Full evaluation summaries were provided directly to district coordinators for dissemination across district coaches. The SWIF survey was collected at the end of the year and the Attrition Survey was collected throughout the calendar year as participants from exiting schools were identified.

Florida's PBS Project has provided external funds to school districts to help support the completion of evaluation activities. Funding was distributed directly to the district. When reports were successfully completed within the specified time frame, grant funding historically allowed for $200 per school for midyear and $600 per school for end-of-year reports. Schools that did not complete midyear reports could complete end-of-year reports but were not eligible for funding. Schools that moved to inactive status (defined as not actively implementing Tier 1/Universal Level PBS, with confirmation by their PBS district coordinators) were ineligible for funding. The final dollar amount varied from year to year based on the availability of grant funding.

Data on the SWIF and attrition factors were collected outside of the midyear and end-of-year evaluation process. At the end of the school year, all PBS team members were asked to complete the SWIF survey. As an incentive to participate, team members completing the survey were entered into a drawing to receive one of three $100 awards. Team members from schools that discontinued formal participation in PBS with Florida's PBS Project were solicited by email to complete the Web-based Attrition Survey. Team members completing the Attrition Survey were eligible to receive a $25 stipend.

DESCRIPTIVE RESULTS

Table 1 provides a summary of each evaluation question and the data sources used to address the question. The analyses described in this section include data from pre-K, elementary, middle, high, alternative/center, and other (i.e., K–8) schools or a subset of those school types. In some analyses, data from particular school types were not available or applicable. For each question that follows, the schools included in the analysis will be identified.

Implementation Fidelity

"Are Florida schools trained in Tier 1/Universal Level PBS implementing with fidelity?" In each school year between 2004 and 2007, more than 50% of all active PBS schools in Florida implemented Tier 1/Universal Level PBS practices with a satisfactory level of fidelity, as demonstrated by scoring at least a 70 on the BoQ. The implementation level of schools increased each year, with 54% scoring 70 or above in 2004–2005, 63% scoring 70 or above in 2005–2006, and 65% scoring 70 or above in 2006–2007.

"Is there a difference in implementation fidelity across years?" Since the 2004–2005 school year, the average level of implementation fidelity by Florida's schools improved, as demonstrated by incremental increases in average BoQ scores across years. In 2004–2005, the average BoQ score for all of Florida's schools was 66. The average score in both 2005–2006 and 2006–2007 was 75, which falls within the cutoff for high-implementing schools, which requires a BoQ score of 70 or higher.

"Is there a difference in implementation fidelity across school types?" Between the 2004–2005 and 2006–2007 school years, alternative/center schools in Florida reported a higher level of implementation fidelity than did other school types. The BoQ score averages for alternative/center schools were 69, 76, and 78 in the 3 consecutive school years starting in 2004–2005. The standard deviation in those years ranged from 18.0 to 19.8. Elementary schools in Florida were the school type implementing with the next highest level of fidelity, averaging 71.3 on the BoQ across 3 consecutive school years. The standard deviation for those school years was from 18.1 to 19.7. Middle schools averaged 67.3 on the BoQ across the same 3-year span, with standard deviations for each year ranging from 17.8 to 19.1. High schools scored the lowest level, with an average of 66 on the BoQ across the 3 years. They also had the greatest range of standard deviations, from 5.7 to 19.7.

"What issues are related to implementing with fidelity?" The SWIF survey revealed differences in issues identified as helpful or problematic for higher and lower implementing teams (see Table 2). The results of the SWIF survey indicated that, overall, respondents from higher implementing schools identified a greater number of issues as helpful than did respondents from lower implementing schools, whereas the respondents from lower implementing schools identified a greater number of issues as problematic than did respondents from higher implementing schools. Common issues that both high- and low-implementing schools identified as being helpful included "expectations and rules clearly defined" and "administrator commitment." However, factors identified as problematic by high-implementing schools (i.e., adequate funding, staff stability) differed from those identified by respondents from lower implementing schools (i.e., staff time for PBS, staff belief about the effectiveness of PBS).

TABLE 2. School-Wide Implementation Factors by Implementation Level

Type of Factor	Higher Implementing (70+ on Benchmarks of Quality)	Lower Implementing(< 70 on Benchmarks of Quality)
Factors most *helpful* to implementation of school-wide positive behavioral support (SWPBS)	At least 90% of respondents of high-implementing schools identified the following factors as *helpful*: • Expectations and rules defined • Administrator committed to PBS, willing to teach, model, and reward • Representative, committed team • Reward system works • PBS coach's guidance with process • Students' responses to rewards and activities	At least 80% of the respondents of low-implementing schools identified the following factors as *helpful*: • Expectations and rules defined • Administrator willing to reward students • Representative PBS team
Factors most *problematic* to implementation of SWPBS	At least 25% of respondents of high-implementing schools identified the following factors as *problematic*: • Adequate funding • Team recognizes faculty participation • Staff stability from year to year • Student stability from year to year	At least 50% of the respondents of low-implementing schools identified the following factors as *problematic*: • Staff time for PBS • Staff belief about effectiveness of PBS • Staff philosophy • Staff consistency in teaching • Staff consistency in discipline procedures

"Do teams that work well together implement with greater fidelity?" Florida's PBS Project measures the degree to which teams work well together, using the Team Process Evaluation. The state average on all process domains was above 4 on a scale of 1 (*strongly disagree*) to 5 (*strongly agree*). The domains with the highest average scores were "no put downs" and "friendly." The domains with the lowest average scores were "time limits," "summary of outcomes," and "checks for understanding of concepts." Both higher and lower implementing schools scored relatively high on team functioning. The 134 higher implementing teams scored an average of 5 points higher on the Team Process Evaluation ($M = 89$, $SD = 13.2$) than did the 94 lower implementing teams ($M = 84$, $SD = 12.6$).

Impact on Student Behavior

"Do schools implementing Tier 1/Universal Level PBS realize a decrease in ODRs, days of ISS, and days of OSS?" After the initial year of implementation, Florida elementary, middle, and high schools implementing Tier 1/Universal Level PBS realized an overall percentage change in ODRs, days of OSS, and days of ISS. Overall, the average number of ODRs per 100 students after 1 year of implementation was approximately 33% lower than the number of ODRs per 100 students during the average baseline year (see Figure 2). The range of change in ODRs per 100 students across schools was –491.81 referrals to +103.13 referrals, with a

median of –22.76. A paired *t* test was used to ascertain whether the change in number of ODRs, days of ISS, and days of OSS between baseline and Year 1 of implementation was statistically significant. For ODRs per 100 students, statistically significant differences were found between baseline and Year 1. The mean difference between ODRs in baseline and Year 1 was 45.01 ($SD = 101.3$, $p = .001$).

The average reduction in days of ISS per 100 students after 1 year of implementation was 16% (see Figure 2). The range of change in the number of days of ISS per 100 students across schools was –205.28 days per 100 to +72.88 days per 100, with a median of +0.30 days per 100. The average change in days of OSS per 100 students after 1 year of implementation reflected an increase of 2%. The range of change in number of days of OSS per 100 students across schools was –86.53 days per 100 to +164.06 days per 100, with a median of –1.79 days per 100. This analysis does not account for fidelity of implementation and instead reflects the average change across elementary, middle, and high schools for which Florida's PBS Project had both baseline and Year 1 data regardless of implementation level. A *t* test with days of ISS and days of OSS did not reveal a statistically significant difference between baseline and Year 1.

Pre-K, alternative/center, and other (i.e., K–8) schools could not be included in the descriptive analysis of these outcome measures due to factors that lead to extraordinary variability of the data. Alternative/center schools have atypically small

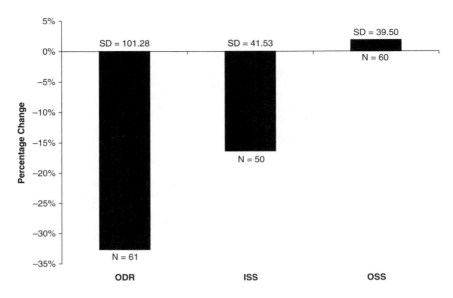

FIGURE 2. Percentage Change in Office Discipline Referrals (ODRs), In-School Suspensions (ISS), and Out-of-School Suspensions (OSS) per 100 Students Before and After 1 Year of Positive Behavior Support Implementation.

populations with high rates of turnover that are often a result of "limited stay" times. Due to the age and developmental stage of students, pre-K programs frequently use alternatives to discipline procedures such as office referrals and suspensions. The school type categorized as "other" for Florida schools captures populations across the standard grade levels, which confounds the descriptive data analysis.

"Do schools implementing Tier 1/Universal Level PBS realize an increase in academic achievement?" From 2004 to 2007, Florida schools trained in the Tier 1/Universal Level of PBS had a higher percentage of students reaching Level 3 (performance on grade level) on the FCAT reading segment (62.67%) when compared to the statewide average (55.67%).

"Is there a difference in outcomes across school types?" Florida's elementary, middle, and high schools implementing Tier 1/Universal Level PBS reported fewer ODRs after their initial year of implementation (see Figure 3). Alternative/center, Pre-K, and other school types were not included in this comparison for the reasons described previously. Both middle and high schools showed similar decreases in ODRs from baseline to Year 1, with middle schools reporting an average of 34% fewer

referrals per 100 students and high schools reporting 33% fewer. Elementary schools realized the smallest decrease in referrals after 1 year of implementation (30%) when compared to the decrease for middle and high schools. Although not represented in Figure 3, middle schools reported the highest average number of referrals overall (285 per 100 students before implementation and 188 per 100 students after implementation; $SD = 186.8$ and 132.5, respectively). High schools reported an average of 179 referrals per 100 students before implementation and 121 referrals after implementation ($SD = 149.2$ and 106.0, respectively). Elementary schools reported the lowest average number of referrals overall (68 per 100 students before implementation and 47 after implementation; $SD = 50.6$ and 32.5, respectively).

Florida's elementary, middle, and high schools implementing Tier 1/Universal Level PBS reported fewer days of ISS during their first year of implementation. Elementary schools reported an average 58% decrease in days of ISS per 100 students ($SD = 40.83$). The range of change in days of ISS per 100 students for elementary schools was −205.28 to +13.72. Middle schools reported an average 8% decrease in days of ISS per 100 students ($SD = 44.51$). The range of change in days of ISS per 100 students for middle schools was −96.26 to +72.88. High schools reported an average decrease of 4%

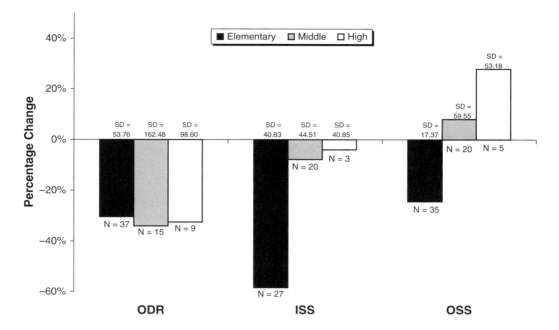

FIGURE 3. Percentage Decrease in Office Discipline Referrals (ODRs), In-School Suspensions (ISS), and Out-of-School Suspensions (OSS) per 100 Students After 1 Year of Implementation (by school type).

(SD = 40.85). There were only three high schools represented in the analysis of change in days of ISS per 100 students. The percentage change for the three high schools was –27.9, –23.5, and +44.9.

Although not depicted in Figure 3, middle schools reported the highest average number of days of ISS, with 98 days per 100 (SD = 77.3) before implementation and 90.7 days per 100 (SD = 73.7) after implementation. Elementary schools reported the lowest average number of days, with 16.5 days per 100 (SD = 44.5) before implementation and 6.9 days per 100 (SD = 8.7) after implementation. High schools reported an average of 54 days per 100 (SD = 41.2) before implementation and 52.6 days per 100 (SD = 23.1) after implementation. The results for high schools should be viewed with caution, as the data set contained only three schools.

Florida's elementary schools implementing Tier 1/Universal Level PBS reported fewer days of OSS during the first year of implementation. Elementary schools reported a decrease in days of ISS, with 24% fewer after 1 year of implementation (SD = 17.37). The range of change in days of OSS per 100 students for elementary schools was –246.4 to +77.4 days per 100 students. Middle and high schools reported an increase in the average number of

days of OSS per 100 students (see Figure 3). Middle schools reported an average increase of 8% in days of OSS per 100 students (SD = 59.55). The range of change in days of OSS per 100 for middle schools was –491.8 to +103.1. High schools reported an average increase of 28% in days of OSS per 100 students (SD = 53.18), ranging from –223.6 to +88.4. It is important to note that these data for high school represent only five schools. Furthermore, a school-level analysis revealed that three of the five high schools realized a decrease in days of OSS after implementing Tier 1/Universal Level PBS.

Although not depicted in Figure 3, middle schools reported the highest average number of days of OSS, with 89.4 days per 100 (SD = 65.0) before implementation and 96.6 days per 100 (SD = 71.7) after implementation. Elementary schools reported the lowest average number of days, with 20.2 days per 100 (SD = 20.4) before implementation and 15.2 days per 100 (SD = 14.7) after implementation. High schools reported an average of 56.6 days per 100 (SD = 30.6) before implementation and 72.4 days per 100 (SD = 42.0) after implementation.

All levels of Florida's schools implementing Tier 1/Universal Level PBS realized an increase in the average percentage of students scoring Level 3 or higher on the reading section of the FCAT after their first year of implementation. Middle schools realized the greatest increase, with 3% more students achieving Level 3 or higher after Year 1 of implementation (SD = 13.1% in baseline and 13.1% in Year 1). Elementary and high schools averaged 1% more students scoring Level 3 or higher (high school SD = 13.9 in baseline and 15.1 in Year 1; elementary school SD = 12.9 in baseline and 13.4 in Year 1).

"Are schools implementing with high fidelity realizing better outcomes than those implementing with low fidelity?" The data indicated that this is true for ODR rates, ISS rates, OSS rates, and reading performance. Overall, higher implementing schools averaged a lower rate of ODRs than did lower implementing schools (see Figure 4). Of the 34 schools for which we have both BoQ and ODR data for 3 consecutive years, in each of the 3 years high-implementing schools reported fewer average number of referrals per 100 students when compared to low-implementing schools. In Year 1, high implementers reported 54.2% fewer ODRs per 100 students, in Year 2 they reported 11.1% fewer ODRs per 100 students, and in Year 3 they reported 38.3% fewer ODRs per 100 students.

Another outcome measure examined in relation to implementation level was the use of suspensions.

For the 3-year period from 2004 to 2007, high-implementing elementary, middle, and high schools realized fewer days of ISS per 100 students than did lower implementing schools. In the 2004–2005 school year, the 37 high-implementing schools had 31.6% fewer days of ISS when compared to the 30 lower implementing schools. For 2005–2006, the 73 high-implementing schools reported 41.6% fewer days of ISS per 100 students than did the 71 low-implementing schools. In 2006-2007, the 106 high-implementing schools reported 26.0% fewer days of ISS per 100 students when compared to the 72 low-implementing schools. For the same sets of schools over the 3-year period from 2004 to 2007, high-implementing schools reported fewer days of OSS per 100 students than did lower implementing schools. In the 2004–2005 school year, high-implementing schools reported 33.8% fewer days of OSS per 100 students when compared to lower implementing schools. For 2005–2006, they reported 21.1% fewer days of OSS per 100 students, and in 2006–2007, they reported 34.3% fewer days of OSS per 100 students.

Schools implementing with higher fidelity had a greater average percentage of students achieving Level 3 or higher on the reading segment of the FCAT. For schools scoring 70 or above on the BoQ, 67.3% of students achieved Level 3 compared to 59% of students in schools with BoQ scores below 70.

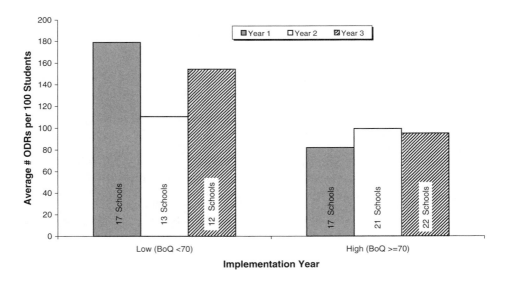

FIGURE 4. Office Discipline Referrals (ODRs) by Implementation Level Across 3 Years of Implementation. Note: BoQ = School-Wide Benchmarks of Quality.

"Do schools with teams that work well together realize better outcomes than those that do not work as well together?" Team functioning across all PBS schools was relatively high (average 87%). Teams functioning above the state average (e.g., 88% or higher) realized 6% fewer ODRs per 100 students than did schools with teams functioning below the state average. Schools scoring below the state average on team functioning averaged 195 referrals per 100 students ($SD = 438.4$), whereas teams scoring above the state average on team functioning averaged 183 referrals per 100 students ($SD = 528.5$).

"Why do schools discontinue implementation of Tier 1/Universal Level PBS?" Items on the Attrition Survey with the highest number of responses revealed three major issues contributing to the schools' decisions to discontinue participation: (a) high rates of administrative and staff turnover in schools, (b) lack of time (administrator, team, staff), and (c) lack of commitment (administrator, team, staff). These data are preliminary while data collection continues as schools drop out of participation in Florida's PBS Project. A summary of a comprehensive dataset for the attrition evaluation is forthcoming.

"Are our consumers satisfied with the training, technical assistance, products, and support received?" Respondents to the SWIF survey responded favorably to the quality of services provided by Florida's PBS Project. More than 82% rated the support from or collaboration with Florida's PBS Project as helpful or somewhat helpful, that staff were professional and respectful, and that materials and resources provided were valuable. More than 70% responded that Florida's PBS Project staff provided good recommendations and technical assistance to help them address district and/or school issues and that staff were effective and efficient in responding to requests for support.

DISCUSSION

This article presents a model for conducting a comprehensive statewide evaluation of training and technical assistance efforts at the Tier 1/Universal Level of PBS. This program evaluation was driven by 12 questions that draw on four types of data (implementation, impact, attrition, and satisfaction) that shaped the evaluation process of Florida's PBS Project. The project assessed the student outcomes of ODRs per 100 students, days of ISS per 100 students, days of OSS per 100 students, and reading achievement to determine the overall impact of the Tier 1/Universal PBS process across hundreds of schools. The evaluation also compared overall student outcomes with the level of fidelity of implementation. The descriptive data indicate the following:

1. The percentage of Florida schools implementing Tier 1 with fidelity has increased in each of 3 years to 65% in 2006–2007.

2. BoQ (fidelity of implementation) scores have increased from the first year of use, indicating overall improvement in fidelity across schools.

3. Measures of team functioning did not effectively differentiate school teams implementing with high or low fidelity or with better or worse outcomes.

4. Teams implementing Tier 1/Universal Level PBS with fidelity saw substantially different effects on all four outcome measures.

5. ODR, ISS, and OSS outcome measures differed considerably depending on the level of school (e.g., elementary, middle, high, etc.).

Although our descriptive results are encouraging, the nature of the sample had some limitations. As the number of schools represented in Florida's PBS database continues to expand, the descriptive differences in the data across hundreds of schools and multiple years will be reported with increasing confidence. And although it is also possible to conduct statistical analyses of the data, the nature of several of the data sets presents some significant challenges. For instance, although fidelity (BoQ) and academic (FCAT) data sets fluctuate within narrow parameters (scores range from 0%–100%), other data sets (ISS, OSS, ODR) have a tremendously large set of parameters that can fluctuate from fewer than 100 per year per school to well over 10,000 per year per school based on circumstances such as the size of the school or the building's discipline policies. The variability in these data sets prohibited the assumptions necessary for the use of parametric statistical analyses (i.e., normal distribution). Given the nature of the sample, the analyses and descriptive data presented in this article are effectual in communicating the results of our study of the relationships between the degree of implementation, implementation factors, outcomes, and team processes at the state, district, and school levels. Although one cannot use these evaluation data to conclude that Tier 1/Universal Level PBS produced a difference in outcomes, the data indicate a clear relationship between implementation fidelity and ODRs per 100 students.

Using Evaluation Data to Affect PBS Practice

This comprehensive evaluation process has resulted in numerous improvements to the training and technical assistance provided by Florida's PBS Project, including the following:

1. Florida's PBS Project provided increased emphasis on the use of the BoQ results for school-level and district-level action planning, recognition of model schools, and improvements in preparation for training activities that resulted in improved implementation fidelity as illustrated by the increase in the average BoQ score each of the past 3 years while at the same time more than doubling the number of participating schools.

2. District coordinators received both individual school data and district average response data from the Team Process Evaluation. If schools across the district were low in any particular area, the district coordinator was encouraged to address that issue during monthly coaches' meetings. PBS Project staff members were also available to provide support to districts with school teams struggling with particular components.

3. Because the average scores for the Team Process Evaluation were more than 87% for both low and high implementers, Florida's PBS Project reviewed the measure to determine whether it is sensitive enough to identify actual differences in high- and low-implementing schools, whether differences actually exist, or whether the items adequately reflect the team variables critical to the Tier 1/Universal Level PBS implementation process. As a result of that review, we no longer require the Team Process Evaluation to be used by schools.

4. The data suggested that Tier 1/Universal Level PBS may have had greater impact on the use of ISS versus the use of OSS at participating schools. Perhaps less-severe problem behaviors are dealt with more effectively through Tier 1/Universal Level PBS strategies, thus reducing ISS, whereas more-severe behavior problems are still occurring at the same rate and are being consequated with the use of OSS. A further analysis of project data may be able to identify the factors related to this difference in ISS and OSS rates.

5. Although the data did not indicate a significant and immediate effect of Tier 1/Universal Level PBS on academic performance, the small increase supports the Florida PBS Project's assertion that Tier 1/Universal Level PBS will not negatively affect a school's academic performance and may in fact produce more significant academic impacts after several years of implementation. These data are used to get buy in at the district and school level from schools that are reluctant to devote time and energy to activities that they perceive to interfere with academic efforts.

6. The data (implementation fidelity, behavioral outcomes, and academic achievement) were not as consistent or significant across the high schools when compared to other school levels. Whereas individual high schools have demonstrated fidelity of implementation and positive student outcomes, only 9% of total trained schools in the state are high schools. In response to the relatively inadequate effectiveness of implementation and outcomes with high schools, Florida's PBS Project began to implement the following strategies: (a) implementing PBS Plus, a 1-year intensive planning process to build administrator and faculty buy in prior to initiating the Tier 1/Universal Level PBS training; (b) training one grade level at a time (e.g., an initial effort at grade-level implementation produced a 93% reduction in ODRs per 100 students after the first year of implementation; English & George, 2008); (c) implementing continued and frequent social skills groups across all students, faculty, and staff; (d) utilizing both internal and external PBS coaches for each site; (e) extended training to accommodate larger school-based teams; (f) encouraging earlier student participation on the school-based teams; and (g) continuously advocating at the district level for administrator stability. As high schools continue to increase in participation and the project continues to expand the data collected, further analyses will be conducted to determine if any of the above strategies may have had an impact on the outcomes.

7. In light of the general acceptance that implementation fidelity was related to student outcomes, we are continuing to explore the specific factors that contribute to successful implementation of Tier 1/Universal PBS. Previous research by Cohen

(2006) indicated that the most important factor in successful PBS implementation is the functioning of the team. As a result, Florida's PBS Project continues to relate team functioning and process variables to implementation fidelity and student outcomes. As a result of this analysis, the project can begin to identify critical team variables that may be affected via statewide training and technical assistance activities.

8. Finally, Florida's PBS Project measurement of helpful and problematic factors to implementation (current and attrition teams) began to identify common variables that facilitate or impede Tier 1/ Universal Level PBS implementation. The identification of systems, training, materials, and so on that facilitate or impede implementation can provide Florida's PBS Project with action plan steps (policy changes, updated training materials, reallocation of resources, etc.) to improve targeted areas each year. Yearly analysis of this survey data should provide information on the success of action plan activities.

State Evaluation Models

Although published evaluation reports of states implementing Tier 1/Universal Level PBS with several hundred schools (Illinois, Maryland, North Carolina, Florida, etc.) are limited, an examination of annual reports from selected state projects responsible for PBS implementation presents a consistent picture of evaluation processes. Each of the above-mentioned states, by and large, follows the template developed by Horner et al. (2005) and evaluates, at a minimum, (a) who is receiving training, (b) whether schools are implementing with fidelity, (c) the impact of PBS on student behavior (e.g., ODR, OSS, ISS, school safety, academics, etc.), and (d) the level of implementation (e.g., sustained, phase of implementation, number of schools implementing, etc.).

However, additional evaluation questions reflect the unique needs of states. Illinois (Eber, Lewandowski, Hyde, & Bohanon, 2008) provides an extensive evaluation of the benefits of PBS for students with complex needs. Maryland (S. Barrett, personal communication, February 21, 2008) identifies the specifics of ODR data across all schools (what, when, where, gender, ethnicity, etc.). And Florida's evaluation includes an analysis of factors related to implementation fidelity and discontinuation of PBS, changes in implementation over

time, and the impact of team work on the fidelity of implementation and outcomes. Thus, it does appear that states that scale up intervention begin to identify some very similar evaluation questions that are consistent from state to state, and they also develop evaluation questions that reflect the unique characteristics of their states (e.g., funding source, mission, etc.).

Florida's evaluation efforts have also taught us some important lessons that may inform the evaluation efforts of other states. First, it is important to "know what you want to know" before collecting data so that you can capture multiple types of student and school outcome measures but not be seduced by the desire to collect more data than necessary. Second, it is important to compare the fidelity of implementation with outcomes to present a strong case for implementing Tier 1/Universal Level PBS with fidelity. Third, additional sources of data can assist the state in determining not just if the Tier 1/Universal Level PBS process is working but why it is or is not working. Qualitative data are necessary for redesigning and adapting the training and technical assistance support provided to schools and districts. Finally, it is essential to address state, district, and school-system issues that might affect implementation success. The development of an effective and efficient data collection and analysis system is one such critical issue that can promote initial success and future expansion.

Future Directions

The questions, data, and processes in this article describe one approach to evaluating Tier 1/Universal Level PBS. As the application of PBS continues to expand through all three tiers of PBS (i.e., Universal, Supplemental/Secondary, Intensive/Tertiary), additional questions (e.g., How many students are receiving Tier 2 and 3 interventions? Are the interventions implemented with fidelity?), data (e.g., How are groups and individuals progress monitored at the school, district, and state levels?), and processes (e.g., How will such data be gathered in an effective and efficient manner and provided back at each level for data-based decision making?) must continue to expand to allow schools, districts, and state education agencies to answer critical evaluation questions. These evaluation efforts will likely produce an array of new tools and measures. As the field of PBS grows, the need to develop tools and assessments that are both reliable and valid is paramount. Future research and evaluation efforts should pay particular attention to procedures that might improve those evaluation tools and assessments (e.g., instrument validation, standardized data collection and summarization procedures, and interpretation guidelines).

Florida's model for evaluation of state, district, and school Tier 1/Universal Level PBS efforts has been presented as one template for evaluation activities that assess multiple variables in various formats. As Tier 1/Universal Level PBS efforts continue to expand across the country at the universal, secondary, and individual levels, the evaluation questions and data sources will continue to grow in number and complexity. We encourage all states and districts to begin framing their critical evaluation questions early in the process and to design data collection and analysis processes to answer those questions in the most effective and efficient manner.

DECLARATION OF CONFLICTING INTERESTS

The authors declared that they had no conflicts of interests with respect to their authorship or the publication of this article.

FUNDING

The authors declared that they received no financial support for their research and/or authorship of this article.

REFERENCES

Barrett, S. B., Bradshaw, C. P. & Lewis-Palmer, T. (2008). Maryland statewide PBIS initiative: Systems, evaluation, and next steps. *Journal of Positive Behavior Interventions, 10*, 105–114.

Chapman, D., & Hofweber, C. (2000). Effective behavior support in British Columbia. *Journal of Positive Behavior Interventions, 2*, 235–237.

Cohen, R. (2006). *Implementing school-wide positive behavior support: Exploring the influence of socio-cultural, academic, behavioral, and implementation process variables.* Unpublished doctoral dissertation, University of South Florida, Tampa.

Cohen, R., Kincaid, D., & Childs, K. (2007). Measuring school-wide positive behavior support implementation: Development and validation of the Benchmarks

of Quality (BoQ). *Journal of Positive Behavior Interventions, 9*, 203–213.

Eber, L., Lewandowski, H., Hyde, K., & Bohanon, H. (2008). *Illinois Positive Behavior Interventions and Supports Network: 2006–2007 progress report.* Retrieved March 11, 2008, from Illinois Positive Behavior Interventions and Supports Web site: *http://www.pbisillinois.org/.*

English, C. L., & George, H. P. (2008). School-wide positive behavior support in schools struggling academically. *Association for Positive Behavior Support Newsletter, 6*(2), 1–3.

Florida Department of Education. (2007). *Assessment and accountability briefing book.* Retrieved August 21, 2008, from *http://fcat.fldoe.org/pdf/BriefingBook07web.pdf.*

George, H., & Kincaid, D. (2008). Building district-level capacity for school-wide positive behavior support. *Journal of Positive Behavior Interventions, 10*(1), 20–32.

George, H. P., Kincaid, D., & Pollard-Sage, J. (2009). Primary tier interventions and supports. In W. Sailor, G. Dunlap, G. Sugai, & R. Horner (Eds.), *Handbook of positive behavior support* (pp. 375–394). Lawrence, KS: Issues in Clinical Child Psychology.

Horner, R. H., Sugai, G., & Lewis-Palmer, T. (2005). *Schoolwide positive behavior support evaluation template.* Retrieved November 2007, from *http://www.pbis.org.*

Irwin, D., & Algozzine, R. (2005). *North Carolina positive behavior supports evaluation report.* Unpublished evaluation report.

Kincaid, D., Childs, K., Blasé, K. A., & Wallace, F. (2007). Identifying barriers and facilitators in implementing schoolwide positive behavior support. *Journal of Positive Behavioral Interventions, 9*, 174–184.

Kincaid, D., Childs, K., & George, H. (2005). *School-wide benchmarks of quality.* Unpublished instrument, University of South Florida, Tampa, Florida.

Kincaid, D., George, H., & Childs, K. (2007). *Florida's Positive Behavior Support Project: Annual report.* Tampa: University of South Florida, Florida's Positive Behavior Support Project.

Lewis-Palmer, T., & Barrett, S. (2007). Establishing and sustaining statewide positive behavior supports implementation: A description of Maryland's model. *Journal of Evidence-Based Practices for Schools, 8*(1), 45–61.

Lohrmann-O'Rourke, S., Knoster, T., Sabatine, K., Smith, D., Horvath, B., & Llewellyn, G. (2000). School-wide application of PBS in the Bangor Area School District. *Journal of Positive Behavior Interventions, 2*, 238–240.

Mass-Galloway, R., Panyan, M. V., Smith, C. R., & Wessendorf, S. (2008). Systems change with school-wide positive behavior supports: Iowa's work in progress. *Journal of Positive Behavior Interventions, 10*, 136–143.

May, S., Ard, W., III., Todd, A. W., Horner, R. H., Glasgow, A., Sugai, G., et al. (2002). *School-wide information system.* Eugene: Education and Community Supports, University of Oregon.

Muscott, H. S., Mann, E., & LeBrun, M. (2007). *Positive*

behavioral interventions and supports in New Hampshire: Effects of large-scale implementation of schoolwide positive behavior support on student discipline and academic achievement. Unpublished manuscript.

Nakusato, J. (2000). Data-based decision making in Hawaii's behavior support effort. Journal of Positive Behavior Interventions, 2, 247–251.

Nersesian, M., Todd, A., Lehmann, J., & Watson, J. (2000). Schoolwide behavior support through district-level systems change. Journal of Positive Behavior Interventions, 2, 244–247.

Office of Special Education Programs, Technical Assistance Center on Positive Behavioral Interventions and Supports. (2008). Retrieved April 10, 2008, from www.pbis.org.

Royse, D., Thyer, B. A., Padgett, D. K., & Logan, T. K. (2001). Program evaluation: An introduction. Belmont, CA: Brookes/Cole.

Sadler, C. (2000). Effective behavior support implementation at the district level: Tigard-Tualatin School District. Journal of Positive Behavior Interventions, 2, 241–243.

ABOUT THE AUTHORS

Karen Elfner Childs is the research and evaluation coordinator for Florida's Positive Behavior Support Project.

Don Kincaid is a research professor at the University of South Florida and principal investigator on several positive behavior support projects.

Heather Peshak George is an assistant research professor at the University of South Florida and co–principal investigator on Florida's Positive Behavior Support Project.

From Childs, K. E., Kincaid, D., & George, H. P. (2010). A model for statewide evaluation of a universal positive behavior support initiative. Journal of Positive Behavior Interventions, 12, 198–210. Copyright 2010 by the Hammill Institute on Disabilities. Reprinted by permission of SAGE.

ILLUSTRATIVE EXAMPLE QUESTIONS

1. What was the purpose of the study?

2. Who were the respondents, and how many Florida schools were involved?

3. In 2006–2007, what percentage of PBIS schools in Florida implemented Tier 1 practices with high implementation fidelity?

4. Did Florida schools implementing Tier 1 practices realize a decrease in office discipline referrals (ODR), in-school suspension (ISS), and out-of-school suspensions (OSS)? If so, how much of a decrease for each?

5. In schools with lower implementation fidelity, name two factors identified in the program evaluation as problematic to implementation of PBIS.

6. Did Florida schools implementing Tier 1 practices realize an increase in academic achievement? If so, how much of an increase?

7. What conclusions did the authors make?

8. What did the study add to the literature?

9. Why is implementation fidelity important? What is the minimum level of fidelity to be considered strong (high implementers)?

10. Was this a comprehensive program evaluation? Given the context of the evaluation, what additional evaluation components would you recommend?

ADDITIONAL RESEARCH EXAMPLES

1. Cohen, M. A., & Piquero, A. R. (2010). An outcome evaluation of the YouthBuild USA Offender Project. Youth Violence and Juvenile Justice, 8, 373–385.

2. Leigh, J. M., Shapiro, E. R., & Penney, S. H. (2010). Developing diverse, collaborative leaders: An empirical program evaluation. Journal of Leadership and Organizational Studies, 17, 370–379.

3. Llosa, L., & Slayton, J. (2009). Using program evaluation to inform and improve the education of young English language learners in U.S. schools. Language Teaching Research, 13, 35–54.

CHAPTER 15
■ ■ ■ ■

Evaluating the Literature

OBJECTIVES

After studying this chapter, you should be able to . . .

1. Describe what is meant by the term *research synthesis* and summarize the two key roles it plays when a new study is designed.
2. Outline the purposes of research syntheses.
3. Explain systematic and unsystematic research syntheses.
4. Characterize the considerations for conducting research syntheses.
5. Illustrate how researchers plan and execute research syntheses.
6. Know when researchers should conduct research syntheses.

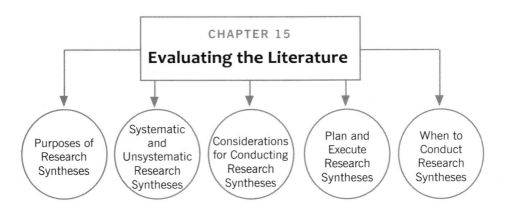

OVERVIEW

We have described the procedures for conducting qualitative and quantitative research throughout this book. These research methods are designed to derive new facts and findings regarding phenomena of interest. Up to this point, we have examined individual research studies in which researchers make hypotheses or ask research questions about the effects of an intervention. So the unit of analysis has been the measure of intervention effects in one particular study. But what about combining, or synthesizing, several studies to determine whether effects of interventions are consistent, or to investigate circumstances in which interventions are effective or ineffective? According to Chalmers, Hedges, and Cooper (2002):

> Science is supposed to be cumulative, but scientists only rarely cumulate evidence scientifically. This means that users of research evidence have to cope with a plethora of reports of individual studies with no systematic attempt made to present new results in the context of similar studies. (p. 12)

Research synthesis involves pulling together the facts and findings from a group of related studies based on different (1) theoretical frameworks, (2) independent variables, (3) dependent measures, (4) research designs, and (5) data analysis procedures. In research synthesis, researchers look at several studies, all of which examine effects of the same or similar interventions. The unit of analysis is the measure of an intervention's effect across multiple studies. We might investigate the effects of a stimulant medication on attention deficit/hyperactivity disorder based on the results of multiple studies (see Faraone, Biederman, & Roe, 2002). Our investigation would "synthesize" results across all studies to arrive at a conclusion about the effects of stimulant medication. Researchers are not limited to effects of an intervention; they may examine several studies investigating characteristics of groups, such as differences between males and females in romantic attachments (see Del Giudice, 2011).

Cooper (2010) describes research synthesis as summarizing "past research by drawing overall conclusions from many separate investigations that address related or identical hypotheses" (p. 4). So research synthesis is an attempt to integrate empirical research for the purpose of creating generalizations (Cooper & Hedges, 2009). Generally, research synthesis brings together in one place the cumulative knowledge on a subject and pinpoints new questions or issues that are unresolved (Cooper, 2010).

Research synthesis plays two key roles in the process of designing any new study. First, although the details of research synthesis may vary across experimental methodologies, all new investigations should build on existing knowledge. The underlying assumption of all research is that new studies incorporate and improve on the findings of earlier work. Research synthesis helps to ensure that gathering new research is a cumulative process rather than simply an exploratory one.

Second, research synthesis enables researchers and other professionals such as policymakers to survey the literature to understand some phenomena more fully. Questions such as "What is known about a problem or issue?"; "What attempts have been made to rectify it?"; "How effective were these attempts?"; "What

---

Research Example

Consider this issue. Think about how you would design a research synthesis to address the question/hypothesis from this research example:

- Research Example: If researchers evaluated the combined findings of previous studies, what would be the effects of full-day compared to half-day kindergarten on academic achievement of children?

The research example appears later in the chapter.

---

factors influenced the effectiveness of the attempts?"; "Should new promising attempts be made?"; and "Should different outcome measures, research designs, and analysis procedures be used?" require a thorough review of the literature or research synthesis. We focus on the research synthesis aspect of reviewing research in this chapter. An illustrative investigation is included at the end of the chapter for critique.

WHAT ARE THE PURPOSES OF RESEARCH SYNTHESES?

The role that research syntheses play in the accumulation of knowledge is important, particularly as the number of specialties in the social sciences increases. Research syntheses involve a broad array of procedures to identify the consistencies and inconsistencies in a group of related research studies. These syntheses integrate research findings for the following four purposes: (1) to establish cause-and-effect relationships; (2) to determine the degree of relationship between two variables; (3) to develop theories; and (4) to assess the external validity of findings. Each of these purposes is described in more detail.

Research synthesis *involves pulling together the facts and findings from a group of related studies.*

Establishing Cause-and-Effect Relationships

The first purpose of a research synthesis is to establish cause-and-effect relationships between variables. If most of the research studies included in the research synthesis have high internal validity, researchers can confidently address whether there is a causal relationship between variables. On the other hand, when most of the research studies included in the research synthesis have low internal validity, researchers are unable to address with confidence whether there is a causal relationship between variables. One of the problems researchers have in conducting a research synthesis is that the degree of confidence that can be placed in a causal inference is dependent on the characteristics of the reviewed studies. In other words, the extent to which we can establish a causal relationship between variables with a research synthesis is established by the underlying research studies. For example, Horner, Carr, Strain, Todd, and Reed (2002) summarized research published between 1996 and 2000 on behavioral interventions for children with autism spectrum disorder. They found 41 studies for which internal validity was strong, thus allowing examination of cause-and-effect relationships. Most common problem behaviors were tantrums, aggression, and self-injury. Generally, studies applied procedures to decrease problem behavior of children with autism based on either stimulus change, reinforcement, extinction, and punishment or combinations of procedures. They found that behavioral intervention was reasonably effective at reducing problem behaviors of children with autism spectrum disorder. Reductions of 80% or greater in problem behavior were reported in one-half to two-thirds of the studies. Researchers concluded that a substantial database indicates reduction of problem behaviors using behavioral intervention in children who experience autism spectrum disorder.

Determining the Degree of Relationship between Two Variables

The second purpose of a research synthesis is to determine the degree of relationship between two variables. Recall that much research in education and psychology is based on research methods aimed at identifying relationships between two variables. A research synthesis can bring together all of the studies that have been conducted and identify the degree of relationship between two variables. Hattie and Marsh (1996) conducted a research synthesis to determine the degree of relationship between research and teaching in universities. The analysis of 58 studies revealed that the relationship between research and teaching was zero, meaning that faculty members who do research are not necessarily good teachers, and faculty who do not do research are not necessarily poor teachers.

Developing Theories

The third purpose for a research synthesis is to develop and confirm theories. A research synthesis can aggregate findings from a number of studies to test theoretical relationships that are rarely tested with a primary research study. It can bring together and test a variety of alternative hypotheses, providing a broader basis from which to develop or confirm theoretical frameworks. For example, Breault and Breault (2010) noted the lack of theoretical base regarding school and university partnerships in professional development schools. Although considerable research had been conducted, little research informed collaborative efforts for leadership preparation. Breault and Breault conducted an extensive literature review of 250 studies across 15 years. They identified 49 exemplary studies and themes involving resources, change, and relationships. They concluded that (1) resources in partnerships become significant elements in terms of use and flexibility; (2) the nature of change in a partnership is more idiosyncratic, because of diverse stakeholders involved; (3) relationships are a vital element in the success or failure of a partnership; (4) partnerships should develop enabling bureaucracies to promote meaningful engagement among partners; and (5) organizational theory offers valuable insights regarding partnerships.

Assessing the External Validity of Findings

The final purpose for a research synthesis is to assess the extent to which the findings from research can be generalized to a larger set of participants, experimental procedures, and situations beyond those of the original research studies. A research synthesis can better address the extent to which results can be generalized than any individual study. A research synthesis can also provide a sense of the external validity of some effect by analyzing findings from a number of studies. All research syntheses by design are used to explore the generalization of findings. For example, Kim and Horn (2010) conducted a research synthesis of evidence regarding the effectiveness of sibling-implemented interventions to teach skills to siblings with disabilities. The literature search spanned 1975 to 2008 and resulted in eight studies meeting inclusion criteria. All eight studies were single-case designs (24 total subjects across studies). Siblings with disabilities included those with intellectual disabilities, autism spectrum disorder, and other impairments. Skills taught included social interaction, sharing, turn taking, offering assistance, and domestic tasks (e.g., bed making, table setting), among others. Six of the eight studies assessed generalization of the sibling-implemented interventions to other settings, tasks, or peers. While sibling-implemented interventions were effective, research was not sufficient to allow researchers to make claims about the external validity of findings.

WHAT ARE SYSTEMATIC AND UNSYSTEMATIC RESEARCH SYNTHESES?

Research syntheses can be organized into two categories: unsystematic and systematic.

Unsystematic Research Syntheses

Traditionally, research syntheses have been unsystematic and subjective in nature. Few, if any, formal procedures and practices have been used by researchers to review the literature. Often, research syntheses have raised more issues than they resolve. Unsystematic research syntheses tend to be less scientifically oriented, because no formal guidelines guide the review. They are typically based on a restrictive sample of studies, including the use of somewhat haphazard strategies for reviewing the research.

Furthermore, researchers tend to rely heavily on their own judgment to guide the review. In short, unsystematic research syntheses tend to be inefficient in integrating the findings of a group of related research studies that may differ greatly with regard to participants, independent and dependent variables, and experimental situations. Often, such reviews are conducted not to create research generalizations but to articulate an author's particular position on an issue.

Systematic Research Syntheses

In contrast, systematic research syntheses parallel the methodologies used in original research studies, in that researchers conducting research syntheses use a set of standard procedures to guide their efforts. In this way, the procedures are much more systematic in nature. Indeed, the research synthesis process has taken a quantum leap forward since the 1970s, when Glass (1976) not only coined the term *meta-analysis* (i.e., statistical analysis and integration of the findings from an exhaustive collection of the results from primary research studies) but also established procedures for conducting systematic research syntheses. Since that time there have been several detailed conceptualizations of how to conduct systematic research syntheses (e.g., Cooper, 2010; Dunst & Trivette, 2009; Hunter & Schmidt, 2004; Littell, Corcoran, & Pillai, 2008; Suri & Clarke, 2009). Research syntheses and meta-analyses are not without critics who challenge the claim that these procedures provide a superior way to summarize research findings (Shercliffe, Stahl, & Tuttle, 2009).

Systematic research syntheses differ from unsystematic ones in that researchers use a set of agreed-upon procedures and practices to review the literature. Although the procedures may vary (e.g., narrative rather than quantitative), systematic research syntheses essentially include (1) formulation of a research question or questions; (2) specification of the procedures used to select the research studies; (3) enumeration of the study characteristics examined (e.g., research design, participants, independent variables); (4) description of the procedures used to analyze the results of the research studies; and (5) neutral representation of the results.

Comparison of Unsystematic and Systematic Research Syntheses

Although we may assume that whereas systematic research syntheses are quantitative in nature, unsystematic research syntheses are qualitative, this is not necessarily the case. Rather, systematic research syntheses simply involve the use of specified procedures and practices. The use of statistical analysis procedures represents only a particular methodology (i.e., meta-analysis) for integrating the results of research studies. Table 15.1 summarizes the similarities and differences between unsystematic and systematic research syntheses. The first column lists some of the key characteristics of the two types of research syntheses; the second and third columns outline the similarities and differences between the two.

Further inspection of Table 15.1 shows that unsystematic and systematic research syntheses typically differ on only two characteristics. The coverage of the research studies is the first characteristic where differences are noted. Systematic research syntheses tend to be exhaustive in the coverage of the research literature, or if they are not, they clearly specify the procedures for including and excluding research studies. In contrast, unsystematic research syntheses are not exhaustive and may not specify the selection procedures. The second characteristic where differences are noted between the two approaches is the stance taken by the researchers. Researchers conducting systematic research syntheses tend to take a nonjudgmental stance, whereas those conducting unsystematic research syntheses tend to take a particular position.

WHAT ARE THE CONSIDERATIONS FOR CONDUCTING RESEARCH SYNTHESES?

Planning and carrying out research syntheses require four considerations: (1) identifying primary sources, (2) identifying secondary sources, (3) overcoming selection biases, and (4) focusing the literature search.

TABLE 15.1. Comparison of Unsystematic and Systematic Research Syntheses

Characteristic	Unsystematic	Systematic
Focus	Identification of results Identification of methods Identification of practices Identification of theories	Identification of results Identification of methods Identification of practices Identification of theories
Goal	Integration of results Generalization of results Resolution of conflicts Identification of central issues	Integration of results Generalization of results Resolution of conflicts Identification of central issues
Perspective	Judgmental	Nonjudgmental
Coverage	Selected	Exhaustive Selected with identified criteria Representative
Organization	Historical Conceptual Methodological Practices	Historical Conceptual Methodological Practices
Audience	Area-related scholars General scholars Practitioners Policymakers General public	Area-related scholars General scholars Practitioners Policymakers General public

Identifying Primary Sources

Research may be found in the *primary sources* that include descriptions of actual studies published in professional journals. Dissertations and theses, as well as government reports, foundation reports, and papers from scholarly meetings or conferences are also considered primary sources. Another primary source called *grey literature* is defined as literature produced for government, academics, business, and industry in print and electronic formats but is not controlled by commercial publishers (McAuly, Pham, Tugwell, & Moher, 2000). Table 15.2 presents the types of grey literature and associated descriptions. Although researchers conducting a research synthesis primarily use secondary sources (described in what follows) to identify

TABLE 15.2. Types of Grey Literature

Type	Description
Dissertations, theses, and course papers	• Includes doctoral dissertations, master's theses, honors theses, and research studies completed for a course.
Paper presentations	• Includes papers presented at international, national, state, and local professional meetings and conventions. Also includes invited conferences and colloquia.
Technical reports	• Includes unpublished technical reports prepared for research funded by the government or private agencies.
Interim reports	• Includes unpublished progress reports submitted at regular intervals during ongoing research funded by the government or private agencies.
Rejected manuscripts	• Includes completed studies that have been rejected for publication.
Uncompleted research manuscripts or reports	• Includes studies that are completed but not yet formally presented or submitted for publication.

studies, the references in primary sources can be used to identify other, relevant studies to include (often called an *ancestral search*).

Identifying Secondary Sources

Research may also be found in **secondary sources** that cite, review, and organize the material from primary studies; that is, secondary sources are "once removed" from the actual research investigations. Secondary sources include (1) review journals (e.g., *Review of Educational Research, Sociology Review,* and *Psychological Bulletin*); (2) periodical reviews (e.g., *Encyclopedia of Educational Research*); and (3) information services or abstract and citation archives (e.g., *Child Development Abstracts and Bibliography, Current Index to Journals in Education, Research in Education,* and *Psychological Abstracts*).

Researchers use secondary sources to find primary sources. These information services are computerized and enable researchers to conduct efficient syntheses.

Overcoming Selection Biases

Identifying studies to be included in research syntheses is the time when the most serious form of bias can occur. Selection bias is a problem, because it is difficult to know exactly whether all of the relevant studies have been identified and included in the research synthesis. Although it is virtually impossible to identify every relevant study on a particular topic to be included in a research synthesis, it is critical that researchers provide a complete description of the procedures used to locate the studies included in the review. A complete description of these procedures helps critical research consumers to assess the representativeness and completeness of the research synthesis. This description also enables critical research consumers to assess the generality of the results. Polman, de Castro, Koops, van Boxtel, and Merk

> **Secondary sources** *cite, review, and organize material from primary studies; they include review journals, periodical reviews, and information services or abstract and citation archives.*

(2007) provide an example of the procedures used to locate the studies in a research synthesis that pertain to services available to postsecondary students with learning disabilities:

> We aimed to include all empirical studies involving the relation between reactive and proactive aggression in children and adolescents conducted between January 1950 and July 2003. Reactive aggression was defined as aggression that occurs as an angry defensive response to a presumed threat and proactive aggression as planned cold-blooded behavior in order to take possession of things or to dominate or intimidate (Dodge, 1991). Four sources were used to identify potentially eligible studies. First, a large set of studies was retrieved by searches in online databases such as PsycINFO (*http://www. psycinfo.com*), Web of Science (*http://www.isinet.com*), ERIC [Educational Resources Information Center] (*http://www.ericnet.com*), and Dissertation Abstracts International (*http://wwwlib. umi.com/dxweb/gateway*). The keywords used in the search were "reactive aggression" and "proactive aggression," and additionally "hostile aggression" and "instrumental aggression." Second, bibliographies of retrieved studies were examined for possible related eligible studies. Third, to include a representative sample of unpublished papers in the meta-analysis, the program book of the International Society for Research in Aggression conference in Montreal, Canada (2002) was searched. Fourth, the authors contacted researchers in the field to find other relevant studies. This exhaustive search resulted in 124 titles. (p. 525)

Focusing the Literature Search

Carefully focusing a literature search is important if researchers are to achieve a research synthesis that accurately reflects accumulated knowledge underlying the phenomenon of interest. Failure to plan and execute a literature search carefully may result in one or more problematic outcomes. First, the literature search may be too broad, requiring researchers to review and reject a large number of unrelated studies, which is not only time-consuming but also frustrating. Second, the literature search may be poorly focused, either neglecting important sources or attempting to accomplish too much. Thus, carefully planning and executing a literature search eliminates wasted time, excessive costs, and irrelevant or missed primary studies.

HOW DO RESEARCHERS PLAN AND EXECUTE RESEARCH SYNTHESES?

Figure 15.1 depicts the eight steps for planning and executing a research synthesis: (1) formulating a precise research question, (2) defining critical terms, (3) formulating a literature search framework, (4) searching the literature, (5) coding study characteristics, (6) determining the magnitude of intervention outcomes, (7) relating study characteristics to intervention outcomes, and (8) reporting the results.

Formulating a Precise Research Question

The first step in planning and executing a research synthesis is to formulate a precise research question that provides structure and guides the planning and execution of the literature search. Failure to formulate a precise

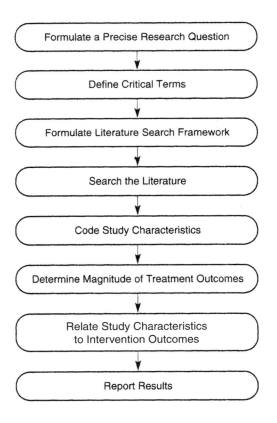

FIGURE 15.1. Steps in planning and executing a review of the literature.

research question often leads to a weak or unfocused attempt to search the literature. A wide range of questions can guide the literature search. Some common questions asked by researchers are as follows:

1. What is the average effect of the independent variable?

2. With whom is the independent variable effective?

3. Are particular versions of the independent variable effective?

4. Are particular versions of the independent variable more acceptable to key stakeholders?

5. What combination of independent variable and individuals is more effective?

6. Under what conditions is the independent variable effective?

7. How should the independent variable be implemented to ensure its effectiveness in a particular situation?

8. What is the degree of relationship between the independent and dependent variable?

9. What theoretical model is most predictive?

10. What is the relationship between study characteristics and intervention outcomes?

In addition to formulating a precise research question, it is important for researchers to determine whether the goal of the research synthesis is to test a specific hypothesis or to explore available information (Cooper, 2010). As with hypothesis testing in primary studies, researchers assert a particular outcome before searching the literature. They select and review only those primary studies that explore the particular hypothesis of interest.

In contrast, some researchers do not state a hypothesis before doing an exploratory literature search; they examine the empirical evidence in the literature, then work backwards to draw a conclusion. Researchers select a wide range of primary studies that explore the phenomenon under study. They cast a wide net when searching for primary studies to include in the literature search, then synthesize the primary studies to draw conclusions.

An example to illustrate hypothesis-testing and exploratory research questions when examining the relationship between teacher expectations and academic achievement of elementary-age children follows. "Is there a positive relationship between teacher expectations and the academic achievement of elementary-age children?" is an example of a hypothesis-testing research question. In this case, researchers would select and review primary research studies that have specifically explored the relationship between teacher expectation and the academic achievement of elementary-age children.

"What is the relationship between teacher expectations and the academic achievement of elementary-age children?" is an example of an exploratory research question. In this case, researchers would select and review all of the primary research studies that have explored the effects of teacher expectations on the academic achievement of elementary-age children.

Defining Critical Terms

Once researchers have formulated a precise research question, the next step is to identify the critical terms that describe the phenomenon under study. This description of terms enables researchers to identify the relevant primary studies that target the phenomenon of interest. Defining these terms improves the precision with which relevant primary studies are identified.

Researchers begin by identifying each key conceptual term involving the phenomenon of interest and its synonyms (related terms that have the same or nearly the same meaning). Using the example of the relationship between teacher expectations and the academic achievement of elementary-age children, three primary concepts can be identified: teacher expectations, academic achievement, and elementary-age children. Once these key conceptual terms have been identified, researchers must look carefully at the terms used by other researchers and information services to describe each of these concepts. Table 15.3 presents the relevant terms that researchers and information services (e.g., EBSCO Host, ERIC, PsycINFO, PsycARTICLES, Psychology and Behavioral Sciences Collection, Digital Dissertations, Web of Science, Google

TABLE 15.3. Relevant Terms for Teacher Expectations, Academic Achievement, and Elementary-Age Children

Teacher expectations	Academic achievement	Elementary-age children
• Teacher expectations • Self-fulfilling prophecy • Teacher attitudes • Teacher characteristics • Teacher influence • Teacher response • Teacher–student relationships	• Educational attainment • Student promotion • Academic ability • Academic aptitude • Academic standards • Academic achievement • Academic failure • Achievement rating • Achievement gains • Grades/grading • Report cards • Student characteristics	• Children • Elementary education • Elementary schools

Scholar) have used to describe *teacher expectations, academic achievement,* and *elementary-age children.* Information services produce a wide range of documents (e.g., primary research studies, conference proceedings, general papers, and position papers). These services can be searched by using a variety of search fields, such as descriptor or subject terms, keyword, author, title, publication date, abstract, and publisher.

Information services rely on a standardized terminology or set of terms to describe concepts in the literature. If a term is not included in the set of terms used to describe a concept, it will not help researchers to identify primary studies exploring the phenomenon of interest. Each information service relies on a different set of terms to describe the same concept. In most databases, these terms are referred to as *subject terms.* Thus, a set of terms used by one information service will yield a different set of primary studies than that used by another service. Because information services do not use the same standardized terms and cover the

same journals, one method for identifying subject terms is to refer to the thesaurus of each service (e.g., *Thesaurus of Psychological Index Terms, Thesaurus of ERIC Descriptors,* and the *Thesaurus of Sociological Indexing*). Table 15.4 presents examples of descriptors used in Psychological Abstracts, ERIC, and Sociological Abstracts for teacher expectations, one of the concepts in our example.

In addition, researchers can identify and verify key terms using a number of primary studies within the literature that explore the phenomenon of interest. They can examine these primary studies to identify the standardized terms used by the information services to index the studies. A comparison of the standardized terms across a number of primary studies provides a solid list of key and subject terms to use in the literature search. Additionally, one can identify key terms by conducting a free-text search of the literature exploring the phenomenon of interest, which allows researchers to search the entire literature base and determine whether a term

TABLE 15.4. Descriptors Used in *Psychological Abstracts,* ERIC, and *Sociological Abstracts* for "Teacher Expectations"

Psychological Abstracts	*Sociological Abstracts*	ERIC
• Teacher expectations • Teacher attitudes • Teacher characteristics • Teacher–student interaction	• Teacher expectations • Effective schooling • Student resistance • Teacher–student opinions/ expectations	• Teacher expectations • Self-fulfilling prophecy • Teacher attitudes • Teacher characteristics • Teacher influence • Teacher response • Teacher–student relationships

appears anywhere within the given abstract of a study. Free-text searching identifies any primary study that includes the term in the title or abstract. Once a related article is found using the free-text method, the researcher can usually view the record for the item and see what subject terms have been assigned. Running a new search using those terms is likely to produce better results. Many databases also suggest subject terms once a search has been conducted.

Formulating a Literature Search Framework

After subject terms have been identified and verified, researchers must develop a strategy for linking these terms. Although information services differ somewhat with regard to how searches are constructed, they all use Boolean rules or logical operators for linking terms. The logical operators and associated descriptions used by information services are listed in Table 15.5.

Inspection of Table 15.5 reveals that how we use Boolean rules or logical operators in a search strategy greatly affects the particular primary studies identified. For example, using OR in the search *educational attainment* OR *academic ability* OR *academic aptitude* OR *academic achievement*, identifies primary studies indexed using the terms or any combination of the terms, creating a broader search with more results. In contrast, using AND in the search *educational attainment* AND *academic ability* AND *academic aptitude* AND *academic achievement*, identifies only indexed primary studies using all four terms. The AND operator can be used to narrow searches and produces fewer results. Researchers must carefully plan how they use the logical operators to link terms together. Each information service provides a guide to its services. For databases, detailed explanations are offered within the "help" option. Additionally, many libraries provide technical assistance to researchers formulating and conducting a search strategy.

Figure 15.2 depicts a search strategy for our example on the effects of teacher expectations on the academic achievement of elementary-age children. The alternative terms associated with each of the key concepts (i.e., *teacher expectations*, *academic achievement*, and *elementary-age children*) are linked with OR to allow the use of each alternative term. Additionally, we linked the three key concepts with AND (symbolized by the arrows) to identify primary studies that have addressed all three of the key concepts.

TABLE 15.5. Boolean Rules or Logical Operators Used by Information Services

Operator	Use in search	Effect on search	Example
AND	• Use AND to search for documents that include all terms linked by AND.	• Using AND to combine terms reduces the number of documents identified. AND is used to combine terms that have different meanings and narrows the search.	• A search on terms *teacher expectations* AND *academic achievement* AND *elementary students* would identify documents in which all of the terms appeared in each document.
OR	• Use OR to search for documents that are about any of the terms being linked by OR.	• Using OR to combine terms increases the number of documents identified. OR is used to combine terms that have similar meaning and broadens the search.	• A search on terms *teacher expectations* OR *teacher attitudes* OR *teacher–student relationship* would identify documents in which at least one of the terms appeared in each document.
NOT	• Use NOT to eliminate documents containing a specific term.	• Using NOT to combine terms reduces the number of documents identified. NOT is used to eliminate terms that have similar meaning to the term(s) of interest and narrows the search.	• A search on terms *teacher expectations* NOT *teacher attitudes* NOT *teacher–student relationship* would identify documents in which no mention was made of the terms *teacher attitudes* and *teacher–student relationships*.

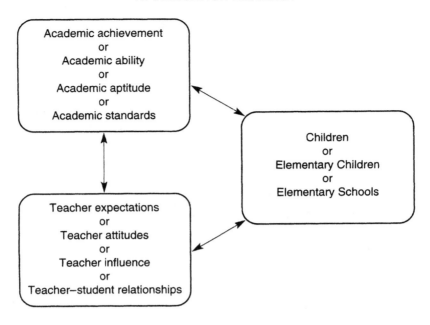

FIGURE 15.2. Example of a search strategy using logical operations.

Another strategy for identifying related studies is to follow the "chain of references" from relevant resources. For example, tracking the sources listed in reference sections and works cited pages of relevant articles can be helpful in locating important or relevant works.

Searching the Literature

Once they formulate a search strategy, researchers conduct a literature search. Indeed, formulating a strategy and searching the literature are directly connected to one another. Researchers may have to reformulate their search strategies many times once they begin to search the literature, because it is difficult to identify all of the relevant research studies. Nevertheless, the goal of researchers is to achieve an accurate and impartial description of the study findings. Conducting such a review of the literature can be done in two ways. The first is to conduct an exhaustive literature search that attempts to identify all primary sources and grey literature exploring the phenomenon of interest. An exhaustive literature search is especially appropriate when researchers are interested in conducting an exploratory research synthesis.

Including a wide range of primary and grey literature sources can enhance degree of confidence in the findings.

The second way to conduct a literature search, selecting a subsample of studies exploring the phenomenon of interest, is appropriate when researchers face an enormous number of studies; it is appropriate for both hypothesis-testing and exploratory literature searches. Of course, it is critical that the process used to select a subsample of studies does not introduce any bias into the search. Because it is difficult to assess the potential bias introduced into such a literature search, researchers, at a minimum, must fully describe the selection criteria they use to both include and exclude studies in the review.

Researchers typically employ a number of approaches to select a subsample of studies. A common approach is to stratify them on a number of key categories (e.g., type of experimental design and geographic location) that must be represented in the study. Researchers then select studies from each category to include in the literature search. Selecting studies from each category is especially useful when key study characteristics are related in some fashion to outcomes. For example, it might be useful to categorize studies into primary grades (K–3) and intermediate grades (4–6) in our example of the effects of teacher expectations on the academic achievement of elementary-age children, then select a sample of representative studies from each of the categories.

Another approach to select a subsample of studies is to use only published studies, eliminating from review any grey literature. Including only published investigations has some advantages. On the one hand, the search process is simplified, since such studies are much easier to find. Also, selected studies tend to be more technically sound, because they have undergone a peer review process. On the other hand, including only published studies may introduce *publication bias* (Rothstein, Sutton, & Borenstein, 2006), which centers on the reality that statistically significant findings are more likely than nonsignificant findings to be submitted and accepted for publication. Thus, literature searches that include only published studies may overestimate the effects of the independent variable.

A final approach for selecting a subsample of studies is to use a panel of experts (Prout & Nowak-Drabik, 2003). Researchers and other specialists with expertise in the phenomenon of interest are either polled to identify the studies or asked to critique the studies included in the literature search. The advantage is that a panel of experts has knowledge of the strengths and weaknesses of different types of studies. Using our example of the effects of teacher expectations on the academic achievement of elementary-age children, a panel of experts on teacher expectations would not only be able to identify the relevant studies but also provide information on study characteristics that might influence the outcomes. Of course, it is important that the panel include a range of professionals to help reduce the potential biases of expert judgment.

Most databases provide a free user account that usually requires a username and password, allowing the researcher to save specific articles and/or search within that database. Saving searches within databases eliminates repetitive searches, especially since these types of searches can produce a substantial number of results using either the exhaustive or subsample

method. The literature searcher should save and organize the results of the search.

There are no set guidelines for searching the literature, because the strategies vary depending on the nature of the search. The goal, depending on the purpose of the review of the literature, is to identify both primary sources and grey literature exploring the phenomenon of interest. The first step is to begin at an academic library that provides adequate electronic sources for conducting a review of the literature. These sources include library resources and databases, references in reviews of the literature, and bibliographic information series. Most academic libraries at colleges and universities are members of interlibrary services, so even if a library does not have access to a particular journal or study, it can be retrieved through interlibrary agreements. Electronic resources and databases vary in name and purpose. The most common databases in education include EBSCO Host and ERIC. Research on topics related to psychology (including educational psychology) can be found in PsycINFO, PsycArticles, Psychology and Behavioral Sciences Collection, JSTOR, and Sociological Abstracts. Google Scholar is a popular database for both education and psychology, although it is not as versatile when it comes to dynamic or complex searches. Researchers use these sources to identify relevant studies from both primary sources and grey literature. Searching typically involves entering a primary search term, then specifying secondary terms, document types (research, case studies, etc.), publication dates (e.g., recent or exhaustive), and other limiters. A researcher can begin broadly (specifying only a primary term) to see what is available in the literature, or narrowly to see whether a specific article or area of research can be found. Once they get started, researchers almost undoubtedly refine search activities by using different terms not originally anticipated, searching specific journals, and so forth. You will want to keep notes detailing your search, so that you can write a description and justification of your navigation in the literature review. Second, researchers retrieve studies and search references found in the first set of studies to identify additional studies. Third, researchers retrieve the identified studies and repeat the retrieval process, until the same studies are identified again and again. These three steps can be accomplished by working from the Internet, although there may be some compromises. For example, some articles may be available only by paying a fee. Others may not be found. If you are working online and encounter problems finding articles, it is advisable to visit an academic library to speak to a representative of the reference section. If working in a rural area, call or e-mail the reference desk representative for assistance. This process leads to a relatively complete list of studies exploring the phenomenon of interest.

Determining High-Quality Research in an Online Search

Regardless of the database used, a search will generate a list of published studies in numerical order. But the numbers do not provide a rank of quality. In fact, the numerical rank reflects only the number of times your search terms were found in the articles. Frequency of match with your terms does not serve as an indicator of research quality. What do you do to ensure quality? How do you reduce or modify your list to retain only quality research? We conducted an informal poll of faculty members available in a particular department to answer this question. Here's what they told us.

1. Discuss your findings with experts on the particular topic. Contact scholars and researchers and ask them to distinguish the credible research.

2. If a journal represents an association or organization in a professional field, it will have a strong peer-review process that rejects low-quality research. Therefore, determine whether you have located research from journals representing associations or organizations (i.e., *flagship* journals).

3. Journals have impact factors, which are ratings of "impact and influence metrics" listed at Web of Knowledge (*http://wokinfo.com*). Examine impact factors of journals with your research.

4. Check for listings of top journals in particular professional fields. Are studies you found published in any of these journals?

5. Look for the number of citations of a particular article. Large numbers of citations suggest that the research is highly influential, controversial, or available many years for citation. To what extent have your research studies been cited?

6. Read the article yourself and critically analyze it. (We knew we would hear this given that we were asking faculty members in a research department.)

Coding Study Characteristics

Researchers conducting a research synthesis must choose the study characteristics and develop methods that interest them to ensure that the information is reliably obtained from each primary study. A well-designed method for identifying study characteristics is an important step in the search process. Although there is no single set of prescribed guidelines for determining which study characteristics to include in a research synthesis, researchers typically code key study characteristics, such as (1) study identification (e.g., author, year, and source of publication); (2) setting (e.g., scope of sampling; population characteristics such as minorities, special populations, and SES level of the community or school; ecological characteristics such as school setting); (3) participants (i.e., specific characteristics of the sample(s) and/or subsample(s), including demographic characteristics such as SES level, education, age, and gender); (4) methodology (e.g., research design, attrition, experimental procedures); (5) independent variable or intervention (e.g., theoretical framework, description of experimental conditions both for the experimental and control groups, duration of independent variable, who delivered the independent variable, verification of the independent variable); (6) research quality (i.e., threats to internal and external validity); (7) dependent variable (e.g., relevance, reliability and validity, time frame); and (8) outcomes (e.g., effect size, statistically significant findings, author's conclusions).

Although each category of key study characteristics should be considered when conducting a review of the literature, it is not necessary to use all of them. The particular categories, and factors within categories, should be selected on the basis of the research domain for the particular phenomenon of interest. The process of identifying study characteristics is ongoing, and researchers should make changes when necessary. It is not uncommon to make several adjustments in study characteristics extracted from the primary studies.

Study characteristics to be extracted from the primary studies are then coded on a coding form. Taking the time to construct a coding form and training the coders is not only important to the quality of the research synthesis but also necessary to manage the large amount of generated information effectively. The coding of study characteristics is more accurate if the coding forms are clear and organized to facilitate coding. Paper-and-pencil coding forms can be used. However, computer database programs are more desirable, because they allow researchers to rearrange and organize the information to facilitate interpretation of the studies. Figure 15.3 presents an example of a coding form for a research synthesis on the use of self-management procedures with students with behavioral disorders (Nelson, Smith, Young, & Dodd, 1991). The form depicts the major study characteristics extracted from each of the studies included in the literature search.

Training Coders

Researchers conducting a research synthesis must train the individuals who will be coding the information extracted from each of the studies. The goal of the training is to teach coders how to use the coding forms and procedures (e.g., identification of threats to internal validity) in the same way. The procedure for training coders parallels the procedure for training observers in single-case research. Stock (1994) recommends the following 10 steps for training coders:

1. An overview of the review of the literature is provided by the principal investigator.

2. Each item on a coding form and its associated description is read and discussed.

3. The process for using the coding forms is described.

4. A sample of five to 10 studies is chosen to test the coders and coding forms.

5. A study is coded independently on the coding forms by everyone.

6. Coded forms are compared, and discrepancies are identified and resolved.

7. The coding form is revised as necessary.

8. Another group of studies is coded and reviewed, and so on. Steps 4 through 8 are repeated until consensus is achieved.

9. Reliability of the coders is then checked throughout the review process. (Intercoder reliability is established in the same way as interobserver agreement.)

10. Frequent meetings are conducted with coders to discuss progress and any problems.

Determining the Magnitude of Intervention Outcomes

Although not all research syntheses are concerned with determining the magnitude of intervention outcomes, a majority is initiated to determine the effectiveness of an independent variable or the degree of relationship between two variables. Thus, it is not surprising that most advances in research syntheses have centered on the use of quantitative procedures to determine the magnitude of intervention outcomes to aid in the integration of studies. The development of quantitative procedures is not surprising given the level of debate that occurs when research syntheses are based on the professional judgment of researchers regarding the magnitude of the intervention. This is not to say that professional judgment is useless in considering the magnitude of intervention effects. Rather, the limitation of such an approach rests on the sheer magnitude of the task. Researchers find it difficult to absorb and transmit the findings from a large number of primary research studies without some reliance on statistical methods.

Researchers conducting research syntheses using experimental studies typically have access to a least one of three types of information they can use to determine the efficacy of the

Study Identification Number: _____

Publication Form: _____Journal _____Book _____Thesis _____Paper Presentation _____Other

Citation: _____

Participants

Age of Participants: _____ Major Diagnosis: _____

Other Characteristics of Participants (e.g., SES, IQ): _____

Setting: _____General Education Classroom _____Special Education Classroom _____Both

Design

Type

_____Group: _____

_____Single-Subject: _____

_____Other: _____

Selection of Subjects

_____Random: _____

_____Intact Groups: _____

_____Convenience: _____

_____Other Nonrandom:

Independent Variable(s)

Description: _____

Duration: _____ Implemented by Experimenter: _____Yes _____No _____Unknown

Dependent Variable(s)

Description: _____

Reliability/Interobserver Agreement: _____

Threats to Internal and External Validity

_____Internal Validity: _____

_____External Validity: _____

Outcome

_____Statistical Analysis: _____

_____Visual Analysis: _____

Comments: _____

_____

_____

FIGURE 15.3. Example of coding form.

independent variable. These three types include (1) information that can be used to compute effect size estimates (e.g., means, standard deviations, proportions, correlations, and test statistics); (2) whether the findings are statistically significant (i.e., p values); and (3) information about the direction of the effects of the independent variable (i.e., positive effect, negative effect, and no effect). These types of information can be rank-ordered on the degree of precision they provide researchers regarding the effectiveness of the independent variable. If the first type of information is available, then researchers should compute effect size estimates. The use of statistical significance is appropriate for the second and third types of information. Additionally, the proportion of overlapping data is a measure to determine statistically the effectiveness of an independent variable in single-case studies. In the remainder of this section, we describe each of these measures.

Statistical Significance

Experimental research methods and statistical analysis procedures in education and psychology rely heavily on statistical significance testing. Recall that statistical significance refers to a difference between sets of scores, at some level of probability, that is the result of one variable influencing another rather than a function of chance due to sampling or measurement error (Gall, Gall, & Borg, 2010). If the findings are statistically significant, researchers typically conclude that the independent variable is effective (produced effects) or that the two variables are related.

Examining the obtained p value provides a way of interpreting effectiveness of the independent variable or degree of relationship. Researchers almost always report the decision yielded by the test of statistical significance, that is, whether the test statistic did or did not exceed a conventional critical value (i.e., the point at which the null hypothesis is rejected), such as $p < .05$, $p < .01$, or $p < .001$, or in the form of an actual p value. Regardless of the form, researchers conducting research syntheses identify whether the findings are statistically significant at some established critical value such as

$p < .05$. Thus, these researchers can generally conclude that an independent variable is effective or that two variables are related if a study yields a test statistic that exceeds the established critical value in a positive direction (or negative direction, in the case of relationship studies). Researchers can use the information obtained from statistical significance testing to synthesize the research literature in several ways. We discuss two possible methods—vote counting and combining significance tests.

Vote Counting

In this case, researchers can use a vote-counting procedure to integrate the studies in a review. **Vote counting** is a method of integrating studies in a research synthesis to provide information on the results of statistical significance testing. Three possible outcomes with regard to the relationship between the independent and dependent variables are noted: (1) The relationship is statistically significantly positive; (2) the relationship is statistically significantly negative; or (3) there is no discernible relationship. The number of studies falling into each of these categories is tallied. If a majority of studies falls into any one of these three categories, this category is declared the winner, because it is assumed that the category provides the best estimate of the direction of the true relationship between the independent and dependent variables.

1. Studies that provide information on the results of statistical significance testing are examined.

2. Three possible outcomes with regard to the relationship between the independent and dependent variables are noted: (a) The relationship is statistically significantly positive; (b) the relationship is statistically significantly negative; and (c) there is no discernible relationship.

> **Vote counting** *is a method of integrating studies in a research synthesis to provide information on the results of statistical significance testing.*

3. The number of studies falling into each of these categories is tallied.

4. If a majority of studies fall into any one of these three categories, this category is declared the winner, because it is assumed that the category provides the best estimate of the direction of the true relationship between the independent and dependent variables.

It is important to note that a research synthesis using a vote-counting procedure is limited in several respects. First, vote-counting procedures do not incorporate sample size into the vote (Bushman & Wang, 2009). Recall that the probability of obtaining a statistically significant finding increases as the sample size increases. Thus, studies with large samples are more likely to result in the conclusion that there is a statistically significant relationship between the independent and dependent variables when in fact there is not. Second, although the vote-counting procedure provides information on which of the three possible outcomes is the winner, it does not provide information on the magnitude of that outcome. Third, the vote-counting procedure tends to have *low power* (i.e., ability to detect intervention effects) for the range of sample sizes and intervention effects most common in the social sciences (Bushman & Wang, 2009). It often fails to detect small to medium intervention effects. Finally, the power of the vote-counting procedure tends to be near zero as the number of studies to be integrated in the literature search increases (Bushman & Wang, 2009).

Combining Significance Tests

Combining significance tests is another procedure for using the results of tests of statistical significance to determine whether an intervention is effective. Procedures for combining significance tests effectively deal with previously identified problems of the vote-counting procedure. However, these procedures require that researchers report the actual obtained p value rather than general information on whether the test of statistical significance met a conventional critical value of $p < .05$, $p < .01$, or $p < .001$.

These procedures also require that one know the sample size (this was not the case with the vote-counting procedure).

There are numerous methods for combining each study's test of statistical significance into an overall pooled test (Lipsey & Wilson, 2001). One method for combining tests of statistical significance is adding Z scores. Z scores from each individual study are added up across studies. The obtained sum is then divided by the square root of the number of studies. The probability level associated with combined Z scores provides an estimate of the overall level of significance for all of the studies included in the research synthesis. The probability level associated with the combined Z scores can be obtained by looking at a table of normal deviations that contains critical values associated with Z scores.

As with the vote-counting procedure, there are a number of potential problems associated with procedures for combining tests of statistical significance. First, although these procedures provide an overall estimate of the intervention effect, they do not enable researchers to examine the distribution of the findings across study characteristics. This understanding enables researchers to examine conditions under which the independent variable is effective or the relationship between two variables exists.

Second, errors in interpretation of the overall combined test of statistical significance are never known. For example, researchers conducting a research synthesis might conclude that the effect of the independent variable is greater than zero, or that there is a relationship between two variables because the null hypothesis was rejected, when in fact it should have been accepted (*Type I error*). Alternatively, researchers may incorrectly conclude that the intervention had *no* effect or that there was *no* relationship between two variables because the null hypothesis was accepted (*Type II error*). Finally, the potential of publication bias is increased when researchers use procedures for combining tests of statistical significance, since there is a tendency for studies that achieve statistical significance to be published, whereas statistically nonsignificant studies are not (Rothstein et al., 2006).

An example is provided to compare the method of adding Z scores and the vote-counting procedure described earlier. The reported p

values of .12, .01, .72, .07, and .17 and associated Z scores of 1.17, –2.33, –0.58, 1.48, and 0.95 were obtained for five studies. Using the vote-counting procedure, we would conclude that there is no intervention effect, because only one of the p values is statistically significant at the $p < .05$ level (i.e., .01). In contrast, computing the combined Z scores for the obtained studies using the method of adding Z scores (sum of the Z scores divided by the square root of the number of studies) yielded a combined Z score of 2.39, $p = .009$. We would conclude that the intervention was effective. This example illustrates how the conclusions drawn by researchers are dependent on the particular procedures they use to determine whether an independent variable was in effect or that there was a relationship between two variables.

Effect Size

Introduced in Chapter 4, effect size is currently the most common measure used by researchers conducting reviews of the literature. It provides much more information than statistical significance. Tests of statistical significance only provide information regarding the probability that the obtained differences between experimental and control groups are due to sampling and measurement error. **Effect size** goes beyond statistical significance by providing information regarding the *magnitude* of the differences between the experimental and control groups or the degree of relationship between two variables. This distinction is important because tests of statistical significance are heavily influenced by sample sizes. Extremely small differences in very large experimental and control samples can be statistically significant even though they may not be socially significant (i.e., how valuable an intervention is). Statistical significance and effect size are related to each other in the following way: Statistical significance = effect size × sample size. This direct relationship shows that any nonzero effect size will reach statistical significance given a sufficiently large sample size.

The effect size is a standardized measure of the difference between the experimental and control groups. The most common use of the effect size is to compare the mean scores of the experimental and control groups. The estimate of the effect size is then the difference between the two groups' means divided by the control group's standard deviation. The control group's standard deviation is believed to provide the best estimate of variance in the population. This measure of effect size is known as Glass's delta (see Table 15.6). The formula is as follows:

$$\Delta = \frac{M_1 - M_2}{SD_c}$$

where M_1 is the mean of the experimental group, M_2 is the mean of the control group, and SD_c is the standard deviation of the control group.

It is important to note that some researchers suggest making a number of adjustments in the computation of effect sizes to provide estimates of the standard deviation in the population and to control for sample size. For example, many computations of effect sizes use a pooled standard deviation rather than the control group's standard deviation, because they believe it provides a better estimate of the standard deviation in the population (e.g., Means, Toyama, Murphy, Bakia, & Jones, 2009). The computational formula for obtaining a pooled sample standard deviation is as follows (Cooper & Hedges, 2009):

$$SD = \sqrt{\frac{(n_e - 1)(SD_e)^2 + (n_c - 1)(SD_c)^2}{n_e + n_c - 2}}$$

where SD is pooled standard deviation, n_e is the sample size for the experimental group, n_c is the sample size for the control group, SD_e is the standard deviation for the experimental group, and SD_c is the standard deviation for the control group.

Parametric Effect Sizes

Parametric effect sizes available to researchers conducting research syntheses. There are two families of parametric effect sizes: r and d (Cooper, 2010). These two families of effect sizes directly align with the purpose of the studies being included in the research synthesis. The r family of effect sizes is used in cases in which

---

Effect size *refers to a statistical procedure for determining the magnitude of the difference between two or more groups.*

TABLE 15.6. Common r-Type and d-Type Effect Sizes and Associated Formulas and Parameters Estimated

Effect size	Type	Formula	Parameter estimated
r	r	$\dfrac{\Sigma Z_x Z_y}{N}$	Population correlation between variables x and y
Z_r	r	$\frac{1}{2}\log_e \dfrac{[1+r]}{[1-r]}$	Population Fisher Z_r transformations of population correlations
Cohen's q	r	$Z_{r1} - Z_{r2}$	Difference between Fisher Z_r transformations of population correlations
Glass's Δ	d	$\dfrac{M_1 - M_2}{SD \text{ of control group}}$	Difference between population means divided by the standard deviation of the population control group
Hedges's g	d	$\dfrac{M_1 - M_2}{\text{pooled } SD}$	Difference between population means divided by average population standard deviation
d'	d	$p_1 - p_2$	Difference between population proportions

the goal of the synthesis is to determine the magnitude of a relationship between two variables. The d family of effect sizes is used when the goal of the synthesis is to determine the magnitude of the difference between the means of experimental and control conditions, for example. However, researchers often encounter situations in which there is a mixture of r and d effect sizes. This mixture is not a problem, because there are procedures for converting these effect sizes into one particular effect size. Table 15.6 presents descriptions and formulae for some of the most common r and d effect sizes used by researchers to conduct reviews of the literature. See Cooper (2010), Lipsey and Wilson (2001), and Morris and DeShon (2002) for in-depth discussions of effect sizes.

Meaning of Effect Sizes

The meaning of effect sizes can be translated into notions of overlapping distributions of scores and comparable percentiles (Cooper, 2010). For example, say the obtained effect size for a hypothetical study on the effects of a Direct Instruction reading program on improving the phonemic awareness of young children versus a literature-based reading program is 1.00. This positive effect size indicates that the average child in the Direct Instruction condition shows

phonemic awareness one standard deviation above that of the average child in the literature-based reading condition. A negative effect size would indicate that the average child in the literature-based reading condition is one standard deviation below the average Direct Instruction child. In this example, phonemic awareness of only 16% of the children in the Direct Instruction reading condition is worse than the average child in the literature-based reading condition. Figure 15.4 depicts the outcomes for this hypothetical study. Additionally, effect sizes that approach or equal zero may also occur; in this case, Direct Instruction and literature-based reading produced comparable student outcomes.

Effect sizes may also be meaningful without comparison to a control group. One approach is to compare relative effect sizes for different interventions or different study characteristics. For example, Rosenshine and Meister (1994) compared the effect sizes obtained with reciprocal teaching interventions across a number of study characteristics. They compared the obtained effect sizes for type of student by outcome measure in an attempt to examine whether certain students improved in comprehension by type of comprehension measure used (i.e., standardized or experimenter-developed tests; see Table 15.7). (Rosenshine and Meister made a number of comparisons in their research syntheses.) These

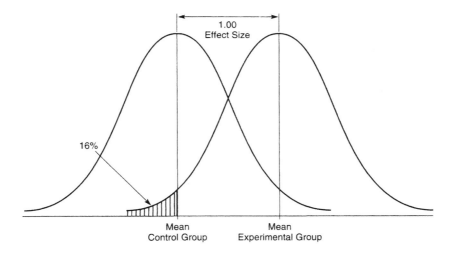

FIGURE 15.4. Illustrative example for interpreting effect sizes.

comparisons enable critical research consumers to examine the relative effects of these factors.

Problems Associated with Effect Sizes

Finally, it is important to understand the problems associated with the use of effect sizes. The first is that researchers conducting primary research studies use a number of different dependent measures, so figuring out the meaning of effect sizes across multiple studies is not easy. Calculating and combining effect sizes are easiest when the same dependent measure is used by researchers. Researchers calculating effect sizes must consider whether it is reasonable to combine effect sizes across different dependent measures.

Related to this issue, the second problem focuses on the fact that researchers conducting primary research studies use a number of dependent measures within a study; that is, one study yields multiple effect sizes. One approach to this problem is to compute separate effect sizes within a study. Although such an approach uses all of the information available from a study, it may weight the results of the study more heavily than studies that have used one or two dependent measures. The common approach to this problem is to treat each study as a unit of analysis and compute an average effect size across the dependent measures.

The final problem is that a number of primary research studies do not provide all of the information necessary to compute an effect size. These studies cannot be included in the research synthesis. Of course, this may eliminate studies that might provide valuable information, and this is why some authors suggest that

TABLE 15.7. Median Effect Sizes for Type of Student by Type of Test

Type of student	Standardized tests	Experimenter-developed tests
All students	.32 (4)	.85 (5)
Good–poor students	.29 (2)	.88 (3)
Below-average students	.08 (4)	1.15 (2)

Note. Numbers in parentheses refer to the number of studies used to compute median effect sizes. From Rosenshine, B., & Meister, C. (1994). Reciprocal teaching: A review of the research. *Review of Educational Research, 64*, 479–530. Copyright 1994 by the American Educational Research Association. Reprinted by permission of SAGE.

researchers conducting reviews of the literature combine narrative and quantitative approaches (e.g., Dochy, Segers, Van den Bossche, & Gijbeis, 2003).

Recall the research question about comparing the effects of full-day kindergarten with half-day kindergarten posed earlier in this chapter? Read on to see how your design compares to how the actual study was designed.

Research Example: Research Synthesis

A meta-analysis of 40 studies investigated the effects of full-day kindergarten compared to half-day kindergarten on childrens' academic achievement, attendance, self-confidence, ability to work and play, positive attitude toward school, and behavior problems (Cooper, Allen, Patall, & Dent, 2010). It should be noted that this research synthesis was one of many meta-analyses on the effects of full-day kindergarten. Several previous studies are noteworthy (e.g., Clark & Kirk, 2000; Education Commission of the States, 2004; Le, Kirby, Barney, Setodji, & Gershwin, 2006). In this meta-analysis, Cooper et al. (2010) examined not only academic achievement but other variables such as attendance and self-confidence. To conduct the literature search, researchers first searched six databases (e.g., ERIC, PsycINFO) for terms. This process yielded 655 potential document records. To be included, a study had to have (1) focused on differences between full- and half-day kindergarten, (2) included a measure of academic achievement or readiness, and (3) included measures of student development or well-being. These criteria reduced the number of studies to 40. Researchers next recorded data on each study (e.g., research design, characteristics of kindergarten programs, setting and sample, outcome measures). Effect size was estimated by using standardized mean difference. Results indicated that an overall effect size for achievement in full-day kindergarten was 0.24, which was statistically significant ($p < .001$). Of 152 unadjusted effect sizes across studies, 128 were positive, 23 were negative, and one was exactly zero. However, improved academic achievement disappeared by third grade. The data indicated a small positive association between full-day kindergarten and attendance,

self-confidence, and ability to work and play with others. Cooper et al. (2010) echoed sentiments of previous researchers (Clark & Kirk, 2000) that a more important variable than full-day versus half-day kindergarten is what children do during the day.

Evaluating Literature in Single-Case Designs: Measures for Overlapping Data across Conditions

As discussed in previous chapters, single-case researchers often rely on visual analysis. Generally, researchers compare a participant's target behavior across conditions (e.g., baseline and intervention) and examine changes in level or trend of behavior (also the rapidity of behavior change; see Chapter 11 for more information). However, in recent years, a growing number of single-case researchers has called for *measures of overlapping data* across conditions, defined as a quantifiable index of the degree to which data points overlap between conditions. There are several reasons for the trend toward measures for overlapping data, but the most powerful one is the call within educational research for evidence-based practice with effect size–like measures to quantify the effectiveness of interventions (Gast, 2010; Kazdin, 2008; Parker, Vannest, & Davis, 2011).

It should be noted that these measures are not the single-case equivalent of effect sizes. That is, degree of overlap does not yield the same outcome as $M_1 - M_2$ divided by the standard deviation. The intent is generally the same as effect size, but the numerical outcome will be different, because most measures of overlap do not take into account the magnitude of the difference between conditions. Yet measures of overlap are common tools in research synthesis of single-case designs. Several researchers have used measures of overlap to conduct meta-analyses across single-case studies (e.g., Bellini, Peters, Benner, & Hopf, 2007; Graham & Perin, 2007).

Types of Measures of Overlapping Data. We offer a brief description of overlapping data here. However, it is beyond the scope of this book to provide a detailed description. The reader is referred to other sources (Gast, 2010; Parker et al., 2011; Wolery, Busick, Reichow, & Barton, 2010). We describe three common measures of overlapping data: (1) percentage of nonoverlapping data (PND; Scruggs, Mastropieri, & Casto, 1987), (2) percentage of data points exceeding the median (PEM; Ma, 2006), and (3) pairwise data overlap squared (PDO^2; Parker & Vannest, 2009). PDO^2 has also been referred to as percentage nonoverlap of all pairs, or NAP.

PND. PND is defined as the number of intervention data points that exceed the highest baseline data point in the expected direction divided by the total number of data points in the intervention condition (Scruggs et al., 1987). To calculate PND, the researcher considers two conditions: the baseline followed by an intervention, and the intended direction of behavior change (i.e., the desired direction). Let's say the intended direction of change is to increase the level of behavior in an intervention. The researcher (1) identifies the highest datum in baseline, (2) draws a horizontal line (parallel to the *x* axis) from that baseline datum through the data in the intervention condition, (3) counts the number of data points in the intervention that are higher than the highest datum in baseline (i.e., nonoverlapping, or therapeutic), (4) divides that count by the total number of data points in intervention, and (5) multiples by 100 to produce

a percentage score. The larger the PND, the greater the effects of the intervention. In cases where the researcher seeks to decrease behavior in intervention, he/she modifies Step 3 above by counting the number of data points in intervention that are lower than the lowest datum in baseline.

Consider an illustrative example to help understand how PND scores are computed. Figure 15.5 presents the results from a hypothetical study using an A-B design on the effectiveness of a reading instruction strategy. Using the computation procedures outlined earlier, there are eight data points in the expected direction, six of which exceed baseline data. The resulting PND for this hypothetical study would be computed as $6 \div 8 \times 100 = 75\%$.

PEM. PEM is defined as the number of data points that exceed the *median* baseline data point in the expected direction divided by the total number of intervention data points in the intervention condition. To calculate PEM for an intervention to increase behavior, a researcher (1) calculates the median for baseline, (2) draws a horizontal line at the level of the baseline median through the data in the intervention condition, (3) counts the number of data points in the intervention that are higher than the baseline median, and (4) divides the total count by

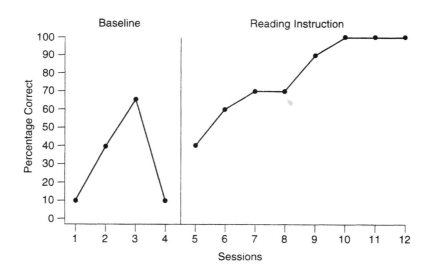

FIGURE 15.5. Illustrative example for computing PND.

the total number of data points in intervention times 100.

Using Figure 15.5, a hypothetical study using an A-B design, PEM can be calculated. The researcher must first calculate the median for baseline. Baseline values are 10, 10, 40, and 65%. Because there are an equal number of data points (4), the researcher first calculates the median by finding the mean between the two middle numbers in the distribution. The two middle numbers in the distribution are 10 and 40, so the median is (10 + 40)/2 = 25. When the researcher draws a horizontal line at the level of the baseline median through the data in the intervention condition, there are no data points overlapping. Therefore, PEM = 100%, that is, the percentage of data points that exceed the median is 100%.

PDO². PDO² (pairwise data overlap squared) involves pairwise comparisons of data points in baseline and intervention. To calculate PDO², the researcher first considers each datum in baseline. For each datum, the researcher counts the number of data points in the intervention condition that are higher than the baseline datum (assuming the desired direction of change is to increase the behavior). This process is repeated for all baseline data points. Next, the researcher (1) sums all higher intervention data points from the pairwise comparison, (2) counts the number of total data points in baseline and the number of total data points in the intervention condition, (3) multiplies the two counts to determine the total number of pairwise comparisons, (4) divides the sum of higher data points from the pairwise comparison (step 1) by the total number of pairwise comparisons (step 3), and (5) squares the quotient. The result is an index of the pairwise data that overlap.

Returning to Figure 15.5, PDO² can be calculated using the same data. The researcher begins by counting the number of data points in the intervention that are higher than each baseline datum. Considering the first datum (10%), eight data points in intervention are higher. Considering the second (40%), seven data points in the intervention are higher (the Session 5 point of 40% is tied). Considering the third (65%), six data points in the intervention are higher (Session 5 and Session 6 data are lower). Considering

the fourth (10%), eight data points in intervention are higher. The sum of the higher data points in the pairwise comparison is 8 + 7 + 6 + 8 = 29. Next, the researcher multiplies the number of baseline and intervention data points to determine the total pairwise comparisons: 4 in baseline × 8 in intervention = 32. The researcher now divides the sum of higher data points (29) from the pairwise comparison by the total number of pairwise comparisons (32) (29 ÷ 32 = .906). Finally, the researcher squares the quotient, so .906 × .906 = .821. Therefore, PDO² = 82.1%.

Comparisons of Measures of Overlapping Data. Wolery et al. (2010) used visual analysis to examine 160 single-case graphs with two adjacent conditions. Four judges agreed on 94 graphs that showed a change in data pattern, and on 27 graphs that showed no change in data pattern. The 121 graphs with agreement across all four judges were then subjected to measures of overlapping data (PND, PDO², PEM). Wolery et al. used the guidelines suggested by Scruggs and Mastropieri (1994) to categorize levels of effects. Measures from 0.90 to 1.00 were considered *very effective interventions*, 0.70 to 0.89 were considered *effective interventions*, and less than 0.70 were considered *questionable or ineffective interventions*. Using this three-part categorization and four measures, PND and PDO² were almost identical in categorizing the effectiveness of interventions. They were also more conservative in identifying interventions as very effective. However, PEM reported much higher percentages of very effective interventions. This finding replicates others (Parker & Hagan-Burke, 2007; Parker & Vannest, 2009), as well as our earlier examples, and suggests that PEM overestimate effects, especially in graphs with a greater number of overlapping data points. The findings regarding PND and PDO², replicated by Parker et al. (2011), suggest that these measures of overlapping data produce similar results.

Weaknesses in Overlap Measures. Wolery et al. (2010) described several weaknesses in overlap measures, four of which are noted here. First, overlap methods are based only on level of data, not trend. Second, the number of data points in an intervention condition influences the percentage of overlap. The size of the effect increases as the number of intervention data points increases. Third, overlap methods are not an estimate of the magnitude of effects (i.e., effect size) between conditions. Fourth, overlap methods fail to use the replication logic inherent in single-case research. That is, functional relations between variables develop through replication with consistent results, not through a high percentage score. Wolery et al. argue that current overlap measures are unacceptable, and call for a common metric for use in single-case measures of overlapping data.

Single-Case Designs: Statistical Analysis or Visual Analysis

Applied behavior analysis has much to contribute to educational and psychological research, and the practice is squarely based on empirical demonstration and replication. However, visual analysis relies on a separate method for evaluation of data and does not interface with the standards currently set by evidence-based practices. Horner et al. (2005) have called for implementation of quality indicators in single-case research to demonstrate the evidence on which the practice is based. But the separation in methodology between statistical analysis and visual analysis is based deeply in underlying philosophies. As stated by Gast (2010),

> Philosophical differences between two experimental paradigms in psychology lie at the core of the dissatisfaction with single-case meta-analysis. Group-based approaches focus on aggregated differences between two groups (nomothetic approach), single-case research designs focus on the intensive study of the individual (idiographic approach) and, opponents to single-subject meta-analysis argue, belie statistical summary. (p. 437)

In fact, Skinner (1963) described the philosophical differences between statistical and visual methods, saying that with direct observation and visual analysis

> the effect is similar to increasing the resolving power of a microscope: a new subject matter is suddenly open to direct inspection. Statistical methods are unnecessary. When a variable is changed and the effect on performance observed, it is for most

purposes idle to prove statistically that a change has indeed occurred. (p. 508)

Once again, critical research consumers need to weigh the advantages and disadvantages of overlap measures, effect sizes, and meta-analysis in single-case research. For single-case research to become a contributing partner of evidence-based practice, it needs the quality indicators recommended by Horner et al. (2005). Whether it also needs statistical measures is a question that will be debated for years to come.

Relating Study Characteristics to Intervention Outcomes

One of the most important steps in conducting a research synthesis is to examine whether particular study characteristics are related to intervention outcomes. This step directly builds on the fifth step in the review process: coding study characteristics. It should be clear by now that relatively few research syntheses yield orderly outcomes or are conducted to construct an average summary of the intervention effects (i.e., to emphasize an intervention's average impact without concern about how study characteristics are related to intervention outcomes). Indeed, study of conflicting results provides researchers an opportunity to understand better those factors that influence effects of the independent variable or the relationship between two variables. Questions such as "Does the effectiveness of a new instructional approach depend on the level of training or duration of the instruction provided?" are critical to understanding better the effectiveness of the intervention.

Variation of an Intervention

We examine why there are variations in the effectiveness of an intervention before looking at some procedures for relating study characteristics to intervention outcomes: Although there are explainable variations in the levels of participants in primary research studies, the main interest of researchers conducting a research synthesis is those contextual variables at the study level that may influence the findings. Contextual variables (i.e., characteristics of the intervention and research methodology) such as the duration of the intervention, who implemented the intervention (e.g., experimenter vs. practitioner), level of training, and type of experimental design or dependent variable may affect the findings. This examination of contextual variables is why a research synthesis may be more useful than even the most carefully conducted primary research study. It is virtually impossible for one primary study to incorporate all of the potential contextual variables into the design. In contrast, a research synthesis enables researchers to look at which contextual variables explain differences in the effectiveness of a particular intervention.

Approaches to Relate Study Characteristics to Intervention Outcomes

As with estimating the magnitude of the effects of the intervention or degree of relationship between two variables, researchers can use a number of approaches to relate study characteristics to intervention outcomes. Regardless of the approach, the goal is to assess whether variations in intervention outcomes across investigations are a function of sampling fluctuation or are due to specific effects of independent variables or components of independent variables.

Professional Judgment. The first approach to relating study characteristics to intervention outcomes centers on the professional judgment of researchers. As with estimating the magnitude of the intervention effects, researchers conducting the research synthesis examine how study characteristics are related to differences in the intervention effects. It is difficult at best for researchers to absorb and relate study characteristics on the magnitude of the intervention effects from a large number of primary research studies without some reliance on statistical methods.

Statistical and Graphic Methods. When indices of intervention effects (e.g., effect sizes, correlations) have been computed for each of the primary studies, all of the standard descriptive statistical methods, such as averages, measures of variability, and frequency distributions, can help to relate study characteristics to intervention outcomes. In addition, graphic

representation of the indices of the magnitude of intervention effects is one approach used by researchers to relate study characteristics to intervention effects. Researchers using this approach construct a graphic representation of the effect size obtained for each of the primary studies. A common approach is to construct frequency distributions of the obtained effect sizes. If the frequency of effect sizes is normally distributed, then one may assume that there is a single intervention outcome that is representative of the population of studies (see Figure 15.6). If the frequency of effect sizes is not normally distributed (e.g., bimodal distribution), one may assume that there are distinct clusters of outcomes.

Figure 15.7 presents an illustrative example in which there appear to be three distinct clusters of effect sizes across studies. These graphs highlight how a simple graphic display of obtained effect sizes can clarify whether there may be some study characteristics related to these distinct clusters of intervention outcomes. Researchers then attempt to identify differences in study characteristics associated with each of the distinct clusters of intervention outcomes. Of course, it is important to keep in mind that these frequency distributions of effect sizes are only descriptive in nature. They do not provide a statistical test of the distribution of the population. Rather, they provide information suggesting that some study characteristics are related to intervention outcomes.

A **box-and-whiskers display** (Tukey, 1991) is another graphical presentation approach that can be used to explore the relationship between study characteristics and intervention outcomes more fully. A box-and-whiskers display uses a schematic box plot with some auxiliary features to depict the distribution of effect sizes. Figure 15.8 presents an illustrative example of a box-and-whiskers display depicting the relationship between some key study characteristics and intervention outcomes. The central box or rectangle (i.e., hinges) marks off, roughly, the first and third quartiles, or approximately the mid-50% of the distribution. The asterisk represents the median, with 25% of those inside the box on either side of it (median). In our example, the hinges (ends of the box or rectangle) for short duration of intervention are approximately .01

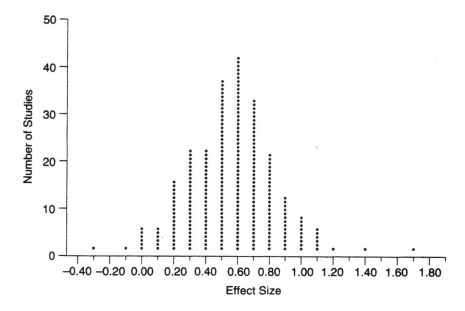

FIGURE 15.6. Illustrative example of normally distributed effect sizes indicating a single treatment outcome.

and .22. The median (represented by the asterisk) is approximately .18. The lines emanating from both ends of the box measure the distance to the "inner fence." The inner fence is one and one-half times the length of the box, or 150% of the "hinge" length (this length is arbitrarily chosen). The line at the end depicts the inner fence (−.24 and .52), and data points that lie outside the inner fences are considered outliers. Outliers should be looked at cautiously, because they may be a function of unexplainable factors such as measurement reporting errors, misprints, or miscalculations.

Inspection of Figure 15.8 reveals that there are only two outliers of concern. We could eliminate the outliers and recalculate the average effect size or, because of the small number, include them in the research synthesis. In this case, it would not really matter because there are relatively few outliers compared to the overall number of effect sizes. If there were a small number of effect sizes, it might be important to eliminate the outliers and recalculate the average effect size, because they would have a greater effect on the outcome. Additionally, there is little overlap in the distributions of effect sizes for the short- and long-duration studies. This finding suggests that the duration of intervention has an effect on the intervention outcomes. Studies that employ longer interventions tend to produce more powerful intervention outcomes.

A statistical approach to determining whether the studies in a research synthesis share one common intervention outcome or whether outcomes are influenced by contextual factors is to test for the homogeneity of effect sizes. There are several methods for calculating a homogeneity statistic for the obtained effect sizes in a research synthesis (see Glass, McGaw, & Smith, 1981; Hedges & Vevea, 1998). The idea behind each of the homogeneity statistics is straightforward. If individual effect sizes vary little from the overall mean effect size, then the obtained homogeneity statistic will be small. Small observed values indicate homogeneity

> A **box-and-whiskers display** *uses a schematic box plot with some auxiliary features to depict the distribution of effect sizes.*

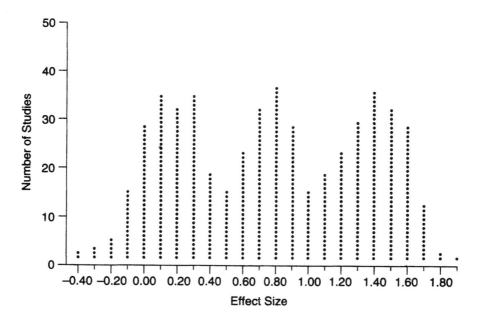

FIGURE 15.7. Illustrative example of effect sizes that are not normally distributed, indicating that there are clusters of treatment outcomes.

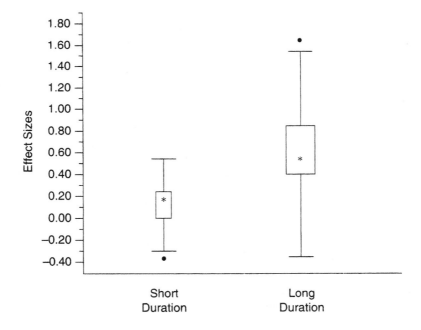

FIGURE 15.8. Illustrative example of box-and-whiskers plot depicting distributions associated with some primary study characteristics.

(sameness) among the obtained effect sizes. Homogeneity suggests that the obtained effect sizes are representative of one intervention outcome for the population. On the other hand, if the individual effect sizes vary dramatically from the overall mean effect size, then the obtained homogeneity statistic will be large. Large observed values indicate significant heterogeneity among the obtained effect sizes. This finding indicates that we need to explore the relationship between study characteristics and intervention outcomes further.

Although tests of the homogeneity of obtained effect sizes in a research synthesis are useful, it is important to be cautious about accepting the absence of statistically significant heterogeneity as definitive. A test of homogeneity may not be powerful enough to identify real differences in intervention outcomes. Thus, tests of homogeneity signal one that there may be variation in intervention outcomes across studies rather than offer the conclusion that the obtained effect sizes are representative of one intervention outcome in the population. In other words, researchers should still explore the relationship between study characteristics and intervention outcomes when tests of homogeneity are statistically nonsignificant.

Finally, all of the standard inferential statistical methods, such as any of the correlational techniques (e.g., Pearson's product moment correlation, point-biserial, and multiple regression) and analysis of variance, are available to help researchers relate study characteristics to intervention outcomes (see Glass et al., 1981; Hedges & Vevea, 1998). For example, researchers conducting research syntheses often correlate study characteristics with intervention outcomes. Smith and Glass (1977) employed correlation methods to relate study characteristics to intervention outcomes in their groundbreaking meta-analysis of the effectiveness of psychotherapy. Although many of the obtained correlations between study characteristics were generally small, some were statistically significant, suggesting (1) a relationship between the intelligence of clients and intervention outcomes; (2) a relationship between the similarity of the therapist and clients in terms of ethnicity, age, and social level and intervention outcomes; (3) a relationship between the reactivity of the dependent measure and intervention outcomes; and (4) a relationship between the age of clients and intervention outcomes.

Reporting the Results

Reporting the results of a research synthesis parallels the process of doing so for primary research studies. Whether presenting the results of a narrative or quantitative review, or some combination of the two, researchers should follow the standard presentation formation for primary research studies: (1) introduction, (2) method, (3) results, and (4) discussion (see Chapter 16 for an in-depth description of these article sections). Additionally, it is critical that the research synthesis be thorough and clearly written. Journal editors indicate that they seek clarity in these syntheses with regard to the purpose and problem definition, thoroughness and clarity in the presentation of methods and findings, and clarity in the researcher's conclusions (Cooper, 2010; Creswell, 2009; Gall et al., 2007). Specifically, Coelho and LaForge (2000) state that research syntheses are typically evaluated by journal editors and reviewers on five criteria: (1) accuracy of information; (2) reasonableness of conclusions based on appropriate data analysis; (3) contribution that the manuscript offers to the field; (4) readability, grammar, and style; and (5) organization in terms of logic and standard format.

Introduction

The goal of the introduction is to set the research synthesis within the field of inquiry. The introduction typically begins by describing the broad scientific question that is being addressed and its importance within the field of inquiry. The introduction should also indicate why the research synthesis is needed (e.g., the first review of its kind, some unresolved controversy in the field, previous research syntheses included only a portion of the primary studies). It is important that researchers specify the problems addressed by research syntheses in detail. Finally, the introduction should indicate what critical research consumers will gain from the review and provide an overview of the research synthesis.

Method

The method section should describe the procedures to conduct the research synthesis in detail. Although the specific procedures may vary, method sections often include operational definitions of the concepts under review, a description of the literature search methods and scope, criteria for including and excluding primary studies, a description of the study characteristics and data gleaned from each of the primary studies, procedures for determining the accuracy of data collection methods (e.g., interrater agreement), and methods for determining the magnitude of the intervention effect and relating study characteristics to intervention outcomes. Additionally, if the specific procedures used in the research synthesis differ substantively from those published elsewhere, differences should be discussed in detail.

Results

The results section presents the findings of each aspect of the research synthesis. It typically begins with a description of the results of the synthesis (i.e., studies included in the research synthesis). Researchers sometimes include two lists of studies in the reference section. One list gives the primary studies used in the synthesis, and the second presents methodological or other articles referenced in the text. This format enables critical research consumers to identify primary studies included in the research synthesis with ease.

A results section should also include a description of relevant study characteristics such as experimental conditions, participants, and dependent measures that are relevant to the purpose of the research synthesis. Researchers often provide summary tables or graphical presentations of study characteristics to help critical research consumers better understand the primary studies included. The amount of information that researchers present regarding study characteristics may depend on the journal space that editors allow.

Finally, the results section should present a detailed description of the primary findings. The primary findings should also be tabled or presented in a graphic format. Researchers

sometimes include both primary study characteristics and results on the same table. However, depending on the complexity of the research synthesis, researchers sometimes present the findings separately from the study characteristics. The results should include a description of both the pooled intervention outcomes (i.e., average intervention outcome) and relationships between study characteristics and intervention outcomes.

Discussion

The discussion section should set the findings of the research synthesis within the context of the field of inquiry. Its focus should be related to the purpose of the review. For example, if the purpose is to assess the overall cost-effectiveness of a particular intervention, the discussion should focus on the economic impact of the intervention outcome. The discussion should clarify implications of findings regarding the relationship between study characteristics and intervention outcomes. Finally, the discussion should address implications of the findings for future research.

Analysis of Data

This section considers threats to the validity of research syntheses and errors associated with searching and selecting primary research studies, coding study characteristics, and drawing conclusions.

Threats to the Validity of Research Syntheses

Research syntheses rely heavily on the conceptual and interpretive skills of researchers. Although recent developments have reduced the scope of error and bias associated with the research synthesis, all approaches are subject to the fallibility of individuals conducting the review. Thus, it is critical that researchers and critical research consumers alike assess the validity of research syntheses, because they are the main sources of assessment relative to the accumulation of knowledge in a given field, impacting future research, policy, and practice. Research syntheses tend to have a greater impact on a field than does any one primary research study.

The validity of a research synthesis is dependent on the way it is conducted and disseminated. At three points in time in conducting a research synthesis, researchers can make errors that affect its validity: (1) searching and selecting primary research studies, (2) coding study characteristics, and (3) drawing conclusions. Hunter and Schmidt (2004) detail errors that researchers make at each of these points in time when conducting a research synthesis. Although it is difficult for critical research consumers to scrutinize research syntheses fully to ensure their validity, it is important to be aware that syntheses are *not* different than primary studies. They are also subject to error at every stage of their development and execution. Thus, researchers who conduct research syntheses need to avoid making these errors, and critical research consumers who use these syntheses should look closely to see whether these errors have been made.

Errors Associated with Searching and Selecting Primary Research Studies

There are two types of errors that researchers can make when searching and selecting primary research studies. The first centers on the exclusion of primary studies that fall within the declared scope of the review. The outcome of this error is that conclusions made by researchers conducting the research synthesis are not based on the entire defined field of inquiry. Inclusion of the missing primary research studies may contradict the findings of those studies based on them. This type of error should become less a problem as tools for conducting literature searches and developing bibliographies become more advanced. However, these advancements will not eliminate mistakes of researchers conducting research syntheses in the use of technologies.

The second type of error focuses on the failure of researchers to discriminate between good and poor research. Some researchers equally weight the findings from good and poor research. The outcome of this error is that conclusions are not balanced, because the findings from good and poor research are given equal status. Weighting the findings from good research more heavily than those from poor research may lead to conclusions that contradict those made if good and poor research are given equal status. Weighting the findings from good research more heavily is important, because not all research on the same phenomena is of equal quality.

Errors Associated with Coding Study Characteristics

The procedures used to code study characteristics is the second point in the review process at which errors can affect the validity of the research synthesis. This is the point at which the variety of errors made by researchers conducting the research synthesis is greatest (Hunter & Schmidt, 2004). It is critical that researchers use procedures to ensure the accuracy of their procedures for coding study characteristics. There are four types of errors that researchers can make at this point in the review process. The first type of error centers on the inaccurate coding or recording of the study characteristics, such as the sampling, methods, designs, procedures, and contexts of the primary research studies. For example, some researchers report the opening statement regarding sample size and fail to recognize that attrition occurred. Errors in the coding of study characteristics can lead to misclassification of primary research studies, so that they do not share essential characteristics that are supposed to make them comparable to other studies. Making studies comparable is critical, because one of the key aspects of conducting a research synthesis is to determine the relationship between study characteristics and intervention outcomes.

The second type of error focuses on double-counting the findings from one primary research study, which gives it more weight in the research synthesis. This type of error occurs in two ways. First, many primary research studies include more than one intervention outcome. As mentioned earlier, researchers typically eliminate this problem by computing an average intervention outcome for the study. However, researchers may not compute an average intervention outcome in all cases. Second, a primary research study can be included more than once in a research synthesis, because researchers often report the findings from a study several times. For example, it is not uncommon for researchers first to report the findings from a primary research study in a conference paper, prior to publishing it in a peer-reviewed journal. Researchers often make this mistake, because it is difficult to detect, especially when titles and lists of authors often change. Thus, it is critical that researchers and critical research consumers alike look closely to ensure that multiple reporting of primary studies is not included in a research synthesis.

The third type of error centers on the failure of researchers to detect the faulty conclusions of authors of primary research studies. Researchers do not always accurately or fully report the findings in their conclusions in primary research studies. Researchers conducting research syntheses risk continuing the misrepresentation of findings if they uncritically accept the conclusions of the authors of the primary research studies. The original authors, who may be biased to the extent of selectively incorporating only expected findings in their conclusions, may contribute to this error.

The final type of error focuses on the suppression of contrary findings. Primary research studies may contain findings that contradict conclusions supported by researchers conducting the research synthesis. This is not to say that the primary studies do not contain findings that support the conclusions of researchers conducting the research synthesis. Rather, the findings in the primary studies that contradict such conclusions may be suppressed or ignored.

Errors Associated with Drawing Conclusions

The conclusions drawn are the final point in the review process at which errors can affect the validity of the research synthesis. It is at this point in time that the errors detailed earlier fully impact the research synthesis. Errors made at this point are a function of those made at earlier stages. All of the previous errors affect the conclusions made by researchers. There is little question that valid conclusions cannot be made from inaccurate assessments of the primary studies or when the review excludes findings that are relevant to the phenomena under study.

WHEN SHOULD RESEARCHERS CONDUCT RESEARCH SYNTHESES?

Research syntheses are important in that they allow us to integrate large amounts of information. Recall from Chapter 1 that replications are critical to the scientific process. Research syntheses may allow us to combine the results of past investigations, many of which are replications. Questions referring to topics such as the effectiveness of certain types of instruction, limitations in our current knowledge level, or directions for future research may be answered with research syntheses. Finally, there are four instances in which one would wish to complete a research synthesis: (1) to establish causal relationships between variables; (2) to determine the degree of relationship between two variables; (3) to develop and confirm theories; and (4) to assess the extent to which the findings from research can be generalized to a larger set of participants, experimental procedures, and situations beyond those of the original research studies.

SUMMARY

❖ Research synthesis involves pulling together the facts and findings from a group of related studies based on different (1) theoretical frameworks, (2) independent variables, (3) dependent measures, (4) research designs, and (5) data analysis procedures.

❖ Research synthesis plays two key roles in the process of designing any new study: (1) to ensure that new research is a cumulative process rather than simply an exploratory one and (2) to enable researchers and other professionals, such as policymakers, to survey the literature to understand some phenomena more fully.

❖ Research syntheses integrate research findings for the following four purposes: (1) to establish cause-and-effect relationships; (2) to determine the degree of relationship between two variables; (3) to develop theories; and (4) to assess the external validity of findings.

❖ Unsystematic research syntheses tend to be less scientifically oriented; no formal guidelines are used to guide reviews, because (1) they are typically based on a restrictive sample of studies, and (2) researchers tend to rely heavily on their own judgment to guide the review. Such reviews are conducted not to create research generalizations but to articulate an author's particular position on an issue. Systematic research syntheses, on the other hand, parallel the methodologies used in original research studies. The procedures are much more systematic in nature and rely on a set of agreed-upon procedures and practices to review the literature. Although the procedures may vary, systematic research syntheses essentially include (1) the formulation of a research question or questions, (2) specification of the procedures used to select the research studies, (3) enumeration of the study characteristics examined, (4) a description of procedures used to analyze results of the research studies, and (5) neutral representation of the results.

❖ Overall, unsystematic and systematic research syntheses typically differ on only two characteristics: (1) the coverage of the research studies, and (2) the stance taken by the researchers.

❖ Planning and carrying out research syntheses require four considerations: (1) identifying primary sources, (2) identifying secondary sources, (3) overcoming selection biases, and (4) focusing the literature search.

❖ There are eight steps for planning and executing a research synthesis: (1) formulating a precise research question, (2) defining critical terms, (3) formulating a literature search framework, (4) searching the literature, (5) coding study characteristics, (6) determining the magnitude of intervention outcomes (e.g., statistical significance, vote counting, combining significance tests, effect size, parametric effect sizes, measures of overlapping data across conditions for single-case data), (7) relating study characteristics to intervention outcomes, and (8) reporting the results.

❖ There are three points in time in the process of conducting a research synthesis when researchers can make errors that affect its validity: (1) searching and selecting primary research studies, (2) coding study characteristics, and (3) drawing conclusions.

❖ Research syntheses may allow us to combine the results of past investigations, many of which are replications. Questions referring to topics such as the effectiveness of certain types of instruction, limitations in our current knowledge level, or directions for future research may be answered with research syntheses. There are four instances when we wish to complete a research synthesis: (1) to establish causal relationships between variables; (2) to determine the degree of relationship between two variables; (3) to develop and confirm theories; and (4) to assess the extent to which the findings from research can be generalized to a larger set of participants, experimental procedures, and situations, beyond those of the original research studies.

DISCUSSION QUESTIONS

1. What are the differences between systematic and unsystematic research syntheses?

2. Should more confidence be placed in a systematic research synthesis than in an unsystematic one? Why or why not?

3. What are the advantages and disadvantages of conducting a systematic as opposed to an unsystematic research synthesis?

4. What steps should we go through to conduct the research synthesis?

5. How would you come up with terms to use in searching the literature for a systematic research synthesis?

6. What are the differences between an exploratory research synthesis and a hypothesis-testing research synthesis? Explain.

7. What process should we use to conduct an exhaustive search of the literature? What is an advantage and a disadvantage of conducting an exhaustive search?

8. What is meant by the term *effect size*? In your answer, explain how an effect size is interpreted.

9. What are the issues related to single-case design studies when conducting a research

synthesis? Are there any good solutions to these issues?

10. What factors might affect the validity of the research synthesis? Describe each.

ILLUSTRATIVE EXAMPLE

Reading Comprehension Instruction for Students with Learning Disabilities, 1995–2006: A Meta-Analysis

Sheri Berkeley
University of Georgia, Athens, GA

Thomas E. Scruggs and Margo A. Mastropieri
George Mason University, Fairfax, VA

Abstract. *Meta-analysis procedures were employed to synthesize findings of research for improving reading comprehension of students with learning disabilities published in the decade following previous meta-analytic investigations. Forty studies, published between 1995 and 2006, were identified and coded. Nearly 2,000 students served as participants. Interventions were classified as fundamental reading skills instruction, text enhancements, and questioning/strategy instruction—including those that incorporated peer-mediated instruction and self-regulation. Mean weighted effect sizes were obtained for criterion-referenced measures: .69 for treatment effects, .69 for maintenance effects, and .75 for generalization effects. For norm-referenced tests, the mean effect size was .52 for treatment effects. These outcomes were somewhat lower than but generally consistent with those of previous meta-analyses in their conclusion that reading comprehension interventions have generally been very effective. Higher outcomes were noted for interventions that were implemented by researchers. Implications for practice and further research are discussed.*

Keywords. *reading comprehension, learning disabilities, meta-analysis*

A large part of academic learning occurs through reading. Reading is not only the ability of a student to accurately and fluently decode words but also the ability to gain meaning through the text that he or she reads (Sideridis, Mouzaki, Simos, & Protopapas, 2006). Although the goal of the reading process is to extract meaning from text, many factors can impede a student's reading comprehension, such as failure to strategically process information and appropriately use background knowledge while reading, lack of metacognitive awareness of learning, knowledge of vocabulary and common text structures (i.e., narrative text structure, expository text structure), poor reading fluency, and passive reading (Gersten, Fuchs, Williams, & Baker, 2001). These challenges are even more significant for students who have learning disabilities (LD) that further affect their acquisition of reading comprehension skills (e.g., Mastropieri, Scruggs, & Graetz, 2003).

Interest in reading comprehension instruction increased substantially after Delores Durkin (1978–1979) wrote about the need for appropriate reading comprehension instruction. Over the past few decades, a substantial number of research studies documenting the efficacy of various strategies for improving reading comprehension for students with LD have been published, as have extensive narrative reviews of this research (e.g., Gersten et al., 2001; Kim, Vaughn, Wanzek, & Wei, 2004; Mastropieri et al., 2003; Vaughn, Gersten, & Chard, 2000; Vaughn, Levy, Coleman, & Bos, 2002). For example, Gersten et al. (2001) described the effectiveness of different interventions when they were employed with various types of text (e.g., narrative vs. expository) and suggested that teaching students to self-regulate their learning was a strategy with potential for improving task persistence and improving reading comprehension. Kim et al. (2004) particularly focused on the effectiveness of graphic organizers in the context of reading comprehension, whereas Mastropieri et al. (2003) specifically focused on reading comprehension instruction for secondary students and paid particular attention to peer tutoring, spatial organization, and computer-assisted instruction. All previous reviews emphasized the overall effectiveness of reading comprehension instruction.

In addition to these narrative reviews, a number of comprehensive quantitative syntheses ("meta-analyses") of research on reading comprehension instruction for students with LD have been conducted. Talbott, Lloyd, and Tankersley (1994) conducted a meta-analysis of 48 relevant research studies (published between 1978 and 1992), using methods described by Glass, McGaw, and Smith (1981), and calculating mean difference effect sizes using the experimental-control mean difference, divided by the control group standard deviation. Differences among categories were evaluated using F ratios. Talbott et al. reported an overall effect size of 1.13 from 255 effect sizes calculated from 48 studies. Of the named interventions, cognitive-behavioral treatments (including self-questioning, self-monitoring, and self-recording) were associated with the descriptively highest effect sizes, followed in turn by "pre- or mid-reading" treatments (e.g., previews or story questions) and cognitive interventions (e.g., specific schema or rules, advance organizers, outlines). In addition, these authors concluded that mean effect sizes were higher for lower level comprehension measures, when researchers delivered the treatment, and when the treatment was compared to a no-treatment control condition.

Mastropieri, Scruggs, Bakken, and Whedon (1996) calculated 205 effect sizes from 68 studies (published between 1976 and 1995), using the procedures recommended by Glass et al. (1981; also see Mastropieri & Scruggs, 1997), and reported an overall standardized mean effect size of .98. Comparing outcomes descriptively, these authors reported that the largest effects were attributed to cognitive strategies (similar to the "cognitive-behavioral" category of Talbott et al., 1994), such as summarizing, activating background knowledge, self-monitoring, and self-questioning. Lower but still substantial effects were obtained for studies using text enhancements (similar to the "cognitive" category of Talbott et al., 1994), such as highlighting, illustrations, embedded questioning,

illustrations, followed finally by skills training and reinforcement (e.g., reinforcement, repeated readings, vocabulary instruction). Higher effects were also observed for criterion-referenced measures (i.e., curriculum or teacher- or researcher-developed comprehension measures) rather than norm-referenced tests and for treatments delivered by researchers rather than teachers (cf. Talbott et al., 1994).

Swanson and colleagues (Swanson, 1999; Swanson & Hoskyn, 2000; Swanson, Hoskyn, & Lee, 1999) conducted a large-scale meta-analysis of intervention research with students with LD in a variety of instructional domains, calculating 1,557 effect sizes from 180 studies, removing "outliers," and weighting each effect size by the reciprocal of the sampling variance (Hedges & Olkin, 1985), which had the effect of somewhat lowering mean effect sizes. Studies were not included if interventions were not implemented over a period of 3 days or more. Differences among categories were evaluated using homogeneity tests (Hedges & Olkin, 1985). Using these criteria, 175 effect sizes from 58 studies (reported between 1972 and 1997) were directly relevant to reading comprehension instruction and, with all effect sizes averaged within studies, yielded an overall weighted mean effect size of .72. Mean effect sizes were higher for treatments that employed combinations of direct instruction and strategy instruction and for treatments that employed criterion-referenced rather than norm-referenced measures. Effect sizes larger than .80 have been considered large (e.g., Cohen, 1988), and each of the above meta-analyses yielded overall mean effect sizes near to or above this standard, suggesting that reading comprehension instruction in general can have a substantial impact on student learning.

Overall, these three meta-analyses, covering very similar publication time periods but employing somewhat different methods, arrived at very similar conclusions: that is, that reading comprehension instruction was overall very effective and that structured cognitive strategies were associated with the highest effect sizes. There was also some agreement that researcher-delivered treatments and criterion-referenced, rather than norm-referenced, tests were associated with higher effect sizes. All three meta-analyses also agreed that length of treatment was not observed to be reliably associated with mean effect size. Although these three investigations arrived at very similar conclusions, there was some individual disagreement; for example, two studies observed no reliable differences among grade levels, whereas Talbott et al. (1994) reported higher effect sizes for senior high school students.

In a recent related research synthesis, Gajria, Jitendra, Sood, and Sacks (2007) summarized 29 research studies on improving comprehension of expository text by students with LD (reported between 1982 and 2004) and reported mean unweighted effect sizes of 1.06 for text enhancements, 1.64 for single comprehension strategies, and 2.11 for multiple comprehension strategies. Although these effect sizes were larger than those of previous research synthesis efforts, they are not directly comparable to the previous meta-analyses because the selection criteria were more restrictive in some areas (e.g., only studies involving expository text were selected) and broader in other areas (e.g., studies on text comprehension were included that would not have been classified as "reading comprehension" by standards of the previous meta-analyses). In addition, this investigation included only a relatively small number of reading comprehension studies conducted in the past decade. Gajria et al. compared their outcomes descriptively and concluded higher effect sizes were observed when participants had higher mean IQ scores, when interventions were implemented in special education classrooms, when materials were specifically designed for the study, and when researchers were the primary treatment delivery agents. Therefore, it can be concluded that there has been no comprehensive review exclusively targeting the reading comprehension literature published in recent years. This in part provides a justification for the present investigation.

The variation in overall obtained mean effect sizes from previous meta-analyses of reading comprehension, from 0.72 (Swanson, 1999) to 0.98 (Mastropieri, Scruggs, Bakken, et al., 1996) to 1.13 (Talbott et al., 1994), is no doubt because of a variety of factors, including differences in criteria and procedures for study selection; differences in procedures for coding, calculating, and analyzing effect sizes; and differences in procedures for data analysis of obtained outcomes. This observed variability underlines the importance of using comparable outcomes (i.e., effect sizes) as a guideline to, rather than a precise indicator of, overall treatment effectiveness. Cook and Leviton (1980) noted, "While qualitative reviews may be equally prone to bias, the descriptive accuracy of a point estimate in meta-analysis can have mischievous

consequences because of its apparent 'objectivity,' 'precision,' and 'scientism'" (p. 455). Keeping this caveat in mind, meta-analysis can be very informative regarding the value of different interventions and in fact has been very valuable in the past in discriminating effective from ineffective treatments throughout the history of special education (Forness, 2001).

The purpose of the present research synthesis was to determine whether reading comprehension instructional research conducted since the time of the earlier meta-analyses, or more specifically since the Mastropieri, Scruggs, Bakken, et al. (1996) investigation, has resulted in comparable outcomes. We were interested to know whether obtained effect sizes from more recent research are generally comparable to previous research and whether other differences would be observed, for example, differences in types of treatments. For this reason, intervention categories used a decade ago (i.e., Mastropieri, Scruggs, Bakken, et al., 1996) were replicated in the current meta-analysis.

METHOD

Search Procedures

The PsycINFO, ERIC, Expanded Academic, Social Sciences Citation Index, EBSCO, and Digital Dissertation online databases were used to locate studies using combinations of the following keywords: *reading disabilities, learning disabilities, reading comprehension*, and *strategies*. Ancestry searches were conducted of both identified studies as well as several other literature reviews concerning reading comprehension and students with LD (i.e., Gajria et al., 2007; Gersten et al., 2001; Kim et al., 2004; Mastropieri et al., 2003; Swanson, 1999; Vaughn et al., 2002; Vaughn, Gersten, et al., 2000). In addition, to ensure a thorough search, professional journals in the field of special education that commonly publish studies with LD participants were hand searched for additional relevant studies (e.g., *Exceptional Children, Learning Disabilities Research and Practice, Journal of Learning Disabilities, Learning Disability Quarterly, Journal of Special Education*, and *Remedial and Special Education*).

Criteria for Inclusion

Studies were included in this meta-analysis if (a) participants in the study were between kindergarten and Grade 12, (b) the intervention study was primarily designed to improve student reading comprehension and specified reading comprehension outcomes, and (c) data were disaggregated for students with disabilities. Studies were included when participants were specifically identified as having LD (students described as reading disabled or dyslexic were considered synonymous with LD for the purposes of this synthesis). In some cases, a small number of the participants were identified as "at risk" or with other high-incidence disabilities (e.g., Mastropieri et al., 2001); these studies were included when at least two thirds of the participants were identified as having LD. This was the case in 8 of the 40 studies. In an effort to be comprehensive, studies were included regardless of duration. Finally, studies were included if sufficient data were provided to calculate an effect size.

Studies were excluded if the study was published prior to 1995 or was written in a language other than English. Studies that primarily focused on characteristics of students with LD in the area of reading were also not included in this synthesis (e.g., Carr & Thompson, 1996; Jenkins, Fuchs, van de Broek, Espin, & Deno, 2003), nor were single-participant studies (e.g., Dowrick, Kim-Rupnow, & Power, 2006; Gardill & Jitendra, 1999) or master's theses (e.g., Heise, 2004) included.

Coding Instruments, Conventions, and Procedures

A coding instrument and coding conventions were developed for this review, including (a) study identification information (e.g., first author, publication outlet, year of publication), (b) characteristics of the sample (e.g., total number of special education students, percentage of male students, mean IQ, achievement description, mean age, grade level, school location), (c) description of interventions (e.g., treatment delivery, teacher type, type of training passages, time and duration of intervention, use of classroom peers, use of self-regulation components), (d) design features (e.g., study design, fidelity measure, intervention type), and (e) effect sizes (e.g., effect size category and relevant effect sizes and variances). Coding conditions were established for each variable. All coders, trained in coding procedures and conventions, regularly met to conduct reliability checking and discuss and resolve coding discrepancies. An initial reliability check, by two independent coders, of a randomly selected subset of reports representing 15% of the total number of studies yielded an initial reliability coefficient of .92. All discrepancies were resolved to 100% agreement.

Interventions on reading comprehension were classified into categories similar to those employed by Mastropieri, Scruggs, Bakken, et al. (1996): questioning/strategy instruction (classified as "self-questioning" in Mastropieri, Scruggs, Bakken, et al., 1996), text structure, fundamental reading skills (classified as "basic skills" in Mastropieri, Scruggs, Bakken, et al., 1996), and "other." Studies were categorized as questioning/strategy instruction if the primary purpose was to teach students strategies or involved direct questioning of students while reading or if the intervention was designed to assist students with becoming independent at self-questioning while reading. Interventions were categorized as text enhancements if the primary purpose of the intervention was to supplement or enhance the text to increase comprehension. Studies were considered to be fundamental reading skill interventions if they focused on training of basic skills (including, e.g., phonological awareness and/or phonics skills) and specifically assessed the impact of this training on reading comprehension. Interventions were classified as "other" if they could not be collapsed into one of the other categories.

Because different types of effect size measures can yield very different values, and to preserve the independence of data in the analyses (Hedges & Olkin, 1985), for each study, one effect size (the effect size that most closely represented the central purpose of the research) was calculated for the treatment effect for criterion-referenced measures (teacher or researcher developed), and one effect size was calculated for any norm-referenced tests. These categories were not combined in the final analysis. In addition, if studies included measures of generalization and/or maintenance, one effect size was computed for each. Again, these categories were not combined in the final analysis. Effect size calculations, employing Hedges's d statistic (Hedges & Olkin, 1985), were computed using a statistical software package (MetaWin; Rosenberg, Adams, & Gurevitch, 2000). However, in instances where information needed to be calculated by hand (e.g., when deriving from a reported F statistic), at least two coders calculated the effect size to ensure accuracy.

Where differences were observed for different levels of a given variable, homogeneity tests were computed using MetaWin (Rosenberg et al., 2000) to compare mean effect sizes when the comparison was appropriate and a sufficient number of cases was present. These tests employed the cumulative effect size, the calculation of which employs large-sample theory, which states that studies with larger sample sizes will be associated with lower variances and therefore provide more accurate estimates of the "true" population effect size. A weighted average was employed to estimate the cumulative effect size, where each effect size is weighted by the reciprocal of its sampling variance, $w_i = 1/v_i$ (Cooper, 1998; Hedges & Olkin, 1985; for relevant equations, see Rosenberg et al., 2000, pp. 22–23). This weighted cumulative effect size is reported for all subsequent analyses and presented in tables along with associated 95% confidence intervals (Thompson, 2006). Furthermore, cross-validation procedures were conducted to determine whether these differences were robust across levels of other significant variables or whether observed differences appeared to systematically vary with levels of another variable.

In the present meta-analysis, we employed procedures designed to maximize the validity of our outcomes. Concerned about the possible compromising effects of combining different numbers of effect sizes for different studies (i.e., that some studies would be inappropriately weighted differently than others), we wished to calculate only one effect size per study. However, we were also concerned that by combining criterion-referenced (e.g., teacher made) and norm-referenced measures (where effect sizes from norm-referenced measures are typically smaller), we would unfairly advantage studies that employed criterion-referenced measures. In addition, we anticipated that generalization and maintenance measures could be expected to vary in effectiveness and at any rate address different research questions, so we did not wish to combine these effects. Therefore, we calculated one effect size each, respectively, for criterion-referenced and norm-referenced measures and for treatment, maintenance, and generalization measures, and we evaluated the effects of each separately. Furthermore, rather than combining all possible effects in one mean effect size, we selected the outcome most closely related to the research question (e.g., score on story retells rather than consumer satisfaction); and we combined measures when there was more than one single appropriate effect size (e.g., story retells and comprehension questions). Therefore, for a given study, more than one multiple effect size may have been calculated,

but these were analyzed separately as (a) criterion-referenced treatment measures, (b) norm-referenced treatment measures, (c) criterion-referenced maintenance measures, (d) norm-referenced maintenance measures, or (e) criterion-referenced generalization measures (there were no norm-referenced generalization measures identified). For data analysis, we calculated weighted effect sizes with the Hedges d statistic and compared differences among categories of effects with homogeneity tests (Cooper, 1998; Hedges & Olkin, 1985). These techniques are generally thought to lead to more precise estimates of overall treatment effectiveness (Rosenberg et al., 2000). When differences were observed, we employed cross-validation procedures to determine whether observed differences were robust across levels of other, potentially compromising variables.

RESULTS

Overall Characteristics of the Data Set

The final sample consisted of 40 experiments from 40 studies published between 1995 and 2006. Studies were located in 16 publication outlets, including doctoral dissertations ($n = 10$) and professional journals ($n = 30$): *Journal of Learning Disabilities, Learning Disability Quarterly, Remedial and Special Education, Journal of Special Education, American Education Research Journal, Learning Disabilities Research and Practice, Exceptional Children, Annals of Dyslexia, Brain and Language, Exceptionality, Learning Disabilities: A Multidisciplinary Journal, Information Technology in Childhood Education Annual, Journal of Adolescent and Adult Literacy, Elementary School Journal*, and *Contemporary Educational Psychology*. The data set included 1,734 participants with a mean age in months of 150.50 ($SD = 26.35$). The average percentage of male students per study was 67.19% ($SD = 11.54$). Of the 40 studies, 25 reported the IQ of students; participants in these investigations had a mean IQ of 91.23 ($SD = 7.83$). Achievement scores from a variety of different measures were reported in 33 investigations (82.5%). These measures ranged from formal norm-referenced measures such as standard scores from the *Woodcock Reading Mastery Test* and grade equivalents on the *Gates–MacGinitie Reading Test* ($n = 25$) to criterion-referenced measures such as an informal reading inventory ($n = 3$) to more informal reports such as the number of years below grade level ($n = 5$). All studies included students with LD, although

8 also included a minority of other students (e.g., attention-deficit/hyperactivity disorder, remedial reading).

In all, 15 studies included elementary-age students, 18 included middle school students, 6 included high school students, and 1 included students in a residential facility for adjudicated youth. Treatments were delivered in large groups (42.5%), small groups (35.0%), and one-to-one settings (22.5%); one study did not clearly report the treatment setting. Interventions were delivered by researchers (40.0%; including authors of the study [28.0%], graduate students with LD certification and/or experience [10.0%], and a "trained researcher" [2.0%]), teachers (47.5%; including special education teachers [25.0%], general education teachers [10.0%], both [10.0%], and unspecified [7.5%]), technology (7.5%), tutors (2.5%), and parents (2.5%).

Interventions lasted a mean of 29.82 sessions (SD = 36.27), with a range of 1 to 155. On average, intervention sessions were 49.68 min in length, with a minimum of 20 min and a maximum of 140 min per session. Most studies utilized comparable amounts of instructional time in intervention and comparison conditions ($n = 22$); however, several studies utilized no comparison, a true control (no instruction), or differing amounts of instructional time ($n = 11$). In addition, several studies were unclear about the amount of time instruction occurred in the comparison condition ($n = 7$). Peers were used in interventions in 35% of investigations, and self-regulation components were included in 25% of investigations.

The most prevalent research design was experimental designs with random assignment of participants to condition (52.5%), followed by quasi-experimental designs with matching or nonrandom assignment (40.0%), and pre-post designs with the pretest as comparison (7.5%). Criterion-referenced tests were employed most frequently as the dependent measure (75.0%). Norm-referenced tests were employed in 37.5% of the studies. Maintenance was assessed in 17.5% of the studies using criterion-referenced measures, but with only one norm-referenced measure of maintenance. Generalization was assessed in 20.0% of studies, in all cases with criterion-referenced measures. The majority of research comparisons consisted of treatment versus an instructional control (65.0%), followed by alternate treatment comparison group (27.5%) and pretest measure (7.5%). Study descriptions of instructional control included true controls

with no instruction ($n = 7$), nonreading instruction including study skills and vocabulary instruction ($n = 2$), read-only controls with and without accompanying questions and/or repeated reading ($n = 6$), and "typical" classroom instruction ($n = 11$). Descriptions of "typical" classroom instruction ranged from very vague (e.g., "typical school based reading program" and "reading instruction in normal fashion") to fairly specific (e.g., "systematic reading instruction by regular special education teacher focusing on decoding and comprehension strategies" and "students reading silently from basal texts, followed by teacher-led, large group discussion").

Type of Effect Size

Weighted mean effect sizes ($N = 59$) were calculated separately for treatment, maintenance, and generalization effects and for norm-referenced versus criterion-referenced tests (because these typically yield effect sizes of different magnitude). Because research studies frequently reported more than one of these measures, analyzing these measures separately allowed us to evaluate their relative effects without sacrificing independence of individual observations. The overall weighted effect size, for criterion-referenced measures, was 0.69 for treatment effects, 0.69 for maintenance effects, and 0.75 for generalization effects (M = 0.70 across all criterion-referenced measures). For norm-referenced tests, the mean effect size was 0.52 for treatment effects. Only one instance of a maintenance norm-referenced test ($ES = 0.22$) and no instances of a generalization norm-referenced test were observed ($M = 0.50$ across all norm-referenced measures). These effect sizes, along with the number of samples and corresponding confidence intervals, are reported in Table 1.

TABLE 1. Hedges's d by Type of Effect

Type of Effect	n	ES_w	95% CI
Treatment CRT	29	0.69*	0.56 to 0.83
Maintenance CRT	7	0.69*	0.38 to 1.00
Generalization CRT	8	0.75*	0.47 to 1.03
Treatment NRT	14	0.52*	0.33 to 0.70
Maintenance NRT	1	0.22	—

Note. n of effect sizes = n of studies; ES_w = weighted effect size; CI = confidence interval; CRT = criterion-referenced test; NRT = norm-referenced test.

*Within-category (Q_w) statistical significance, $p < .05$.

Comparisons of Effect Sizes for Intervention Treatments

Across all effect types, 27 studies were categorized as questioning/strategy instruction (67.5%), 6 studies were categorized as text enhancements (15.0%), 5 studies were categorized as fundamental reading skills training (12.5%), and 2 studies were categorized as "other" (5.0%). Associated weighted mean effect sizes, along with the number of samples and corresponding confidence intervals, are reported in Table 2.

Questioning/Strategy Instruction

Interventions in this category included direct questioning of students while reading, teaching students comprehension strategies (including questioning strategies), and assisting students with becoming independent at self-questioning while reading. Some examples of teacher-directed questioning include elaborative interrogation where, in this case, students read passages about animals and were trained to ask themselves why certain facts (e.g., that camels have long eyelashes) may be true (Mastropieri, Scruggs, Hamilton, et al., 1996); a guided reading approach for identification of story themes (Williams, 1998); main idea strategy instruction with self-monitoring training where students assessed their ability to apply the main idea strategy (Jitendra, Hoppes, & Xin, 2000); peer-assisted learning strategies where peers question each other on the main topic, relevant information, and text summary (e.g., Saenz, Fuchs, & Fuchs, 2005); and text structure analysis, where students were trained to identify the type of text structure in paragraphs (*main idea*, with a summary idea and supporting statements; *list*, with information presented in a list format; and *order*, with listed information presented in a specific order) to facilitate comprehension (Bakken, Mastropieri, & Scruggs, 1997).

Text Enhancements

Examples of interventions in this category included in-text question placement with and without feedback (Peverly & Wood, 2001), graphic organizers designed for both narrative (Boyle, 1996) and expository text (DiCecco & Gleason, 2002), technology including hypermedia (MacArthur & Haynes, 1995), and video vocabulary instruction for text enhancement (Xin & Rieth, 2001).

Fundamental Reading Skills

These investigations utilized packaged intervention programs and had very low student to teacher ratios during implementation. The programs included (a) the Behavioral Reading Therapy Program (Burns & Kondrick, 1998), (b) the Failure Free Reading Program (Rankhorn, England, Collins, Lockavitch, & Algozzine, 1998), (c) the Auditory Discrimination in Depth Program (Torgesen et al., 2001), (d) Embedded Phonics (Torgesen et al., 2001), and (e) the Dyslexia Training Program (Oakland, Black, Stanford, Nussbaum, & Balise, 1998).

Other Interventions

These interventions included a schoolwide cooperative learning program (Stevens & Slavin, 1995)

TABLE 2. Hedges's *d* (Treatment Effects) by Type of Intervention and Treatment Delivery

	Criterion-Referenced Tests			Norm-Referenced Tests		
	n	ES_w	95% CI	n	ES_w	95% CI
Type of intervention						
Questioning/strategy instruction	22	0.75*	0.58 to 0.92	8	0.48	0.18 to 0.77
Text enhancements	6	0.62*	0.24 to 1.00	2	0.46	−2.98 to 3.90
Fundamental reading skills instruction	1	1.04	—	4	0.82	0.25 to 1.40
Other intervention	1	0.07	—	1	0.25	—
Treatment delivery						
Researchers	15	0.83*	0.62 to 1.04	4	0.52	−0.05 to 1.10
Teachers	12	0.56	0.33 to 0.79	7	0.51	0.23 to 0.78
Adult tutors	1	0.42	—	1	0.80	—
Technology	2	0.66	−2.90 to 4.72	2	0.32	−3.11 to 3.76

Note. n of effect sizes = n of studies; ES_w = weighted effect size; CI = confidence interval.
*Within-category (Q_w) statistical significance, $p < .05$.

and an evaluation of a program with multiple components (Project Read; Laub, 1997).

Outcomes

Type of measure, mean weighted effect sizes, and frequencies and confidence intervals associated with these interventions are reported in Table 2. For criterion-referenced measures, overall, the two interventions with the largest number of effect sizes—questioning/strategy instruction and text enhancements—were associated with mean weighted effect sizes that were moderate to large in magnitude. The effect for fundamental reading skills was large, and a small effect was noted for "other"; however, each of these latter outcomes was associated with only a single effect size and was therefore not included in the analysis. Overall, outcomes by intervention type were not statistically different according to a homogeneity test, $Q(1, N = 28) = 0.60$, $p = .71$. Significant heterogeneity was found within each of the questioning/strategy instruction and text enhancements categories, suggesting considerable variability was associated with each of these treatments.

On norm-referenced tests, mean outcomes were also similar, although lower overall as expected, and paralleled effect sizes from criterion-referenced measures, as shown in Table 2. Descriptively, highest effect sizes were associated with fundamental reading skills instruction, followed by questioning/strategy instruction, and text enhancements. These differences, however, were not statistically significant according to a homogeneity test, $Q(2, N = 14) = 2.71$, $p = .40$. Neither were significant differences observed within any of the treatment categories. Outcomes on criterion-referenced measures for generalization ($M = 0.75$) and maintenance effects ($M = 0.69$) were associated with too few cases of text enhancement or fundamental reading skills treatments for statistical comparisons to be made. However, it was interesting to note that mean effect sizes for these measures were very similar to treatment effects.

Extreme Cases

Extreme cases (studies very high or very low effect sizes) were closely examined in an attempt to explain the variability within specific categories. In the questioning/strategy instruction category, five studies were associated with very high effect sizes (> 2): Bakken et al. (1997), Jitendra et al. (2000),

Miranda, Villaescusa, and Vidal-Abarca (1997), Williams (1998), and Esser (2001). All of these studies included teaching students to ask and answer questions about the main idea and all but Williams (1998) included some form of self-monitoring. In addition, both Miranda et al. (1997) and Esser (2001) included attribution retraining components. Only one text enhancement study was associated with a very high effect size: Peverly and Wood (2001).

Three questioning/strategy instruction studies (Johnson, Graham, & Harris, 1997; Klingner & Vaughn, 1996; Vaughn, Chard, Bryant, Coleman, & Kouzekanani, 2000) and one fundamental reading skills study (Rabren, Darch, & Eaves, 1999) were associated with negative effect sizes. Johnson et al. (1997) had negative effect sizes both immediately following treatment and on a generalization measure; however, because of the comparison involved with this study, this outcome may be misleading. The purpose of this investigation was to investigate additional benefits of adding explicit self-regulation procedures (goal setting and/or self-instruction) to story grammar strategy taught using a self-regulated strategy development instructional model. Although all students benefited from strategy instruction, differential benefits were not found for the additional self-regulation procedures investigated. Findings from the Klingner and Vaughn (1996) study also may be misleading because of the nature of the comparisons. The purpose of this study was to investigate outcomes of reciprocal teaching in different peer arrangements (cross-age tutoring and cooperative learning). Like the Johnson et al. study, students improved after the intervention, but an advantage was not found between instructional conditions with varying peer tutoring arrangements. A study conducted by Vaughn, Chard, et al. (2000) also resulted in negative effect sizes. This study incorporated peer tutors using collaborative strategic reading (CSR). The intervention was implemented by general education classroom teachers, and the researchers indicated that a limitation of the study was that CSR was a more complex intervention than the comparison condition and took considerably longer for teachers to teach students and integrate into reading practice. In addition, the sample in this study included students whose fluency was far below grade level and therefore may have benefited to a lesser degree from the complex reading comprehension strategies taught. Finally, two questioning/strategy instruction studies (Abdulaziz, 1999; Mastropieri, Scruggs, Hamilton, et al., 1996) and one "other" study (Laub, 1997) were associated with small effect sizes (< 0.2). Both of these questioning/strategy instruction studies investigated elaborative interrogation for improving reading comprehension.

Comparisons of Effect Sizes for Instructional Variables

Delivery Agent

Outcomes were evaluated for differences among treatment delivery agents (e.g., researcher, adult tutor, teacher) and are presented in Table 2. For criterion-referenced measures of treatment effects, the mean effect size for researchers (0.83) was higher than the mean effect size for teachers (0.56). Although these differences fell slightly short of statistical significance, $Q(1, N = 26) = 3.64$, $p = .056$, cross-validation procedures revealed that the effect of delivery agent was quite robust across levels of other study categories and explained much of the observed differences in other comparisons, as described in the following sections. Substantial heterogeneity was found within researcher-delivered treatments, however, indicating considerable variability within this category. Statistical differences by treatment delivery agents were not observed for norm-referenced measures of treatment effects ($p = .92$).

Grade Level

As seen in Table 3, mean treatment effects for criterion-referenced measures for middle and high school students (0.80) were larger than mean

effects for elementary school students (0.52). These means were statistically different according to a homogeneity test, $Q(1, N = 30) = 4.07$, $p = .04$. Similar significant differences were also observed for maintenance, $Q(1, N = 7) = 22.03$, $p < .01$, and generalization measures, $Q(1, N = 8) = 24.59$, $p < .01$, although in these latter two cases the total number of studies was limited. Significant heterogeneity was found within many of these categories. In any case, cross-validation procedures revealed that the apparent difference in mean effect size by grade level was not a reliable effect and could be explained by the influence of researcher-delivered treatments in different grade levels. Grade-level effects were not observed when collapsed across different levels of delivery agents. Neither were grade-level differences significant for norm-referenced tests ($p = .68$).

Setting

Outcomes were evaluated for differences among different types of setting (one to one, small group, classrooms) and are presented in Table 4. Differences among weighted means by setting were statistically different for criterion-referenced treatment measures, $Q(2, N = 30) = 10.53$, $p < .01$ (although significant heterogeneity was observed within categories) but not for norm-referenced tests ($p = .93$). Differences among settings types, when observed, could be explained by the differential presence of positive researcher-delivered treatments in the small group category; teacher-delivered treatments did not vary appreciably by setting.

TABLE 3. Hedges's *d* by Grade Level and Type of Measure

	Criterion-Referenced Tests			Norm-Referenced Tests		
	n	ES_w	95% CI	*n*	ES_w	95% CI
Treatment measures						
Elementary	9	0.52*	0.26 to 0.77	7	0.55	0.25 to 0.86
Middle or high	21	0.80	0.62 to 0.98	8	0.48	0.20 to 0.77
Maintenance measures						
Elementary	4	0.26*	−0.23 to 0.76	1	0.22	—
Middle or high	3	1.53*	0.58 to 2.47	—	—	—
Generalization measures						
Elementary	2	−0.34	−3.52 to 2.84	—	—	—
Middle or high	6	1.07	0.72 to 1.42	—	—	—

Note. n of effect sizes = *n* of studies; ES_w = weighted effect size; CI = confidence interval.
*Within-category (Q_w) statistical significance, $p < .05$.

TABLE 4. Hedges's *d* (Treatment CRT) by Setting, Passage Type, Duration, and Design

	Criterion-Referenced Tests			Norm-Referenced Tests		
	n	ES_w	95% CI	*n*	ES_w	95% CI
Setting						
One to one	6	0.50*	0.09 to 0.91	4	0.53	−0.15 to 1.21
Small group	12	1.00*	0.75 to 1.26	5	0.58	0.14 to 1.03
Classroom	12	0.55	0.34 to 0.77	6	0.48	0.17 to 0.78
Passage type						
Narrative	7	0.62*	0.30 to 0.94	4	0.88	0.36 to 1.40
Expository	15	0.71*	0.50 to 0.92	7	0.32	−0.02 to 0.65
Both	6	1.00	0.57 to 1.43	2	0.72	−2.45 to 3.50
Unknown	2	0.26	−2.61 to 3.14	2	0.28	−2.27 to 2.82
Treatment duration						
Short (< 1 week)	7	0.48*	0.13 to 0.82	—	—	—
Medium (> 1 week and < 1 month)	20	0.84*	0.66 to 1.03	7	0.49	0.14 to 0.84
Long (> 1 month)	3	0.50	−0.17 to 1.17	8	0.53	0.27 to 0.79
Study design						
Experimental	20	0.90*	0.71 to 1.09	5	0.38	−0.10 to 0.86
Quasi-experimental	9	0.46	0.22 to 0.70	8	0.45	0.18 to 0.72
Pre–post	1	0.27	—	2	0.98	−1.74 to 3.69

Note. n of effect sizes = *n* of studies; ES_w = weighted effect size; CI = confidence interval; CRT = criterion-referenced test.
*Within-category (Q_w) statistical significance, *p* < .05.

Type of Passage

Weighted mean effect sizes by type of passage are presented in Table 4. Weighted means associated with passage types approached but did not attain statistical significance for criterion-referenced measures, $Q(3, N = 30) = 7.25$, $p = .07$; however, expository text was associated with lower mean effect sizes than other measures on norm-referenced tests, $Q(3, N = 15) = 9.08$, $p = .03$. Within-category heterogeneity was not significant for any individual group. However, these effects were inconsistent across delivery agents and contained limited numbers of observations.

Duration of Treatment

Mean weighted effect sizes for criterion-referenced measures and norm-referenced tests by treatment duration are reported in Table 4. For criterion-referenced measures, mean weighted treatment effect sizes were highest for treatments of medium duration (more than 1 week but less than 1 month). Differences among treatments of varying length were statistically different according to a homogeneity test, $Q(2, N = 30) = 6.68$, $p = .04$. However, differences on norm-referenced tests by study duration

were not statistically significant ($p = .83$). That treatments of moderate length were associated with higher effect sizes than either shorter or longer treatments is not easily explained; however, cross-validation procedures indicated that this finding was robust across levels of other variables, including delivery agent and setting. Because researchers were not intervention agents in any longer-term treatments, however, it is possible that this variable played some role in the observed outcomes.

Other Variables

Correlations were calculated between criterion-referenced treatment effect sizes and other study variables. It was found that weighted effect size was not significantly correlated with the percentage of male participants in the sample or the mean reported sample IQ (*p* values > .34). Comparisons were also made between studies that included only students with LD and a smaller number of studies that also included a minority of students who were not characterized as having LD. The average mean treatment effect size for criterion-referenced measures for studies including only students with LD ($M_{es} = 0.63$, $n = 24$) was smaller than the average effect size for studies that also included a minority of students (in any case, no more than one third) without LD ($M_{es} = 0.88$, $n = 6$), although this difference was not significant according to a homogeneity test, $Q(1, N = 30) = 2.56$, $p = .11$. Examination of these outcomes by delivery agent revealed that descriptive differences were associated with differential effectiveness of researcher-implemented treatments in the studies that included mixed samples.

Comparisons of Effect Sizes Related to Study Quality

Study Design

Table 4 displays mean weighted effect sizes by study design. For criterion-referenced tests, studies with experimental (i.e., randomized) designs were associated with higher effect sizes than studies with quasi-experimental designs. Differences among study designs were found to be statistically different according to a homogeneity test, $Q(1, N = 29) = 9.94$, $p < .01$. This observed outcome appeared to be the consequence of disproportional numbers of researcher-delivered experimental treatments, with higher than average effect sizes in these investigations. No significant difference on norm-referenced tests was observed between experimental designs and quasi-experimental designs ($p = .75$), which were associated with smaller numbers of observations and larger confidence intervals. The small number of pre-post designs ($n = 3$) were associated with a descriptively lower than average effect size for experimental measures and higher than average effect sizes for norm-referenced measures. However, none of these studies were extreme cases ($ES = 0.27$, $ES = 0.98$, $ES = 0.97$).

Fidelity of Implementation

Studies were coded for reported treatment fidelity measures. For criterion-referenced treatment measures and norm-referenced treatment measures, comparisons between weighted means for studies reporting and not reporting fidelity of treatment measures were not statistically significant (p values = .70 and .87, respectively).

Use of Classroom Peers

Many studies that investigated questioning/strategy instruction also included peer mediation or self-regulation components. Peer tutoring is designed to increase academic engagement and ownership of learning by students (Mastropieri, Scruggs, & Berkeley, 2007). Several of these peer tutoring interventions incorporated components of questioning/strategy instruction (e.g., activating prior knowledge, making predictions, summarizing, identifying main ideas, clarifying, questioning, and analyzing text structure). These studies were also classified as questioning/strategy instruction. Examples include (a) peer-assisted learning strategies (Calhoon, 2005; D. Fuchs, Fuchs, Mathes, & Simmons, 1997; L. S. Fuchs, Fuchs, & Kazdan, 1999; Saenz et al., 2005), (b) CSR (Bryant et al., 2000; Vaughn, Chard, et al., 2000), (c) the Text Content and Structure Program (Lovett et al., 1996), (d) reciprocal teaching (e.g., Klingner & Vaughn, 1996), and (e) classwide peer tutoring (Mastropieri et al., 2001).

Effects for use of classroom peers are presented in Table 5 for criterion-referenced and norm-referenced treatment measures. The weighted mean treatment effect size from criterion-referenced measures in studies employing classroom peers was only slightly smaller than the mean weighted effect size from studies not employing classroom peers. These differences were not statistically significant according to a homogeneity test, $Q(1, N = 30) = 0.20$, $p = .65$. Significant heterogeneity was observed among outcomes of treatments that did not include peer mediation. On norm-referenced measures, the weighted mean treatment effect size for studies employing peers was also descriptively smaller than that for studies not employing peers, although these differences also were not statistically significant, $Q(1, N = 14) = 0.53$, $p = .47$.

Self-Regulation

Several studies also included some type of self-regulation component. Examples include (a) self-regulated strategy development combined with story grammar marker for narrative text (Johnson et al., 1997), (b) attribution retraining combined with a combination of questioning strategies (Manset-Williamson & Nelson, 2005; Miranda et al., 1997), (c) self-regulation strategies combined with reading comprehension strategies (Manset-Williamson & Nelson, 2005), (d) self-regulation and the "RAP" strategy (Katims & Harris, 1997), and (e) self-monitoring combined with a main idea strategy (Jitendra et al., 2000).

Table 5 displays mean weighted effect sizes, with associated frequencies and confidence intervals,

TABLE 5. Hedges's *d* (Treatment Effects) by Peer Mediation and Self-Regulation Components

	Criterion-Referenced Tests			Norm-Referenced Tests		
	n	ES_w	95% CI	*n*	ES_w	95% CI
Peer mediation component						
Yes	10	0.65	0.39 to 0.91	6	0.45	0.12 to 0.78
No	20	0.72*	0.54 to 0.89	9	0.58	0.30 to 0.85
Self-regulation component						
Yes	8	0.92*	0.59 to 1.26	3	0.54	−1.29 to 2.37
No	22	0.62*	0.46 to 0.78	10	0.34	−0.08 to 0.76

Note. n of effect sizes = *n* of studies; ES_w = weighted effect size; CI = confidence interval.
*Within-category (Q_w) statistical significance, $p < .05$.

for studies incorporating and not incorporating a self-regulation feature. As can be seen, studies incorporating a self-regulation feature were associated with higher weighted mean effect sizes than were those that did not incorporate self-regulation. These differences approached, but did not reach, statistical significance according to a homogeneity test, $Q(1, N = 30) = 3.52$, $p = .06$. The mean for the self-regulation effects was lowered somewhat by the treatment outcome of a study by Johnson et al. (1997), which did not employ a true control condition (all conditions received strategy instruction) and in which the gain for students receiving strategy instruction plus instruction in self-instruction and goal setting was negative compared to students receiving strategy instruction alone. The effect for goal setting and self-instruction was positive for a generalization measure in this same investigation. However, overall only two studies assessed generalization effects for treatments involving self-regulation, and the difference between these and generalization effects for treatments that did not involve self-regulation was not significant ($p = .79$).

DISCUSSION

The overall findings of this investigation are that interventions on reading comprehension were generally very effective, for both criterion-referenced measures ($M_{es} = 0.70$) and norm-referenced tests ($M_{es} = 0.52$). The overall mean effect size, for both types of measures across treatment, maintenance, and generalization outcomes, was 0.65, a figure most similar to that (0.72) reported by Swanson (1999) for reading comprehension intervention studies reported between 1972 and 1997. Overall effect sizes reported by Talbott et al. (1994), and Mastropieri, Scruggs, Bakken, et al. (1996) were

larger (1.13 and 0.98, respectively) but nonetheless also revealed the overall effectiveness of reading comprehension interventions. Although the present results are based on different investigations reported since the previous meta-analyses, one reason the present outcomes most closely resemble those reported by Swanson may be that some similar procedures were employed, for example, in employing only one effect size per study for analysis (although we computed these separately for different outcomes) and using weighted effect sizes, which in these investigations had the effect of generally lowering effect size values. Furthermore, the Talbott et al. metaanalysis included effect sizes as large as 15.1 standard deviation units, which may have inflated the overall obtained mean to some extent.

The general conclusion that can be drawn from the present investigation is that an additional decade of research has demonstrated the continuing effectiveness of a wide variety of reading comprehension interventions, including fundamental reading instruction, text enhancements, and questioning/strategy instruction. In response to a possible concern that these generally positive findings represent a kind of "dodo bird verdict," where "everybody has won and all must have a prize" (Carroll, 1865/1995, p. 33; see Parloff, 1984; Rosenzweig, 1936; Swanson & Sachse-Lee, 2000), it should be considered that meta-analytic techniques have also underscored the ineffectiveness of many other types of special education interventions, including perceptual training ($M_{es} = 0.08$), diet interventions ($M_{es} = 0.12$), and modality training ($M_{es} = 0.14$; Forness, 2001).

The present investigation also supported previous findings that structured cognitive strategies were very effective; however, in the present investigation these effects were not greater than other types of intervention, such as text enhancements (cf. Mastropieri, Scruggs, Bakken, et al., 1996). Furthermore, a variety of additional study characteristics, such as peer mediation and self-regulation, although useful in individual studies, did not exert a differential effect on overall study outcomes.

Large confidence intervals reveal variability within the data set. In many cases this had to do with the effectiveness of the control condition, not necessarily the fact that the intervention was not effective. Variability is commonly observed in meta-analysis, and it may be because of a number of factors. For example, another previously reported finding supported by the present investigation is that interventions implemented by researchers resulted in reliably higher effect sizes than interventions implemented by teachers or other school personnel. This finding, reported in previous meta-analyses (Gajria et al., 2007; Mastropieri, Scruggs, Bakken, et al., 1996; Talbott et al., 1994; also see Mastropieri, Scruggs, Berkeley, & Graetz, in press), was seen to be robust across a variety of potentially compromising variables, such as setting, design, and grade level. Although the precise reasons for this outcome are not known for certain, one possibility is that researchers implemented treatments with more precision and intensity, not necessarily because they were better teachers but rather because they were more familiar with the particular strategy in question and how it should best be implemented. If this explanation is true, it suggests that, with additional training and perhaps more "ownership" of the instruction by teachers, these strategies could be even more effective.

The influence of this "intervention agent" variable also explained several of the other statistically "significant" findings. That is, the observed differences among different levels of variables such as grade level, passage type, duration of treatment, study design, and inclusion of small numbers of students without LD could be explained at least to some extent by the presence of differential numbers of researcher-implemented treatments within different levels of other variables. Although significant heterogeneity was also observed within researcher-delivered interventions, the overall effect was apparently sufficiently robust to have influenced these other variables. In general, it could be stated that statistical significance testing was less useful than cross-validation procedures in identifying important variables in this investigation. Further complicating statistical significance testing was the fact that comparisons were

underpowered as a consequence of small sample sizes.

In addition to the similarities, differences were observed in the type of investigations that were reported over the past decade. In the present set of research reports, we observed proportionally more norm-referenced measures; more whole class and general education classroom (and fewer individually administered) interventions; more teacher-implemented, rather than researcher-implemented, treatments; fewer behavioral treatments; and more peer-mediated interventions than those identified in previous meta-analyses. Thus, it appears that more recent research on reading comprehension has moved into larger, whole class settings, implemented more often by teachers and classroom peers, and has nevertheless documented overall effective outcomes.

IMPLICATIONS FOR RESEARCH TO PRACTICE

The results of the present meta-analysis, taken together with the results of previous synthesis efforts on the same topic, now including approximately 100 independent investigations, suggest that a variety of interventions are very effective in improving reading comprehension of students with LD; on criterion-referenced and norm-referenced measures; including cognitive strategies, text enhancements, and behavioral treatments; in a variety of classroom settings; and across different treatment durations. These substantial effect sizes suggest that, compared to traditional instruction, reading comprehension can be greatly improved by the application of these treatments.

Although the types of treatments in these investigations varied considerably, most had in common an effort to teach students to *attend more carefully* or to *think more systematically* about text as it was being read. This was true to some extent whether the treatment involved basic reading skills training; whether it involved highlighting, outlining, illustrating, and spatial or semantic feature organization of text; or whether students were asked to summarize text, predict outcomes, provide main ideas, analyze text structure, or provide explanations for provided information. Particularly given the commonly observed failures of students with LD to spontaneously employ such strategies (e.g., Scruggs, Bennion, & Lifson, 1985), the greatest overall implication is that systematically employing virtually any or all of these techniques is very likely to improve students' ability to construct meaning from text.

Unfortunately, observational studies suggest that very little specialized strategy instruction is presently taking place, particularly in general education settings, even when special education teachers are present. Scruggs, Mastropieri, and McDuffie (2007) recently summarized qualitative studies of coteaching practice and concluded that systematic, strategic instruction intended to improve learning of academic skills or content was observed only infrequently in these inclusive settings. Empirically validated strategies, however effective in research studies, are of little use if they are not systematically implemented in a variety of classroom settings.

Future research could provide more evidence on the effects of longer term implementations of reading comprehension instruction on norm-referenced measures of reading and the effectiveness of combinations of these treatments. Researchers also could investigate the reasons behind the observed "researcher-implementation" effect by studying this variable directly or noting in teacher implementation studies any observed barriers to systematic implementation. Finally, because these interventions are apparently infrequently implemented in inclusive environments, future research could address why strategy instruction is not commonly implemented in general education classrooms and what steps could be taken to improve current practice. At present, however, it does appear that the knowledge exists for greatly improving reading comprehension skills of students with LD.

DECLARATION OF CONFLICTING INTERESTS

The authors declared no potential conflicts of interest with respect to the authorship and/or publication of this article.

FINANCIAL DISCLOSURE/FUNDING

The authors received no financial support for the research and/or authorship of this article.

REFERENCES

References marked with an asterisk indicate studies included in the meta-analysis.

*Abdulaziz, T. M. (1999). The role of elaborative interrogation in acquiring knowledge from expository prose passages for students with learning and behavior disorders. *Dissertation Abstracts International, 61*(01A), 132. (UMI No. 9957697)

*Bakken, J. P., Mastropieri, M. A., & Scruggs, T. E. (1997). Reading comprehension of expository science materials and students with learning disabilities: A comparison of strategies. *Journal of Special Education, 31*, 300–325.

*Boyle, J. R. (1996). The effects of cognitive mapping strategy of the literal and inferential comprehension of students with mild disabilities. *Learning Disability Quarterly, 12*, 86–99.

*Boyle, J. R. (2000). The effects of a Venn diagram strategy on the literal, inferential, and relational comprehension of students with mild disabilities. *Learning Disabilities: A Multidisciplinary Journal, 10*, 5–13.

*Bryant, D. P., Vaughn, S., Linan-Thompson, S., Ugel, N., Hamff, A., & Hougen, M. (2000). Reading outcomes for students with and without reading disabilities in general education middle-school content area classes. *Learning Disability Quarterly, 23*, 238–252.

*Burns, G. L., & Kondrick, P. A. (1998). Psychological behaviorism's reading therapy program: Parents as reading therapists for their children's reading disability. *Journal of Learning Disabilities, 31*, 278–285.

*Calhoon, M. B. (2005). Effects of a peer-mediated phonological skill and reading comprehension program on reading skill acquisition for middle school students with reading disabilities. *Journal of Learning Disabilities, 38*, 424–433.

Carr, S. C., & Thompson, B. (1996). The effects of prior knowledge and schema activation strategies on the inferential reading comprehension of children with and without learning disabilities. *Learning Disability Quarterly, 19*, 48–61.

Carroll, L. (1995). *Alice's adventures in wonderland.* London: Anness. (Original work published 1865)

Cohen, J. (1988). *Statistical power analysis for the behavioral sciences* (2nd ed.). New York: Academic Press.

*Conklin, J. T. (2000). The effect of presentation media on student reading comprehension. *Dissertation Abstracts International, 61*(09A), 3512. (UMI No. 9988426)

Cook, T. D., & Leviton, L. C. (1980). Reviewing the literature: A comparison of traditional methods with meta-analysis. *Journal of Personality, 4*, 449–472.

Cooper, H. (1998). *Synthesizing research: A guide for literature reviews* (3rd ed.). Thousand Oaks, CA: Sage.

*DiCecco, V. M., & Gleason, M. M. (2002). Using graphic organizers to attain relational knowledge from expository text. *Journal of Learning Disabilities, 35*, 306–320.

Dowrick, P. W., Kim-Rupnow, W. S., & Power, T. J. (2006). Video feedforward for reading. *Journal of Special Education, 39*, 194–207.

Durkin, D. (1978–1979). What classroom observations reveal about reading comprehension instruction. *Reading Research Quarterly, 15*, 481–553.

*Esser, M. M. S. (2001). The effects of metacognitive strategy training and attribution retraining on reading comprehension in African-American students with learning disabilities. *Dissertation Abstracts International, 67*(7-A), 2340. (UMI No. 3021672)

*Fagella-Luby, M. (2006). Embedded learning strategy instruction: Story-structure pedagogy in secondary classes for diverse learners. *Dissertation Abstracts International, 67*(2-A), 516. (UMI No. 3207952)

Forness, S. R. (2001). Special education and related services: What have we learned from meta-analysis? *Exceptionality, 9*, 185–197.

*Fuchs, D., Fuchs, L. S., Mathes, P. G., & Simmons, D. C. (1997). Peer-assisted learning strategies: Making classrooms more responsive to diversity. *American Educational Research Journal, 34*, 174–206.

*Fuchs, L. S., Fuchs, D., & Kazdan, S. (1999). Effects of peer-assisted learning strategies on high school students with serious reading problems. *Remedial and Special Education, 20*, 309–318.

Gajria, M., Jitendra, A. K., Sood, S., & Sacks, G. (2007). Improving comprehension of expository text in students with LD: A research synthesis. *Journal of Learning Disabilities, 40*, 210–225.

Gardill, M. C., & Jitendra, A. K. (1999). Advanced story map instruction: Effects on the reading comprehension of students with learning disabilities. *Journal of Special Education, 33*, 2–17, 28.

Gersten, R., Fuchs, L. S., Williams, J. P., & Baker, S. (2001). Teaching reading comprehension strategies to students with learning disabilities: A review of research. *Review of Educational Research, 71*, 279–321.

Glass, G. V., McGaw, B., & Smith, M. L. (1981). *Meta-analysis in social research.* Beverly Hills, CA: Sage.

Hedges, L., & Olkin, I. (1985). *Statistical methods for meta-analysis.* New York: Academic.

Heise, K. (2004). The effects of the Read Naturally program on fluency, accuracy, comprehension, and student motivation in students with learning disabilities. *Masters Abstracts International, 42*(06), 1957. (UMI No. 1419865)

Jenkins, J. R., Fuchs, L. S., van de Broek, P., Espin, C., & Deno, S. L. (2003). Accuracy and fluency in list and context reading of skilled and RD groups: Absolute and relative performance levels. *Learning Disabilities Research and Practice, 18*, 237–245.

*Jitendra, A. K., Hoppes, M. K., & Xin, Y. P. (2000). Enhancing main idea comprehension for students with learning problems: The role of a summarization strategy and self-monitoring instruction. *Journal of Special Education, 34*, 127–139.

*Johnson, L., Graham, S., & Harris, K. R. (1997). The effects of goal setting and self-instructions on learning a reading comprehension strategy: A study with students with learning disabilities. *Journal of Learning Disabilities, 30*, 80–91.

*Katims, D. S., & Harris, S. (1997). Improving the reading comprehension of middle school students in inclusive classrooms. *Journal of Adolescent and Adult Literacy, 41*, 116–123.

*Kim, A. (2002). Effects of computer-assisted collaborative strategic reading on reading comprehension for high-school students with learning disabilities.

Dissertation Abstracts International, 64(11A), 4009. (UMI No. 3110632)

*Kim, A., Vaughn, S., Klingner, J. K., Woodruff, A. L., Reutebuch, C. K., & Kouzekanani, K. (2006). Improving the reading comprehension of middle school students with disabilities through computer-assisted collaborative strategic reading. *Remedial and Special Education, 27*, 235–249.

Kim, A., Vaughn, S., Wanzek, J., & Wei, S. (2004). Graphic organizers and their effects on the reading comprehension of students with LD: A syntheses of research. *Journal of Learning Disabilities, 37*, 105–118.

*Klingner, J. K., & Vaughn, S. (1996). Reciprocal teaching of reading comprehension strategies for students with learning disabilities who use English as a second language. *Elementary School Journal, 96*, 275–293.

*Laub, C. M. (1997). Effectiveness of Project Read on word attack skills and comprehension for third and fourth grade students with learning disabilities. *Dissertation Abstracts International, 36*(01), 0036. (UMI No. 1386289)

*Lovett, M. W., Borden, S. L., Warren-Chaplin, P. M., Lacerenza, L., DeLuca, L., & Giovinazzo, R. (1996). Text comprehension training for disabled readers: An evaluation of reciprocal teaching and text analysis training programs. *Brain and Language, 54*, 447–480.

*MacArthur, C. A., & Haynes, J. B. (1995). Student Assistant for Learning from Text (SALT): A hypermedia reading aid. *Journal of Learning Disabilities, 28*, 150–159.

*Manset-Williamson, G., & Nelson, J. M. (2005). Balanced, strategic reading instruction for upper-elementary and middle school students with reading disabilities: A comparative study of two approaches. *Learning Disability Quarterly, 28*, 59–74.

Mastropieri, M. A., & Scruggs, T. E. (1997). Best practices in promoting reading comprehension in students with learning disabilities. *Remedial and Special Education, 18*, 197–213.

Mastropieri, M. A., Scruggs, T. E., Bakken, J. P., & Whedon, C. (1996). Reading comprehension: A synthesis of research in learning disabilities. In T. E. Scruggs & M. A. Mastropieri (Eds.), *Advances in learning and behavioral disabilities: Intervention research* (Vol. 10, pt. B, pp. 201–227). Oxford, UK: Elsevier.

Mastropieri, M. A., Scruggs, T. E., & Berkeley, S. (2007). Peers helping peers. *Educational Leadership, 64*(5), 54–58.

Mastropieri, M. A., Scruggs, T. E., Berkeley, S., & Graetz, J. (in press). Does special education improve learning of secondary content? A meta-analysis. *Remedial and Special Education.*

Mastropieri, M. A., Scruggs, T. E., & Graetz, J. E. (2003). Reading comprehension instruction for secondary students: Challenges for struggling students and teachers. *Learning Disability Quarterly, 26*, 103–116.

*Mastropieri, M. A., Scruggs, T. E., Hamilton, S. L., Wolfe, S., Whedon, C., & Canevaro, A. (1996). Promoting thinking skills of students with learning disabilities: Effects on recall and comprehension of expository prose. *Exceptionality, 6*, 1–11.

*Mastropieri, M. A., Scruggs, T. E., Mohler, L., Beranek,

M., Boon, R., Spencer, V., et al. (2001). Can middle school students with serious reading difficulties help each other and learn anything? *Learning Disabilities Research and Practice, 16,* 18–27.

*Miranda, A., Villaescusa, M. I., & Vidal-Abarca, E. (1997). Is attribution retraining necessary? Use of self-regulation procedures for enhancing the reading comprehension strategies of children with learning disabilities. *Journal of Learning Disabilities, 30,* 503–512.

*Mothus, T. G. (1997). The effects of strategy instruction on the reading comprehension achievement of junior secondary school students. *Dissertation Abstracts International, 42*(01), 44. (UMI No. 766434601)

*Newbern, S. L. (1998). The effects of instructional settings on the efficacy of strategy instruction for students with learning disabilities. *Dissertation Abstracts International, 59*(05A), 1527. (UMI No. 9832950)

*Oakland, T., Black, J. L., Stanford, G., Nussbaum, N. L., & Balise, R. R. (1998). An evaluation of the dyslexia training program: A multisensory method for promoting reading in students with reading disabilities. *Journal of Learning Disabilities, 31,* 140–147.

Parloff, M. B. (1984). Psychotherapy research and its incredible credibility crisis. *Clinical Psychology Review, 4,* 95–109.

*Peverly, S. T., & Wood, R. (2001). The effects of adjunct questions and feedback on improving the reading comprehension skills of learning-disabled adolescents. *Contemporary Educational Psychology, 26,* 25–43.

*Rabren, K., Darch, C., & Eaves, R. C. (1999). The differential effects of two systematic reading comprehension approaches with students with learning disabilities. *Journal of Learning Disabilities, 32,* 36–47.

*Rankhorn, B., England, G., Collins, S. M., Lockavitch, J. F., & Algozzine, B. (1998). Effects of the failure free reading program on students with severe reading disabilities. *Journal of Learning Disabilities, 31,* 307–312.

*Rooney, J. (1997). The effects of story grammar strategy training on the story comprehension, self-efficacy and attributions of learning disabled students. *Dissertation Abstracts International, 58*(5-A), 1642. (UMI No. 9732965)

Rosenberg, M. S., Adams, D. C., & Gurevitch, J. (2000). *MetaWin: Statistical software for meta-analysis.* Sunderland, MA: Sinauer Associates.

Rosenzweig, S. (1936). Some implicit common factors in diverse methods of psychotherapy. *American Journal of Orthopsychiatry, 6,* 412–415.

*Saenz, L. M., Fuchs, L. S., & Fuchs, D. (2005). Peer-assisted learning strategies for English language learners with learning disabilities. *Exceptional Children, 71,* 231–247.

Scruggs, T. E., Bennion, K., & Lifson, S. (1985). Learning disabled students' spontaneous use of test-taking skills on reading achievement tests. *Learning Disability Quarterly, 8,* 205–210.

Scruggs, T. E., Mastropieri, M. A., & McDuffie, K. A. (2007). Coteaching in inclusive classrooms: A metasynthesis of qualitative research. *Exceptional Children, 73,* 392–416.

Sideridis, G. D., Mouzaki, A., Simos, P., & Protopapas, A.

(2006). Classification of students with reading comprehension difficulties: The roles of motivation, affect, and psychopathology. *Learning Disability Quarterly, 29,* 159–180.

*Stevens, R. J., & Slavin, R. E. (1995). The cooperative elementary school: Effect on student achievement and social relations. *American Educational Research Journal, 32,* 321–351.

Swanson, H. L. (1999). Reading research for students with LD: A meta-analysis of intervention outcomes. *Journal of Learning Disabilities, 32,* 504–532.

Swanson, H. L., & Hoskyn, M. (2000). Intervention research for students with learning disabilities: A comprehensive meta-analysis of group design studies. In T. E. Scruggs & M. A. Mastropieri (Eds.), *Advances in learning and behavioral disabilities: Vol. 14. Educational interventions* (pp. 1–153). Oxford, UK: Elsevier.

Swanson, H. L., Hoskyn, M., & Lee, C. (1999). *Interventions for students with learning disabilities: A meta-analysis of treatment outcomes.* New York: Guilford.

Swanson, H. L., & Sachse-Lee, C. (2000). A meta-analysis of single-subject research for students with LD. *Journal of Learning Disabilities, 33,* 114–136.

Talbott, E., Lloyd, J. W., & Tankersley, M. (1994). Effects of reading comprehension interventions for students with learning disabilities. *Learning Disability Quarterly, 17,* 223–232.

Thompson, B. (2006). Research synthesis: Effect sizes. In J. Green, G. Camilli, & P. B. Elmore (Eds.), *Handbook of complementary methods in education research* (pp. 583–603). Washington, DC: American Educational Research Association.

*Torgesen, J. K., Alexander, A. W., Wagner, R. K., Rashotte, C. A., Voeller, K. K. S., & Conway, T. (2001). Intensive remedial instruction for children with severe reading disabilities: Immediate and long-term outcomes from two instructional approaches. *Journal of Learning Disabilities, 34,* 33–58.

*Ugel, N. S. (1999). The effects of a multicomponent reading intervention on the reading achievement of middle school students with reading disabilities. *Dissertation Abstracts International, 61*(01A), 118. (UMI No. 9959597)

*Vaughn, S., Chard, D. J., Bryant, D. P., Coleman, M., & Kouzekanani, K. (2000). Fluency and comprehension interventions for third-grade students. *Remedial and Special Education, 21,* 325–335.

Vaughn, S., Gersten, R., & Chard, J. D. (2000). The underlying message in LD intervention research: Findings from research synthesis. *Exceptional Children, 67,* 99–114.

Vaughn, S., Levy, S., Coleman, M., & Bos, C. S. (2002). Reading instruction for students with LD and EBD: A synthesis of observation studies. *Journal of Special Education, 36,* 2–13.

*Williams, J. P. (1998). Improving the comprehension of disabled readers. *Annals of Dyslexia, 48,* 213–238.

*Xin, J. F., & Rieth, H. (2001). Video-assisted vocabulary instruction for elementary school students with learning disabilities. *Information Technology in Childhood Education Annual, 1,* 87–103.

ABOUT THE AUTHORS

Sheri Berkeley, PhD, was an assistant professor in the Department of Communication Sciences and Special Education at the University of Georgia in Athens, GA, at the time of writing. She is now an assistant professor in the College of Education and Human Development, George Mason University in Fairfax, VA.

Thomas E. Scruggs, PhD, is university professor and director of the PhD in education program, College of Education and Human Development, George Mason University in Fairfax, VA.

Margo A. Mastropieri, PhD, is university professor, College of Education and Human Development, George Mason University in Fairfax, VA.

From Berkeley, S., Scruggs, T. E., & Mastropieri, M. A. (2010). Reading comprehension instruction for student with learning disabilities, 1995–2006: A meta-analysis. *Remedial and Special Education, 31*, 423–436. Copyright 2010 by the Hammill Institute on Disabilities. Reprinted by permission of SAGE.

ILLUSTRATIVE EXAMPLE QUESTIONS

1. What is the purpose of the research synthesis?
2. What descriptors were used by the authors? In your response, indicate what types of studies were reviewed.
3. What study characteristics did the authors extract from the primary studies?
4. What was the average effect size obtained?
5. What did the authors conclude about the effects of reading comprehension?
6. How did authors address the issue of mixed quality across studies?
7. To what population of individuals would you be willing/able to generalize the results of this review of the literature? Explain.
8. Given the variation in studies reviewed, what is your impression of the authors' conclusions?
9. What threats to the validity of this review of the literature should concern critical research consumers?
10. Although your review of one study is insufficient, what is your opinion of the meta-analysis technique? State reasons for your opinion.

ADDITIONAL RESEARCH EXAMPLES

1. D'Agostino, J. V., & Powers, S. J. (2009). Predicting teacher performance with test scores and grade point average: A meta-analysis. *American Educational Research Journal, 46*, 146–182.

2. Jeynes, W. H. (2005). A meta-analysis of the relation of parental involvement to urban elementary school student academic achievement. *Urban Education, 40*, 237–269.

3. Rakes, C. R., Valentine, J. C., McGatha, M. B., & Ronau, R. N. (2010). Methods of instructional improvement in algebra: A systematic review and meta-analysis. *Review of Educational Research, 80*, 372–400.

PART VII

.....

Action Research

CHAPTER 16

■ ■ ■ ■

Action Research

Moving from Critical Research Consumer to Researcher

OBJECTIVES

After studying this chapter, you should be able to . . .

1. Explain the advantage of a practitioner conducting his/her own research.
2. Define the term *action research*.
3. Describe the characteristics of action research.
4. Illustrate how quantitative methods are used in action research.
5. Outline how qualitative methods are used in action research.
6. Characterize how single-case methods are used in action research.
7. Depict how survey, historical, and program evaluation methods are used in action research.
8. Explain the ethical principles and codes of conduct for research.
9. Describe how one writes a research article.
10. Specify how articles are submitted for publication.
11. Characterize how one should conduct action research.

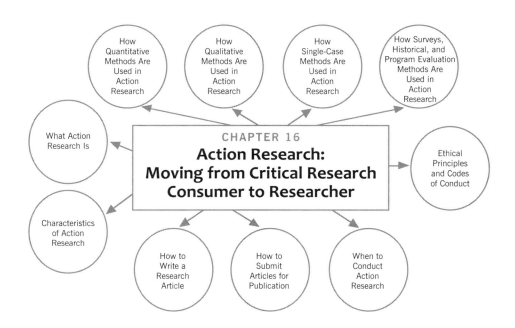

OVERVIEW

Throughout this text, we have described procedures that directly impact researchers and critical research consumers alike. The focus has been on what researchers do and why. Our goal has been to help you become aware of the complexities of research in such a way as to aid you in becoming a critical research consumer. But researchers are not the only ones capable of conducting research. When you become a critical research consumer, you can also begin to produce research. Thus, we now turn our attention to making critical research consumers the actual researchers.

Becoming a researcher is not easy for many direct care providers because of the sheer amount of time needed to conduct, write, and publish research findings. Many individuals see this as more of a burden than a benefit. However, the question to address is what type of research is a critical research consumer capable of doing given the constraints of his/her particular situation?

We have to keep in mind that research informs practice. A practitioner who conducts research may be in a central position to improve practice. So questions emerge. What are the necessary skills needed to conduct, write, and publish findings when critical research consumers are immersed in providing direct services to others? What must teachers, psychologists, and other care providers do to show that what they are doing is actually working?

This chapter describes the practice of action research. Action research is usually associated with qualitative methods; however, we believe this is shortsighted. Teachers, psychologists, and other professionals use other research methods in an applied setting as well. Part of conducting any type of research is a concern with research ethics. Thus, research ethics is discussed later in the chapter. Additionally, if teachers, psychologists, and other professionals are interested in publishing the results of their action research, they should possess some understanding of the publication process. This chapter covers how to write an action research article and how to go about getting it published. Finally, an illustrative action research investigation is presented at the end of the chapter for critique.

Research Examples

Consider these issues. Think about how you would design research to address the questions/hypotheses from these research examples:

- Research Example 1: How do researchers design action research to identify variables accounting for underachievement of male students in elementary, middle, and high schools?
- Research Example 2: How do researchers design action research to decrease disruptive behaviors of a 12-year-old in the classroom?

These research questions are answered later in the chapter.

WHAT IS ACTION RESEARCH?

According to Stringer (2007), **action research** is "a systematic approach to investigation that enables people to find effective solutions to problems they confront in their everyday lives" (p. 1). Action research has gained popularity in the last few years but has been around for some 50 years (Stringer, 2007). Elden and Chisholm (1993) indicate that Kurt Lewin introduced the term "action research" in 1946, which Lewin described as "a way of generating knowledge about a social system while, at the same time, attempting to change it" (p. 121). Action research may be conducted by a person in a particular situation or by persons who have a major role in the design and implementation of the investigation in that setting.

For example, if research were conducted in the classroom, a teacher would be acting as the researcher. Action research could also involve the teacher helping a researcher design and conduct the investigation. In other words, the participants of action research can be involved in the research process *with* researchers. Additionally, professionals can collaborate to conduct action research, such as when several teachers from a school district get together, discuss, and actually pursue action research questions of interest (Stringer, 2007). This collaborative effort is different from having a researcher come into the classroom and take data, without the help of the teacher. As described by Elden and Chisholm (1993):

> Lewin (1946) and most subsequent researchers have conceived of AR [action research] as a cyclical inquiry process that involves diagnosing a problem situation, planning action steps, and implementing and evaluating outcomes. Evaluation leads to diagnosing the situation anew based on learnings from the previous activities cycle. A distinctive feature of AR is that the research process is carried out in collaboration with those who experience the problem or their representatives. The main idea is that action research uses a scientific approach to study important organizational or social problems with the people who experience them. (p. 124)

Thus, when individuals plan for the collection of data, actually collect the data, and then evaluate or analyze the data to improve their situation, they are conducting action research.

Action research should also contain data that are collected frequently throughout the experimental period (e.g., grading period). For example, suppose a teacher were concerned with the effectiveness of her approach to teaching spelling in the third grade. The teacher could use her method of instruction as the independent variable and the percentage of words spelled correctly as the dependent measure. She could then track students' acquisition of spelling words throughout the semester. If the students' spelling skills improve, the teacher is more confident in her instructional approach. If the student performance does not improve greatly, she knows this during the grading period and can adjust to her instructional approach. *Data-based decision making* is another term that has been used for this practice in fields such as special education and rehabilitation: that is, we make changes in how we teach (instruction) based on how our students are doing (assessment).

Although action research may contribute to our understanding of a phenomenon, its sole purpose is not to control for threats to internal or external validity. The purpose of action research is primarily to determine what is occurring in a particular setting, how it affects participants and/or professionals, and why it occurs. The level of internal validity is usually limited, because the level of experimental control necessary to control for all threats to internal validity may not be possible. In addition, information on the external validity of a single investigation is also limited, because the variables to be taken into consideration (different participants, different teachers, different dependent variables/measures) are not controllable. The focus is on the particular context in which the research takes place.

Dimensions of Action Research

The five dimensions of action research (Chisholm & Elden, 1993) include (1) the complexity of the system levels (from last complex and restricted to the particular group under study to most complex across societies); (2) the level of organization in the system (from loosely organized, with unclear values and unclear goals, to tightly organized, with clarity of roles and shared values); (3) the openness of the research process (from open, in which the action research process is discovered, to closed, in which the action research is predetermined); (4) the intended outcomes of the research (from basic, in which there is a change in the key parameters within the system, to complex, in which there is a change in the existing parameters of an organization); and (5) the role of the researcher (from collaboratively managed, in which the researcher and system members make decisions together to researcher-dominated, in which the researcher is in control of the project).

Thus, it is difficult to determine exactly what does and does not constitute "pure" action research. The important consideration is that action research investigations are not all the same, and they vary in important ways. For example, quantitative, qualitative, single-case, survey, historical, and program evaluation research methods can all be used in action research.

Action research *involves application of the scientific method to everyday problems in the classroom or other applied settings; personnel are involved directly with the implementation of the research.*

WHAT ARE THE CHARACTERISTICS OF ACTION RESEARCH?

There are five characteristics of action research (see Figure 16.1): (1) purposes and value choice, (2) contextual focus, (3) change-based data and sense making, (4) participation in the research process, and (5) knowledge diffusion (Elden & Chisholm, 1993). However, all of these characteristics must be present for an investigation to be considered action research. The extent to which each characteristic is present across investigations will vary.

Purposes and Value Choice

"Action research adds solving problems to the scientific enterprise. It rejects the idea that science is completely value free" (Elden & Chisholm, 1993, p. 126). Thus, the primary goal of action research is to solve problems in real-life situations. Also, action research indicates that persons conducting the research usually have something at stake in the outcomes of that research. In action research, teachers' obvious stake is to have their students learn what they need to function effectively in society. Additionally, teachers have an involvement with their students that prevents them from remaining totally objective and separated. However, this situation can be seen as an advantage. When we realize that our values can and do affect how we see the world, we can take these values into consideration when interpreting research results. This realization is important for teachers and practitioners. Perhaps more important than anything else, action research can help practitioners understand their values and how these values affect what they are doing.

Contextual Focus

Action research is also context-bound: It occurs in the real world and addresses real-life problems or situations. The problems or situations to be addressed in action research are defined by those who are already a part of the context, such as classroom teachers. Action researchers set out to solve a problem or to answer a research question, then attempt to fit the solution or answer within a theory. This sequence of events is the reverse of much of quantitative research, in which theory is developed first and research is an attempt to verify predictions based on the theory. The ultimate outcome of action research is the process through which the action researcher must go to obtain a solution. The gathering of data allows action researchers to learn more about their settings, students/participants, and themselves.

Change-Based Data and Sense Making

The data collected in action research are obtained in a systematic fashion, similar to that of researchers conducting field research. The goal for action researchers is to generate the data, then make interpretations, with the ultimate goal of making changes in their practice. Thus, the manner in which the data are collected must be logical and follow accepted methods of data gathering. For example, if action researchers are using qualitative methods, triangulation should be obtained. After the data are collected, action researchers should relate the findings to a theory or theories, in much the same manner as conventional qualitative researchers. The data gathered by action researchers and their conclusions based on the data can be as legitimate as those of other researchers.

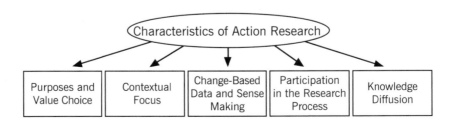

FIGURE 16.1. The five characteristics of action research.

Participation in the Research Process

In action research, the researcher(s) are participants in the process. Action researchers are part of the context being investigated; thus, they are also being investigated. Unlike other research, action research may involve investigation of one's self in a wider context. For example, if a classroom teacher uses a qualitative research method to investigate how students react to new classroom rules, she should measure her own responses to the changes in the rules as well. Additionally, since the teacher probably developed the rules with the help of her students, her action of setting up the new rules is under investigation. Thus, the teacher is determining how her actions affect others in the classroom context.

Knowledge Diffusion

A final characteristic of action research is that solutions to problems through the use of action research are disseminated in some manner. Dissemination of information obtained from action research occurs on a continuum. At one end, dissemination occurs when action researchers inform other teachers and/or staff of what was found. At the other end, action researchers determine how the problem and solution add to current knowledge and theory. Once this is done, action researchers write up the results for publication (this process is discussed later in this chapter). Somewhere in between, action researchers can present the findings at local, regional, or national meetings. The point here is that action research is typically disseminated in some way once the information has been gained and the solution to a problem has been found.

HOW ARE QUANTITATIVE METHODS USED IN ACTION RESEARCH?

The use of quantitative research designs is not as common in action research as in other research approaches, since much of quantitative research does not necessarily incorporate all of the characteristics outlined earlier. Quantitative research methods usually require at least two groups of participants (e.g., two classrooms). It is possible

for two or more teachers to get together, design a quantitative research investigation, and compare their respective classrooms, but this is not likely. Action research is usually conducted by one teacher in one classroom.

Teachers are also not likely to develop formal research hypotheses and approach the phenomenon in a deductive manner. Teachers are more likely to ask questions such as "I wonder what would happen if . . . ?" or "I wonder how effective this procedure is?" It is also unlikely that most teachers and practitioners have the degree of information about educational and psychological theories that is normally required to develop a hypothesis.

A final difficulty for teachers using quantitative research in the classroom is the need for ongoing data collection or assessment throughout the experimental period. Quantitative research requires, at a minimum, a posttest or a set of pretest–posttest assessments. Unfortunately, a research design that calls for only posttest or pretest–posttest assessments does not provide the necessary information to teachers. If teachers and practitioners conduct action research, they are doing so to improve their own performance and/or the performance of the students they serve. For example, if teachers have access to only one assessment or measure after the grading period, it is too late to help their students. Ongoing assessments aid teachers in making needed adjustments throughout the grading period.

Quantitative research methods are not commonly used in action research. Yet they can provide comparative information because, in some cases, large groups of individuals can be studied and compared.

HOW ARE QUALITATIVE METHODS USED IN ACTION RESEARCH?

Qualitative methods seem to be ideally suited to action research. Qualitative research occurs in a natural context and requires ongoing or at least frequent contact with participants. There is no need for qualitative research to be driven by some preconceived hypothesis, so experimental conditions do not need to be established. Action researchers are able to generate a great deal of information about the individuals they serve and make decisions as time passes. They are not restricted to a single dependent variable; thus, action researchers can take into consideration a greater variety of variables than can quantitative researchers.

Those who wish to conduct action research using qualitative designs can be somewhat flexible in how they approach the research. Action researchers should have an idea of what they research. Many times, the research is conducted to solve problems such as classroom disruptions. At other times, action research is conducted to find out how students like to be instructed. Once a reason for collecting data has been identified, action researchers should determine how the data are to be collected.

For example, in the classroom environment, an ethnographic-type approach, albeit on a much smaller scale, is acceptable. The teacher is part of the classroom culture. Participant observations can be conducted, and the teacher can collect field notes in the form of journal entries throughout the day or at the end of the day. The teacher can also use interviews to gain more specific information from specific students. Interviews with students who are especially open and honest can be extremely valuable. In order to gain triangulation, the teacher can ask both the students and others in the setting, such as paraprofessionals or peer tutors, to make daily journal entries. Over a period of time, the information obtained by the teacher can aid in the improved classroom management and/or the learning situation.

The main advantage of qualitative research methods in action research is that the action researcher is already a part of the culture to be studied. The disruptions to daily activities are minimal, since an outsider is not required. Additionally, the information gained allows action researchers to reflect on critical variables in their environment. A potential problem in qualitative research is the large amount of effort it takes to gather and assess the obtained data. Action researchers should have considerable skill in qualitative methods. Additionally, action researchers must be cautioned against making cause-and-effect claims using qualitative methods. Although action researchers may believe or hypothesize that one variable is responsible

for another, the type of experimental rigor required to make such statements is difficult to achieve in such an applied context. In order to make cause-and-effect statements, additional constraints must be placed on those conducting the research and on participants. The following research example illustrates an action research investigation using both quantitative and qualitative data.

Recall the research question about male underachievement posed earlier in this chapter? Read on to see how your design compares to how the actual study was designed.

Research Example 1: Action Research with Qualitative and Quantitative Methods

Action research involving both quantitative and qualitative methods examined male underachievement in elementary, middle, and high schools (Clark, Lee, Goodman, & Yacco, 2008). Research has documented that some male students lag far behind female students, earning lower grades and dropping out of school at higher rates (e.g., Clark, Oakley, & Adams, 2006). Students in one particular school district were split evenly according to gender. Ethnic composition of students included about 50% European American, 37.2% African American, 5.2% Hispanic, 3.5% Asian American, and 4% other. In this study, quantitative data were obtained from school records to document disparities between male and female students. In elementary, middle, and high schools, males were more likely than females to have 15-plus unexcused absences, discipline referrals, and referrals to special education. In middle and high schools, males were more likely to have lower GPAs. Qualitative data were obtained to account for the documented differences in males and females. Researchers conducted semistructured interviews with five school-level teachers, five school counselors, and five administrators. Qualitative themes were coded, and revealed that interviewees perceived that boys had underdeveloped organizational skills, did not carry daily planners, rarely turned in homework, appeared more influenced by media (especially sports-related media), and lacked adult role models at school and at home. Interviewees provided recommendations for teachers, counselors, and administrators (e.g., provide hands-on, kinesthetic experiential activities in classroom lessons; focus on positive reinforcement and respect to motivate male students to stay in school; set high academic expectations).

HOW ARE SINGLE-CASE METHODS USED IN ACTION RESEARCH?

Although action research is considered by many to be the domain of qualitative methods, single-case research methods are also well-suited to applied settings. For example, teachers and practitioners can use single-case research methods to determine the effectiveness of both behavior management procedures and skills development programs. However, they should be careful when determining the type of design to use. The most basic design (i.e., A-B) can easily assess a program. But, as you know, researchers are unable to determine causal effects using an A-B design. Action researchers will most likely not use the A-B-A design, which is limited in terms of ethical concerns (see Chapter 11), as well as practical problems (i.e., returning to baseline levels). Action researchers who use an experimental single-case design to determine a cause-and-effect relationship will most likely use a multiple-baseline design. Remember, single-case designs do not require single subjects but single entities. These single entities can contain several individuals, such as a group of students. Other usable designs include the changing-criterion design and the alternating treatments design. For example, the alternating treatments design can be used to compare two or more skills development or behavior management programs directly.

In order to use single-case designs, action researchers must plan ahead. The independent and dependent variables must be determined and defined. The measures must be designed and checked for interobserver agreement by some other person in the setting, such as a peer tutor, student, therapist, or instructional aide. Finally, data must be gathered on an ongoing basis.

There are several advantages of using single-case research methods in action research. First, data-based decisions can be made on an ongoing basis. Second, cause-and-effect relationships can be determined with most of the research methods. Finally, experimental control can be achieved with a small number of students.

A disadvantage of the single-case approach is that one or a small number of dependent variables is typically included. Other important information may be overlooked when action researchers focus on a single dependent variable. What could and probably should occur is to combine single-case methods with qualitative methods. Action researchers can collect not only objective data in a single-case fashion but also qualitative data through interviews and participant observations, as long as the qualitative methods are conducted throughout the baseline and intervention conditions.

The following research example illustrates the use of action research incorporating single-case methodology. Additionally, qualitative information has been gathered to assess the impact of the program on classroom personnel.

Recall the research question posed earlier in this chapter about a 12-year-old with disruptive behavior? Read on to see how your design compares to how the actual study was designed.

Research Example 2: Action Research with Single-Case Methods

The study by Martella et al. (1993) is an example of action research using a single-case design. This study was previously described as a single-case, multiple-baseline design across settings (with changing criteria) research example in Chapter 13. In that investigation, a student teacher in a classroom was involved with a 12-year-old student who had mild intellectual disability and a high level of disruptive behaviors. The classroom teacher and the student teacher developed the intervention package with the help of the other researchers. The classroom staff implemented the self-monitoring program, collected the data, and were involved in the interpretation of the results. In the self-monitoring activity, the student kept track of his negative statements, while staff independently recorded the same behaviors. The student and staff compared their counts of negative behaviors at the end of certain periods. Low counts of negative behaviors and agreement with staff on the number of counts resulted in the student accessing privileges. The results demonstrated that the student's disruptive behaviors (i.e., negative statements) decreased when the self-monitoring program was implemented. The teacher and the student teacher reported an improved classroom environment, and the student began to interact with other students more appropriately. Other students became more accepting of the target student. Martella and colleagues concluded that the self-monitoring program aided in improving the classroom environment for all students.

HOW ARE SURVEY, HISTORICAL, AND PROGRAM EVALUATION METHODS USED IN ACTION RESEARCH?

The following research methods are not typically considered types of action research; however, we describe how teachers and practitioners can use each method when conducting action research.

Survey Research

Teachers and practitioners can use surveys when they want to learn important information about students or parents that cannot be obtained in another fashion. For example, suppose a teacher wanted to determine parents' levels of satisfaction with the social and/or academic progress of their children. Constructing a simple open-ended survey would allow parents to describe areas of satisfaction and those in need of improvement. Another example might involve a secondary teacher whose students with impairments are about to make the transition into employment situations. He may need to survey potential employers to prepare his students better for future employment situations. Finally, school counselors could distribute surveys to recruiters at a number of colleges and universities to determine the expectations for college entrance. Thus, surveys could provide valuable information from sources that are critical in the lives of students. Also, publication of this information would help to inform other professionals in the field.

Historical Research

Teachers and practitioners may use historical research when attempting to determine the best way to approach the education of certain students. For example, detailed information is kept in files for students with special needs as part of their individualized educational programs. Once this information is obtained from historical search, more informed plans for the educational future of these students can be made. Teachers may also wish to determine why a particular form of instruction is used today. Many educational practices seem to come and go in a cyclical pattern. Reading instruction is an example. A teacher may want to determine how students learned to read in the past and compare those methods with the reading methods used today. This information can aid the teacher in understanding why she is expected to teach or facilitate reading in a certain manner.

Program Evaluation

We have all experienced program evaluations to some extent. The emphasis on standardized tests to measure the cognitive and intellectual achievement of students is an example of this. These standardized tests are measures of how the educational system is meeting the expectations of the community. Many action research investigations are a type of program evaluation but on a much smaller scale. For example, a teacher sets out to determine whether his academic program is working as intended by looking at test scores; talking with students, parents, and other teachers; and observing students during academic and social activities. In this way, he is evaluating his program. Reflective teaching is essentially an activity in program evaluation, though not usually as formal. Thus, program evaluations are used on an ongoing basis by teachers and practitioners who want to improve the academic, social, and behavioral performance of their students.

WHAT ARE THE ETHICAL PRINCIPLES AND CODES OF CONDUCT FOR RESEARCH?

Once we have determined that action research is warranted, ethical concerns should be considered. (*Note.* The following descriptions of ethical concerns are also pertinent to other types of research for all researchers. Ethical principles are presented here to aid action researchers and all other researchers in carrying out successful research projects.)

All participants in an investigation have certain rights that must not be violated when a researcher conducts research. In many circumstances, researchers need to have the research approved by an **institutional review board (IRB)**. An IRB must be established by any institution receiving federal funding. For instance, public school districts across the country have IRBs (usually called *research committees* or *human subjects committees*). Sometimes districts go together to form an IRB across multiple districts. The primary purpose of an IRB is to protect the rights of persons involved in research. Rights of research participants relate to (1) comparison of benefits to risks in regard to participating in the study; (2) involvement of vulnerable populations, such as individuals with disabilities and children; (3) freedom from coercion; (4) informed consent prior to participation; (5) ability to withdraw without penalty; (6) confidentiality of records; and (7) privacy (see Figure 16.2).

The IRB comprises a group of professionals who assess the level of risk to participants in an investigation and make sure that ethical safeguards are in place, such as informed consent (discussed later). According to federal definitions and regulations governing research, IRBs must be formed by all universities receiving federal funds and conducting research. These definitions were developed in the 1960s and 1970s. In 2005, these definitions were updated in the "Federal Policy for the Protection of Human Subjects; Notices and Rules" published by the Federal Register (2005).

The more action researchers know about research ethics and human rights protections, the better able they are to protect the rights of the participants. Thus, it would be fruitful for those interested in conducting research to be familiar with the ethical standards of the American Educational Research Association (AERA; 2004) and the "Ethical Principles of Psychologists and Code of Conduct" of the American Psychological Association (APA; 2010). The following are brief discussions of the concerns of the AERA and APA.

AERA Ethical Standards

The AERA has 45 ethical standards organized into six topics: (1) responsibility to the field; (2) research populations, educational institutions, and the public; (3) intellectual ownership; (4) editing, reviewing, and appraising research; (5) sponsors, policymakers, and other users of research; and (6) students and student researchers. Individuals interested in conducting action research should read and understand the AERA standards. Table 16.1 presents the preamble for each of the six topics.

APA Codes of Conduct

The APA has put forth codes of conduct for psychologists. These codes can be modified to fit the ethical requirements for action researchers. The APA codes overlap to a certain extent with AERA standards. The APA stresses eight ethical standards: (1) general; (2) evaluation, assessment, or intervention; (3) advertising and other public statements; (4) therapy; (5) privacy and confidentiality; (6) teaching, training supervision, research, and publishing; (7) forensic activities; and (8) resolving ethical issues (see Figure 16.3). Standards (2), (5), (6), and (8) are especially relevant to the conduct of research.

As with the AERA standards, those who are interested in conducting action research should review the APA standards in depth. The APA also includes six general principles that should guide one who considers conducting research (see Figure 16.3). These principles include (1) competence, (2) integrity, (3) professional and scientific responsibility, (4) respect for people's rights and dignity, (5) concern for other's welfare, and (6) social responsibility. These principles are discussed next.

Competence

Individuals conducting research should be competent to carry out all aspects of the investigation. Competence should be demonstrated

> **Institutional review board (IRB)** *comprises a group of professionals who assess the level of risk to participants in a study and make sure that ethical safeguards are in place.*

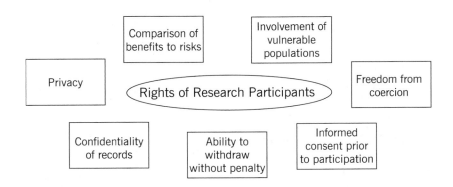

FIGURE 16.2. The rights of research participants protected by the IRB.

TABLE 16.1. Preambles from the Ethical Standards of the American Educational Research Association

I. Guiding Standards: Responsibilities to the Field (12 standards)

Preamble.   To maintain the integrity of research, educational researchers should warrant their research conclusions adequately in a way consistent with the standards of their own theoretical and methodological perspectives. They should keep themselves well informed in both their own and competing paradigms where those are relevant to their research, and they should continually evaluate the criteria of adequacy by which research is judged.

II. Guiding Standards: Research Populations, Educational Institutions, and the Public (10 standards)

Preamble.   Educational researchers conduct research within a broad array of settings and institutions, including schools, colleges, universities, hospitals, and prisons. It is of paramount importance that educational researchers respect the rights, privacy, dignity, and sensitivities of their research populations and also the integrity of the institutions within which the research occurs. Educational researches should be especially careful in working with children and other vulnerable populations. These standards are intended to reinforce and strengthen already existing standards enforced by institutional review boards and other professional associations.

III. Guiding Standards: Intellectual Ownership (2 standards)

Preamble.   Intellectual ownership is predominantly a function of creative contribution. Intellectual ownership is not predominantly a function of effort expanded.

IV. Guiding Standards: Editing, Reviewing, and Appraising Research (6 standards)

Preamble.   Editors and reviewers have a responsibility to recognize a wide variety of theoretical and methodological perspectives and, at the same time, to ensure that manuscripts meet the highest standards as defined in the various perspectives.

V. Guiding Standards: Sponsors, Policy Makers, and Other Users of Research (9 standards)

Preamble.   Researchers, research institutions, and sponsors of research jointly share responsibility for the ethical integrity of research, and should ensure that this integrity is not violated. While it is recognized that these parties may sometimes have conflicting legitimate aims, all those with responsibility for research should protect against compromising the standards of research, the community of researchers, the subjects of research, and the users of research. They should support the widest possible dissemination and publication of research results. AERA should promote, as nearly as it can, conditions conducive to the preservation of research integrity.

VI. Guiding Standards: Students and Student Researchers (6 standards)

Preamble.   Educational researchers have a responsibility to ensure the competence of those inducted into the field and to provide appropriate help and professional advice to novice researchers.

Note. Excerpted from American Educational Research Association (2004).

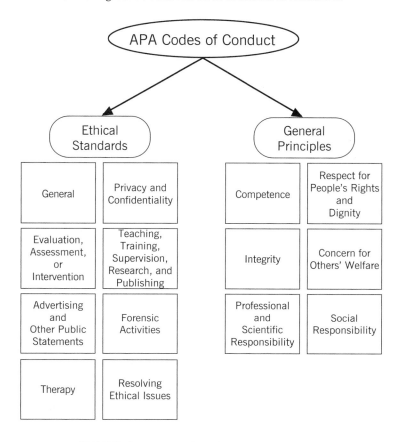

FIGURE 16.3. APA codes of conduct in research.

in several areas. For example, a teacher who attempts a classroom management system and wishes to demonstrate its effectiveness should have the knowledge and skills necessary to implement the strategy. Similarly, a math teacher who plans to use a certain mathematics curriculum and conduct action research on its effects should be well versed in that particular curriculum. The competence needed here is the same as that required for a teacher or practitioner in general. If teachers are to provide effective instruction, then they should have the necessary skills to do so. Likewise, if psychologists are to provide counseling or assessment services, they should be skillful in the implementation of their services. Additionally, competence in using programs in a setting can determine the success the program achieves and, ultimately, the conclusions made by the teacher or practitioner. If

teachers and practitioners who conduct action research for purposes described earlier are not competent in delivering the program, they may incorrectly conclude that the program is not effective, when it in fact could have been effective if implemented by a competent person (Type II error).

Competence also refers to the use of research methods. Teachers and practitioners (i.e., action researchers) should be competent in data collection and evaluation methods. If action researchers are unable to obtain adequate data and/or make reasonable conclusions based on the data, valuable information could be lost. Finally, it is critical that action researchers and researchers using all other methods remain current in their chosen fields. For example, teachers should be aware of advances in education to determine whether the planned investigation is part of best practice.

Integrity

Research integrity refers to "the degree to which researchers adhere to the rules, laws, regulations, guidelines, and commonly accepted professional codes and norms of their respective research areas" (Steneck, 2000, p. 2). A variety of actions compromise research integrity, some of which we discuss here. For example, researchers must avoid being disrespectful to participants. When conducting research, it is critical that action researchers honor participants' rights. Rosenthal (1994b) describes the concern of *hyperclaiming* when recruiting participants, or at least gaining the support of administrators and parents in the research project. Hyperclaiming is a problem when action researchers tell interested parties that the research is likely to achieve goals that are unlikely. For example, if a teacher wishes to determine whether a reading program successfully improves reading skills, a claim that the research will tell him/her how best to teach reading is not accurate. A single investigation with only one instructional method cannot achieve this claim. It is more ethical to tell interested parties what will be obtained; in this example, we would expect the investigation to determine whether students exposed to the reading instruction demonstrate improved skills.

Additionally, teachers and practitioners should not coerce individuals they are serving. First, teachers and practitioners should not coerce individuals to become involved in the research project. These individuals should not be threatened in any way if they choose not to participate. Second, individuals participating in the study should not receive compensation that is excessive, such as grants or large monetary payments. Third, individuals should be allowed not to participate or to withdraw from research without any negative consequences. Fourth, individuals should not be influenced in either overt or subtle ways to behave in any particular manner to affect research results.

Another concern related to integrity is what Rosenthal (1994b) called *causism*, which refers to claiming that a causal relationship will be revealed. In the preceding example, the teacher who claimed that the reading program would definitely cause improved reading performance would most likely be making an unfounded claim. At best, the teacher can state that students' reading skills may improve during the reading instruction. If the teacher wanted to determine whether the reading program actually was responsible for the improvement, she would need to use a high-constraint research method.

Professional and Scientific Responsibility

Researchers should be accountable for all aspects of their research and uphold the highest possible professional standards. Action researchers should consult with other professionals on research-related concerns. For example, if other teachers in the school have particular expertise in assessment, action researchers should seek out help from those individuals when designing the investigation. Additionally, action researchers must ensure that the research does not interfere with their normal responsibilities and the progress of those they serve.

Respect for People's Rights and Dignity

Action researchers should always protect the rights of participants in an investigation in terms of privacy, confidentiality, self-determination, and autonomy. It is unethical to distribute the assessment scores of students to individuals not associated with the education of these students. If data are collected as part of an action research investigation, teachers and practitioners must ensure that identifying information of participants does not go beyond the boundaries of the setting, such as a classroom. For example, a teacher who makes a presentation of the results of an investigation should never use actual names of the students. Researchers commonly use pseudonyms and/or convert actual student names to numbers.

Children and/or authorized adults should provide their consent to participate in the investigation. An IRB is concerned with the method of obtaining informed consent. Informed consent documents should be easy to read and understood by the parties. Figure 16.4 is an example of an informed consent letter to parents. This letter is similar to one used in a federally funded grant sponsored by a university. If parents are non-English-speakers, the informed consent documents should be written in their language. Teachers should be aware of cultural and individual differences, such as gender, race, and religion, when developing programs and obtaining informed consent. For example, a teacher who wishes to determine the effectiveness of a social skills curriculum should be sensitive to cultural practices that may make some of the required skills objectionable. Additionally, non-English-speaking parents or research participants who have questions about a research project should have their questions answered by an interpreter who is fluent in the same language.

Another concern has to do with deception. There may be times when research questions or procedures require that participants be denied complete information (i.e., they are deceived). For example, Martella, Marchand-Martella, and Agran (1992) used deception in several generalization assessments of individuals with developmental disabilities in employment settings. The researchers used contrived situations to make the environments look as if something could cause an injury (e.g., water on a kitchen floor). The participants were not told that the situations were simulated. The researchers assessed whether participants responded in a manner to avoid injury by telling a supervisor and/or removing the safety hazard. They received permission to use deception, but only if there was an exceptionally low probability of injury, and if participants were debriefed afterward. The use of deception was acceptable in the investigation, since the occurrence of injuries was overall very low. Thus, the simulations helped to decrease the frequency of potentially injury-producing situations. Individuals serving on IRBs understand that some research can only be conducted when information is withheld from participants or false information is initially provided. However, an IRB typically requires full justification and evidence that there are benefits inherent in a participant's involvement in the research that outweigh the deception. For example, in the study by Martella et al., participants learned to respond to safety hazards in a variety of employment environments. Although they were not informed about the hazards when they entered the study, they gained an important skill.

Deception should only be used if there is no other way to gather the data, and the data to be gathered are important to our knowledge and understanding of a phenomenon. Teachers and practitioners rarely encounter situations where deception is needed. If these situations are encountered, appropriate permission from human rights committees, advocacy groups, parents, administrators, and so on, should be sought.

Concern for Others' Welfare

Action researchers must be concerned with the welfare of study participants. Teachers and practitioners may be required to have the IRB review a proposed research investigation. A critical concern for the IRB is that the welfare of participants be considered. A concern is the potential for adverse effects on participants involved in the investigation. Action researchers should act to minimize the possibility of harm to participants. For example, it would not be permissible to use a withdrawal design for problem behaviors in the classroom if a participant has the potential to harm him-/herself or others.

For researchers, the point is to view one's research from the standpoint of the participant. Several questions need to be answered from the participant's point of view:

1. How was the participant contacted regarding the prospect of participation? Was it someone familiar to the participant or was it the researcher? If the researcher, was he/she familiar to the participant or someone who gained access to individual records? If it was someone who gained access to records, was access granted by the parent/legal guardian a priori?

2. How was the participant selected? What criteria were used? Were these criteria communicated to the participant or the participant's parent/legal guardian?

> **Research integrity**, according to Steneck (2000), refers to the degree to which researchers adhere to the rules, laws, regulations, guidelines, and commonly accepted professional codes and norms of their respective research areas.

Dear Parent:

(Name and affiliation) is conducting a research study to find out (*describe study's purpose*). Your son or daughter has been asked to take part to see if (*describe why child is being asked to participate*). There will be about (*specify number*) participants in this study at (*specify locations*).

Procedures: If you agree to be in this research study, your son or daughter will be involved in the following activities. First, (*describe what the participant will be asked to do from start to finish*). This process will take (*specify time*) minutes. The process will be repeated (*specify how many sessions*).

New findings: During the course of this research study, you will be informed of any significant new findings (either positive or negative), such as changes in the risks or benefits resulting from participation in the research, or new alternatives to participation that might cause you to change your mind about continuing in the study. If new information is obtained that is useful to you, or if the procedures and/or methods change at any time throughout this study, you will be asked to participate again.

Risks: The researcher predicts that risks of participation in this study are no greater than those encountered in regular school-related activities.

Unforeseeable risks: Since this is an assessment that takes place during school activities, there may be some unknown risks. To minimize the effects of unforeseeable risks, your son or daughter will be under supervision of the researcher and the researcher will remain in frequent communication with the teacher (*modify this section as necessary*).

Benefits: There may or may not be any direct benefit to you and your son or daughter from these procedures. Your son or daughter may (*describe benefits that are likely to be realized by all participants*).

Explanation and offer to answer questions: (*Name of researcher or qualified research assistant*) has explained this research study to you. If you have other questions, concerns, complaints, or research-related problems, you may reach (*researcher's name and contact information—include multiple forms of contact such as phone and mailing address*).

Extra cost(s): There will be no costs for participating in this study.

Voluntary nature of participation and right to withdraw without consequence: Participation in this research study is entirely voluntary. You may refuse to allow your son or daughter to participate or withdraw **at any time without consequence or loss of benefits**. On the other hand, your son or daughter may be withdrawn from this study without your consent by the investigator if the assessment is not completed.

Confidentiality: Research records will be kept confidential, consistent with federal and state regulations. Only (*researcher's name*) will have access to records. They will be kept in a password-protected file on (*researcher's name*) password-required computer. Participants will be assigned a code that will be used in place of names on all records and computer files. Participants' names and their corresponding codes will be stored in a separate password-protected file on (*researcher's name*) password-required computer to ensure the confidentiality of records. The computer file and the file with names and corresponding codes will be kept for no more than three years (*or specify other time period*) after the end of this study. The results of this study may be published and/or presented at meetings but without naming your son or daughter as a participant.

IRB approval statement: The Institutional Review Board (IRB) for the protection of human participants at (*specify organization*) has reviewed and approved this research study. If you have any pertinent questions or concerns about your rights or think the research may have harmed your son or daughter, you should contact the IRB Administrator at (*specify IRB's contact information in multiple forms*). If you have a concern or complaint about the research and you would like to contact someone other than the researcher, you may contact the IRB Administrator.

(continued)

FIGURE 16.4. Informed consent letter to parents.

Copy of consent: You have been given a photocopy of this Informed Consent. Please retain the copy for your files.

Investigator statement: "I certify that the research study has been explained to the individual, by me or my research staff, and that the individual understands the nature and purpose, the possible risks and benefits associated with taking part in this research study. Any questions that have been raised have been answered."

Signatures:

_____
(Researcher)

By signing below I agree to have my son or daughter participate.

_____   _____
Signature of Parent/Guardian   Date

Child's Assent

By signing below I agree to participate.

_____   _____
Signature of Child   Date

FIGURE 16.4. *(continued)*

3. Were the purpose, potential risks, and procedures of the study explained in detail? Did the participant or the participant's parent/legal guardian have all questions answered?

4. After the study was explained, did the participant or the participant's parent/legal guardian have an opportunity to decline participation?

5. Following an explanation of the research, was the participant or the participant's parent/legal guardian informed about how to get in touch with the researcher or the IRB if questions arose?

6. During the study, did the participant or the participant's parent/legal guardian have opportunities to withdraw from participation? Also, during the study, were questions promptly answered by the researcher?

7. Were changes in purpose, potential risks, or procedures during the study communicated to the participant or the participant's parent/legal guardian?

8. Will the participant or the participant's parent/legal guardian be satisfied at the end of the study that the benefits outweighed the risks, and that participating in this study was worth the time and effort?

Social Responsibility

Action researchers have a responsibility to inform others if their findings can contribute to educational practice. Those who inform others of the findings should follow accepted methods of dissemination. Rosenthal (1994b) cautions against several practices that may be viewed as unethical. First, *fabricating data,* a practice that cannot be tolerated, means "inventing" data or changing values of data to support a particular viewpoint. Inventing or changing data amounts to research fraud, which is viewed extremely negatively by research professionals (Kennedy, 2003). Researchers have forfeited their careers by engaging in research fraud. Strict policies of universities and other institutions of higher education regarding research fraud impose extremely stiff consequences (often suspension or expulsion). Another ethical problem is dropping data that contradict a researcher's theory or prediction. This practice involves eliminating or not considering data that fail to support one's hypothesis. One form of data dropping occurs when researchers reject data from outliers—in other words, when a single case is quite different from other cases and eliminated because it is not representative of the overall sample. For example, suppose a teacher wants to determine how well a self-management strategy works in keeping students on task during a 20-minute daily academic activity. The teacher defines what on-task behavior means and sets out to measure the on-task rate of each student in the class. The teacher divides the class into four cooperative learning groups, with five members per group. The self-management system is then presented to each group in a multiple-baseline fashion; that is, the first group receives the program, then the second, then the third, and so on. Throughout the self-management program, the teacher sees measurable improvement in the on-task duration of each of the groups. Few students are off task; in fact, the average time on task for each group is at least 18 minutes during the 20-minute daily activity by the end of the semester. The teacher concludes that the average student on-task rate improved when the self-management program was provided. However, two students in the first group and one in the third group were off task much more than the other children. In fact, by the end of the semester, the three students never exhibited 10 minutes of on-task behavior. There was no overall improvement in their on-task performance. Thus, the teacher chose to delete their data to come up with the reported 18 minutes of on-task time.

Rosenthal (1994b) indicates that data dropping may be acceptable in some very limited cases, but the practice occurs more when the outliers are bad for the researcher's theory or expectations. Thus, Rosenthal indicated that if outliers are omitted from consideration, the researcher should point this out and possibly report in a footnote what the results would have been if the outliers had been considered. Furthermore, although we highly discourage it, data dropping might involve excluding a subset of data in the analysis (Rosenthal, 1994b). For example, suppose a teacher wishes to determine the effects of improving the self-esteem of students through self-esteem-building exercises. Thirty of the students go through the self-esteem-building exercises throughout the semester. The self-esteem of 20 of the children improves as assessed through journal entries of the students, but 10 of the children feel like failures throughout the term. If the teacher does not recognize that many of the students feel bad

about themselves and concludes that the self-esteem-building exercises improve students' self-esteem, his/her ethics are questionable. The teacher, ethically, should consider and comment on all students' perceptions, or at least, pick representative journal entries from all of the students.

There are different views about data dropping in the research community. We oppose the practice and view it as unethical. Regardless of one's view, we offer a very important caveat: if data are dropped, then report it and explain the rationale for doing so. Dropping data without providing a rationale looks very suspicious and could result in serious consequences to the researcher.

Ethical Conduct of Action Researchers

Teachers and practitioners conducting action research should seek approval from an IRB to conduct the investigation. Under federal regulations, there are exemptions for some types of research; however, these exemptions are not in effect for children/students. Therefore, teachers and practitioners should always consult with an administrator or supervisor before attempting a research project. Most importantly, teachers and practitioners should ensure that they engage in ethical practice when conducting the research. Participants' rights and welfare should be of primary concern. Also, teachers and practitioners should maintain professionalism when conducting the investigation and reporting their results.

HOW DOES ONE WRITE A RESEARCH ARTICLE?

There may be times when teachers want to write up the results of their action research because they see the information as being important for other professionals. The dissemination of the results of one's action research can inform other professionals to improve their instruction. One journal in special education (i.e., *Teaching Exceptional Children* [TEC]) is intended for the dissemination of approaches that work in the classroom. Many of the authors are teachers, and teachers collaborate with college/university faculty as members of the journal's editorial board. Therefore, TEC encourages teachers to conduct action research and publish their findings.

Once the decision has been made to disseminate the findings, action researchers need to determine to which journal to send the manuscript. The decision should be based on the journal's readership. For example, if an action researcher wishes to have other secondary-level teachers read her report, she should target a journal that secondary teachers typically read. Another consideration action researchers must take into account is the requirements a journal may have for article submissions. Most journals want authors to use a limited amount of jargon. Others may want authors to present a certain type of data (i.e., quantitative vs. qualitative). Journals may also require authors to submit a certain number of copies to the journal editor, and to write in a certain style (e.g., APA publication manual, 2010). Finally, if action researchers wish to have their articles peer reviewed, they should seek out refereed journals. If they would rather their articles not be peer reviewed or they wish to submit to a journal or magazine that does not have a peer review process, action researchers should seek out a nonrefereed publication.

Contents

Whether presenting the results of a narrative or quantitative review, or some combination of the two, action researchers may follow the standard presentation format for primary research studies: (1) title page; (2) abstract; (3) introduction; (4) method; (5) results; (6) discussion; (7) references; and (8) additional sections, such as tables, figures, footnotes, and acknowledgments (see Figure 16.5). Numerous examples of research articles appear throughout this text. The following is a brief description of each of the sections of a research article an action researcher may wish to include in a write-up of an investigation. The length of each section depends on two primary variables. First, length depends on how much information the action researcher wishes to place in each section. The rule of thumb is to describe one's research with enough specificity that a reader could replicate the entire research

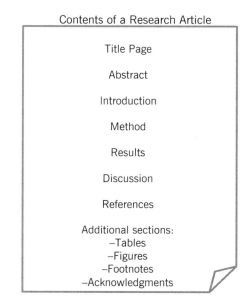

FIGURE 16.5. Standard presentation format for primary research studies.

study, step-by-step. Second, the length of each section depends on what the reviewers and/or editor deem to be acceptable. We have experienced having an editor request that we cut a 30-page manuscript down to 15 pages, but with additional information requested. The message from the editor is sometimes, in effect, "Say more but write less." Please be aware, however, that the format and sections contained in all articles are not the same. The formats and sections vary across types of research methods used (e.g., qualitative or quantitative), journals, and the purpose of the article (e.g., a formal research project description or an informal write-up of what was done).

Title Page

The title page is the first page of a manuscript. The title should be concise yet provide enough information to indicate the topic of the article. The title page should contain (in the following order) the title, action researcher's name, and affiliation. Additionally, an author note is placed on the title page under the affiliation. Other information, such as a running head, may also be included. The running head is an abbreviation of the title. Two or three words usually suffice. For example, for the title "Problem-Solving Training on the Work Safety Skills of Individuals in Supported Employment," the running head could be "Problem-Solving," "Problem-Solving Skills," or "Work Safety."

Abstract

The abstract, essentially a summary of the paper, is usually the last major part of the article to be written. Action researchers should be cautious about pasting sentences or paragraphs from parts of the article into the abstract. We have found that the abstract is best written after one reads the article, sets it aside, then attempts to describe the article in one's own words. Abstracts are typically short—less than 150 words or less than a half page in length. The abstract is typically a single paragraph that contains information about the topic, what was done, the results, and conclusions, implications, or limitations contained in the discussion. The abstract usually does not contain any citations, since it is only a summary of the article.

Although the abstract is typically less than a page in length, it is a critical part of the article. Many potential readers determine whether they want to take time to read the entire article based on what is contained in the abstract. It makes a first impression. Therefore, the abstract should contain enough information and be written in an engaging style that will catch the reader's eye.

Introduction

The goal of the introduction is to set the research investigation within the field of inquiry. The introduction typically begins by describing the scientific question that is addressed and its importance within the broad context of the field of inquiry. The introduction should also indicate why the research investigation is needed: Research on the phenomenon may be new to the literature; there may be some controversy in the field unresolved by research investigations; or the investigation replicates previous research in a direct, systematic, or clinical manner. It is important that action researchers specify the problem addressed by the investigation in detail.

We have found that it is best to think of the information in the introduction as an inverted pyramid (see Figure 16.6). At the top, the information is very broad and general. For example, in an investigation of teaching individuals to solve problems encountered on a daily basis, the beginning of the introduction might be a general description of what constitutes problem solving. As we move down the inverted pyramid, the topic becomes more focused. For example, we begin to focus on a certain type of problem-solving training, such as a brainstorming, or a generation of alternative approaches versus a single-solution approach to solving problems. Then we discuss weaknesses in the current research, such as questions left unanswered (e.g., Do individuals who go through a problem-solving program generalize or transfer the skills to "real-life" situations?). In essence, we need to justify the importance of the investigation or indicate what we are going to contribute to the literature. In the final stage of the introduction, at the apex of the inverted pyramid, we describe our research question or hypothesis. We also indicate the purpose of the investigation, such as "The purpose of this investigation is to measure the generality of a problem-solving program from situations presented during training to actual problem situations." The purpose statement should inform the reader of what to expect in the rest of the article.

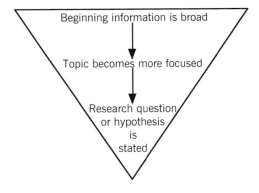

FIGURE 16.6. The introduction written in an inverted pyramid style.

Method

The method section should describe in detail the procedures used to conduct the investigation. Although the specific procedures may vary, method sections often include a description of the participants (e.g., characteristics, grade level, age, testing information such as intelligence), the setting used in the investigation (e.g., the physical layout of a classroom), the dependent variable on which the study is based (e.g., reading skill) and dependent measure (e.g., percentage of comprehension questions correct or participant attitudes of their reading performance), measurement procedures (e.g., standardized tests given, types of interviews used, methods of observations, frequency of assessments), procedures for implementing the independent variable (e.g., reading method used, design utilized), and methods of analyzing the data (e.g., type of research design, inferential statistical methods, qualitative interpretive methods, visual inspection of graphs).

Results

The results section presents the findings of each aspect of the review of the literature. The results section typically begins with a description of the results of the investigation (e.g., what was found statistically, what the triangulation methods found overall). Results sections should not include the action researcher's interpretation of the results. The results are presented in an objective manner, informing the reader of what was found during the data analysis. The results section may include summary tables or graphical presentations of results to help the reader better understand what is read. If figures or tables are used, the narrative is essentially a summarization of the figures or tables.

Discussion

The discussion section is possibly the most important section from a conceptual level. It is in this section that action researchers interpret their results (i.e., what they mean). Action researchers should set the findings of their investigation within the context of the field of inquiry. In other words, the results of the investigation are placed within the context of current knowledge in the field. Therefore, action researchers should revisit some of the information in the introduction. For example, suppose that the investigation is on the use of self-monitoring in the classroom to help decrease a student's inattentive behavior. In the introduction, the action researcher indicates that a great deal of research demonstrates that self-monitoring is effective with students who have behavior problems, but there is a lack of research on the effects of self-monitoring on attention difficulties in a classroom environment. In the discussion section, the action researcher revisits this and indicates that we now have information about the effects of self-monitoring on maintaining attention in a classroom environment.

Weaknesses of the research should also be addressed in the discussion section. For example, suppose that in a qualitative investigation on whether students find a self-monitoring program helpful in maintaining their attention on a task, there is a problem with gaining multiple viewpoints for triangulation (e.g., an aide forgot to keep a journal of student comments). Once difficulties are noted, the action researcher could indicate ways that these difficulties may be avoided in the future, such as having a daily reminder or an aid to journal student comments.

Finally, the discussion should include implications of the findings for future research. Action researchers should indicate "where we go from here." Based on action researchers' knowledge about the subject matter from the literature review in the introduction, they should have some idea of the weak areas in their research. They may also describe related issues of interest. For example, although self-monitoring has been shown to be effective for a wide range of behaviors, there is a paucity of investigations that examine how well students monitor their own behaviors. Many graduate students seeking ideas for research topics read discussion sections to find interesting issues identified by previous researchers. In this way, a line of research continues to move forward.

The discussion section should be written in a manner that captures the reader's attention.

It should prompt thoughts about where we go from here in terms of the topic of interest. Since this is the final narrative section of the article, the discussion section should provide a summary of what was discussed previously.

References

The reference section should contain all of the sources of information (e.g., articles, books, presentations) throughout the article. Most references come from the introduction. In a reference section, only sources that are cited within the article should be included.

Tables

As indicated earlier, tables may be included in the results section to display data in a visual format. Tables may also be placed in the method section to provide more detailed information about procedures or participants (e.g., intelligence scores, ages, settings). Tables should be as concise as possible. They should be organized in a manner that makes them easy to read and interpret.

Figures

If figures are used in the article, they should provide information that is easy to interpret. Figure captions are placed directly beneath the figure. Many journals have standards that should be met for graphic displays of data. Action researchers should consult the journal or specific style guide for more information on graphing requirements, such as those presented in Chapters 11 and 12.

Respectful Language

When writing an article, action researchers should use language considered respectful to person, gender, and culture, making a clear attempt not to offend individuals based on their gender, ethnicity, culture, or label. First, individuals involved in investigations should be called participants rather than subjects. The term *participant* indicates that the individual is free to participate or not participate versus being "subjected" to an intervention.

Second, any overgeneralizations or stereotyping should be avoided. For example, if participants in a study are low readers, it would be inappropriate to indicate that low reading performance is expected for individuals from a particular ethnic group or gender.

Third, always use the label or description of an individual *after* the person, not before. For example, use of "the mentally ill" or "intellectually disabled" is not considered respectful. It is more appropriate to use *person-first language*, such as, "individuals with mental illness" or "individuals with intellectual disabilities."

Finally, gender-specific language should be avoided or, if used, action researchers should justify its use. For example, always using "he" or "his" throughout the manuscript is not acceptable unless action researchers indicate that since they are discussing the topic of hyperactivity and since most children with hyperactivity are male, gender-specific language is used. The use of "he or she" is an acceptable substitute if it is used sparingly, since it can become awkward if overused. Using a more generic pronoun such as, "the teacher is teaching the students" is preferable to "the teacher is teaching her students." According to the APA publication manual (2010), going back and forth between "he" and "she" indicates that "he" or "she" is generic, which is not true. A final alternative is to turn singular language into plural such as "a good teacher keeps the attention of her students" to "good teachers keep the attention of their students."

HOW ARE ARTICLES SUBMITTED FOR PUBLICATION?

Once articles are written, action researchers then submit the manuscript to editors who consider publication. Journals have different submission requirements, such as page length and number of copies. Once an article is received, editors determine whether it is worth publishing if the journal is nonrefereed (i.e., not reviewed by peers). If the journal is refereed, the editors send the manuscript to reviewers. Reviewers are either individuals who comprise editorial boards or outside "guest" reviewers who have little or no formal association with the journal. Reviewers are typically experts in the field of education or psychology and/or the topic selected, such as reading. The number of reviewers varies from journal to journal. Whereas some journals have as many as five reviewers, others may have as few as one or two. The review process typically lasts approximately 3 months but it can take a much longer or shorter time. Reviewers can be "blind" to the names of the action researchers (authors) or they may know their names. Reviewers look for aspects of research covered throughout this text. Thus, if action researchers select journals that require a certain methodology (e.g., quantitative) and they complete different types of investigations (e.g., qualitative), their manuscripts may not be reviewed kindly. Reviewers are also concerned with the internal and external validity of the investigation, as well as the writing style.

Once the review process is finished, editors collect the reviews and make their decision. The editors' job is to summarize the reviews for the authors. Researchers are typically sent copies of the reviews; they usually are not given the names of their reviewers. At least four decisions are possible (see Figure 16.7). First, the editor may accept the manuscript as is; this is the exception rather than the rule. Second, the editor may recommend the manuscript for publication with revisions. Once the revisions are completed as specified by the editor, the manuscript is usually formally accepted. Third, the editor may recommend that the manuscript be revised and resubmitted for review. If this occurs, the manuscript may need to go through the entire review process again. Finally, the editor may reject the manuscript for consideration of publication.

If a manuscript is rejected for publication, action researchers should be persistent and not give up. They should take the reviewers' suggestions and revise the manuscript, then submit the manuscript to another journal, if they still believe it is worth publishing. Perseverance often pays off when attempting to get a manuscript in print. However, even if the manuscript does not get into a journal, action researchers should accept the feedback as an opportunity to improve on future action research they may conduct. Most reviewers attempt to provide feedback in order to help authors. The difficulty is getting used to receiving feedback from people one does not know. Action researchers should not take ownership of the manuscript. They should look at feedback not as criticism but as an opportunity to learn and improve in the future research they may conduct.

WHEN SHOULD ONE CONDUCT ACTION RESEARCH?

The obvious advantage of action research is that teachers and practitioners can inform their own practice. For example, action research aids teachers in reflective teaching, in that it helps them to determine how to improve instruction. Another advantage concerns the concept of replications and external validity. It is acceptable to think of action research as a type of systematic or clinical replication process, in that other persons are conducting the research, in different contexts (in applied settings) and with different participants. Additionally, the dependent measures may be different from those used by the researcher in the original investigation. Therefore, action research can be thought of as a way to expand scientific knowledge to other situations and individuals, which is critical for a demonstration of external validity.

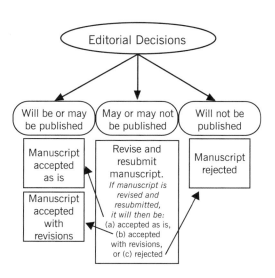

FIGURE 16.7. Possible editorial decisions for submitted articles for publication.

The opportunity for individuals in the field to publish is professionally beneficial. Teachers and practitioners working in applied settings should consider becoming actively involved in advancing our knowledge. The simplest way to do this is to stay current with the research in our chosen profession. In order to become adequate researchers, we must be critical research consumers. The second way we contribute to the knowledge in our profession is to conduct our own research. We have heard many teachers state that they teach one way or the other because they "know" it is the best way. If this is the case, then the possibility of validating their belief is at their fingertips. Additionally, it may be possible to learn something new about how best to approach the instruction of students, something that may be different from how one normally approaches instruction.

If teachers and practitioners consider conducting research in their respective applied settings, they must be aware of ethical safeguards from their professional organizations, school districts, and building administrators. Once action researchers are confident that ethical safeguards have been satisfied, they can conduct the investigation. Once the investigation is completed, action researchers should try to disseminate their findings. Dissemination can occur through several avenues, such as presentations at local, regional, or national conferences or professional meetings; brief descriptions in newsletters; or through publications in nonrefereed or refereed journals. If action researchers feel they would like to publish the results of the investigation, they should seek out an appropriate outlet and determine the journal's requirements. Finally, once the outlet has been determined, action researchers can write the manuscript and submit it for publication.

The exciting part about writing and submitting our own work for publication is that we can obtain recognition for our work. It is satisfying to have a colleague read an article you authored. It is even more satisfying to have a colleague approach you and say, "I read your article, and when I tried your intervention in my class, it really worked!" More importantly, the feedback we receive from the process of seeking to publish our own work can be critical to professional development. Other professionals have an opportunity to view our work and understand our thinking. We may have our thinking validated or criticized. Either way, we receive feedback that helps to shape our future thinking and cannot help but make us improved professionals. We can advance our profession by working together to become critical consumers of research.

SUMMARY

❖ A practitioner who conducts research may be in a central position to inform and improve practice.

❖ Action research involves application of the scientific method to everyday problems in the classroom or other applied setting by personnel involved directly with the implementation of the research. There are five dimensions of action research: (1) the complexity of the system levels, (2) the level of organization in the system, (3) the openness of the research process, (4) the intended outcomes of the research, and (5) the role of the researcher.

❖ There are five characteristics of action research: (1) purposes and value choice, (2) contextual focus, (3) change-based data and sense making, (4) participation in the research process, and (5) knowledge diffusion.

❖ Quantitative research methods are not commonly used in action research, because they are not as adaptable as qualitative methods to the day-to-day operations of the classroom environment. However, teachers and practitioners can conduct quantitative research if they wish to provide comparative information by using large groups of individuals.

❖ Qualitative methods seem to be ideally suited to action research, because they occur in the natural context and require ongoing or at least frequent contact with participants. The main advantage of using qualitative research methods is that the action researcher is already a part of the culture to be studied, so an outsider is not required. The information gained allows action researchers to reflect on critical variables in their environment.

❖ Single-case research methods are also well suited to applied settings. There are three advantages of using single-case research methods in action research: (1) Data-based decisions can be made on an ongoing basis, (2) cause-and-effect relationships can be determined with most of the research methods, and (3) experimental control can be achieved with a small number of students.

❖ Teachers and practitioners can use surveys to learn important information about students or parents that cannot be obtained in another fashion. Teachers and practitioners may use historical research when attempting to determine the best way to approach the education of certain students. Teachers and practitioners can use program evaluations on an ongoing basis to improve the academic, social, and behavioral performance of their students.

❖ All participants in an investigation have certain rights that must not be violated when researchers conduct research. In many circumstances, researchers need to have the research approved by an IRB. The primary purpose of an IRB is to protect the rights of persons involved in research. The AERA ethical standards contain 45 standards organized into six topics: (1) responsibility to the field; (2) research populations, educational institutions, and the public; (3) intellectual ownership; (4) editing, reviewing, and appraising research; (5) sponsors, policymakers, and other users of research; and (6) students and student researchers.

❖ The APA codes of conduct for psychologists, which can be modified to fit the ethical requirements for action researchers, stress eight ethical standards: (1) general; (2) evaluation, assessment, or intervention; (3) advertising and other public statements; (4) therapy; (5) privacy and confidentiality; (6) teaching, training supervision, research, and publishing; (7) forensic activities; and (8) resolving ethical issues.

❖ The APA also includes six general principles that should guide those who consider conducting research: (1) competence, (2) integrity, (3) professional and scientific responsibility, (4) respect for people's rights and dignity, (5) concern for other's welfare, and (6) social responsibility.

❖ Action researchers may follow the standard presentation format for primary research studies: (1) title page; (2) abstract; (3) introduction; (4) method; (5) results; (6) discussion; (7) references; and (8) additional sections such as tables, figures, footnotes, and acknowledgments. When writing an article, language considered respectful to person, gender, and culture should be used.

❖ Journals have different submission requirements, such as page length and number of copies. Once articles are received, editors determine whether the articles are worth publishing, if the journals are nonrefereed (i.e., not reviewed by peers). If the journals are refereed, the editors send the manuscripts to reviewers. There are four possible decisions: (1) Accept the manuscript as is; (2) recommend the manuscript for publication with revisions; (3) recommend the manuscript be revised and resubmitted for review; and (4) reject the manuscript for consideration of publication.

❖ Action research should be conducted when teachers and practitioners wish to inform their own practice. Action research aids reflective teaching in that it helps teachers to determine how to improve instruction. Action research may also be an external validity aid, because it may be considered a form of replication.

DISCUSSION QUESTIONS

1. What does the term *action research* mean? Why should practitioners consider conducting action research?

2. How is action research different from other forms of research? How is it similar? In your answer, describe the characteristics of action research.

3. Is qualitative research the only form of action research? Explain your answer.

4. Is it unethical to treat students as experimental subjects? In your answer, describe why practitioners should be aware of research ethics when conducting action research.

5. What are AERA and APA ethical guidelines? In your answer, describe each of these guidelines.

6. Should practitioners get permission to conduct research in their applied settings, and if so, from whom?

7. What are the components of a research article? In your answer, summarize each component.

8. What is the publication process? How would you explain the importance of this process?

9. What is the difference between refereed and nonrefereed journals? In which one would you place more confidence and why?

10. What are the issues related to language use in an article? Why is it important to be sensitive to these issues?

ILLUSTRATIVE EXAMPLE

Learning from Young Adolescents: The Use of Structured Teacher Education Coursework to Help Beginning Teachers Investigate Middle School Students' Intellectual Capabilities

Hilary G. Conklin
DePaul University, Chicago, IL

Todd S. Hawley
Kent State University, Kent, OH

Dave Powell
Gettysburg College, Gettysburg, PA

Jason K. Ritter
Duquesne University, Pittsburgh, PA

Abstract. *In this article, the authors discuss a case study in which beginning teachers interviewed young adolescents as part of structured teacher education coursework designed to challenge teachers' low expectations for young adolescents. Based on pre- and postsurveys, pre- and post–focus group interviews, classroom field notes, and teachers' written analysis papers, the authors' data suggest that the coursework helped to shape changes in beginning teachers' views of young adolescents' analytical capabilities and social studies knowledge. However, these shifts in teachers' thinking about young adolescents' capabilities did not translate into shifts in the teachers' ideas about middle school social studies instruction. The authors argue that carefully structured coursework like this interview project holds promise for helping beginning teachers develop new understandings about learners, but attention to students' abilities must also be accompanied by attention to teachers' purposes and pedagogical understandings.*

Keywords. *pedagogy of teacher education, teacher learning, social studies education, middle school education*

Of the many challenges teacher educators face, one of the most persistent and vexing is that of helping beginning teachers hold high expectations for their students. For many years, researchers have documented how teachers' low expectations of their students' capabilities shape the learning opportunities made available to their students. For example, an important body of research illustrates that students living in poverty and students of color often have teachers who hold lower expectations for their achievement and provide them with schoolwork that is less demanding than the work given to their wealthier and White peers (e.g., Rist, 2000; Sleeter, 2008).

Teachers' low expectations for students, however, have been a problem not just for students living in poverty and students of color. Some scholars in the field of social studies education, for instance, have found that elementary students are often shortchanged because their teachers believe they lack either the intellectual capacity or the appropriate level of development to take part in social studies learning that requires higher order thinking (Hinde & Perry, 2007; James, 2008; VanSledright, 2002). Other scholars have noted that elementary learners possess important historical reasoning skills that educators often do not recognize (e.g., Barton, 1997; Barton & Levstik, 1996) and are capable of engaging in more sophisticated learning than teachers often assume (e.g., McBee, 1996).

Indeed, as suggested by scholars in both social studies education (e.g., Barton, 2008; Grant, 2003; Newmann, 1991) and the field of education more broadly (e.g., Bruner, 1960), students of any age have the ability to engage in higher order thinking. Students in social studies classrooms at any grade level are capable of engaging in tasks that require them to interpret, analyze, evaluate, and synthesize knowledge—tasks such as crafting position papers on U.S. foreign policy (King, Newmann, & Carmichael, 2009), discussing controversial public issues (Hess, 2002), and constructing historical arguments and interpretations based on primary source evidence (Levstik & Barton, 1996; Van-Sledright, 2002).

Unfortunately, the middle school years (Grades 6–8) provide another case of teachers' expectations and students' capabilities conflicting in ways that do not serve young adolescents' intellectual potential well. Researchers have found that schoolwork typically does not provide enough cognitive challenge for young adolescents (Eccles et al., 1993; Eccles, Lord, & Midgley, 1991; Jackson & Davis, 2000). Similarly, studies have shown that many teachers prepared in secondary teacher education programs, including social studies programs (Conklin, 2007, 2008; Yeager & Wilson, 1997), hold low expectations for the kind of intellectual work middle school students can accomplish (Lexmond, 2003).

The middle school years also have the distinction of being associated with young adolescents' raging hormones, a social construction (cf.

Saltman, 2005) that many adults assume precludes students from engaging in anything that involves their minds (cf. Lesko, 2005). Yet researchers have offered powerful documentation that middle school students can engage in challenging learning (e.g., Brodhagen, 1995; Gersten, Baker, Smith-Johnson, Dimino, & Peterson, 2006; Hess, 2002). Nevertheless, the prevailing wisdom among many teachers—and indeed among the general populace—seems to be that young adolescents' immaturity should simply be managed as well as possible and teachers should do their best to provide middle school students with essential factual information so that they can do more challenging work when they get to high school (e.g., Conklin, 2007, 2008).

How, then, might teacher education challenge this conventional wisdom so that middle school students have more opportunities to engage in intellectually demanding learning? In the field of social studies education, many authors have examined the role that teacher education can play in helping beginning teachers learn teaching strategies that require students to engage in intellectually challenging work (e.g., Fehn & Koeppen, 1998; James, 2008; Parker & Hess, 2001; Yeager & Wilson, 1997). For example, Fehn and Koeppen (1998) studied how a social studies methods course could help secondary teachers use document-based history instruction in their teaching, whereas Parker and Hess (2001) investigated how their secondary social studies methods course helped prospective teachers learn to lead good discussions. Although these studies have illuminated important ways for teacher educators to improve novice teachers' acquisition of challenging teaching strategies, the studies have focused less on novice teachers' understanding of the learners they will teach.

Additional research in social studies education has addressed this issue by examining teacher educators' efforts to help beginning teachers learn more about their students' prior knowledge and capabilities. Barton, McCully, and Marks (2004) provided beginning elementary teachers with opportunities to interview and learn from their students, whereas Seixas (1994) implemented a similar intervention with his beginning secondary teachers. In both cases, the interview assignments offered beginning teachers important insight into the prior knowledge and reasoning skills that students bring to their learning; however, in none of these studies did authors focus specifically on beginning teachers' understanding of the capabilities of young adolescents in the context of social studies instruction.

Thus, in this article, we report on our effort to help beginning teachers learn from young adolescents in a teacher education course in the American South. In particular, we discuss findings from a case study in which beginning secondary social studies teachers interviewed young adolescents with the goal of unearthing and possibly challenging the teachers' beliefs about middle school students' capabilities in social studies. The research question that guided our inquiry was, how can structured coursework influence beginning teachers' views of middle school students' intellectual capabilities and interests in social studies? For the purposes of this article, we focus on the role of the structured coursework in shaping beginning teachers' views of young adolescents' intellectual capabilities.

We situate our work in the field of social studies education in part because we are all social studies teacher educators. In addition, social studies education warrants attention because it continues to fall short of its tremendous potential for engaging students and developing citizens who can analyze information, make informed decisions, and think for themselves in a complex democracy—those higher order thinking skills that make for intellectually challenging learning. Social studies has earned a reputation for being one of students' least favorite subjects (e.g., Goodlad, 1990) because it is persistently taught as a regurgitation of facts, devoid of the controversy and challenging questions that engage students. As American society faces escalating dropout rates and school disengagement, especially among poor students and students of color (Bridgeland, DiIulio, & Morison, 2006), engaging and challenging our emerging citizens through social studies education during their middle school years is of paramount importance.

THEORETICAL FRAMING

Learning to teach is a complex and challenging process that necessitates that teacher educators attend to numerous dimensions of how teachers learn. As part of learning to teach, beginning teachers need to develop a particular vision of teaching practice; understandings of subject matter, learners, and modes of instruction; conceptual and practical tools for teaching (Grossman, Smagorinsky, & Valencia, 1999); particular dispositions; and a set of practices that will enable them to enact their vision of good teaching (Hammerness, Darling-Hammond, & Bransford, 2005).

In this project, we focus on teachers' understandings of their students and of modes of instruction that support a particular vision of social studies teaching and learning. Our course the intervention was designed to support a vision of intellectually demanding social studies teaching and learning, a conception that is characterized by students' engagement in challenging instruction that emphasizes higher order thinking skills and prepares students for critical democratic citizenship (Dinkelman, 1999; Newmann, King, & Carmichael, 2007; Parker, 2003). Such instruction involves students in the active construction of knowledge (Grant, 2003; King et al., 2009) through challenging tasks that require them to develop reasoned conclusions, interpret primary sources or evidence, and construct informed arguments. Tasks like these require a deep factual and conceptual knowledge base (King et al., 2009) but also take advantage of students' higher order reasoning capabilities of analyzing, evaluating, interpreting, and synthesizing information.

To enact such instruction, in turn, middle school social studies teachers need not only a strong conceptual understanding of social studies content (e.g., VanSledright, 2002; Wilson, 1991) but also a strong understanding of young adolescents' capabilities, curiosities, and prior knowledge (Beane, 1993; Brodhagen, 1995; Hammerness et al., 2005; Jackson & Davis, 2000). Teachers with these understandings of young adolescents can then implement instruction that capitalizes on the thinking that young adolescents bring to the classroom. Such teachers would understand that young adolescents, like all students, are able to develop informed opinions about public issues or historical dilemmas, reason about those problems, and construct possible solutions to them. Furthermore, teachers would recognize that young adolescents are often very interested in complex social issues, such as injustice, poverty, politics, and violence (cf. Beane, 1993).

To help teachers develop these understandings, the teacher learning theory guiding this project suggests that teacher educators need to provide learning opportunities that engage teachers as learners, uncover their existing conceptions of teaching, learning, and students, and build on their prior knowledge and understandings to facilitate the learning of new beliefs and practices

(Borko & Putnam, 1996; Feiman-Nemser & Remillard, 1995; Hammerness et al., 2005). Such learning can be facilitated by carefully structuring and scaffolding learning experiences, helping teachers learn in the context of classroom practice, and providing opportunities for reflection and collaboration with others (Hammerness et al., 2005).

Having teachers conduct carefully designed interviews with young adolescents holds promise for shaping teachers' learning for a number of reasons. Given the need for teachers to develop an understanding of their students' prior knowledge, thinking, and experiences (Hammerness et al., 2005), a structured interview provides teachers with contextualized student responses that provide insight into these domains. By helping teachers analyze these responses with carefully selected questions, teacher educators can help beginning teachers learn "in and from practice" (Ball & Cohen, 1999), a process that may cause teachers to reconsider their original expectations for student learning (Ball & Cohen, 1999). Finally, sharing the results of their interviews can provide beginning teachers with opportunities to learn collectively by reflecting on their findings with each other (Ball & Cohen, 1999; Hammerness et al., 2005).

METHOD

Course Context and Coursework

In the fall of 2007, the first author taught a master's-level course titled Problems of Teaching Secondary Social Studies at a research university in the American South. The course was required for students seeking the Social Studies Education Program's master of arts in teaching (MAT; with initial certification) and master of education (MEd) degrees. Therefore, the course included full-time graduate students who were pursuing teacher certification as well as first-year, full-time social studies teachers and full-time graduate students who had previously earned teaching certification at the undergraduate level. Thus, all of the students were "beginning teachers" at the secondary level (Grades 6–12), although they had varying levels of experience in classrooms and prior teacher education coursework.

As part of the design of the course, the first author planned a set of required course experiences intended to help the beginning teachers develop a better understanding of young adolescents' intellectual interests and capabilities in social studies.

Drawing on the methods of Barton et al. (2004) and previous research of one of the authors (Conklin, 2008, 2009), students were required to complete the following series of assignments:

- A pre- and postsurvey designed to assess the teachers' ideas about young adolescents' capabilities in social studies and the best approaches for teaching students at this age
- A structured interview with two to four young adolescents (ages 10–15)[1] about their social studies interests and understandings
- A reading that documented the ability of young adolescents to engage in complex historical learning (Gersten et al., 2006)
- An in-class discussion in which teachers compared their interview findings with one another
- A written analysis paper that discussed the influence of these interventions on their thinking

We describe the rationale for and further details about each of these course experiences in the context of the data collected for the study.

Data Sources

All 17 teachers enrolled in the course were asked to participate in the study; 13 teachers agreed and submitted some or all of the coursework described above as data for this study. All 13 agreed to submit their analysis papers and observations of their participation in the class discussion, and 12 of these 13 agreed to submit their surveys as data. Of the 13 participants, 7 were female, 2 were African American, and the remaining participants were White.[2]

The 13 participants had limited teaching experience, and most had limited experience with education coursework. Of these 13, 11 were earning their initial teaching certificates (MAT), whereas the other 2 were in the MEd program and had thus earned teaching certificates as undergraduates. During the semester of study only 1 of the participants, an MEd student, taught full-time; he was a ninth grade social studies teacher in his second year of teaching. One of the MAT students had also spent one year as a full-time high school social studies teacher without certification. All of the other participants were either completing their first social studies part-time field experience in a middle or high school ($n = 8$) or had completed a part-time field experience and a full-time student teaching field experience (n = 3). The three participants who had completed student teaching had also completed a required social studies methods class and other required certification coursework, whereas the other 9 were enrolled in the required methods class and other certification courses during the semester of the study.

A subset of these 13 participants agreed to take part in videotaped focus group interviews prior to and following completion of the coursework. Of the 13 participants, 9 took part in the initial focus group interview, and 8 of those participants (4 female, 4 male) took part in the subsequent focus group interview. Thus, data sources for the study included pre- and postsurveys, pre– and post–focus group interviews, field notes from the in-class discussion, and teachers' written analysis papers.

The initial survey, which was administered before participants engaged in any of the structured coursework, provided baseline data on what beginning teachers thought about young adolescents' capabilities and the best approaches to teaching students at this age prior to completing the coursework. The survey included 14 questions that investigated the teachers' prior experiences working with young adolescents and teaching social studies, their views on the most important reasons for students to learn social studies, their beliefs about young adolescents' interests in social studies issues, how capable young adolescents are of engaging in particular social studies discussion topics in meaningful ways, the best instructional approaches for teaching young adolescents, and the cognitive level of assessment that would be most appropriate for young adolescents.[3] These questions were taken from a survey designed for a previous study on the preparation of middle school social studies teachers (Conklin, 2008, 2009); the original survey was carefully developed based on data from a pilot study (Conklin, 2007) and on survey items used in another teacher learning study (Kennedy, Ball, & McDiarmid, 1993).

The initial focus group interviews, which were conducted during the week following the initial survey administration, provided an alternative form of baseline data that allowed beginning teachers to elaborate on and explain their survey responses. These interviews provided further insight into the teachers' interpretation of the survey questions and their ideas about young adolescents' capabilities and also allowed beginning

teachers to think further about their initial ideas through discussion with two or three of their peers. To minimize the problems caused by the instructor being in the position of both researcher and course evaluator, the focus group interviews were conducted by the second, third, and fourth authors. Thus, both the initial surveys and focus groups provided us with insight into the teachers' initial ideas about young adolescents, which gave us a comparison point from which to track any possible changes in ideas after they completed the coursework.

The interview assignment was designed to give the beginning teachers an opportunity to learn directly from young adolescents about their understandings, insights, and capabilities in the context of social studies. Although the interviews themselves were not a data source, this course requirement provided the primary substance for teachers' subsequent reflection and learning. Among the 15 questions for the teachers to ask young adolescents, the assignment included, for example, a task that required young adolescents to arrange three historical photographs in chronological order and elicited students' reasoning for arranging the photos in the order they did. We purposely selected three photographs from distinct historical eras (1862, 1906, 1963) that included a range of contextual clues that we anticipated would fuel young adolescents' reasoning. The interview assignment also included brief case examples of public issues for young adolescents to discuss, including whether school uniforms are a good idea and whether citizens younger than 18 should be allowed to vote. We deliberately scaffolded the teachers' asking of these questions so that, for example, the teachers first asked students to discuss advantages and disadvantages of school uniforms before asking students their opinion on the issue. The interview assignment also included questions designed to elicit young adolescents' views on social studies topics they would like to know more about, national and global issues that they felt were important, and the kind of instruction that helps them learn in social studies. All of these questions were designed to elicit what young adolescents did understand and care about in social studies and the reasoning, insight, and intellect they brought to bear in thinking about these issues.

To facilitate implementation of the interviews, we provided teachers with a written set of student interview questions and photocopies of the three historical photographs; we also included "interviewing tips" for the teachers, suggesting, for example, that interviewers ask for clarification if they did not understand a response. In addition, the protocol included directions for each section of the interview, such as, "Explain to students that you want to find out what they think about social studies and what they are interested in. . . . Ask if they have any questions before you start." We handed out this protocol and the accompanying assignment description three weeks before the teachers were to conduct their interviews and provided class time to discuss the assignment and respond to any questions the teachers had.

After the teachers completed their interviews, an in-class discussion gave teachers the opportunity to share what they learned from their interviews, first in small groups and then as a whole class. We provided a written set of questions to guide the small group discussions, including questions such as the following: What initial conclusions have you come to based on these interviews? What is the evidence you are using to draw these conclusions? and How does the Gersten et al. (2006) reading inform what you learned from your interviews? Because the Gersten et al. article provided compelling research evidence that middle school students with learning disabilities could engage in complex historical learning, we believed that discussing such evidence would help the beginning teachers make connections between the insights they had gleaned through their student interviews and the intellectually challenging forms of instruction described in the reading. Furthermore, by comparing their findings with others, we anticipated that the teachers might learn more about middle school student capabilities. To track each participant's learning during this in-class discussion, the second, third, and fourth authors each sat in with one of the small groups and recorded field notes to document the individual teachers' contributions; the authors also recorded field notes during the whole-class discussion to capture the teachers' large-group conversations.

At the end of the class discussion, the teachers completed the postsurvey. Their responses provided data that were directly comparable to the initial survey, thereby giving us the opportunity to document any changes in their responses following the coursework. We also asked the teachers to rank the top three influences (e.g., survey, interview, Gersten et al. reading, etc.) from the interview project on their view of middle school students' ideas and thinking about social studies.

The following week, teachers submitted their written analysis papers. These provided all beginning teachers the opportunity to reflect on, document, and analyze what they had learned from the interviews they had conducted. The assignment asked them to provide contextual information about the students they interviewed (e.g., how they selected the students, whether they interviewed the students individually or in pairs, etc.), identify three or four main conclusions they had reached (with supporting examples from the students' responses), compare their findings to those of their classmates, and draw on their conclusions to suggest implications for how they might approach teaching social studies at the middle and high school levels. The analysis papers provided written, elaborated evidence of the teachers' thinking following the interviews. Finally, after they had submitted their papers, those beginning teachers who took part in the final focus group interviews had the opportunity to elaborate on and explain their postsurvey responses as well as think further about what they had learned from the coursework through discussion with others.

Data Analysis

We began data analysis by compiling the survey data to form a general profile of the participants' beliefs before and after completing the coursework. To analyze the qualitative data, we coded all written documents and wrote ongoing analytical memos to make sense of these data sources (Glesne & Peshkin, 1992). The audio portions of the video data were transcribed and subsequently coded, along with the analysis papers and the field notes from the class discussion, using codes that corresponded with the central elements of the teacher learning theory that guides the study and the research question. These codes included, for example, participants' experience with middle school students and with teaching social studies, middle school students' capabilities, and middle school students' interests. After coding the data, we wrote analytical memos that synthesized themes from each code prior to and after the coursework. We examined each code across cases to find patterns in participants' ideas as well as notable differences in the ways participants made sense of young adolescents' capabilities in social studies.

Limitations

To contextualize the findings of our study, it is important to point out several limitations of our study design. First, this is a small case study with a small number of participants at one institution; it is not clear the extent to which the findings we report might play out in other contexts with other beginning teachers. Second, we do not know the role that other coursework or experiences might have played in these beginning teachers' learning. It may be the case that concurrent coursework in social studies teaching methods or other learning theories, for example, facilitated some teachers' learning in this study. Although we did ask in the postsurvey and in the final focus group interviews about the role of other influences on the teachers' views of middle school students, we did not investigate these influences beyond the teachers' own reports. Third, it is possible that the shifts in teachers' thinking that we discuss below are attributable to their desire to please the course instructor and report findings that would earn them a good grade. Although the focus group interviews were intentionally not conducted by the instructor and the mixed conclusions that some teachers drew suggest that they were not necessarily trying to please the instructor, this is an important consideration to keep in mind. Fourth, because we conducted our postsurvey and final focus group interviews within a week of the culmination of the coursework, we do not know whether this coursework had any lasting effect on teachers' beliefs. Finally, the results of this study do not speak to how these beginning teachers might take up their views in teaching practice. Changing teachers' views is only one small piece of learning to teach, and it is not clear from this study how these teachers' new ideas about young adolescents' capabilities might shape their social studies instruction.

RESULTS

Initial Views

Prior to the coursework, these beginning teachers held varied conceptions of young adolescents' capabilities in social studies and the instructional approaches that might correspond with those capabilities. Many of the participants initially expressed skepticism that young adolescents could do much more than learn factual knowledge, suggesting that higher order thinking should be reserved

primarily for the high school years. For example, in the initial focus group, Isaac explained,[4]

> I think a lot of higher level social studies gets into the abstraction of . . . certain concepts like citizenship . . . and supposedly, psychologically, I didn't think those skills were developed until a little bit after middle school age, so I just wouldn't think that the high level stuff would be as attainable.

Explaining her response to a survey question that asked about the best approach to teaching seventh grade social studies, Leah expressed a similar perspective:

> As far as controversial public issues and examining stuff like that . . . engaging minds. I think that usually works better when you are older and have been able to really live life a little more to formulate your own opinions, and I just think that maybe the goal of history in middle school is to prepare them for higher level work by giving them basic facts and helping them to start learning to build their own opinions.

Many of these initial views were rooted in participants' own recollections of being in middle school and in a developmental and psychological view that challenging, conceptual thought, as Isaac expressed it, "just comes with maturity." Similarly, many expressed the stereotypical images of the tumult of the middle school years and a perspective that suggests young adolescents have few interests in learning. Dustin, for example, acknowledging that he had only his own middle school experience to draw on, observed that the middle school years are "an emotional time of your life" and a "mixed up stage."

Although many of these beginning teachers did have a skeptical view of young adolescents' capabilities going into the project, several saw greater intellectual potential in students at this age. Katherine, for example, expressed her desire to challenge middle school students, a desire that appeared to be rooted in her own experience in a middle school in which, as she explained, "a lot was expected of me." Chad also referenced his recent observations in a sixth grade classroom and hypothesized that students "are capable of a lot more than we probably think they are capable of."

Peter and Anne expressed the most confidence in young adolescents prior to the coursework and indicated their awareness of how stereotypes of the middle school years shape societal views of what young adolescents can and cannot accomplish. In response to the interview prompt "tell me what you think about middle school students," Peter responded, "Initially, right when it comes out . . . puberty, hormones raging, that kind of stereotypical view of middle school students." Anne, who was participating in the same focus group interview, followed up Peter's response by adding, "I think they get a bad rap. I feel bad for them. People . . . if you say you want to teach middle school are like, 'God, why? They are awful.' "

Both Peter and Anne initially believed that middle school students had high levels of unrealized capability in social studies. As Peter noted, "Teachers don't necessarily tap into [middle school students' capabilities] . . . but I think there is the potential." Anne shared a similar view based on her observations of middle school classrooms. As she explained, "I don't really know what their capabilities are because I haven't really seen them be challenged. . . . I would assume that they would be capable of more advanced things than they are taught." Compared with their peers, Peter and Anne seemed to have spent more time with young adolescents prior to this initial interview: Peter, who had recently completed the undergraduate teacher certification program, had spent two field experiences in middle school settings and also had a nephew in middle school. Anne also explained that she had worked with middle school students in social settings. Peter made the observation that challenging middle school students might be difficult work for teachers but noted, "We shouldn't limit middle school students because of our own limitations as teachers or people." Thus, the beginning teachers' initial ideas about young adolescents covered a spectrum of perspectives.

Changes in Ideas about Young Adolescents' Thinking

Based on these initial views, our data suggest that the structured coursework led to changes in many of the teachers' ideas about young adolescents' reasoning abilities and their social studies understandings. Although the interview project did not produce universally powerful results, following the coursework many of these teachers saw greater potential in young adolescents' higher order thinking skills than they had previously imagined and also developed new understandings about the nature of students' social studies knowledge.

Young Adolescents' Reasoning Abilities

Following the coursework—after each beginning teacher had conducted interviews with young adolescents, read the article by Gersten et al. (2006), and talked with their peers about their findings and conclusions—the in-class discussion,[5] post-surveys, individual analysis papers, and post-focus group interviews indicated that all but one of these beginning teachers showed some sign of seeing more potential in young adolescents' analytical and reasoning capabilities in social studies, even if they already held high expectations for students at this age. Isaac explained in his analysis paper a sentiment that reflected the views of most of his classmates: "After having completed the assignment—even though their overall knowledge may be limited—I believe the cognitive abilities of middle school students are underrated and often go unchallenged." The majority of these beginning teachers, like Isaac, concluded that young adolescents had stronger analytical capabilities than they had previously imagined.

The survey responses provided one indicator that some of the teachers had shifted in their thinking about young adolescents' capabilities. For example, comparing the survey responses prior to the coursework to those following the coursework, three more beginning teachers responded that the statement "middle school students are capable of remarkable intellectual work" was "extremely true" in the postsurvey (see Table 1). Meanwhile, four more responded that seventh graders are "extremely capable" of discussing topics such as "whether students should be allowed to wear hats in school or not" in meaningful ways (see Table 2). In addition, four more teachers responded that a more challenging assessment involving either

TABLE 1. Beginning Teachers' Views of Middle School Students' Capability for "Remarkable Intellectual Work"

How true do you think the following statement [is]? Middle school students are capable of remarkable intellectual work.	Presurvey (N = 12)	Postsurvey (N = 12)
Not at all true	0	0
Slightly true	0	0
Moderately true	1	2
Quite true	6	2
Extremely true	5	8

TABLE 2. Beginning Teachers' Views of Seventh Graders' Capability for "Meaningful Discussion"

How capable do you think 7th graders are of discussing the following [topic] in a meaningful way? Whether students should be allowed to wear hats in school or not.	Presurvey (N = 12)	Postsurvey (N = 12)
Not at all capable	0	0
Slightly capable	1	1
Moderately capable	1	0
Quite capable	9	6
Extremely capable	1	5

analysis or evaluation would be appropriate for seventh grade students after they had completed this course intervention (see Table 3).

Although the survey data do not provide evidence that all of the teachers shifted in their thinking, data from the focus group interviews

TABLE 3. Beginning Teachers' Views on Appropriate Middle School Assessments

Suppose you are teaching a mini-unit on the qualifications for becoming a U.S. president to a group of 7th grade students. Which of the following types of assessments would you choose as the most intellectually appropriate for your 7th grade students?	Presurvey (N = 12)	Postsurvey (N = 12)
A basic level cognitive assessment that requires *summarizing information.* (Example: students summarize the qualifications necessary for becoming a U.S. president.)	5	1
A mid-level cognitive assessment that requires *analyzing and comparing information.* (Example: students compare and contrast several candidates' qualifications for becoming a U.S. president.)	3	6
A high-level cognitive assessment that requires *evaluating information.* (Example: students construct an argument about the value of the current qualifications for becoming a U.S. president.)	4	5

and analysis papers suggest that many of these beginning teachers did, indeed, begin to think differently about young adolescents' capabilities following the coursework. Many of the participants expressed pleasant surprise that young adolescents could do more than they anticipated, as Kelly and Ben noted in their analysis papers. For instance, Kelly wrote, "I really think that we underestimate middle school students and the level of material that they are able to understand along with their analytical skills." Ben echoed this point when he explained, "Middle school students are very capable of complex reasoning skills. . . . I am thoroughly surprised by how much these middle school kids knew."

Similarly, Dustin concluded in his post–focus group interview that one of the most important things he learned from this interview project was that "middle schoolers can think. They are not things you can just put information into. They do have the ability to analyze . . . you can actually engage them in higher order things." These comments are representative of all but one of the participants' ideas from the focus group interviews and analysis papers and indicate that, after having completed the coursework, these beginning teachers believed that young adolescents possess higher order reasoning and thinking skills.

Many of the teachers particularly noted young adolescents' reasoning abilities as they worked to put the series of historical photographs in chronological order. For example, in her analysis paper, Maria wrote,

One of the first things I noticed during the interview is that each of these girls noticed in the photographs I presented specific and what I considered obscure details, at least what I thought was obscure for their age. Both girls placed the photos in incorrect chronological order; however, most interestingly, they had really reasonable arguments for doing so.

Leah, too, found the young adolescents' work with the pictures notable because she felt that students were making judgments based on their analysis of the pictures. In her post–focus group interview, Leah observed,

I think mine were actually better at analyzing the pictures, too, because . . . they were talking about the Civil War picture, "Well, that has to be older than this one because that has cars, and there weren't cars during the Civil War."

Thus, the historical photographs and the numerous context clues within them seemed to provide a helpful tool for young adolescents to showcase their reasoning skills and for the teachers to observe this reasoning in action.

Even those beginning teachers who began the coursework with high expectations for young adolescents—Peter and Anne—found evidence not only to support their prior convictions but actually to strengthen their views of young adolescents' capabilities in social studies. Peter interviewed one 10-year-old and one 14-year-old and noted that he was impressed to see how the 10-year-old relied on contextual clues to sort the photographs, even though he did not have background knowledge to help him put the pictures in chronological order. Similarly, Anne observed that she had confirmed her hunch that young adolescents had untapped intellectual capability and even saw greater potential than she expected. As she explained in her paper,

> Both girls had superior reasoning skills. They gave answers that indicated they had considered the questions and provided well-thought, articulate answers. I was surprised by the girls' exemplary answers; the caliber of their logic really exceeded my expectations. . . . I was impressed by the way that Gabby addressed issues like individuality and social interaction in relation to [school] uniforms.

Thus, even for these teachers who already held high expectations for young adolescents, the specific tasks and discussion prompts required by the interview project appeared to be productive in facilitating new observations about young adolescents' thinking abilities.

Although almost all of these participants developed new ideas about young adolescents' strong intellectual capabilities, Christine was the one notable exception. In contrast to her peers, Christine was the only participant who showed evidence of becoming less impressed with what young adolescents could do. Among the focus group participants, Christine was the only teacher who, on her postsurvey, selected an assessment that required lower order thinking than her previous response to the middle school assessment question. In her analysis paper, Christine also responded to what she saw as the superficial nature of young adolescents' thinking. She wrote,

> All three students correctly placed the pictures in chronological order, but their reasons for doing so

were rather shallow or inaccurate. All three students seemed to place the pictures primarily by identifying the absence or presence of things by saying that they did not "have up to date stuff," that there was "no technology," they did not "have jobs back then," or they "look[ed] poor." While the students' picture placement was correct, their interpretations were not fully developed.

This comment stands in contrast to comments such as Maria's and Peter's above in which they are most impressed with students' use of contextual clues to arrange the photographs, even when the students' reasoning did not lead them to the correct chronological order. Although Maria and Peter appeared to see the potential in young adolescents' insights, Christine seemed to be able to see only what the students could not do.

Young Adolescents' Fragmented Knowledge

Although Christine was alone in not seeing greater potential in young adolescents' reasoning and analytical capabilities following this coursework, several teachers made similar observations about the social studies knowledge young adolescents possess. Almost all of the teachers observed that the young adolescents they interviewed did not have extensive "foundational" social studies knowledge. Dustin, for example, explained in his post–focus group interview,

> They don't have that fundamental stuff that you can really build on. . . . I still would like to be able to engage them more in some of the higher order ideas. I think they are very capable of doing so. But I've still got to build that fundamental knowledge somewhere.

Several of the teachers noted young adolescents' lack of knowledge beyond their immediate community. In her paper, for example, Leah wrote,

> Middle school students know very little about important national and international events [and] are primarily concerned with the things that affect them most. . . . I was impressed with the ability to answer questions about the pictures, but I was concerned with some of the inaccuracies about the historical content.

These comments are representative of the teachers' agreement that, as Isaac noted, young adolescents' "overall knowledge may be limited."

Although the participants as a group took note of young adolescents' factual errors or limited knowledge, as Leah's comment above suggests, some of the teachers viewed this fragmented knowledge as more problematic than others did. Later in her paper, Leah elaborated on her concern about young adolescents' limited knowledge. She explained,

> They were very good at explaining their views on the voting age. However, both students had a harder time explaining, or even identifying, their knowledge and opinions on national and world levels. Both seemed to have picked up on some "buzz words," such as "global warming," "Iraq," "immigration," and "China," that they had maybe heard from their parents or the news but didn't know much about. For some questions, the only reply was "I don't know." While they were able to vocalize their opinions on some issues, they tended to be on more of a superficial level, instead of having put much real thought into it.

Like Christine, Leah revealed her more negative judgment about what she saw as the superficiality of the young adolescents' knowledge—a perspective she expressed more bluntly during the in-class discussion when she referred to the students she interviewed as "dumb as bricks." As the tone of these comments suggests, then, these teachers drew different implications from the conclusion that young adolescents had strong reasoning abilities but fragmented knowledge.

Contradictory Instructional Conclusions

Although most of the teachers shifted toward seeing greater reasoning potential among young adolescents, these shifts did not necessarily correspond to a new belief that teachers should engage young adolescents in teaching that asks them to use these analytical skills. The survey responses provide one window into the conclusions participants drew from the project about their teaching. For example, Table 4 reveals that the beginning teachers' ideas about the best approach to teaching seventh grade social studies remained mostly unchanged, and half of this group continued to respond that a fact-oriented approach to teaching social studies would be best for seventh graders. Although these compiled survey responses mask some changes in the teachers' ideas, the eight focus group participants' survey responses reveal that although three teachers answered this question differently on their postsurvey, the other five

TABLE 4. Beginning Teachers' Selections of Best Approaches to Teaching Seventh Grade Social Studies

Three teachers—Pat, Lou, and Chris—describe their approach to teaching 7th grade social studies. Which of these teachers do you think has the BEST understanding of how to teach social studies to middle school students?	Presurvey (N = 12)	Postsurvey (N = 12)[a]
Pat: "In my class, students discuss controversial public issues, examine primary sources, and analyze social problems. These are the things that engage middle school minds."	4	5
Lou: "In my class, I work hard at helping students learn some of the fundamental ideas and events from our history. I want to give them the critical background knowledge that will enable them to do high level work when they get to high school."	6	6
Chris: "In my class, I want to make social studies come alive by getting students involved in hands-on activities. For example, I have my students make food from different cultures and build models of historical structures like the Roman Coliseum."	2	2

[a]One participant selected both Pat and Chris on the final survey.

responded with the same teacher they had selected before the coursework.

The teachers' analysis papers and focus group interview responses provide further insight into the stability of these responses and reveal the nature of teachers' differing conclusions. In some cases, the beginning teachers drew the conclusion that if young adolescents have strong higher order thinking capabilities and fragmented content knowledge, it is the responsibility of teachers to facilitate their learning so that they can make connections and integrate their knowledge. For example, Peter wrote, "Teachers must realize that students will have a fragmented notion of history (how can we not?), but that is okay and we must work with students' knowledge towards powerful teaching." Similarly, in her analysis paper, Maria explained,

The minds of children are struggling to make sense of what they see. Without someone paying attention to this and helping to inform their conclusions it seems there are many opportunities for students to draw misdirected conclusions. . . . I believe it is the responsibility of social studies teachers to find out what questions may be looming and provide legitimate sources for students to turn to in their search for clarity. . . . Some students know little or nothing about specific current events, they are always listening and formulating opinions based upon the information they do encounter in the media or from overhearing adult conversations. . . . They should be given an opportunity in their class to discuss their concerns and teachers should show their students how to marshal the evidence they need to make sense of their world.

These comments are representative of those participants—fewer than half of the group—who concluded that social studies teachers should use instruction that takes advantage of and builds on young adolescents' strong reasoning capabilities, a conclusion that is consistent with the goals of our project.

However, although some of the teachers, like those above, appeared to develop a consistent set of ideas about the need for challenging middle school students in social studies teaching, some of the other teachers' conclusions appear contradictory. That is, they spoke of the need for teachers to capitalize on young adolescents' reasoning capabilities yet selected a fact-oriented approach to teaching middle school social studies as best. Dustin provides one interesting case of these seemingly contradictory conclusions. He wrote in his paper,

I think that it is clear that these students, even by the sixth grade, are able to do more than "memorize" things. They should be given the opportunity to further develop their critical thinking and analysis skills, thereby learning both the conceptual/foundational content that I can further build on in high school as well as some of the "higher order superstructure." Just because these kids are young does not mean that they cannot perform some impressive tasks. . . . I think that, at times, we as teachers just assume that younger students cannot do "higher order" activities and thereby create a self-fulfilling prophecy.

Although Dustin articulates ideas that are in many ways consistent with Pat's intellectually challenging approach to teaching, surprisingly Dustin maintained his selection of Lou, the teacher with a fact-oriented approach to teaching, as the best teacher on the postsurvey.

Although Dustin's surprising teacher selection could simply represent a different interpretation of the survey question, some of the other teachers came to conclusions that we found similarly perplexing. Anne spoke and wrote about how impressed she was with young adolescents' reasoning skills and noted in her paper that middle school students "are capable of informed discussion," can form "pro/con arguments about topics and reach conclusions that were supported by ideas and not feelings," love to "discuss and debate," and should be given more "agency." She also expressed her dismay that many of her classmates maintained low expectations for young adolescents. However, she changed her survey response from Pat on the presurvey to Lou on the postsurvey and explained,

I felt that they were really good at conversing and socially talking about the issues . . . but when it came down to . . . say dates and times, that's really lacking. I saw that need in them so that's why I was more inclined to say Lou.

Some of the other beginning teachers developed conclusions similar to Anne's but seemed even more strongly convinced that the interview project supported a need to focus on more factual instruction in the middle grades. Leah's comment is representative of the conclusion that several of her peers reached:

[In terms of] the most important reason for students to learn social studies . . . at first, I had thought . . . they need to learn to think historically and analyze and everything. But then I realized that some of these kids don't actually know enough about the facts to be able to analyze it. And so I think maybe you need to make sure that they have a really good foundation of facts before you try to push them to analyze anything.

Although Dustin's comment above suggests his view that students might indeed learn content *through* instruction that demands higher order thinking, Anne's and Leah's comments indicate that they do not make a connection between engaging students in interpretation and analysis and the use of social studies content.

Finally, some of these teachers concluded that the young adolescents they interviewed were not representative of young adolescents in general and tempered their conclusions with skepticism that perhaps they had only interviewed the "good kids." Ben, for example, wrote,

We all agreed that we do not give middle school kids enough credit and often do not recognize their great capacity for learning. However, all of us felt that the teachers that had provided these students for us had picked them out, not only because they were well behaved, but also because they were above average students. I cannot help but wonder how our findings would have been different had we interviewed some different students from different backgrounds.

Similarly, Chad concluded that the remarkable responses of one of the young adolescents he interviewed represented that particular student's exceptionality. He explained,

> It became ever apparent to me that there is definitely a need for gifted classes so that students like Will can be challenged. . . . I have come to realize that though there is tremendous potential for discussion amongst all of the students, a student such as Will could discourage students like Sarah or John to talk in class even though they have great ideas.

These teachers were hesitant to draw conclusions about instruction that would be applicable for all young adolescents.

By contrast, Dustin felt confident that his conclusions could hold across a range of students. He noted in his paper,

> My belief that middle school students possess the ability to reason and analyze from evidence seemed quite well supported across grade levels in our discussion Monday night. . . . I think this is especially significant for my sample because while many of the subjects interviewed by others in class seemed to be the "advanced" students, my sample was deliberately selected to include a wide variety of intellectual capability, so perhaps these findings can be generalized beyond the "gifted few."

Dustin's comment points to the potential importance of the teachers interviewing young adolescents whom they view as "typical" or otherwise more representative of other young adolescents in general.

DISCUSSION

The structured coursework described in this article suggests some reason for cautious optimism as well as the need for additional work on the part of teacher educators. These data point to the interview assignment with young adolescents as a useful tool for helping beginning teachers recognize intellectual capabilities in middle school students that many of them had not previously recognized; however, the study also suggests that focusing beginning teachers' attention on students' abilities must also be accompanied by attention to the purposes of teaching and pedagogical practices.

The data gathered both before the course intervention and after suggest that the interview project had some success in shifting teachers' thinking toward seeing young adolescents as more intellectually capable. Most of the teachers who participated in the study attributed their change in thinking to the required coursework, particularly the structured interview. Kelly, for example, noted that she "was shocked at just how capable" students were and added, "If we hadn't had these questions, I would have never known this." Isaac expressed a similar sentiment when he said that "interviewing middle school students . . . just seeing it firsthand kind of made a big difference, and then . . . completing the survey before and after . . . as I was taking it . . . I was aware of how my perspective shifted." The structured interview task, then, appears to be one way in which teachers can learn "in and from practice" (Ball & Cohen, 1999) and develop new understandings about learners and their thinking (Hammerness et al., 2005).

Although the results of the study indicate that the coursework showed potential for shifting teachers' views of young adolescents' intellectual capabilities and, in some cases, shaping new commitments to teaching middle school students, these teachers' varied conclusions and sometimes inconsistent reasoning about instruction suggest that such coursework experiences alone may be insufficient for helping teachers develop commitments to teaching young adolescents in ways that capitalize on their intellectual potential. In fact, our interview project addressed only a very small piece of the large body of tools, practices, and understandings that beginning teachers require to enact complex forms of teaching (Hammerness et al., 2005): The interview assignment primarily targeted beginning teachers' ideas about young adolescents and their capabilities as learners. It may be that our intervention would have been more successful if we had addressed not only teachers' understandings of students but also their understanding of engaging forms of social studies instruction along with conceptual and practical tools that would have given them frameworks in which to situate their understandings (Grossman et al., 1999; Hammerness et al., 2005).

Indeed, implicit in the design of this coursework was an assumption that teachers' belief in young adolescents' reasoning capabilities would translate into a commitment to social studies instruction that would capitalize on and further those reasoning abilities. Yet our research suggests that helping teachers learn that young adolescents are capable of sophisticated thinking is insufficient if the teachers do not also have strong understandings about corresponding teaching practices. Although other parts of the course offered an implicit vision of intellectually demanding social studies teaching, we did not provide the participants with a common set of structured experiences to help them develop an understanding of how to link such instruction to their sense of students' capabilities.

Our findings also suggest that our course intervention might have been more powerful if we had provided the teachers with conceptual tools (Grossman et al., 1999; Hammerness et al., 2005) to help them consider the role that teachers can play in facilitating learning. For example, past research on students' historical thinking reveals that young students typically have understandings of historical time in "broad sequences rather than precise dates," whereas "older students often recognize broad historical themes and patterns even when their knowledge of specific details is vague or inaccurate" (Barton, 2008, p. 241). However, Barton (2008) explains that this research also illustrates that, "none of these patterns is inevitable . . . nor are they a direct function of age; rather, instruction that specifically addresses diversity or historical time can enhance students' understanding of these elements of the subject" (p. 241). The beginning teachers in our study might have profited from explicit engagement with the principle that it is up to teachers to provide opportunities that build on and further students' existing understandings.

In addition, the social studies research literature suggests that we may have needed to address the issue of purpose more explicitly. That is, some researchers (e.g., Barton & Levstik, 2004; Grant, 2003) have argued that teachers require a strong vision of their goals for social studies education, and these goals must require a type of instruction that corresponds with these goals. For example, Barton and Levstik (2004) contend that if a teacher's larger purpose in teaching social studies is helping students contribute to a participatory,

pluralistic democracy, then these goals necessitate that students learn to reason, examine multiple viewpoints, and investigate different kinds of evidence. Thus, it may be that we needed to focus more on our teachers' purposes for teaching social studies so that we could help them make connections among purpose, practice, and student capabilities.

How, then, might these assignments be adjusted for the future? First, for teachers such as Christine who seem particularly inclined toward viewing students in terms of what they cannot do, teacher educators might need to point out the perils of deficit thinking and help them develop ways of seeing students in terms of their strengths (cf. Ayers, 1993). Perhaps our assignment should have explicitly directed teachers to focus on what students do know rather than what they do not. Next, we may have needed to help these teachers learn about intellectually demanding social studies teaching practices explicitly to illuminate the kinds of practices that both help students develop a deep factual and conceptual knowledge base and take advantage of their higher order reasoning capabilities (King et al., 2009). We might ask teachers, for instance, to read King et al.'s (2009) article on authentic intellectual work and accompany this reading with a task or video case analysis that asks them to evaluate the kind of intellectual work being asked of middle school students. Similarly, we might read the children's story *Fish Is Fish* (Lionni, 1970), a book that illustrates how learners construct knowledge through the lens of their prior knowledge, and discuss the implications of this idea for teaching and learning. We might also have included a prompt on the analysis paper assignment that directed teachers to "discuss the kind of social studies instruction that would capitalize on and build upon young adolescents' reasoning abilities, taking into account class readings and experiences on different forms of social studies instruction." Finally, to address the issue of purpose, it may have been helpful to engage teachers in an examination of different possible purposes for teaching social studies and the particular teaching practices that these purposes would require, as Barton and Levstik (2004) discuss.

To implement all of these adjustments requires considerable time, and it is possible that our particular course context was not well suited for such a comprehensive approach. It is well established that teachers' existing beliefs can be very difficult to change (e.g., Borko & Putnam, 1996), and the limited number of class sessions we were able to devote to this project was likely insufficient to challenge all of the beliefs we needed to tackle. Indeed, one of the challenges we faced in conducting this project was the variation in prior knowledge and experiences of the beginning teachers enrolled in this course: some had already taken methods courses whereas others had not, and some had already spent considerable time examining the possible purposes for teaching social studies whereas others had not. A project such as ours might be better suited for a methods course in which learning about purposes, practices, and students' abilities can be the central focus. Alternatively, the challenges we faced may speak to the need for teacher educators to work together across courses to develop more coherent teacher education experiences.

CONCLUSIONS AND IMPLICATIONS

These data suggest that carefully planned and implemented teacher education has the potential to play an important role in shaping teachers' views of young adolescents' capabilities in social studies. In particular, helping beginning teachers learn more about young adolescents' curiosity, prior knowledge, and intellectual potential may be one critical component of preparing social studies teachers who can and do engage and challenge young adolescents' minds. The interview assignment and related coursework we describe suggest one pedagogical approach teacher educators might use to help beginning teachers focus on and learn about the intellectual interests and abilities of their students.

At the same time, our findings point to the importance of teacher educators attending to the multiple facets of teacher learning and creating learning opportunities for beginning teachers that address these multiple dimensions in a coherent manner. Addressing only one aspect of teacher learning may lead to productive change but also unintended consequences. Our study suggests that when teacher educators develop experiences for beginning teachers targeted at particular goals, they must take into account the complexities of teacher learning and make efforts to provide teachers with the requisite understandings and tools as well as carefully designed opportunities to synthesize their learning from these experiences.

Thus, we must carefully construct learning experiences that will help teachers learn about and make connections among purposes of social studies teaching, particular instructional practices that support those purposes, and the student capabilities that they can build on through those instructional practices. Furthermore, although we may want beginning teachers to construct and "discover" their own conclusions through the assignments we provide, we need to pose questions that will help them link ideas that may not be obviously linked in their minds. We cannot assume that they possess the same frameworks for instruction that guide our own thinking—such as the connection between students' reasoning abilities and higher order instruction. These frameworks are part of what they need to learn, and it is our responsibility to help them learn these frameworks.

In sum, our study suggests that teacher educators must be exceptionally thoughtful and rigorous in the design and implementation of teacher education practice and also in the study of these efforts. This research illustrates the value of studying our interventions for illuminating both the ways in which our efforts achieve their intended outcomes and the ways in which they fall short. Careful study of teacher education practice can continue to help us understand the complexities of our responsibilities as teacher educators and envision how we might improve our instruction to serve beginning teachers and, in turn, the young people they serve.

NOTES

1. For the purposes of the assignment, we defined "young adolescent" as students aged 10 to 15 who are "typically in Grades 6 to 9." We adopted this definition to include Grade 9 to make it less burdensome for the full-time high school teachers to complete the interview assignment.

2. The gender and racial/ethnic categorizations are the authors' description. We did not ask participants for these demographic data.

3. For the purposes of this article, we include data from those survey questions that are representative of and most relevant to participants' learning about young adolescents' intellectual capabilities.

4. All participant names are pseudonyms.

5. Although we did draw on the in-class discussion data for our analysis, for the purposes of this article we draw primarily on data from the postsurveys, analysis papers, and post–focus group interviews because these sources provided the clearest examples to represent our findings.

ACKNOWLEDGMENTS

We are very grateful to the participants who were willing to take part in this study. We also would like to thank Keith Barton for his valuable feedback on an earlier version of this article.

DECLARATION OF CONFLICTING INTERESTS

The author(s) declared no potential conflicts of interests with respect to the authorship and/or publication of this article.

FUNDING

The author(s) received no financial support for the research and/or authorship of this article.

REFERENCES

Ayers, W. (1993). *To teach: The journey of a teacher*. New York: Teachers College Press.

Ball, D. L., & Cohen, D. K. (1999). Developing practice, developing practitioners: Toward a practice-based theory of professional education. In L. Darling-Hammond & G. Sykes (Eds.), *Teaching as the learning profession: Handbook of policy and practice* (pp. 3–32). San Francisco: Jossey-Bass.

Barton, K. C. (1997). "I just kinda know": Elementary students' ideas about historical evidence. *Theory and Research in Social Education, 25*, 407–430.

Barton, K. C. (2008). Research on students' ideas about history. In L. S. Levstik & C. A. Tyson (Eds.), *Handbook of research in social studies education* (pp. 239–258). New York: Routledge.

Barton, K. C., & Levstik, L. S. (1996). "Back when God was around and everything": The development of children's understanding of historical time. *American Educational Research Journal, 33*, 419–454.

Barton, K. C., & Levstik, L. S. (2004). *Teaching history for the common good*. Mahwah, NJ: Erlbaum.

Barton, K. C., McCully, A. W., & Marks, M. J. (2004). Reflecting on elementary children's understanding of history and social studies: An inquiry project with beginning teachers in Northern Ireland and the United States. *Journal of Teacher Education, 55*(1), 70–90.

Beane, J. A. (1993). *A middle school curriculum: From rhetoric to reality* (2nd ed.). Columbus, OH: National Middle School Association.

Borko, H., & Putnam, R. T. (1996). Learning to teach. In D. C. Berliner (Ed.), *Handbook of educational psychology* (pp. 673–708). New York: Simon & Schuster.

Bridgeland, J. M., DiIulio, J. J., Jr., & Morison, K. B. (2006). *The silent epidemic: Perspectives of high school dropouts* (Report by Civic Enterprises in association with Peter D. Hart Research Associates). Seattle, WA: Bill & Melinda Gates Foundation.

Brodhagen, B. (1995). The situation made us special. In M. W. Apple & J. A. Beane (Eds.), *Democratic schools* (pp. 83–100). Alexandria, VA: Association for Supervision and Curriculum Development.

Bruner, J. (1960). *The process of education*. New York: Vintage.

Conklin, H. G. (2007). Methods and the middle: Elementary and secondary preservice teachers' views on their preparation for teaching middle level social studies. *Research in Middle Level Education Online, 31*(4). Retrieved from http://www.nmsa.org/portals/0/pdf/publications/RMLE/rmle_vol31_no4.pdf.

Conklin, H. G. (2008). Promise and problems in two divergent pathways: Preparing social studies teachers for the middle school level. *Theory and Research in Social Education, 36*(1), 36–65.

Conklin, H. G. (2009). Purposes, practices, and sites: A comparative case of two pathways into middle school teaching. *American Educational Research Journal, 46*(2), 463–500.

Dinkelman, T. (1999). Critical reflection in a social studies methods semester. *Theory and Research in Social Education, 27*(3), 329–357.

Eccles, J. S., Lord, S., & Midgley, C. (1991). What are we doing to early adolescents? The impact of educational contexts on early adolescents. *American Journal of Education, 99*, 521–542.

Eccles, J. S., Midgley, C., Wigfield, A., Buchanan, C. M., Reumann, D., Flanagan, C., et al. (1993). Development during adolescence: The impact of stage–environment fit on young adolescents' experiences in schools and in families. *American Psychologist, 48*(2), 90–101.

Fehn, B., & Koeppen, K. (1998). Intensive document-based instruction in a social studies methods course and student teachers' attitudes and practice in subsequent field experiences. *Theory and Research in Social Education, 26*(4), 461–484.

Feiman-Nemser, S., & Remillard, J. (1995). Perspectives on learning to teach. In F. Murray (Ed.), *The teacher educator's handbook: Building a knowledge base for the preparation of teachers* (pp. 63–91). San Francisco: Jossey-Bass.

Gersten, R., Baker, S. K., Smith-Johnson, J., Dimino, J., & Peterson, A. (2006). Eyes on the prize: Teaching complex historical content to middle school students with learning disabilities. *Exceptional Children, 72*(3), 264–280.

Glesne, C., & Peshkin, A. (1992). *Becoming qualitative researchers: An introduction*. White Plains, NY: Longman.

Goodlad, J. I. (1990). *Teachers for our nation's schools*. San Francisco: Jossey-Bass.

Grant, S. G. (2003). *History lessons: Teaching, learning, and testing in U.S. high school classrooms*. Mahwah, NJ: Erlbaum.

Grossman, P., Smagorinsky, P., & Valencia, S. (1999). Appropriating tools for teaching English: A theoretical framework for research on learning and teaching. *American Journal of Education, 108*, 1–29.

Hammerness, K., Darling-Hammond, L., & Bransford, J.

(2005). How teachers learn and develop. In L. Darling-Hammond & J. Bransford (Eds.), *Preparing teachers for a changing world: What teachers should learn and be able to do* (pp. 358–389). San Francisco: Jossey-Bass.

Hess, D. E. (2002). Discussing controversial public issues in secondary social studies classrooms: Learning from skilled teachers. *Theory and Research in Social Education, 30*(1), 10–41.

Hinde, E. R., & Perry, N. (2007). Elementary teachers' application of Jean Piaget's theories of cognitive development during social studies curriculum debates in Arizona. *Elementary School Journal, 108*(1), 63–79.

Jackson, A., & Davis, G. A. (2000). *Turning points 2000: Educating adolescents in the 21st century.* New York: Teachers College Press.

James, J. H. (2008). Teachers as protectors: Making sense of preservice teachers' resistance to interpretation in elementary history teaching. *Theory and Research in Social Education, 36*(3), 172–205.

Kennedy, M. M., Ball, D. L., & McDiarmid, G. W. (1993). *A study package for examining and tracking changes in teachers' knowledge.* East Lansing: Michigan State University, National Center for Research on Teacher Education.

King, M. B., Newmann, F. M., & Carmichael, D. L. (2009). Authentic intellectual work: Common standards for teaching social studies. *Social Education, 73*(1), 43–49.

Lesko, N. (2005). Denaturalizing adolescence: The politics of contemporary representations. In E. R. Brown & K. J. Saltman (Eds.), *The critical middle school reader* (pp. 87–102). New York: Routledge.

Levstik, L. S., & Barton, K. C. (1996). *Doing history: Investigating with children in elementary and middle schools.* Mahwah, NJ: Erlbaum.

Lexmond, A. J. (2003). When puberty defines middle school students: Challenging secondary education majors' perceptions of middle school students, schools, and teaching. In P. G. Andrews & V. A. Anfara Jr. (Eds.), *Leaders for a movement: Professional preparation and development of middle school teachers and administrators* (pp. 27–52). Greenwich, CT: Information Age.

Lionni, L. (1970). *Fish is fish.* New York: Pantheon.

McBee, R. H. (1996). Can controversial topics be taught in the early grades? The answer is yes! *Social Education, 60*(1), 38–41.

Newmann, F. M. (1991). Promoting higher order thinking in social studies: Overview of a study of sixteen high school departments. *Theory and Research in Social Education, 19*(4), 324–340.

Newmann, F. M., King, M. B., & Carmichael, D. L. (2007). *Authentic instruction and assessment: Common standards for rigor and relevance in teaching academic subjects.* Des Moines: Iowa Department of Education.

Parker, W. (2003). *Teaching democracy: Unity and diversity in public life.* New York: Teacher's College Press.

Parker, W., & Hess, D. E. (2001). Teaching with and for discussion. *Teaching and Teacher Education, 17,* 273–289.

Rist, R. (2000). Student social class and teacher expectations: The self-fulfilling prophecy in ghetto education. *Harvard Educational Review, 70*(3), 257–301.

Saltman, K. J. (2005). The social construction of adolescence. In E. R. Brown & K. J. Saltman (Eds.), *The critical middle school reader* (pp. 15–20). New York: Routledge.

Seixas, P. (1994). Preservice teachers assess students' prior historical understanding. *Social Studies, 85,* 91–94.

Sleeter, C. (2008). Preparing White teachers for diverse students. In M. Cochran-Smith, S. Feiman-Nemser, & J. McIntyre (Eds.), *Handbook of research on teacher education: Enduring issues in changing contexts* (3rd ed., pp. 559–582). New York: Routledge.

VanSledright, B. (2002). *In search of America's past: Learning to read history in elementary school.* New York: Teachers College Press.

Wilson, S. M. (1991). Parades of facts, stories of the past: What do novice history teachers need to know? In M. M. Kennedy (Ed.), *Teaching academic subjects to diverse learners* (pp. 99–116). New York: Teachers College Press.

Yeager, E., & Wilson, E. (1997). Teaching historical thinking in the social studies methods course: A case study. *Social Studies, 88*(3), 121–127.

ABOUT THE AUTHORS

Hilary G. Conklin is an Assistant Professor of Social Studies Education at DePaul University. Her research interests include teacher learning, the preparation of middle school social studies teachers, and the pedagogy of teacher education.

Todd S. Hawley is an Assistant Professor in the Department of Teaching, Learning, and Curriculum Studies at Kent State University. His research focuses on rationale-development as a core theme of graduate and undergraduate social studies teacher education.

Dave Powell is an Assistant Professor in the Education Department at Gettysburg College, where he teaches courses in social studies methods, secondary methods, educational psychology, teacher action research, and history.

Jason K. Ritter is Assistant Professor of Social Studies Education in the Department of Instruction and Leadership at Duquesne University, Pittsburgh, PA, 15282. His scholarly interests include social studies, teacher education, professional development, democratic citizenship, and qualitative research.

ILLUSTRATIVE EXAMPLE QUESTIONS

1. What is the purpose of the article?
2. What type of research approach is used?
3. How is information gathered in the interviews?
4. How is information gathered in the focus groups?
5. Describe the findings as reported by the researchers.
6. What do the authors report as implications for teacher education?
7. Describe how the action research approach is applied to this study.
8. Discuss the practice of including interview excerpts from individual interviewees in the research article. Is it an effective way to convey themes derived from the study? Are there any potential problems with the practice of including interview excerpts?
9. Do the authors arrive at reasonable findings? How do you know?
10. Do you think the findings yield any additional recommendations that the authors could have made regarding implications for practice, policy, and research?

ADDITIONAL RESEARCH EXAMPLES

1. Lane, K. L., Wehby, J. H., Robertson, E. J., & Rogers, L. A. (2007). How do different types of high school students respond to school-wide positive behavior support programs? *Journal of Emotional and Behavioral Disorders, 15*, 3–20.

2. Little, M. E., & King, L. M. (2008). Using online modules to bridge research to practice in classrooms. *Teacher Education and Special Education, 31*, 208–223.

3. Louis, K. S., Thomas, E., Gordon, M. F., & Febey, K. S. (2008). State leadership for school improvement: An analysis of three states. *Educational Administration Quarterly, 44*, 562–592.

Glossary

A-B design: A single-case design that combines the "A" condition or baseline/preintervention measurements with a "B" condition to determine the effectiveness of an intervention.

A-B-A/withdrawal design: A single-case design that combines the "A" condition or baseline/preintervention measurements with a "B" condition or intervention to determine the effectiveness of the intervention; the "B" condition is followed by a second "A" condition.

A-B-A-B design: A single-case design that combines the "A" condition or baseline/preintervention measurements with a "B" condition or intervention to determine the effectiveness of the intervention, returns to a second "A" condition, then ends with a return to the "B" intervention.

A-B-C-B design: A single-case design that combines the "A" condition or baseline/preintervention measurements with a "B" condition or intervention; the first two conditions are followed by a "C" condition to allow for the control of extra attention a participant may have received during the "B" condition.

Action research: Research that involves application of the scientific method to everyday problems in the classroom or other applied settings; personnel are involved directly with the implementation of the research.

Alpha level: Statistical significance level chosen before data are gathered and analyzed for failing to accept (or to reject) the null hypothesis; also called the Type I error rate.

Alternating treatments design: A single-case design presents two or more conditions in rapidly alternating succession (e.g., on alternating days) to determine differences between the conditions; also called the multielement design.

Alternative hypothesis: States that there are no differences between two groups of data.

Analysis of covariance (ANCOVA): Used to control for initial differences between or among groups statistically before a comparison is made; makes groups equivalent with respect to one or more control variables (potential explanatory variables).

Analysis of variance (ANOVA): A powerful parametric test of statistical significance that compares the means of two or more sets of scores to determine whether the difference between them is statistically significant at the chosen alpha level.

Applied research: Research that attempts to solve real-life problems or study phenomena that directly impact what practitioners or laypeople do by using a theory developed through basic research.

Arithmetic mean (or average): Obtained by summing the scores for a data set and dividing by the number of participants or entities in that data set; takes into account all scores in the data set.

Attenuation: The lowering of the correlation coefficient because of the unreliability of the measure.

Authority: Information is gathered based on the views of "experts" in the field.

B-A-B design: A single-case design in which the "B" condition or intervention is followed by an "A" condition or baseline/preintervention, then ends with a second "B" condition.

Backward elimination multiple regression: This procedure starts with all of the independent variables in the regression model and sequentially removes each one if it meets established criteria for removal and if the independent variable does not meet the established criteria for removal, it remains in the regression model.

Baseline: In single-case designs, "A" refers to the baseline, the level at which the participant performs a behavior without the intervention; the repeated measurement of a behavior under natural conditions.

Basic research: Research that focuses on more theoretical issues; used to develop a new theory or refine an existing one.

Beta (β): Significance level for accepting (or failing to reject) the null hypothesis; also called the Type II error rate.

Beta weights: Standardized regression coefficients (i.e., the regression coefficients that would be obtained if independent variables were equal to one another in terms of means and standard deviations) that enable direct comparisons of the relative relationship of each of the independent variables and the dependent variable.

Boolean rules: *See* Logical operators.

Box-and-whiskers display: A display using a schematic box plot with some auxiliary features to depict the distribution of effect sizes.

Canonical correlation: Correlation procedure used when researchers are interested in determining the relationship between a *set* of independent variables and a *set* of dependent variables.

Carryover effects: Occur when an intervention used in one experimental condition influences behavior in an adjacent condition, not because the interventions are equal in effectiveness or one intervention was clearly less effective than the other, but because the effectiveness of one intervention improves or harms the performance of the other intervention.

Case study designs: A type of field-oriented investigation that involves an in-depth study of a single participant or group of participants; considered to be qualitative in nature.

Causal–comparative research: A research method involving comparison of two groups drawn from the same population that differ on a critical variable but are otherwise comparable. Causal–comparative research seeks to determine whether two or more groups differ on some critical variable.

Causism: Making claims that a causal relationship will be found.

Chain sampling: *See* Snowball sampling.

Changing-criterion design: A single-case experimental design achieved by following the initial baseline with a series of intervention phases with successive and gradually changing criteria.

Chi-square test (χ^2): A nonparametric test of statistical significance that compares the number of participants, objects, or responses that fall into two or more categories, each with two sets of data to determine whether the difference in the relative frequency of the two sets of data in a given category is statistically significant at the chosen alpha level.

Clinical replication: An investigation that involves the combination of two or more independent variables to form an intervention package.

Closed-ended questions: In surveys or interviews, respondents are asked to select their answers from among those provided by the researchers.

Cluster sampling frames: In survey research, sampling frames in which the sampling is done in two or more stages (i.e., cluster sampling); in the first stage(s), researchers sample something other than the individuals to be surveyed; in one or more stages, these primary units are sampled from which a final sample is selected.

Coefficient of alienation: The proportion of variance of one variable that is *not* predictable from the variance of another variable; calculated as the square root of $1 - r^2$.

Coefficient of determination: The proportion of predictable variance obtained by squaring the obtained correlation coefficient r^2 and multiplying it by 100; allows one to state that a certain percentage of the variance of one variable is predictable from the variance of the other variable.

Coefficient of equivalence (or alternative or parallel forms reliability): A measure of the magnitude of the relationship between participants' scores on two analogous forms of the measurement device.

Coefficient of internal consistency: The tendency of different items to evoke the same response from any given participant on a single administration of the measurement device.

Coefficient of stability (or test–retest reliability): A magnitude of relationship measure determined by administering the measurement device to a sample of individuals, then readministering the device to the same sample after some time delay.

Comparison group: In causal–comparative research, the group that does not possess the subject or organismic characteristic under study.

Complete observer observation: Similar to the types of observations used in single-case investigations; when one is a complete observer, there is an attempt to remain separated from the subject matter.

Complete participant observation: Observers become involved with participants as if they are part of the group; participants usually do not know they are being observed.

Concurrent validity: A type of criterion-related validity that determines the extent to which the measurement device may be used to estimate an individual's present standing on a criterion variable.

Confirming and disconfirming cases (sampling technique): In qualitative research, confirming and disconfirming cases involve the attempt to confirm what was found during the exploratory state of the investigation; once some conclusions have been drawn from the data (in field work or from other sources, such as stakeholders), these conclusions should be confirmed or disconfirmed by sampling cases that either confirm or disconfirm the earlier interpretations.

Construct validity: The extent to which a measurement device can be shown to measure a hypothetical construct.

Content validity: The representativeness of the sample of items included in the measurement device.

Contextual variable: Characteristics of the intervention and research methodology, such as the duration of the intervention, who implemented the intervention (e.g., experimenter vs. practitioner), level of training, and type of experimental design or dependent variable, that may affect the findings.

Contingency coefficient: Correlation coefficient that assesses the relationship between nominal variables.

Control group: In a controlled experiment, the group that receives no treatment or a treatment different from that of the experimental group.

Convenience sampling: Selecting participants for a sample because they are easy to access.

Convenience sampling frames: In survey research, sampling frames in which the individuals sampled do something or go somewhere that enables researchers to administer a survey to them; this class of sampling frame differs from the exhaustive sampling frame, in that there is not an advance list from which researchers can sample; rather, the creation of the list or inventory of the members of the population and sampling occur simultaneously.

Correlation coefficient: The statistic that describes the relationship between two variables (is there a relationship between x and y?); a descriptive statistic; a given sample is represented with the italic letter r, and the population value is represented by the Greek letter ρ (rho).

Correlation ratio (η^2): The proportion of the total variability in the dependent variable that can be accounted for by knowing the value of the independent variable in correlational research.

Correlational research: A type of research investigation used to determine the strength of the relationship between/among variables; uses correlation as the statistical method.

Counterbalanced design: A quasi-experimental design in which two or more groups get the same independent variable(s), but the independent variable(s) is/are introduced in different orders.

Covariation: If a researcher applies an intervention to one behavior, there should not be a corresponding change in the other behavior (called covariation).

Criterion: In a changing-criterion design, the level set by the researcher that the participant must attain before moving on to a higher or lower level.

Criterion-referenced test: A test that compares a participant's score to some predetermined standard (criterion) or mastery level.

Criterion-related validity: The extent to which an individual's score on a measurement device is used to predict his/her score on another measurement device.

Criterion sampling: In qualitative research, setting a criterion of performance for individuals; those who meet or surpass the criterion are included in the sample.

Criterion variable: In correlational research, the object of the research (dependent variable)—the variable about which researchers seek to discover more information.

Critical case sampling: Identifying critical cases that are particularly important for some reason.

Critical research consumer: An individual who is able to think critically about research and make conclusions based on the research findings.

Critical thinking: The ability to take a topic, consider both sides of the issue, and make an informed decision on the topic.

Curvilinear relationship: Nonlinear relationship between or among variables as noted on a scattergram used in correlational research.

Data-based decision making: In fields such as special education and rehabilitation, a term used for making changes in how we teach (instruction) based on how our students are doing (assessment).

Data dropping: Data that contradict a researcher's theory or prediction are dropped from the study; outliers are dropped from the study; a subset of data is excluded from analysis.

Deductive logic: Moving from the general to the specific; involves the construction of a theory followed by testing parts of the theory to determine whether results of the testing uphold the theory.

Dependent variable: When trying to determine whether X caused Y, Y would be the effect and, thus, the dependent variable; the variable that is affected by the independent variable (occurs or results from this other variable).

Descriptive research: *See* Naturalistic research.

Descriptive statistics: Allows for the simple and parsimonious mathematical description of a data set, including central tendency, variation, and shape of the distribution.

Descriptive validity: The factual accuracy of the researcher's or observer's account; the concern here is whether the data gathered are contrived or distorted; others should be able to agree that the events or situations occurred.

Deviant case sampling: *See* Extreme case sampling.

Diffusion of treatment: A threat to the internal validity of a study when the independent variable is applied when it is not intended.

Direct instruction: A comprehensive system of instruction that focuses on active student involvement, mastery of skills, empirically validated curricula, and teacher-directed activities.

Direct replication: An investigation conducted in the same manner as a previous experiment.

Directional hypothesis: The population parameter (e.g., mean) that is stated to be greater or smaller than the other population parameter is then tested by collection and analysis of data.

Discriminant function analysis: A type of multiple regression employed when the dependent variable is nominal in nature; the goal is to identify the best set of independent variables that maximizes the correct classification of participants/objects.

Distribution: Any set of scores that has been organized in a way that enables the shape of the data to be seen.

Document analysis: Obtaining data from any number of written or visual sources, such as diaries, novels, incident reports, pictures, advertisements, speeches, official documents, files, films, audiotapes, books, newspapers, and so on.

Ecological validity: Generalizing the results of a study to other environmental conditions.

Effect size: A statistical procedure for determining the magnitude of the difference between two or more groups.

Efficiency evaluation: An assessment to determine whether a program is conducted in a cost-effective way; deals with questions of cost.

Empiricism: Gathering information by gaining knowledge through the observation of our world; it is the information we gain from our senses.

Ethnography: A type of research investigation that involves an intense and in-depth study of an intact cultural group in a natural setting over a prolonged period of time by collecting observational and/or interview data.

Evaluative validity: Making valid statements that fit with the public's evaluation.

Exhaustive sampling frames: In survey research, sampling frames in which the sampling is done from a more or less complete list of individuals in the population to be studied; this typically occurs when the population is small or clearly defined, and the list is used by researchers to select a sample.

Experimental control: Demonstrating that the independent variable produced changes in the dependent variable while decreasing the possibility of extraneous factors producing the results.

Experimenter effects: Are threats in which there is a lack of information that someone other than the person implementing the independent variable will have the same success.

Experimental group: In a controlled experiment, the group that receives the treatment (independent variable).

Experimental research methods: A type of research investigation that is quantitative in nature, typically placing a number of participants into one or several groups; also called group designs; the highest level of constraint research.

External criticism: Authenticity of the information obtained; has to do with the choice of sources historical researchers will read—they must be authentic.

External generalizability: The ability to generalize to other communities or groups.

External validity: Is concerned with the generalizability of a study; asks the question, "What is the generalizability of the results of a study?"

Extraneous variables: Factors not designed (unplanned) to be in a study that may influence the results.

Extreme or deviant case sampling: Selecting cases that are the most outstanding successes or failures related to some topic of interest, because they are expected to yield especially valuable information about the topic of interest.

Fabricating data: "Inventing" data or changing values of data to support a particular viewpoint.

Factor analysis: A multivariate statistical method used to identify unobserved or latent variables; its purpose is to identify a structure or pattern within a set of variables.

Factorial experimental design: A design that assesses the effects of two or more independent variables or the interaction of participant characteristics with the independent variable; used to determine whether the effect of a particular variable studied concurrently with other variables will have the same effect as it would when studied in isolation.

Field notes: Participant observations recorded as facts or direct descriptions of what is seen and/or overheard (this can also be in the form of audio recordings or the observer's thoughts about the events and interviews).

Field-oriented studies: Studies conducted in applied settings wherein the researcher gathers information about a phenomenon (e.g., a person, group of people, or event), as well as all contextual factors that influence the phenomenon.

Formative evaluation: Measures taken during the development of a project to improve effectiveness and use resources efficiently.

Forward selection multiple regression: The first variable entered into the regression model is the one with the largest positive or negative relationship with the dependent variable; if the first variable selected for entry meets the established criterion (alpha level established by the researcher) for inclusion in the model, forward selection continues; if the independent variable does not meet the criterion for inclusion in the model, the procedure terminates with no variables in the regression model; in this case, none of the independent variables is predictive of the dependent variable.

Functional relationship: When a change is produced in the independent variable (intervention), it is reliably followed by changes in the dependent variable.

General interview guide approach: This type of interview involves having an outline of topics to be covered during the interview; however, the order in which the topics are addressed is not set; the questions are not formulated beforehand; the purpose of outlines or guides is to aid interviewers in addressing each of the topics.

Generalizability (generalization): Ability to transfer results of an investigation to other situations/contexts/times.

Grounded theory: A theory that is generated from data during the research process.

Hawthorne effect: Occurs when participants are aware that they are in an experiment and/or are being assessed.

Historical research: Involves a systematic process of researching data from the past that can help us understand what is going on now and what may occur in the future; geared to describe relations, to correct inaccurate conclusions from other historical reports, or to explain what has occurred in the past.

History threat: A threat to the internal validity of a study when anything other than the independent variable occurs between the pretest and the posttest or during implementation of the independent variable and affects a participant's performance.

Homogeneity of variance: Equivalent score variances for the populations under study (an assumption of parametric tests).

Homogeneous sampling: The opposite of maximum variation sampling, in that participants similar to one another are selected to decrease variation within the sample (in qualitative research).

Hyperclaiming: When researchers tell interested parties that the research they are conducting is likely to achieve specific goals that are unlikely.

Hypothesis: A prediction made by researchers about expected results in future investigations of the phenomenon.

Independent variable: When trying to determine whether X caused Y, X is what the researcher manipulates or is interested in observing, and is thus the independent variable; the variable that produces changes in a dependent variable.

Inductive logic: Moving from the specific to the general; used in the formulation of theories after supporting research data are collected in a systematic fashion.

Inferential statistics: Allow for statistical inference; that is, researchers are able to generalize their results to the larger population or make an "inference" about the population based on the responses of the experimental sample.

Informal conversational interview: This type of interview usually occurs with participant observation in the field and is the most open-ended interviewing method; it proceeds as a conversation in which interviewers ask spontaneous questions; there is no structured format, although interviewers should have some notion of the type of information they desire; in some instances, those being interviewed may be unaware of the interview.

Informed consent: Participant recruitments should be voluntary and include a complete understanding of the investigation, risks involved, and requirements imposed by the study; if participants are underage or not competent to provide informed consent, a parent or legal guardian may provide this; informed consent provides the freedom to accept or decline participation in a study after making an informed decision.

Institutional review board (IRB): A group of professionals who assess the level of risk to participants in an investigation and make sure that ethical safeguards are in place. Required by any institution receiving federal funding; as well as by the government for federally funded agencies under federal definitions and regulations governing research by such agencies.

Instrumentation threat: May threaten the internal validity of a study when there is a change in calibration of the instrument used in measurement.

Interaction effect: The effect of an independent variable on a dependent variable that is influenced by one or more other independent variables.

Interaction of personological variables and treatment effects: Occurs when the independent variable has a differential effect on members of the experimental group dependent on their characteristics.

Internal criticism: Accuracy of the information obtained; documents are examined with the intent of making sure they are judged correctly.

Internal generalizability: The ability to generalize within the community or group being investigated to those not directly involved in the investigation.

Internal validity: Indicates a functional relationship between the independent variable and the dependent variable; addresses the question, "Did the treatment make the difference or was the change due to something else?"

Interobserver agreement: A direct comparison of behavior when observers record the occurrence and nonoccurrence of specific behaviors.

Interpretive validity: Concerned with the subjective meanings of objects, events, and behaviors to the individuals engaged in and with the objects, events, and behaviors; specifically relevant to qualitative research.

Interval scale: Scale of measurement that provides equal intervals between equidistant points on a scale yet lacks an absolute zero point.

Intervention: The "B" or intervention condition is the time that the independent variable is in effect; the treatment.

Interview study: A study in which direct interaction between the researcher and participant involves oral questions to the interviewer and oral responses by the participant.

Intuition: Information is gathered based on a "feeling" one gets about a topic.

Kendall coefficient of concordance: Correlation coefficient used when researchers want to establish the relationship among the rankings of several variables.

Kendall part rank correlation: Correlation coefficient used when researchers want to control the influence of a third variable on the relationship between two variables; similar to the part correlation, except that it is appropriate when the variables are measured on at least ordinal scales rather than interval or ratio scales.

Kendall rank correlation coefficient: Referred to as τ, or tau; correlation coefficient that provides a measure of the disparity in the rankings between two variables and is computed by ranking the scores for each of the variables from smallest to largest and computing the Pearson product–moment correlation coefficient on the ranks.

Kruskal–Wallis ANOVA: A nonparametric test of statistical significance that compares the medians or means of three or more sets of scores (at least ordinal scale).

Level of constraint: The degree to which the researcher imposes limits or controls on any part of the research process; involves a continuum from low constraints to high constraints.

Linear relationship: A straight line that can be visualized in the middle of the values of scores running from one corner to another in a scattergram in correlational research.

Literature search: Gathering sources to use in an introduction of a journal article or in a research synthesis.

Logical operators: Terms used in a search strategy when conducting research syntheses that greatly affect the particular primary studies identified; bibliographical services provide guides to their services for these terms.

Main effect: The effect of an independent variable by itself on a dependent variable.

Mann–Whitney *U* test: A nonparametric test of statistical significance that compares the medians or means of two sets of scores to determine whether the difference between them is statistically significant at the chosen alpha level.

Matching: Equating two or more groups of participants on a variable to rule out the variable's influence.

Maturation threat: A threat to the internal validity of a study when due to the passage of time biological or psychological changes take place in participants.

Maximum variation sampling: Capturing and describing the central themes or principle outcomes that cut across a great deal of participant or program variation.

Measurement error: Fluctuations in scores because the measurement device does not measure an attribute the same way every time; unknown and unrepeatable causes of variability in task performance over time and context.

Median: The point at which half of the scores fall above and half fall below; it is not affected by extreme scores in the data set.

Mixed-methods studies: Involve collecting, analyzing, and mixing both quantitative and qualitative methods in a study.

Mode: The most frequently occurring score in a data set.

Mortality: Differential loss of participants due to death, selective elimination of scores of some group members, or withdrawal of participants.

Multielement design: *See* Alternating treatments design.

Multiple-baseline design: An experimental design that starts with measurement of two or more behaviors in a baseline condition, followed by application of an independent variable to one of the behaviors, while baseline conditions remain in effect for other behaviors. The independent variable is then applied in a sequential fashion to other behaviors.

Multiple-probe design: Essentially a multiple-baseline design in which the measurements do not occur on a frequent basis; overcomes the problem of using repeated measurements by probing (assessing) the behavior intermittently; probes are also used in assessing generalization/transfer or maintenance of intervention effects; a single-case design.

Multiple regression: An extension of the correlation coefficient in which the overall and relative degree of relationship between a set of independent variables (nominal, ordinal, interval, or ratio in nature) and a dependent variable (interval or ratio in nature) is determined.

Multiple treatment interference threat: Occurs when multiple independent variables are used together.

Multitreatment design: A single-case design that allows for the comparison of two or more interventions or the additive components of an intervention after baseline data are taken (e.g., A-B-A-C-A or A-B-A-B-BC-B-BC); considered an associate of the withdrawal design.

Narrative: A written representation of observed phenomena.

Naturalistic observation study: A study that involves observing participants unobtrusively in their natural settings; there is no attempt to manipulate what goes on in the setting.

Naturalistic research: A type of research investigation that typically occurs in the participant's natural setting; typically considered qualitative in nature.

Needs assessment: Identifying the level of existing needs within an organization or program; the goal is to look for potential but unavailable services for an identified population of individuals.

Nominal scale: Scale of measurement in which numbers simply act as identifiers, names, or labels.

Nondirectional hypothesis: A difference between two population parameters is stated but no direction is specified before collecting and analyzing the data.

Nonequivalent control-group design: A quasi-experimental design is similar to the pretest–posttest control-group design except for the absence of the random selection of participants from a population and the random assignment of participants to groups.

Nonparametric test: A test of statistical significance that does not rely on assumptions such as the shape or variance of the population scores.

Nonparticipant observation study: A study in which the observer's presence is unknown to the participants.

Nonprobability sampling: The likelihood of any individual, object, or event of the population being selected is unknown.

Normal distribution: A purely theoretical distribution obtained by plotting theoretically obtained probabilities across the whole range of possible values from minus infinity to plus infinity along the horizontal axis.

Novelty and disruption effects: Are threats when participants react to changes in the experimental situation as opposed to the independent variable.

Null hypothesis: A statement that there is no difference between variables being studied or between the values of a population parameter.

Observation study: A study in qualitative research in which an observer or observers work in the field to gather information about a phenomenon.

Observer-as-participant observation: Involves observers remaining separate from participants, but participants are informed that they will be observed; these methods of observation overcome the ethical problem of complete observation; however, observers also risk reactivity on the part of the participants as a result of being aware that they are being observed.

Observer bias: Recording what is seen inaccurately because of a preexisting attitude or experience.

Observer drift: Occurs when observers change the way they employ the definition of behavior over the course of a study.

Observer effects: Problems that may bias the reliability or validity of the data collected by observers.

One-group pretest–posttest design: A preexperimental design that differs from the one-shot case study, in that a pretest measure is administered prior to introduction of the independent variable.

One-shot case study: A preexperimental design in which introduction of an independent variable to a group of participants is followed by measurement of the dependent variable.

Open-ended questions: In surveys or interviews, the respondents are asked to provide their own answers to the questions.

Ordinal scale: Scale of measurement in which numbers represent a rank ordering of those objects/individuals of interest.

Outcome evaluation: Use of person- and organization-referenced outcomes to determine current and desired person- and program-referenced outcomes, the extent to which a program meets goals and objectives, and whether a program has made a difference.

Outlier: An individual or other entity whose score differs considerably from the scores obtained by the other participants or entities of the sample.

Parameter: Numerical description of a population's scores on some characteristic.

Parametric test: A type of test of statistical significance that makes certain assumptions about population parameters, including normal distribution of scores about the mean, equal population variances, and interval or ratio scale data.

Part correlation: A correlation coefficient that establishes the relationship between two variables after the influence or effect of another variable has been removed from one but not both variables.

Partial correlation: Differs from the part correlation in that it enables researchers to establish the relationship between two variables after the influence or effect of a third variable has been removed from both.

Participant-as-observer observation: Involves observers engaging with participants and also informing participants of their intent to observe them.

Participant observation study: A study in which the observer becomes personally acquainted with the participants.

Path analysis: Advanced statistic used to determine the amount of variance in a dependent variable that can be accounted for by a set of independent variables; in contrast to multiple regression, path analysis has the additional aim of determining whether the pattern of shared variances among the independent and dependent variables is consistent with particular causal pathways.

Personological variable: A variable related to characteristics of people in the sample.

Phenomenology: The study of how people come to understand events in their lives.

Phi coefficient: A correlation coefficient that assesses the relationship between nominal variables.

Pilot test: A "trial run" of an investigation to determine potential problems before an investigation is conducted formally; in survey research, finding out how the survey instrument works under realistic conditions.

Population: A group of potential participants, objects, or events to whom or to which researchers want to generalize the results of a study derived from a sample drawn from the population.

Population validity: The ability to generalize results of a study from a sample to a larger group of individuals; includes two types—generalization across participants and interaction of personological variables and treatment effects.

Posttest-only control-group design: A true experimental design similar to the pretest–posttest-only control-group design, with the exception that pretests of the dependent variable are not administered to the experimental and control groups.

Posttest sensitization: Occurs when the posttest makes the independent variable more effective than it would have been without the posttest.

Power: Detecting a difference when one is actually present, or correctly rejecting the null hypothesis; mathematically, Power = 1 − Type II error rate, or β.

Predictive validity: A type of criterion-related validity that determines the extent to which the measurement device may be used to estimate an individual's future standing on a criterion variable.

Predictor variable: In correlational research, the independent variable; variables in which participants' scores enable prediction of their scores on some criterion variable.

Preexperimental design: A research design that differs from true experimental designs and two of the quasi-experimental designs (i.e., counterbalanced and time-series) in that it does not include a control group.

Pretest sensitization: Occurs when the pretest makes the independent variable more effective than it would have been without the pretest.

Pretest–posttest control group design: A true experimental design that includes measurement of the dependent variable before and after implementation of the independent variable.

Primary sources: Sources of information used in historical research, including oral testimony of individuals who were present at the time, documents, records, and relics.

Probability sampling: The likelihood of any one individual, object, or event of the population being selected is known.

Probability value: The level of significance actually obtained; indicated by the symbol p; a higher level of statistical significance corresponds to a lower p value.

Process evaluation: Assessment of the extent to which a program has been implemented, serves the identified population, and operates as expected.

Program evaluation: A systematic process of collecting and analyzing data on the quality or effectiveness of programs, products, or practices for purpose of making decisions.

Proportion of nonoverlapping data (PND): An index of the magnitude of the intervention in research reviews using single-case research; the number of data points that exceed the highest baseline data point in the expected direction divided by the total number of intervention data points in the intervention phase.

Purposeful sampling (or purposive sampling): Deliberately selecting particular persons, events, or settings for the important information they provide.

Qualitative research: Research concerned with understanding the context in which behavior occurs, not just the extent to which it occurs; the assessment may be more subjective, in that the dependent variables are not necessarily defined in observable terms; the data are collected in the natural setting; meanings and understandings are reached by studying cases intensively; inductive logic is used to place the resulting data in a theoretical context.

Quantitative research: Research involving an attempt to gather information in an objective manner; the research is usually conducted in a group format; quantitative research comes from a scientific–rational perspective; the method of gathering data is strictly prescribed, and the resulting data are subjected to a statistical analysis.

Quasi-experimental design: An experimental design in which participants are neither randomly selected from the specified population nor randomly assigned to experimental and control groups.

Random assignment: Every individual, object, or event that comprises a sample has an equiprobability of being included in each group (treatment or control).

Random sample: Every individual, object, or event has an equiprobability of being included in the sample.

Range: The difference between the largest and smallest scores.

Ratio scale: Scale of measurement that provides equal intervals between equidistant points on a scale and has an absolute-zero point.

Rationalism: Information is gathered by interpreting or understanding the world around us through our reasoning processes.

Reactivity: Differences in interobserver agreement that result from observers being aware that their observations will be checked.

Refereed journal: A journal that accepts articles that have undergone a peer-review process; this process typically includes feedback from an editor and members of a review or editorial board.

Regression line (line of best fit): A line drawn on a scattergram to show the general relationship or trend in the data; provides an average statement about how a change in one variable affects another variable.

Reliability: Consistency of results over time.

Replication: The primary method scientists use to determine the reliability and usefulness of their findings and to discover mistakes.

Research integrity: The degree to which researchers adhere to the rules, laws, regulations, guidelines, and commonly accepted professional codes and norms of their respective research areas.

Research question: If a study is not designed to test a hypothesis, a researcher may formulate a question to frame a study (e.g., "Does Direct Instruction produce high reading scores as compared to whole language instruction?").

Research synthesis: Pulling together the facts and findings from a group of related studies based on different (1) theoretical frameworks, (2) independent variables, (3) dependent measures, (4) research designs, and (5) data analysis procedures.

Response rate: The number of people surveyed (or interviewed) divided by the total number of individuals sampled multiplied by 100. The numerator includes all the individuals who were selected and did respond; the denominator includes all the individuals who were selected but did not respond for whatever reason.

Restriction of range: The restricted or abbreviated variability (variance) of one variable reduces the correlation coefficient between the two variables.

Reversal design: A single-case design in which the researcher changes the level of participant behavior during the "B" condition, such as reinforcing behavior that is the opposite of desired behavior rather than simply removing the intervention.

Sample: A subset of the population.

Sampling error: A group's scores may be different each time the group is sampled; the difference between the characteristics of the sample and those of the population.

Sampling frame: The set of people (it is always people in the case of survey research) that has the chance to be selected, given the sampling procedure(s) used by researchers; the population or defined list from which the sample will be drawn.

Sampling politically important cases: A variation of the critical case strategy used in qualitative research; researchers attempt to select a politically sensitive site or analyze a politically sensitive topic; in some cases, researchers may attempt to avoid the politically sensitive site or topic.

Sampling population: The population to which the sample survey results will be generalized.

Scattergram: The plotted scores of two variables on a graph visually depicting the degree of relationship between the two variables or the extent to which they covary.

Science: The search for understanding the world around us; the attempt to find order and lawful relations in the world; a method of viewing the world; the testing of our ideas in a public forum.

Scientific method: A method of gaining information that includes five steps: (1) identifying the problem, (2) defining the problem, (3) formulating a hypothesis or research question, (4) determining observable consequences of the hypothesis or research question, and (5) testing the hypothesis or attempting to answer the research question.

Scientific theory: A theory that is falsifiable or refutable; it must be able to be disproven.

Secondary sources: Sources of information used in historical research, including reports that relay information from people who were present during a historical period, reports from individuals who have read information from the past, and books about the period under question, such as history books and encyclopedias.

Selection threat: A threat to the internal validity of a study when groups of individuals are selected in a differential manner.

Self-management: Procedures designed to help an individual change and/or maintain his/her own behavior (e.g., self instruction involves individuals talking themselves through tasks to complete them correctly and more efficiently).

Significance level (called alpha): This probability enables researchers to interpret how unlikely the difference might be due to sampling or measurement (chance) errors (symbolized α).

Simulation: The creation or recreation of a situation to see how participants react under such circumstances.

Single-case research: A type of research investigation that relies on the intensive examination of a single individual or a group of individuals, uses objective data collection techniques, and may be thought of as a combination of qualitative and quantitative designs.

Snowball sampling: Also called chain sampling; involves asking others who would be a good choice to be involved in the sample.

Social validity: Research is considered to have social validity when society deems it to be important.

Solomon four-group design: A true experimental design that essentially combines the pretest–posttest control-group design and the posttest-only control-group design; two groups serve as experimental groups and two groups serve as control groups.

Spearman rank correlation coefficient: Referred to as ρ; the correlation coefficient that provides a measure of the disparity in the rankings between two variables and is computed by ranking the scores for each of the variables from smallest to largest and computing the Pearson product–moment correlation coefficient on the ranks.

Stakeholders: People who have a vested interest in the design, implementation, and results of an investigation.

Standard deviation: Symbolized as *SD*; a statistic that describes how much the scores are spread out (distributed) around the mean; the larger the standard deviation, the more "spread out" the scores.

Standard error of measurement: An estimate of the variability of an individual's score when the measurement device is administered over and over again.

Standardized open-ended interview: This type of interview involves not only set topics, similar to the general interview guide, but also predeveloped questions that researchers ask throughout the interview; each participant is exposed to the same topics and questions in the same order.

Standardized test: A test that has established procedures for administration, scoring, and interpretation for consistency across testing situations.

Static-group comparison design: A quasi-experimental design that is the same as the posttest-only control-group design except for the absence of the random selection of participants from a population and random assignment of participants to groups.

Statistical regression: A threat to the internal validity of a study that occurs when participants deviate from the norm or are extreme on some attribute.

Statistical significance: The probability that results of a study are likely or unlikely because of chance factors due to sampling or measurement error.

Statistical validity: Occurs when research results reach a certain level of confidence (pertains to the probability of obtaining the results of the investigation by chance and not some systematic variable).

Stepwise selection multiple regression: A combination of the forward selection and backward elimination procedures; stepwise selection is the most commonly used procedure; the first independent variable for consideration in the regression model is selected in the same manner as in the forward selection procedure; if the independent variable does not meet the established criteria for inclusion, the procedure is terminated, with no

independent variables in the regression model; if the independent variable meets the established criteria for inclusion in the regression model, the second independent variable is selected based on the highest partial correlation.

Structural equation modeling (LISREL): Statistical methodology that enables researchers to take a confirmatory approach to correlational research; includes the use of regression models to represent the causal relationships under study; LISREL stands for Linear Structural Relationships, a structural equation modeling computer program.

Summative evaluation: Measures taken to determine the worth of a fully developed program.

Survey: The most widely used research method within and outside the social sciences; used to identify how people feel, think, act, and vote; useful for collecting information from relatively large numbers of dispersed groups of people rather than a small number, as in the case of other research methods.

Synthesis of information: Involves organizing information, making conclusions, and, finally, making generalizations.

Systematic replication: An investigation conducted by different researchers and/or persons implementing the independent variable, involving participants with different characteristics than those in the original investigation and/or in a different setting than the original experiment.

Systematic research syntheses: Paralleling the methodologies used in original research studies, in that researchers conduct research syntheses using a set of standard procedures to guide their efforts; in this way, the procedures are much more systematic in nature.

Systematic variance: Variability we can account for between or among groups of people; this variability makes a group of individuals move in the same direction; may involve the independent variable or extraneous variables.

Tenacity: Information gathered is based on the persistence of a certain belief or way of thought for a long period of time.

Testing threat: A threat to the internal validity of the study when participants show improvement on a posttest simply due to the effects of taking the pretest.

Theoretical validity: Maintaining integrity to ensure accurate interpretation of data; theories go beyond the data in that they attempt to provide an explanation for what is observed; one is concerned with taking descriptions and interpretations, and constructing a grounded theory to help explain the phenomenon.

Theory: A simple guess in which the person stating the theory is making some prediction or explanation; a model derived to help understand a phenomenon; an explanatory system that describes the data gathered.

Time-series design: Quasi-experimental designs involving a series of repeated measurements of a group of research participants.

Triangulation: Collecting data from multiple sources and methods in order to increase the strength of themes, including using both quantitative and qualitative approaches; a combination of data collection methods (e.g., observation, interview, and document analyses) is used, so that the strength of one method can compensate for weakness of another method.

True experimental design: An experimental design that involves random selection of participants from the population to form a sample, random assignment of participants to experimental and control conditions, and equal treatment of both groups with the exception of the implementation of the independent variable.

t-test: A powerful parametric test of statistical significance that compares the means of two sets of scores to determine whether the difference between them is statistically significant at the chosen alpha level.

Type I error: Occurs when researchers incorrectly conclude that the differences between groups are due to chance factors.

Type II error: Occurs when researchers incorrectly conclude that the differences between groups are due to chance factors.

Typical case sampling: Selecting one or more typical cases for a sample; what is typical is decided by significant others (parents, teachers, community leaders, administrators, etc.) in the setting.

Unit of analysis: The focus of the research, such as a group of individuals treated as one case or each individual case.

Unsystematic research syntheses: The few, if any, formal procedures and practices used by researchers to review the literature for research syntheses.

Unsystematic variance: Variability within individuals and/or groups of individuals; it is essentially random; it may involve individual differences or measurement error.

Validity: The degree to which accurate inferences are based on the results of a study; relates to the question, "Does the measure assess what it purports to measure?"

Variability: The amount of dispersion or fluctuation in a set of scores.

Variable: A research expression for the construct or object of interest that varies in observable phenomena.

Variance: Calculated by squaring the standard deviation; a statistic that describes how much the scores are spread out (distributed) around the mean.

Verification of the independent variable: Refers to measuring the extent to which the independent variable was implemented as described.

Vote counting: Method of integrating studies in a research synthesis to provide information on the results of statistical significance testing.

Whole-language approach: A philosophical approach to teaching and learning that emphasizes immersion (in the context of use), collaboration between learners and teachers, writing across the curriculum, and authentic materials and tasks.

Wilcoxon signed rank test: A nonparametric test of statistical significance that compares the medians or means of two sets of scores considered to be related in some fashion.

Withdrawal/A-B-A design: A single-case design that combines the "A" condition or baseline/preintervention measurements with a "B" condition or intervention to determine the effectiveness of the intervention; the "B" condition is followed by a second "A" condition.

References

Abedi, J., & Herman, J. (2010). Assessing English language learners' opportunity to learn mathematics: Issues and limitations. *Teacher's College Record, 112,* 723–746.

Adler-Baeder, F. (2007). *Smart steps: Embrace the journey.* Auburn, AL: National Stepfamily Resource Center.

Agodini, R., & Harris, B. (2010). An experimental evaluation of four elementary school math curricula. *Journal of Research on Educational Effectiveness, 3,* 199–253.

Aldiabat, K. M., & Le Navenec, C. L. (2011). Philosophical roots of classical grounded theory: Its foundations in symbolic interactionism. *The Qualitative Report, 16,* 1063–1080.

Allison, P. D. (1999). *Multiple regression: A primer.* Thousand Oaks, CA: Sage.

American Educational Research Association (AERA). (2004). *Ethical standards of the American Educational Research Association.* Retrieved from *www.aera.net/uploadedfiles/about_aera/ethical_standards/ethical-standards.pdf.*

American Educational Research Association (AERA), American Psychological Association, & National Council on Measurement in Education. (1999). *Standards for educational and psychological testing.* Washington, DC: American Psychological Association.

American Psychological Association. (2010). *Publication manual of the American Psychological Association* (6th ed.). Washington, DC: Author.

American Psychological Association. (2010). *Ethical principles of psychologists and code of conduct.* Washington, DC: Author.

Anastasi, A. (1982). *Psychological testing* (5th ed.). New York: Macmillian.

Anderson, S. W., Damasio, H., Tranel, D., & Damasio, A. R. (2000). Long-term sequelae of prefrontal cortex damage acquired in early childhood. *Developmental Neuropsychology, 18,* 281–296.

Arbuckle, J. L. (1999). *Amos 4.0* [Computer software]. Chicago: Smallwaters.

Ayres, K. M., Langone, J., Boon, R. T., & Norman, A. (2006). Computer-based instruction for purchasing skills. *Education and Training in Developmental Disabilities, 41,* 253–263.

Barclay, L., Herlich, S. A., & Sacks, S. Z. (2010). Effective teaching strategies: Case studies from the alphabetic Braille and contracted Braille study. *Journal of Visual Impairment and Blindness, 104,* 753–764.

Barlow, D. H., Nock, M., & Hersen, M. (2008). *Single case experimental designs: Strategies for studying behavior change* (3rd ed.). New York: Allyn & Bacon.

Barry, C. A. (1998). Choosing qualitative data analysis software: Atlas.ti and Nudist compared. *Sociological Research Online, 3.* Retrieved from *www.socresonline.org.uk/socresonline/3/3/4.html.*

Basham, R. E., Jordan, C., & Hoefer, R. A. (2009). Reliability and validity in quantitative measurement. In B. A. Thyer (Ed.), *The handbook of social work research methods* (pp. 51–64). Thousand Oaks, CA: Sage.

Bassett, R. (2004). Qualitative data analysis software: Addressing the debates. *Journal of Management Systems, 16,* 33–39.

Bast, J., & Reitsma, P. (1998). Analyzing the development of individual differences in terms of Matthew effects in reading: Results from a Dutch longitudinal study. *Developmental Psychology, 34,* 1373–1399.

Belfiore, P. J., Fritts, K. M., & Herman, B. C. (2008). The role of procedural integrity: Using self-monitoring to enhance discrete trial instruction (DTI). *Focus on Autism and Other Developmental Disabilities, 23,* 95–102.

Bellini, S., Peters, J. K., Benner, L., & Hopf, A. (2007). A meta-analysis of school-based social skills interventions for children with autism spectrum disorders. *Remedial and Special Education, 28,* 153–162.

Bentler, P. M. (2000). *EQS 6 structural equations program manual.* Encino, CA: Multivariate Software.

Biemiller, A., & Boote, C. (2006). An effective method for building meaning vocabulary in primary grades. *Journal of Educational Psychology, 98,* 44–62.

Bogdan, R. C., & Biklen, S. K. (1998). *Qualitative research for education: An introduction to theory and methods* (3rd ed.). Needham Heights, MA: Allyn & Bacon.

Bogdan, R. C., & Taylor, S. J. (1975). *Introduction to qualitative methods.* New York: Wiley.

Bornstein, R. F. (1999). Criterion validity of objective and projective dependency tests: A meta-analytic assessment of behavior prediction. *Psychological Assessment, 11,* 48–57.

Box, G. E. P., Hunter, J. S., & Hunter, W. G. (2005). *Statistics for experimenters: Design, innovation, and discovery* (2nd ed.). Hoboken, NJ: Wiley.

Brantlinger, E., Jimenez, R., Klingner, J., Pugach, M., & Richardson, V. (2005). Qualitative studies in special education. *Exceptional Children, 71,* 195–207.

Breault, D., & Breault, R. (2010). Partnership for preparing leaders: What can we learn from PDS research? *International Journal of Leadership in Education, 13,* 437–454.

Brigance, A. (1991). *Revised Brigance Diagnostic Inventory of Early Development.* North Billerica, MA: Curriculum Associates.

Buckley, M. R. (2010). Grounded theory methodology. In C. J. Sheperis, J. S. Young, & M. H. Daniels (Eds.), *Counseling research: Quantitative, qualitative, and mixed methods* (pp. 115–134). Boston: Pearson.

Burke, M. D., Hagan-Burke, S., Kwok, O., & Parker, R. (2009). Predictive validity of early literacy indicators from the middle of kindergarten to second grade. *Journal of Special Education, 42,* 209–226.

Bushman, B. J., & Wang, M. C. (2009). Vote-counting procedures in meta-analysis. In H. Cooper, L. V. Hedges, & J. C. Valentine (Eds.), *The handbook of research synthesis and meta-analysis* (pp. 207–220). New York: Russell Sage Foundation.

Byrne, B. M. (2001). Structural equation modeling with AMOS, EQS, and LISREL: Comparative approaches to testing for the factorial validity of a measuring instrument. *International Journal of Testing, 1,* 55–86.

Campbell, D. T., & Stanley, J. C. (1963). *Experimental and quasi-experimental designs for research.* Boston: Houghton Mifflin.

Cannell, C. F., Marquis, K. H., & Laurent, A. (1977). *A summary of studies of interviewing methodology* (Vital and Health Statistics, Series 2, No. 69; DHEW Publication No. HRA 77–1343). Washington, DC: U.S. Government Printing Office.

Carey, R. F. (1980). Commentary: Empirical vs. naturalistic research? *Reading Research Quarterly, 15,* 412–415.

Carver, R. (1978). The case against statistical significance testing. *Harvard Educational Review, 48,* 378–399.

Carver, R. (1993). The case against statistical significance testing, revisited. *Journal of Experimental Education, 61*(4), 287–292.

Chalmers, I., Hedges, L. V., & Cooper, H. (2002). A brief history of research synthesis. *Evaluation and the Health Professions, 25,* 12–37.

Chandon, P., Morwitz, V. G., & Reinartz, J. (2005). Do intentions really predict behavior?: Self-generated validity effects in survey research. *Journal of Marketing, 69,* 1–14.

Chapman, J. W., & Tunmer, W. E. (1995). Development of young children's reading self-concepts: An examination of emerging subcomponents and their relation with reading achievement. *Journal of Educational Psychology, 87,* 154–167.

Chenail, R. J. (2011). How to conduct clinical qualitative research on the patient's experience. *The Qualitative Report, 16,* 1173–1190.

Chiesa, M. (1994). *Radical behaviorism: The philosophy and the science.* Boston: Authors Cooperative.

Childs, K. E., Kincaid, D., & George, H. P. (2010). A model for statewide evaluation of a universal positive behavior support initiative. *Journal of Positive Behavior Interventions, 12,* 198–210.

Chisholm, R. F., & Elden, M. (1993). Features of emerging action research. *Human Relations, 46,* 275–297.

Cho, J., & Trent, A. (2006). Validity in qualitative research revisited. *Qualitative Research, 6,* 319–340.

Christensen, T. M., & Brumfield, K. A. (2010). Phenomenological designs: The philosophy of phenomenological research. In C. J. Sheperis, J. S. Young, & M. H. Daniels (Eds.), *Counseling research: Quantitative, qualitative, and mixed methods* (pp. 135–150). Boston: Pearson.

Cicchetti, D., Bronen, R., Spencer, S., Haut, S., Berg, A., Oliver, P., et al. (2006). Rating scales, scales of measurement, issues of reliability: Resolving some critical issues for clinicians and researchers. *Journal of Nervous and Mental Disease, 194,* 557–564.

Clark, M. A., Lee, S. M., Goodman, W., & Yacco, S. (2008). Examining male underachievement in public education: Action research at a district level. *NASSP Bulletin, 92,* 111–132.

Clark, M. A., Oakley, E., & Adams, H. (2006). The gender achievement gap challenge. *ASCA School Counselor, 43*(3), 20–25.

Clark, P., & Kirk, E. (2000). All-day kindergarten: Review of research. *Childhood Education, 76*(4), 228–231.

Coelho, R. J., & LaForge, J. (2000). Manuscript characteristics affecting reviewers' decisions for rehabilitation counseling-related journals. *Journal of Rehabilitation, 66,* 4–8.

Cohen, J., Cohen, P., West, S. G., & Aiken, L. S. (2003). *Applied multiple regression/correlation analysis for the behavioral sciences* (3rd ed.). Mahwah, NJ: Erlbaum.

Cohen, L., Manion, L., & Morrison, K. (2007). *Research methods in education* (6th ed.). Oxford, UK: Routledge.

Connors, R. J. (1992). Dreams and play: Historical method and methodology. In G. Kirsch & P. Sullivan (Eds.), *Methods and methodology in composition research* (pp. 15–36). Carbondale: Southern Illinois University.

Cook, T. D., & Campbell, D. T. (1979). *Quasi-experimentation: Design and analysis issues for field settings.* Chicago: Rand McNally.

Cooper, H. (2010). *Research synthesis and meta-analysis: A step-by-step approach.* Thousand Oaks, CA: Sage.

Cooper, H., Allen, A. B., Patall, E. A., & Dent, A. L. (2010). Effects of full-day kindergarten on academic achievement and social development. *Review of Educational Research, 80,* 34–70.

Cooper, H., & Hedges, L. V. (2009). Research synthesis as a scientific process. In H. Cooper, L. V. Hedges, & J. C. Valentine (Eds.), *The handbook of research synthesis and meta-analysis* (2nd ed., pp. 3–16). New York: Russell Sage Foundation.

Cooper, J. O., Heron, T. E., & Heward, W. L. (2007). *Applied behavior analysis* (2nd ed.). Upper Saddle River, NJ: Pearson, Merrill, Prentice Hall.

Corbin, J., & Strauss, J. (2007). *Basics of qualitative research: Techniques and procedures for developing grounded theory.* Thousand Oaks, CA: Sage.

Cozby, P. C. (2008). *Methods in behavioral research* (9th ed.). Boston: McGraw-Hill.

Creswell, J. W. (2009). *Research design: Qualitative, quantitative, and mixed methods approaches* (3rd ed.). Thousand Oaks, CA: Sage.

Creswell, J. W., & Plano-Clark, V. L. (2007). *Designing and conducting mixed methods research.* Thousand Oaks, CA: Sage.

Daniel, L. G. (1998). Statistical significance testing: A historical overview of misuse and misinterpretation with implications for the editorial policies for educational journals. *Research in the Schools, 5*(2), 23–32.

Del Giudice, M. (2011). Sex differences in romantic attachment: A meta-analysis. *Personality and Social Psychology Bulletin, 37,* 193–214.

Dellinger, A. B., & Leech, N. L. (2007). Toward a unified validation framework in mixed methods research. *Journal of Mixed Methods Research, 1,* 309–332.

Denzin, N. K., & Lincoln, Y. S. (Eds.). (2005). *The sage handbook of qualitative research* (3rd ed.). Thousand Oaks, CA: Sage.

De Winter, A. F., Oldehinkel, A. J., Veenstra, R., Brunnekreff, J. A., Verhulst, F. C., & Ormel, J. (2005). Evaluation of non-response bias in mental health determinants and outcomes in a large sample of pre-adolescents. *European Journal of Epidemiology, 20,* 173–181.

Dochy, F., Segers, M., Van den Bossche, P., & Gijbeis, D. (2003). Effects of problem-based learning: A meta-analysis. *Learning and Instruction, 13,* 533–568.

Dodge, K. A. (1991). The structure and function of reactive and proactive aggression. In D. J. Pepler & K. H. Rubin (Eds.), *The development and treatment of childhood aggression* (pp. 201–218). Hillsdale, NJ: Erlbaum.

Drake, S. (1958). Galileo gleanings III: A kind word for Sizzi. *JSTOR, 49*(2), 155–165.

Dunst, C. J., & Trivette, C. M. (2009). Using research evidence to inform and evaluate early childhood intervention practices. *Topics in Early Childhood Special Education, 29,* 40–52.

Education Commission of the States. (2004). *The progress of education reform 2004: Kindergarten: Full-day kindergarten programs improve chances of academic success.* Denver, CO: Author.

Eisner, E. W. (1991). *The enlightened eye: Qualitative inquiry and the enhancement of educational practice.* Upper Saddle River, NJ: Merrill/Prentice Hall.

Elden, M., & Chisholm, R. F. (1993). Emerging varieties of action research: Introduction to the special issue. *Human Relations, 46,* 121–141.

Emerson, E. (2003). Mothers of children and adolescents with intellectual disability: Social and economic situation, mental health status, and the self-addressed social and psychological impact of the child's difficulties. *Journal of Intellectual Disability Research, 47,* 385–399.

Emerson, R. W., Holbrook, M. C., & D'Andrea, F. M. (2009). Acquisition of literacy skills by young children who are blind: Results of the ABC Braille Study. *Journal of Visual Impairment and Blindness, 103,* 610–624.

Erseg-Hurn, D. M., & Mirosevich, V. M. (2008). Modern robust statistical methods: An easy way to maximize the accuracy and power of your research. *American Psychologist, 63,* 591–601.

Faraone, S. V., Biederman, J., & Roe, C. (2002). Comparative efficacy of Adderall and Methylphenidate in attention-deficit/hyperactivity disorder: A meta-analysis. *Journal of Clinical Psychopharmacology, 22,* 468–473.

Faul, F., Erdfelder, E., Lang, A., & Buchner, A. (2007). G*power 3: A flexible statistical power analysis program for the social, behavioral, and biomedical sciences. *Behavior Research Methods, 39,* 175–191.

Federal Register. (2005). *49 CFR Part 11. Federal Policy for the Protection of Human Subjects: Notices and Rules, 70*(120), 36325–36328.

Feeney, T. J., & Ylvisaker, M. (2008). Context-sensitive cognitive-behavior supports for young children with TBI: A second replication study. *Journal of Positive Behavior Interventions, 10,* 115–128.

Ferguson, G. A. (1989). *Statistical analysis in psychology and education* (6th ed.). New York: McGraw-Hill.

Fetterman, D. M. (1989). *Applied social research methods series: Vol. 17. Ethnography step by step.* Newbury Park, CA: Sage.

Feuer, M. J., Towne, L., & Shavelson, R. J. (2002). Scientific culture and educational research. *Educational Researcher, 31,* 4–14.

Fielding, N. G., & Lee, R. M. (1998). *Computer analysis and qualitative research: New technology for social research.* London: Sage.

Finn, C. A., & Sladeczek, I. E. (2001). Assessing the social validity of behavioral interventions: A review of treatment acceptability measures. *School Psychology Quarterly, 16,* 176–206.

Fischer, F. (1998). Beyond empiricism: Policy inquiry in postpositivist perspective. *Policy Studies Journal, 26,* 129–146.

Fitz-Gibbon, C. T. (2003). Milestones en route to evidence-based policies. *Research Papers in Education, 18*, 313–329.

Fleischmann, M., Pons, S., & Hawkins, M. (1989). Electrochemically induced nuclear fusion of deuterium. *Journal of Electroanalytical Chemistry and Interfacial, 261*, 301–308.

Fossey, D. (2000). *Gorillas in the mist.* New York: Houghton Mifflin.

Fowler, F. J. (2009). *Survey research methods* (4th ed.). Thousand Oaks, CA: Sage.

Fraenkel, J. R., & Wallen, N. E. (2000). *How to design and evaluate research in education* (4th ed.). Boston: McGraw-Hill.

Franklin, C., & Jordan, C. (1995). Qualitative assessment: A methodological review. *Families in Society, 76*, 281–295.

Galison, P. (1997). *Image and logic: A material culture of microphysics.* Chicago: University of Chicago.

Gall, M. D., Gall, J. P., & Borg, W. R. (2007). *Educational research: An introduction* (8th ed.). Boston: Pearson Education.

Gall, M. D., Gall, J. P., & Borg, W. R. (2010). *Applying educational research* (6th ed.). Boston: Pearson.

Gardner, H. (2006). *Multiple intelligences: New horizons.* New York: Basic Books.

Gast, D. L. (2010). *Single subject research methodology in behavioral sciences.* New York: Routledge.

Gast, D. L., Wellons, J., & Collins, B. C. (1994). Home and community safety skills. In M. Agran, N. E. Marchand-Martella, & R. C. Martella (Eds.), *Promoting health and safety: Skills for independent living* (pp. 11–32). Baltimore: Brookes.

Gast, D. L., & Wolery, M. (1988). Parallel treatment design: A nested single subject design for comparing instructional procedures. *Education and Treatment of Children, 11*, 270–285.

Gay, L. R., Mills, G. E., & Airasian, P. (2009). *Educational research: Competencies for analysis and applications.* Upper Saddle River, NJ: Merrill/Pearson.

Gersten, R., Fuchs, L. S., Compton, D., Coyne, M., Greenwood, C., & Innocenti, M. S. (2005). Quality indicators for group experimental and quasi-experimental research in special education. *Exceptional Children, 71*, 149–164.

Gilbride, D., Stensrud, R., Vandergoot, D., & Golden, K. (2003). Identification of the characteristics of work environments and employers open to hiring and accommodating people with disabilities. *Rehabilitation Counseling Bulletin, 46*, 130–137.

Glaser, B. G. (2002). Constructivist grounded theory? *Forum: Qualitative Social Research, 3*(3), 1–12.

Glass, G. V. (1976). Primary, secondary, and meta-analysis of research. *Educational Researcher, 5*, 3–8.

Glass, G. V., McGaw, B., & Smith, M. L. (1981). *Meta-analysis in social research.* Beverly Hills, CA: Sage.

Glass, G. V., Wilson, V. L., & Gottman, J. M. (2008). *Design and analysis of time-series experiments.* Charlotte, NC: Information Age.

Good, R. H., & Kaminski, R. A. (2002). *Dynamic indicators of basic early literacy* (6th ed.). Eugene, OR: Institute for the Development of Educational Achievement.

Gould, S. J. (1996). *The mismeasure of man* (2nd ed.). New York: Norton.

Graham, S., & Perin, D. (2007). What we know, what we still need to know: Teaching adolescents to write. *Scientific Studies of Reading, 11*, 313–335.

Graziano, A. M., & Raulin, M. L. (2010). *Research methods: A process of inquiry* (7th ed.). Boston: Pearson.

Greene, J. C., & Caracelli, V. J. (1997). *Advances in mixed-method evaluation: The challenges and benefits of integrating diverse paradigms.* (New Directions for Evaluation, No. 74). San Francisco: Jossey-Bass.

Grimshaw, J. (1993). Effect of clinical guidelines on medical practice: A systematic review of rigorous evaluations. *Lancet, 342*, 1317–1322.

Hagermoser-Sanetti, L. M., Gritter, K. L., & Dobey, L. M. (2011). Treatment integrity of interventions with children in school psychology literature from 1995 to 2008. *School Psychology Review, 40*, 72–84.

Hammond, J. L., Iwata, B. A., Fritz, J. N., & Dempsey, C. M. (2011). Evaluation of fixed momentary DRO schedules under signaled and unsignaled arrangements. *Journal of Applied Behavior Analysis, 44*, 69–81.

Hansen, D. L., & Morgan, R. L. (2008). Teaching grocery store purchasing skills to students with intellectual disabilities using a computer-based instruction program. *Education and Training in Developmental Disabilities, 43*, 431–442.

Hart, J. E., Cramer, E. D., Harry, B., Klingner, J. K., & Sturges, K. M. (2010). The continuum of "troubling" to "troubled" behavior: Exploratory case studies of African American students in programs for emotional disturbance. *Remedial and Special Education, 31*, 148–162.

Hattie, J., & Marsh, H. W. (1996). The relationship between research and teaching: A meta-analysis. *Review of Educational Research, 66*, 507–542.

Hays, D. G., & Wood, C. (2011). Infusing qualitative traditions in counseling research designs. *Journal of Counseling and Development, 89*, 288–295.

Hedges, L. V., & Vevea, J. L. (1998). Fixed- and random-effects models in meta-analysis. *Psychological Methods, 3*, 486–504.

Hemond-Reuman, E., & Moilanen, D. (1992). *The Academic Self-Efficacy Scale.* Unpublished manuscript, Boston College, Chestnut Hill, MA.

Hendrick, C. (1990). Replications, strict replications, and conceptual replications: Are they important? *Journal of Social Behavior and Personality, 5*(4), 41–49.

Henson, R. K. (2001). Understanding internal consistency reliability estimates: A conceptual primer on coefficient alpha. *Measurement and Evaluation in Counseling and Development, 34*, 177–189.

Hernan, M. A., & Wilcox, A. J. (2009). Epidemiology, data sharing, and the challenge of scientific replication. *Epidemiology, 20*, 167–168.

Hewitt, M. (2007). Influence of primary performance instrument and education level on music performance evaluation. *Journal of Research in Music Education, 55,* 18–30.

Holland, P. W., & Thayer, D. T. (2000). Univariate and bivariate loglinear models for discrete test score distributions. *Journal of Education and Behavioral Statistics, 25,* 133–183.

Horner, R. D., & Baer, D. B. (1978). Multiple-probe technique: A variation of the multiple baseline. *Journal of Applied Behavior Analysis, 11,* 189–196.

Horner, R. D., Carr, E. G., Hale, J., McGee, G., Odom, S., & Wolery, M. (2005). The use of single-subject research to identify evidence-based practice in special education. *Exceptional Children, 71,* 165–179.

Horner, R. H., Carr, E. G., Strain, P. S., Todd, A. W., & Reed, H. K. (2002). Problem behavior interventions for young children with autism: A research synthesis. *Journal of Autism and Developmental Disorders, 32,* 423–446.

Horner, R. H., Sugai, G. & Lewis-Palmer, T. (2005). School-wide positive behavior support evaluation template. Retrieved from *http://www.pbis.org.*

Hotelling, H. (1935). The most predictable criterion. *Journal of Educational Psychology, 26,* 139–142.

Howe, K., & Eisenhart, M. (1990). Standards for qualitative (and quantitative) research: A prolegomenon. *Educational Researcher, 19,* 2–9.

Huberty, C. J. (1987). On statistical testing. *Educational Researcher, 16*(8), 1–9.

Huberty, C. J. (1993). Historical origins of statistical testing practices: The treatment of Fisher versus Neyman–Pearson views in textbooks. *Journal of Experimental Education, 61,* 317–333.

Human Services Research Institute. (2001). *Consumer survey phase II technical report.* Retrieved from *www. hsri.org/cip/doc/phaseII_consumer_survey_report_new.pdf.*

Humphreys, P. (2004). *Extending ourselves: Computational science, empiricism, and scientific method.* New York: Oxford University Press.

Hunter, J. E., & Schmidt, F. L. (2004). *Methods of meta-analysis: Correcting error and bias in research findings* (2nd ed.). Thousand Oaks, CA: Sage.

Idrees, I., Vasconcelos, A. C., & Cox, A. M. (2011). The use of grounded theory in PhD research in knowledge management: A model four-stage research design. *Aslib Proceedings: New Information Perspectives, 63,* 188–203.

Jackson, S. L. (2011). *Research methods and statistics: A critical thinking approach* (4th ed.). *www.cengage.com.*

Jankowski, N. W., & Wester, F. (1991). The qualitative tradition in social science inquiry: Contributions of mass communications research. In K. B. Jensen & N. W. Jankowski (Eds.), *A handbook of qualitative methodologies for mass communication research* (pp. 44–74). New York: Routledge.

Jensen, K. B., & Jankowski, N. W. (Eds.). (1991). *A handbook of qualitative methodologies for mass communication research.* New York: Routledge.

Johns, J. (2005). *Basic reading inventory.* Dubuque, IA: Kendall/Hunt.

Johnson, D. H. (1999). The insignificance of statistical significance testing. *Journal of Wildlife Management, 63,* 763–772.

Johnson, N. L., Kemp, A. W., & Kotz, S. (2005). *Univariate frequency distributions* (3rd ed.). Hoboken, NJ: Wiley.

Johnson, R. B., & Onwuegbuzie, A. (2001). Mixed methods research: A research paradigm whose time has come. *Educational Researcher, 33,* 14–26.

Johnston, J. M., & Pennypacker, H. S. (1993). *Strategies and tactics of human behavioral research* (2nd ed.). Hillsdale, NJ: Erlbaum.

Jones, S. R. G. (1992). Was there a Hawthorne effect? *American Journal of Sociology, 98,* 451–468.

Joreskog, K. G., & Sorborn, D. (2001). *LISREL 8: New statistical features.* Hillsdale. NJ: Erlbaum.

Juvonen, J., Wang, Y., & Espinoza, G. (2011). Bullying experiences and compromised academic performance across middle school grades. *Journal of Early Adolescence, 31,* 152–173.

Kaplan, B., & Maxwell, J. A. (2005). Qualitative research methods for evaluating computer information systems. In J. G. Anderson, C. E. Aydin, & S. J. May (Eds.), *Evaluating health care information systems: Methods and applications* (pp. 30–55). Thousand Oaks, CA: Sage.

Kazdin, A. E. (2003). *Research design in clinical psychology.* Boston: Allyn & Bacon.

Kazdin, A. E. (2008). Evidence-based treatment and practice: New opportunities to bridge clinical research and practice, enhance knowledge base, and improve patient care. *American Psychologist, 63,* 149–159.

Kellogg Foundation. (2004). *Logic model development guide: Using logic models to bring together planning, evaluation, and action.* Battle Creek, MI: Author.

Kemper, E. A., Stringfield, S., & Teddlie, C. (2003). Mixed methods sampling strategies in social science research. In A. Tashakkori & C. Teddlie (Eds.), *Handbook of mixed methods in social and behavioral research* (pp. 273–296). Thousand Oaks, CA: Sage.

Kennedy, D. (2003). Research fraud and public policy. *Science, 300,* 393.

Keppel, G. (1973). *Design and analysis: A researcher's handbook.* Englewood, CA: Prentice-Hall.

Keselman, H. J., Huberty, C. J., Lix, L. M., Olejnik, S., Cribble, R. A., Donahue, B., et al. (1998). Statistical practices of educational researchers: An analysis of ANOVA, MANOVA, and ANCOVA analyses. *Review of Educational Research, 68,* 350–386.

Kim, T., & Horn, E. (2010). Sibling-implemented intervention for skill development with children with disabilities. *Topics in Early Childhood Special Education, 30,* 80–90.

Kitchener, R. F. (1994). Semantic naturalism: The

problem of meaning and naturalistic psychology. In W. F. Overton & D. S. Palermo (Eds.), *The nature and ontogenesis of meaning* (pp. 279–293). Hillsdale, NJ: Erlbaum.

Kline, R. (2011). *Principles and practice of structural equation modeling* (3rd ed.). New York: Guilford Press.

Klingner, J. K. (2006). *Why are so many minority students in special education?: Understanding race and disability in schools*. New York: Teachers College Press.

Koenig, A. J., & Farrenkopf, C. (1995). *Assessment of Braille literacy skills*. Houston, TX: Region IV Education Service Center, Special Education Department.

Kubiszyn, T., & Borich, G. (2007). *Educational testing and measurement: Classroom application and practice* (8th ed.). Hoboken, NJ: Wiley.

Lancy, D. F. (1993). *Qualitative research in education: An introduction to the major traditions*. New York: Longman.

Lane, K. L., Bocian, K. M., MacMillian, D. L., & Gresham, F. M. (2004). Treatment integrity: An essential—but often forgotten—component of school-based interventions. *Preventing School Failure, 48*(3), 36–43.

Lane, K. L., Rogers, L. A., Parks, R. J., Weisenbach, J. L., Mau, A. C., Merwin, M. T., et al. (2007). Function-based interventions for students who are nonresponsive to primary and secondary prevention efforts: Illustrations at the elementary and middle school levels. *Journal of Emotional and Behavioral Disorders, 15*, 169–183.

Lawlor, D. A., Smith, G. D., & Ebrahim, S. (2004). Commentary: The hormone replacement–coronary heart disease conundrum: Is this the death of observational epidemiology? *International Journal of Epidemiology, 33*(3), 464–467.

Le, V. N., Kirby, S. N., Barney, H., Setodji, C. M., & Gershwin, D. (2006). *School readiness, full-day kindergarten, and student achievement: An empirical investigation*. Santa Monica, CA: RAND.

Lease, S. H., & Dahlbeck, D. T. (2009). Parental influences, career decision-making attributions, and self-efficacy: Differences for men and women? *Journal of Career Development, 36*, 95–113.

Ledford, J. R., & Wolery, M. (2011). Teaching imitation to young children with disabilities: A review of the literature. *Topics in Early Childhood Special Education, 30*, 245–255.

Lee, V. E., & Bryk, A. S. (1989). Effects of single-sex secondary schools: Response to Marsh. *Journal of Educational Psychology, 81*, 647–650.

Leech, N. L., & Onwuegbuzie, A. J. (2011). Beyond constant comparison qualitative data analysis: Using NVivo. *School Psychology Quarterly, 26*, 20–84.

Leitenberg, H. (1965). Is time-out from positive reinforcement an aversive event?: A review of experimental evidence. *Psychological Bulletin, 64*, 428–441.

Lent, R. W., Brown, S. D., & Hackett, G. (2002). Social cognitive career theory. In D. Brown & Associates (Eds.), *Career choice and development* (pp. 255–311). San Francisco: Jossey-Bass.

Levin, H. M., & McEwan, P. J. (2000). *Cost-effectiveness analysis: Methods and applications* (2nd ed.). Thousand Oaks, CA: Sage.

Lewin, K. (1946). Action research and minority problems. *Journal of Social Issues, 2*(4), 34–46.

Likins, M., Salzberg, C. L., Stowitschek, J. J., Lignugaris/Kraft, B., & Curl, R. (1989). Co-worker implemented job training: The use of coincidental training and quality-control checking on the food preparation skills of trainees with mental retardation. *Journal of Applied Behavior Analysis, 22*, 381–393.

Lincoln, Y., & Cuba, E. G. (1985). *Naturalistic inquiry*. Beverly Hills, CA: Sage.

Lindlof, T. R. (1991). The qualitative study of media audiences. *Journal of Broadcasting and Electronic Media, 35*(1), 23–42.

Lipsey, M. W., & Wilson, D. B. (2001). *Practical meta-analysis*. Thousand Oaks, CA: Sage.

Littell, J. H., Corcoran, J., & Pillai, V. (2008). *Systematic reviews and meta-analysis*. New York: Oxford University Press.

Logan, K. J., Byrd, C. T., Mazzocchi, E. M., & Gillam, R. B. (2011). Speaking rate characteristics of elementary-school-aged children who do and do not stutter. *Journal of Communication Disorders, 44*, 130–147.

Lorenzo, J. M. P., & Garcia Sanchez, I. M. (2007). Efficiency evaluation in municipal services: An application to the street lighting service in Spain. *Journal of Productivity Analysis, 27*, 149–162.

Lourenco, O., & Machado, A. (1996). In defense of Piaget's theory: A reply to 10 common criticisms. *Psychological Review, 103*, 143–164.

Lu, C. J., & Shulman, S. W. (2008). Rigor and flexibility in computer-based qualitative research: Introducing the coding analysis toolkit. *International Journal of Multiple Research Approaches, 2*, 105–117.

Luckerhoff, J., & Guillemette, F. (2011). The conflicts between grounded theory requirements and institutional requirements for scientific research. *The Qualitative Report, 16*, 396–414.

Ma, H. H. (2006). An alternative method for quantitative synthesis of single-subject researches: Percentage of data points exceeding the median. *Behavior Modification, 30*, 598–617.

Maclean, L., Meyer, M., Estable, A., Kothari, A., & Edwards, N. (2010). These data do not compute. In D. L. Streiner & S. Sidani (Eds.), *When research goes off the rails: Why it happens and what you can do about it* (pp. 309–319). New York: Guilford Press.

Maddaus, G., & Stufflebeam, D. (2002). Program evaluation: A historical overview. *Evaluation in Education and Human Services, 49*, 3–18.

Mari, D. D., & Kotz, S. K. (2001). *Correlation and dependence*. London: Imperial College Press.

Marsh, H. W. (1989a). Effects of single-sex and coeducational high schools on achievement, attitudes, behaviors, and sex differences. *Journal of Educational Psychology, 81,* 70–85.

Marsh, H. W. (1989b). Effects of single-sex and coeducational schools: A response to Lee and Bryk. *Journal of Educational Psychology, 81,* 651–653.

Marshall, C., & Rossman, G. B. (2011). *Designing qualitative research* (5th ed.). Thousand Oaks, CA: Sage.

Martella, R. C., Leonard, L. J., Marchand-Martella, N. E., & Agran, M. (1993). Self-monitoring negative statements. *Journal of Behavioral Education, 3,* 77–86.

Martella, R. C., Marchand-Martella, N. E., & Agran, M. (1992). Problem-solving to prevent work injuries in supported employment. *Journal of Applied Behavior Analysis, 25,* 637–645.

Martella, R. C., Nelson, J. R., Marchand-Martella, N., & O'Reilly, M. (2012). *Comprehensive behavior management: Individualized, classroom, and schoolwide approaches* (2nd ed.). Thousand Oaks, CA: Sage.

Mason, R. O., McKenney, J. L., & Copeland, D. G. (1997, September). An historical method for MIS research: Steps and assumptions. *MIS Quarterly,* pp. 307–319.

Maxwell, J. A. (1992). Understanding and validity in qualitative research. *Harvard Educational Review, 62*(3), 279–300.

Maxwell, J. A. (1997). Designing a qualitative study. In L. Bickman & D. J. Rog (Eds.), *Handbook of applied social research methods* (pp. 69–100). Thousand Oaks, CA: Sage.

Maxwell, J. A. (2004). Causal explanation, qualitative research, and scientific inquiry in education. *Educational Researcher, 33*(2), 3–11.

Maxwell, J. A. (2005). *Qualitative research design: An interactive approach.* Thousand Oaks, CA: Sage.

Maxwell, J. A. (2010). Using numbers in qualitative research. *Qualitative Inquiry, 16,* 475–482.

McAuly, L., Pham, B., Tugwell, P., & Moher, D. (2000). Does the inclusion of grey literature influence estimates of intervention effectiveness in meta-analysis? *Lancet, 356,* 1228–1231.

McBurney, D. H., & White, T. L. (2009). *Research methods* (6th ed.). Belmont, CA: Thomson/Wadsworth.

McLean, J. E., & Ernest, J. M. (1998). The role of statistical significance testing in educational research. *Research in the Schools, 5*(2), 15–22.

Means, B., Toyama, Y., Murphy, R., Bakia, M., & Jones, K. (2009). *Evaluation of evidence-based practices in online learning: A meta-analysis and review of online learning students.* Washington, DC: U.S. Department of Education, Office of Planning, Evaluation, and Policy Development.

Medina, M., & Escamilia, K. (1992). English acquisition by fluent and limited Spanish-proficient Americans in a 3-year maintenance bilingual program. *Hispanic Journal of Behavioral Sciences, 14,* 252–267.

Mertens, D. M. (2009). *Research and evaluation in education and psychology: Integrating diversity with quantitative, qualitative, and mixed methods* (3rd ed.). Thousand Oaks, CA: Sage.

Mertler, C. A., & Charles, C. M. (2011). *Introduction to educational research* (7th ed.). Thousand Oaks, CA: Sage.

Messick, S. (1994). *Validity of psychological assessment: Validation of inferences from persons' responses and performances as scientific inquiry into score meaning* (ERIC Research Report RR 94-45). Retrieved from *http://eric.ed.gov/ericwebportal/search/detailmini.jsp?_nfpb=true&_&ericextsearch_searchvalue_0=ED380496&ericextsearch_searchtype_0=no&accno=ed380496.*

Michaels, M. L. (2000). The stepfamily enrichment program: A preliminary evaluation using focus groups. *American Journal of Family Therapy, 28,* 61–73.

Mishler, E. G. (1990). Validation in inquiry-guided research: The role of exemplars in narrative studies. *Harvard Educational Review, 60,* 415–442.

Morgan, D. (1998). Practical strategies for combining qualitative and quantitative methods: Applications to health research. *Qualitative Health Research, 8,* 362–376.

Morgan, P. L., Fuchs, D., Compton, D. L., Cordray, D. S., & Fuchs, L. S. (2008). Does early reading failure decrease children's reading motivation? *Journal of Learning Disabilities, 41,* 387–404.

Morgan, R. L., & Horrocks, E. L. (2011). Correspondence between video-based preference assessment and subsequent community job performance. *Education and Training in Autism and Developmental Disabilities, 46,* 52–61.

Morris, S. B., & DeShon, R. P. (2002). Combining effect size estimates in meta-analysis with repeated measures and independent-groups designs. *Psychological Methods, 7,* 105–125.

Morse, J. M., Barrett, M., Mayan, M., Olson, K., & Spiers, J. (2002). Verification strategies for establishing reliability and validity in qualitative research. *International Journal of Qualitative Methods, 1*(2), 13–22.

Murphy, L. L., Spies, R. A., & Plake, B. S. (2006). *Tests in print VII.* Lincoln: University of Nebraska Press.

National Center for Educational Statistics. (2001, May). *Statistics in brief: Internet access in U.S. public schools and classrooms, 1994–2000.* Washington, DC: Office of Educational Research and Improvement, U.S. Department of Education.

National Research Council. (1998). *Preventing reading difficulties in young children.* Washington, DC: National Academy Press.

National Research Council. (2002). *Scientific research in education.* Washington, DC: National Academy Press.

Neary, A., & Joseph, S. (1994). Peer victimization and its relationship to self-concept and depression among schoolgirls. *Personality and Individual Differences, 16,* 183–186.

Nelson, J. R., Drummond, M., Martella, R. C., & Marchand-Martella, N. E. (1997). The current and future outcomes of interpersonal social interactions: The views of students with behavioral disorders. *Behavioral Disorders, 22,* 141–151.

Nelson, J. R., Smith, D. J., Young, K. R., & Dodd, J. (1991). A review of self-management outcome studies conducted with students that exhibit behavioral disorders. *Behavioral Disorders, 16*, 169–179.

Nevin, A. (2006). *Reviews of single subject research designs: Applications to special education and school psychology.* Miami: Florida International University, College of Education, Department of Educational and Psychological Services.

Oja, H., & Randles, R. H. (2004). Multivariate nonparametric tests. *Statistical Science, 19*, 598–605.

Olivier, A. (2011). Phenomenology of the human condition. *South African Journal of Philosophy, 30*, 184–196.

Olsson, M. B., & Hwang, C. P. (2008). Socioeconomic and psychological variables as risk and protective factors for parental well-being of children with intellectual disabilities. *Journal of Intellectual Disability Research, 52*, 1102–1113.

Onwuegbuzie, A. J., & Johnson, R. B. (2006). The validity issue in mixed research. *Research in the Schools, 13*, 48–63.

Parker, R. I., & Hagan-Burke, S. (2007). Single case research results as clinical outcomes. *Journal of School Psychology, 45*, 637–653.

Parker, R. I., & Vannest, K. J. (2009). An improved effect size for single case research: Nonoverlap of all pairs (NAP). *Behavior Therapy, 40*, 357–367.

Parker, R. I., Vannest, K. J., & Davis, J. L. (2011). Effect size in single-case research: A review of nine nonoverlap techniques. *Behavior Modification, 35*, 303–322.

Patton, M. Q. (1987). *How to use qualitative methods in evaluation.* Newbury Park, CA: Sage.

Patton, M. Q. (1990). *Qualitative evaluation and research methods.* Newbury Park, CA: Sage.

Patton, M. Q. (2002). *Qualitative research: Encyclopedia of statistics in behavioral science.* New York: Wiley.

Pauly, J. J. (1991). A beginner's guide to doing qualitative research in mass communication. *Journalism Monographs* (No. 125).

Payne, L. D., Scott, T. M., & Conroy, M. (2007). A school-based examination of the efficacy of function-based intervention. *Behavioral Disorders, 32*, 158–174.

Perry, J. C., DeWine, D. B., Duffy, R. D., & Vance, K. S. (2007). The academic self-efficacy of urban youth: A mixed-methods study of a school-to-work program. *Journal of Career Development, 34*, 103–126.

Piaget, J. (2002). *Piaget: The language and thought of a child.* London: Routledge Classics.

Pitman, M. A., & Maxwell, J. A. (1992). Qualitative approaches to evaluation: Models and methods. In M. D. LeCompte, W. L. Millory, & J. Preissle (Eds.), *The handbook of qualitative research in education* (pp. 729–770). San Diego: Academic Press/Harcourt Brace.

Plano-Clark, V. L., & Creswell, J. W. (2010). *Understanding research: A consumer's guide.* Boston: Merrill.

Polman, H., de Castro, B. O., Koops, W., van Boxtel, H. W., & Merk, W. W. (2007). A meta-analysis of the distinction between reactive and proactive aggression in children and adolescents. *Journal of Abnormal Child Psychology, 35*, 522–535.

Ponterotto, J. G., & Ruckdeschel, D. E. (2007). An overview of coefficient alpha and a reliability matrix for estimating adequacy of internal consistency coefficients with psychological measures. *Perceptual and Motor Skills, 105*, 997–1014.

Popper, K. R. (1957/1996). Philosophy of science: A personal report. In S. Sarkar (Ed.), *Science and philosophy in the twentieth century: Decline and obsolescence of logical empiricism* (pp. 237–273). New York: Garland. (Reprinted from *British philosophy in the mid-century: A Cambridge symposium*, pp. 155–191, by C. A. Mace [Ed.], 1957.) New York: Macmillian Norwood Russe.

Popper, K. R. (2002). *The logic of scientific discovery.* London: Routledge Classics.

Posavac, E. J., & Carey, R. G. (2003). *Program evaluation: Methods and case studies* (6th ed.) Upper Saddle River, NJ: Prentice Hall.

Potter, W. J. (1996). *An analysis of thinking and research about qualitative methods.* Mahwah, NJ: Erlbaum.

Potvin, P. J., & Schutz, R. W. (2000). Statistical power for the two-factor repeated measures ANOVA. *Behavior Research Methods, Instruments, and Computers, 32*, 347–356.

Presser, S., Couper, M. P., Lessler, J. T., Martin, E., Martin, J., Rothgeb, J. M., et al. (2004). Methods for testing and evaluating survey questions. *Public Opinion Quarterly, 68*, 109–130.

Prout, H. T., & Nowak-Drabik, K. M. (2003). Psychotherapy with persons who have mental retardation: An evaluation of effectiveness. *American Journal on Mental Retardation, 108*, 82–93.

QSR International Pty Ltd. (2008). *NVIVO: Version 8. Reference guide.* Doncaster Victoria, Australia: Author.

Quesenberry, A. C., Hemmeter, M. L., & Ostrosky, M. M. (2011). Addressing challenging behaviors in Head Start: A closer look at program policies and procedures. *Topics in Early Childhood Special Education, 30*, 209–220.

Rafter, J. A., Abell, M. L., & Braselton, J. P. (2002). Multiple comparison methods for means. *SIAM Review, 44*, 259–278.

Reynolds, C. R. (2010). *Behavior Assessment Scale for Children* (2nd ed.). New York: Wiley Online Library.

Roberts, S., & Pashler, H. (2000). How persuasive is a good fit?: A comment on theory testing. *Psychological Review, 107*, 358–367.

Rosenshine, B., & Meister, C. (1994). Reciprocal teaching: A review of the research. *Review of Educational Research, 64*, 479–530.

Rosenthal, R. (1994a). Parametric measures of effect sizes. In H. M. Cooper & L. V. Hedges (Eds.), *The handbook of research synthesis* (pp. 231–243). New York: Sage.

Rosenthal, R. (1994b). Science and ethics in conducting, analyzing, and reporting psychological research. *Psychological Science, 5,* 127–134.

Rosenthal, R., & Rosnow, R. L. (2009). The volunteer subject. In R. Rosenthal & R. L. Rosnow (Eds.), *Artifacts in behavioral research* (pp. 48–93). New York: Oxford University Press.

Rothstein, H. R., Sutton, A. J., & Borenstein, M. (2006). *Chapter 1. Publication bias in meta-analysis.* Wiley Online Library.

Royce, D., Thyer, B., & Padgett, D. (2010). *Program evaluation: An introduction* (5th ed.). Belmont, CA: Wadsworth.

Rozenberg, S., Vasquez, J. B., Vandromme, J., & Kroll, M. (1998). Educating patients about the benefits and drawbacks of hormone replacement therapy. *Drugs and Aging, 13,* 33–41.

Ruse, M. (2009). Chapter 7—Humans. In C. Darwin, *The descent of man* (pp. 1–6). Oxford, UK: Blackwell.

Salvia, J., Ysseldyke, J. E., & Bolt, S. (2009). *Assessment* (11th ed.). Belmont, CA: Wadsworth Cengage Learning.

Sandbek, T. (2010). *The worry free life.* Retrieved January 19, 2011, from *http://theworryfreelife.blogspot.com/2010/02/scientific-illiteracy.html.*

Saunders, T. C., & Holahan, J. M. (1997). Criteria-specific rating scales in the evaluation of high school instrumental performance. *Journal of Research in Music Education, 45,* 259–272.

Schalock, R. L. (2001). *Outcome-based evaluation* (2nd ed.). New York: Kluwer Academic/Plenum.

Schenker, J. D., & Rumrill, P. D. (2004). Causal-comparative research designs. *Journal of Vocational Rehabilitation, 21,* 117–121.

Schroyens, W., & Schaeken, W. (2003). A critique of Oaksford, Chater, and Larkin's (2000) conditional probability model of conditional reasoning. *Journal of Experimental Psychology, 29,* 140–149.

Scruggs, T. E., & Mastropieri, M. A. (1994). Successful mainstreaming in elementary science classes: A qualitative study of three reputational cases. *American Educational Research Journal, 31,* 785–812.

Scruggs, T. E., Mastropieri, M. A., & Casto, G. (1987). The quantitative synthesis of single-subject research: Methodology and validation. *Remedial and Special Education, 8*(2), 24–33.

Seale, C. (1999). *The quality of qualitative research.* London: Sage.

Seidman, I. (2006). *Interviewing as qualitative research: A guide for researchers in education.* New York: Teachers College, Columbia University.

Shadish, W. R., Cook, T. D., & Campbell, D. T. (2001). *Experimental and quasi-experimental designs for generalized causal inference.* Boston: Houghton Mifflin.

Shalock, R. L., Brown, I., Brown, R., Cummins, R. A., Felce, D., Matikka, L., et al. (2002). Conceptualization, measurement, and application of quality of life for persons with intellectual disabilities: Report

of an international panel of experts. *Mental Retardation, 40,* 457–470.

Sheppard-Jones, K., Prout, H. T., & Kleinart, H. (2005). Quality of life dimensions for adults with developmental disabilities: A comparative study. *Mental Retardation, 43,* 281–291.

Shercliffe, R. J., Stahl, W., & Tuttle, M. P. (2009). The use of meta-analysis in psychology: A superior vintage or the casting of old wine in new bottles? *Theory and Psychology, 19,* 413–430.

Shippen, M. E., Crites, S. A., Houchins, D. E., Ramsey, M. L., & Simon, M. (2005). Preservice teachers' perceptions of including students with disabilities. *Teacher Education and Special Education, 28,* 92–99.

Sidman, M. (1960). *Tactics of scientific research: Evaluating experimental data in psychology.* New York: Basic Books.

Silverman, D. (2005). *Doing qualitative research* (2nd ed.). London: Sage.

Sindelar, P. T., Rosenberg, M. S., & Wilson, R. J. (1985). An adopted alternating treatments design for instructional research. *Education and Treatment of Children, 8,* 67–76.

Skinner, B. F. (1963). Operant behavior. *American Psychologist, 18,* 503–515.

Skinner, B. F. (1972). Current trends in experimental psychology. In *Cumulative record: A selection of papers* (3rd ed., pp. 295–313). New York: Appleton–Century–Crofts. (Original work published 1947)

Skogard, L., Torres, E., & Higginbotham, B. J. (2010). Stepfamily education: Benefits of a group-formatted intervention. *The Family Journal, 18,* 234–240.

Slavin, R. E. (1994). *Educational psychology: Theory and practice.* Needham Heights, MA: Allyn & Bacon.

Smith, J. A., Osborn, M., & Flowers, P. (1999). Doing interpretative phenomenological analysis. In M. Murray & K. Chamberlain (Eds.), *Qualitative health psychology: Theories and methods* (pp. 218–240). London: Sage.

Smith, M. L., & Glass, G. V. (1977). Meta-analysis of psychotherapy outcome studies. *American Psychologist, 32,* 752–760.

Smith, S. G., & Cook, S. L. (2008). Disclosing sexual assault to parents: The influence of parental messages about sex. *Violence Against Women, 14,* 1326–1348.

Soodak, L. C., Podell, D. M., & Lehman, L. R. (1998). Teacher, student, and school attributes as predictors of teachers' responses to inclusion. *Journal of Special Education, 31,* 480–497.

Spence, J. C., Burgess, J., Rodgers, W., & Murray, T. (2009). Effect of pretesting on intentions and behaviour: A pedometer walking intervention. *Psychology and Health, 24,* 777–789.

Spies, R. A., & Plake, B. S. (Eds.). (2005). *The sixteenth mental measurements yearbook.* Lincoln: The University of Nebraska Press.

Stake, R. E. (1995). *The art of case study research.* Thousand Oaks, CA: Sage.

Steneck, N. H. (2000). *Assessing the integrity of publicly funded research: A background report for the November 2000 ORI Research Conference on Research Integrity.* University of Michigan: Author.

Stevens, A., & Gillam, S. (1998). Needs assessment: From theory to practice. *British Medical Journal, 316,* 1448–1452. *www.bmj.com/content/316/7142/1448.extract.*

Stock, W. A. (1994). Systematic coding for research synthesis. In H. Cooper & L. Hedges (Eds.), *The handbook of research synthesis* (pp. 125–138). New York: Sage.

Strauss, A., & Corbin, J. (1997). *Grounded theory in practice.* Thousand Oaks, CA: Sage.

Stringer, E. T. (2007). *Action research* (3rd ed.). Thousand Oaks, CA: Sage.

Suddaby, R. (2006). From the editors: What grounded theory is not. *Academy of Management Journal, 49,* 633–642.

Suri, H., & Clarke, D. (2009). Advancements in research synthesis methods: From a methodologically inclusive perspective. *Review of Educational Research, 79,* 395–430.

Tashakkorie, A., & Teddlie, C. (2003). *Mixed methods in social and behavioral research.* Thousand Oaks, CA: Sage.

Teddlie, C., & Yu, F. (2007). Mixed methods sampling: A typology with examples. *Journal of Mixed Methods Research, 1,* 77–100.

Thomas, R. M. (1996). *Comparing theories of child development* (4th ed.). Pacific Grove, CA: Brooks/Cole.

Thompson, B. (2002). What future quantitative social science research could look like: Confidence intervals for effect size. *Educational Researcher, 31,* 25–32.

Tiger, J. H., Hanley, G. P., & Bruzek, J. (2008). Functional communication training: A review and practical guide. *Behavior Analysis in Practice, 1*(1), 16–23.

Tourangeau, R., Rips, L. J., & Rasinski, K. (2000). *The psychology of survey response.* Cambridge, UK: Cambridge University Press.

Tufte, E. R. (1983). *The visual display of quantitative information* (2nd ed.). Cheshire, CT: Graphic Press.

Tukey, J. W. (1991). The philosophy of multiple comparisons. *Statistical Science, 6,* 157–176.

Vennesson, P. (2008). Case studies and process tracing: theories and practices. In D. Della Porta & M. Keating (Eds.), *Approaches and methodologies in the social sciences: A pluralist perspective* (pp. 223–239). Cambridge, UK: Cambridge University Press.

Vermes, G. (1999). *An introduction to the complete Dead Sea Scrolls.* Minneapolis, MN: Augsburg Fortress.

Wagner, M., & Cameto, R. (2009). *Wave 5 Parent/Young Adult Survey: Employment of young adult and postsecondary education at any institution (combined).* Retrieved from *www.nlts2.org/data_tables/index.html.*

Wagner, M., & Cameto, R. (2011, July). *A longitudinal look at the post-high school experiences of young adults with disabilities up to 8 years after high school: Findings from the NLTS-2.* Paper presented at the Office of Special Education Programs (OSEP) Project Directors Meeting, Washington, DC.

Wagner, R. K., Torgesen, J. K., & Rashotte, C. A. (1999). *Technical manual: Comprehensive Test of Phonological Processing.* Austin, TX: Pro-Ed.

Wakeley, A., Rivera, S., & Langer, J. (2000). Can young infants add and subtract? *Child Development, 71,* 1525–1534.

Walker, H. M., Stiller, B., & Golly, A. (1999). First step to success: A collaborative home–school intervention for preventing antisocial behavior at the point of school entry (Young Exceptional Children Monograph Series No. 1). In S. Sandall & M. Ostrosky (Eds.), *Practical ideas for addressing challenging behaviors* (pp. 41–48). Longmont, CO: Sopris West.

Warner, R. M. (2007). *Applied statistics: From bivariate through multivariate techniques.* Thousand Oaks, CA: Sage.

Wechsler, D. (2008). *Wechsler Adult Intelligence Scale* (4th ed.). Retrieved from *www.pearsonassessments.com.*

Weinstein, C. S. (1990). Prospective elementary teachers' beliefs about teaching: Implications for teacher education. *Teaching and Teacher Education, 6,* 279–290.

Whitemore, R., Chase, S. K., & Mandle, L. (2001). Validity in qualitative research. *Qualitative Health Research, 11,* 522–537.

Wiersma, W., & Jurs, S. G. (2009). *Research methods in education* (9th ed.). Boston: Allyn & Bacon.

Williams, R. L. (1974). Black pride, academic relevance, and individual achievement. In R. W. Tyler & R. M. Wolf (Eds.), *Crucial issues in testing* (pp. 219–231). Berkeley, CA: McCutchan.

Willig, C. (2001). *Introducing qualitative research in psychology: Adventures in theory and method.* Philadelphia: Open University Press.

Willingham, D. T. (2005, Summer). Ask the cognitive scientist: Do visual, auditory, and kinesthetic learners need visual, auditory, and kinesthetic instruction? *American Educator.* Retrieved from *www.aft.org/newspubs/periodicals/ae/summer2005/index.cfm.*

Wimmer, R. D., & Dominick, J. R. (1991). *Mass media research: An introduction* (3rd ed.). Belmont, CA: Wadsworth.

Winter, G. (2000). A comparative discussion of the notion of "validity" in qualitative and quantitative research. *The Qualitative Report, 4.* Retrieved from *www.nova.edu/ssss/qr/Qr4-3/winter.html.*

Wolery, M., Busick, M., Reichow, B., & Barton, E. E. (2010). Comparison of overlap methods for quantitatively synthesizing single-subject data. *Journal of Special Education, 44,* 18–28.

Wolery, M., & Garfinkle, A. N. (2002). Measures in intervention research with young children who have autism. *Journal of Autism and Developmental Disabilities, 32,* 463–478.

Wolf, M. M. (1978). Social validity: The case of subjective measurement or how applied behavior analysis is finding its heart. *Journal of Applied Behavior Analysis, 11,* 203–214.

Wolfe, E. W., & Chiu, C. W. T. (1999). Measuring pretest posttest change using the Rasch Rating Scale Model. *Journal of Outcome Measurement, 3,* 134–161.

Wood, J. M., Nezworski, M. T., & Stejskal, W. J. (1997). The reliability of the comprehensive system for the Rorschach. *Psychological Assessment, 9,* 490–494.

Woodcock, R. W. (1987). *Woodcock Reading Mastery Test, Revised.* Circle Pines, MN: American Guidance Service.

Wright, K. B. (2005). Researching Internet-based populations: Advantages and disadvantages of online survey research online questionnaire authoring software packages, and web survey services. *Journal of Computer-Mediated Communication, 10.* Retrieved from *http://jcmc.indiana.edu/vol10/issue3/wright.html.*

Wright, S. (1921). Correlation and causation. *Journal of Agricultural Research, 20,* 557–585.

Wu, C. F., & Hamada, M. S. (2000). *Experiments: Planning, analysis, and parameter design optimization.* Hoboken, NJ: Wiley.

Yin, R. K. (2009). *Case study research: Design and methods* (4th ed.). Thousand Oaks, CA: Sage.

Zimmerman, D. W., & Zumbo, B. D. (2004). The relative power of parametric and nonparametric statistical methods. In G. Keren & C. Lewis (Eds.), *A handbook for data analysis in the behavioral sciences: Methodological issues* (pp. 481–533). Hillsdale, NJ: Erlbaum.

Zuriff, G. (1995). Continuity over change within the experimental analysis of behavior. In J. T. Todd & E. K. Morris (Eds.), *Modern perspectives on B. F. Skinner and contemporary behaviorism* (pp. 171–183). Westport, CT: Greenwood Press.

Author Index

Subject Index

About the Authors

Ronald C. Martella, PhD, BCBA-D, is a professor of special education at Eastern Washington University, where he teaches classes in behavior management and research methodology. Dr. Martella has over 26 years of experience working with at-risk populations. He provides technical assistance to numerous states and districts on positive behavior support (PBS)/behavior management for students with or without disabilities. Dr. Martella has over 150 professional publications, including two six-level supplemental reading programs (*Lesson Connections* and *Core Lesson Connections*) for *Reading Mastery Signature Edition*, a two-level adolescent literacy program (*Read to Achieve*), and a comprehensive reading and language arts intervention system for struggling readers in grades 3 and above (*SRA FLEX Literacy*™). He served on the Washington State PBS Leadership Team as a PBS coach for several schools throughout eastern Washington, and as a consultant for the Washington State Striving Readers Grant that featured the adolescent literacy program he co-wrote.

J. Ron Nelson, PhD, is a professor at the University of Nebraska–Lincoln. Dr. Nelson has over 20 years of experience in the field of special education as a teacher, technical assistance provider, and professor. He has a national reputation as an effective researcher and received the 2000 Distinguished Initial Career Research Award from the Council for Exceptional Children. Dr. Nelson has over 150 publications, including journal articles, book chapters, and books, that focus on serving children at risk of school failure and research issues. He has developed a number of behavior and literacy interventions that have been recognized by the U.S. Department of Education (e.g., the *Think Time Strategy, Stepping Stones to Literacy, Early Vocabulary Connections, Multiple Meaning Vocabulary Program*).

Robert L. Morgan, PhD, is a professor in the Department of Special Education and Rehabilitation at Utah State University, where he serves as Head of the Severe Disabilities Teacher Preparation Program and Chair of the Undergraduate Committee. Dr. Morgan worked in schools, adult residential facilities, and supported employment programs for 11 years. His research interests include transition from school to adult roles and applied behavior analysis. He serves on numerous state and national committees dedicated to personnel preparation in special education and transition specialization.

He has published two books, four book chapters, over 100 journal articles, and 13 educational products.

Nancy E. Marchand-Martella, PhD, BCBA-D, is a professor of special education at Eastern Washington University. Dr. Marchand-Martella has over 26 years of experience working with at-risk populations. For the state of Washington, she served as a consultant for the Washington Improvement and Implementation Network and the Washington State Striving Readers Grant, which featured an adolescent literacy program she co-wrote, and as a Reading First panel member for selecting core, supplemental, and intervention programs for students in grades K–12. Dr. Marchand-Martella has over 160 professional publications, including a two-level vocabulary program (*Multiple Meaning Vocabulary*), two six-level supplemental reading programs (*Lesson Connections* and *Core Lesson Connections*) for *Reading Mastery Signature Edition*, a two-level adolescent literary program focused on comprehending content-area and narrative text (*Read to Achieve*), and a comprehensive reading and language arts intervention system for struggling readers in grades 3 and above (*SRA FLEX Literacy*™).